Contributions Toward Evidence-Based

Psychocardiology

Contributions Toward Evidence-Based

Psychocardiology

A Systematic Review of the Literature

Edited by

Jochen Jordan, Benjamin Bardé,
and Andreas Michael Zeiher

American Psychological Association • Washington, DC

Published by
American Psychological Association
750 First Street, NE
Washington, DC 20002
www.apa.org

To order
APA Order Department
P.O. Box 92984
Washington, DC 20090-2984
Tel: (800) 374-2721; Direct: (202) 336-5510
Fax: (202) 336-5502; TDD/TTY: (202) 336-6123
Online: www.apa.org/books/
E-mail: order@apa.org

In the U.K., Europe, Africa, and the Middle East, copies may be ordered from
American Psychological Association
3 Henrietta Street
Covent Garden, London
WC2E 8LU England

Typeset in Berkeley by World Composition Services, Inc., Sterling, VA

Printer: Maple-Vail Book Manufacturing Group, Binghamton, NY
Cover Designer: Naylor Design, Washington, DC
Technical/Production Editor: Harriet Kaplan

The opinions and statements published are the responsibility of the authors, and such opinions and statements do not necessarily represent the policies of the American Psychological Association.

Library of Congress Cataloging-in-Publication Data

Contributions toward evidence-based psychocardiology : a systematic review of the literature / edited by Jochen Jordan, Benjamin Bardé, and Andreas Michael Zeiher.—1st ed.

p. cm.

Includes bibliographical references and index.

ISBN-13: 978-1-59147-358-9

ISBN-10: 1-59147-358-6

1. Coronary heart disease—Psychological aspects. 2. Heart—Diseases—Psychological aspects. 3. Evidence-based medicine.

I. Jordan, Jochen, 1951- . II. Bardé, Benjamin. III. Zeiher, Andreas Michael.

[DNLM: 1. Coronary Disease—psychology—Meta-Analysis. 2. Evidence-Based Medicine—Meta-Analysis. WG 300 C7635 2006]

RC685.C6C598 2006

616.1'2306—dc22

2005018432

British Library Cataloguing-in-Publication Data

A CIP record is available from the British Library.

Printed in the United States of America
First Edition

Contents

Contributors

Bernhard Badura, PhD, MD, Full Professor, School of Public Health, University of Bielefeld, Bielefeld, Germany

Benjamin Bardé, PhD, Psychoanalytic Practice, Frankfurt am Main, Germany

Jürgen Barth, PhD, Assistant Professor, Department of Rehabilitation Psychology, Institute of Psychology, University of Freiburg, Freiburg, Germany

Jürgen Bengel, PhD, MD, Full Professor, Department of Rehabilitation Psychology, Institute of Psychology, University of Freiburg, Freiburg, Germany

Klaus Bös, PhD, Full Professor, Department of Sport and Exercise Science, University of Karlsruhe, Karlsruhe, Germany

Hans-Günter Budde, PhD, Bad Münster am Stein-Ebernburg, Germany

Ullrich Buss, PhD, Department of Psychosomatic Medicine and Psychotherapy, Georg August University of Göttingen, Göttingen, Germany

Gesine Grande, PhD, Full Professor, Department of Social Work, University of Applied Sciences, Leipzig, Germany

Christoph Herrmann-Lingen, MD, Full Professor, Department of Psychosomatic Medicine and Psychotherapy, University of Marburg, Marburg, Germany

Jochen Jordan, PhD, Professor, Clinic for Psychosomatic Medicine and Psychotherapy, Hospital J. W. Goethe-University Frankfurt, Frankfurt am Main, Germany

Martina Kanning, Department of Sport and Exercise Science, University of Stuttgart, Stuttgart, Germany

Kurt Laederach-Hofmann, MD, PhD, Assistant Professor, Department of General Internal Medicine, University of Bern, Inselspital, Bern, Switzerland

Wolfgang Langosch, PhD, Professor, Cardiac Clinic of Bad Krozingen, Bad Krozingen, Germany

Claudia Lazanowski, PhD, Clinic for Psychosomatic Medicine and Psychotherapy, Hospital J. W. Goethe-University Frankfurt, Frankfurt am Main, Germany

Wolfgang Linden, PhD, Full Professor, Department of Psychology, University of British Columbia, Vancouver, British Columbia, Canada

Nadine Messerli-Buergy, PhD, Department of General Internal Medicine, University of Bern, Inselspital, Bern, Switzerland

Michael Myrtek, MD, Full Professor, Department of Biological and Differential Psychology, University of Freiburg, Freiburg, Germany

Reiner Rugulies, PhD, MPH, Senior Researcher, National Institute of Occupational Health, Copenhagen, Denmark

Wolfgang Schlicht, PhD, Full Professor, Department of Sport and Exercise Science, University of Stuttgart, Stuttgart, Germany

Johannes Siegrist, PhD, Full Professor, Department of Medical Sociology, University of Düsseldorf, Düsseldorf, Germany

Andreas Michael Zeiher, PhD, MD, Full Professor, Medical Clinic III: Cardiology, Hospital J. W. Goethe-University Frankfurt, Frankfurt am Main, Germany

Contributions Toward Evidence-Based

Psychocardiology

INTRODUCTION: A NEW SCIENTIFIC DISCIPLINE

Jochen Jordan and Benjamin Bardé

The collaboration of Jochen Jordan, Benjamin Bardé, and Andreas Michael Zeiher as editors of this book follows many years of clinical cooperation and scientific investigation. During this time, we have been able to pool our joint knowledge as psychosomatic researcher, psychoanalyst, and cardiologist, respectively, and have been struck by a strange and seemingly inexplicable phenomenon: Although research on the psychosocial aspects of coronary heart disease (CHD) and other cardiac diseases has been extensive, perhaps exceeding that for other comparable diseases, the research findings are seldom applied in clinical settings. This apparent paradox exists despite patients' and cardiologists' awareness of the importance of psychosocial factors in the etiology and course of the disease.

Most of the so-called classic risk factors, such as smoking, sedentary lifestyle, and malnutrition, are behavioral lifestyle factors. Changing behaviors is difficult and requires psychological strategies. In recent decades, new findings have provided evidence that additional psychosocial variables, such as depression, anxiety, vital exhaustion, anger and hostility, work stress, social isolation, and negative affectivity are strong predictors for the onset and course of CHD. Although this is common knowledge, and although nearly all scientific societies and major health institutions, including the World Health Organization, emphasize the importance of psychosocial variables, psychologically oriented interventions in both diagnosis and therapy still play only a marginal role in the treatment of cardiac disease worldwide.

Two principal hypotheses have been proposed to explain this phenomenon. First, the diagnostic and therapeutic strategies currently used in interventional cardiology are very different from psychological interventions. Psychological interventions demand patience and time, because they must take into account the patient's life history and previous and existing social attachments as well as his or her unconscious conflicts and contradictory motivations. The processes of transference and countertransference need to be analyzed to help shed light on the patient's mental processes. These qualitatively different types of intervention lead to different types of patient relationships and to difficult interactions between medically oriented and psychologically oriented health care professionals.

The second hypothesis for the lack of psychological intervention in cardiac rehabilitation is that psychosocial knowledge, although extensive, is still controversial. Thus, it is hardly surprising that cardiologists and psychologists disagree on the relative importance of many behavioral issues and are unable to keep current with the vast amount of research available. For example, more than 500 publications exist on the topic of anxiety and depression after the onset of CHD; more than 4,000 empirical studies and 13 meta-analyses have investigated the relationship between psychological factors and high blood pressure; and 27 controlled and prospective studies, numerous intervention studies, and several meta-analyses exist for Type A behavior. Given the plethora of information available, it is perhaps understandable, although unfortunate, that there is no concise and complete textbook or manual for psychocardiology. Existing guidelines, such as those provided in *Behavioral Research in Cardiovascular, Lung, and Blood Health and Disease* (National Heart, Lung, and Blood Institute, 1998), although not universally accepted in the scientific community, are helpful nevertheless. For instance, the National Heart, Lung, and Blood Institute still sees Type A behavior and hostility as independent risk factors, whereas European researchers have abandoned these constructs (see the meta-analysis in chap. 6 of this volume on Type A behavior and hostility as independent risk factors for CHD).

To address this state of affairs, we conducted a comprehensive meta-analytic review of the existing knowledge and systematized it under the aegis of one scientific discipline. Before we discuss the results of our work, a note on terminology: The term *psychocardiology* embraces the psychosocial aspects of the etiology, course, and treatment of cardiac diseases and the corresponding coping processes as well as all psychological interventions in the field of cardiology. Systematic research concerning psychological factors of CHD began in 1923. One of the most important researchers was Flanders Dunbar of the New York Presbyterian Hospital (see chap. 2). Over the past 3 decades, the scope of psychocardiological research has widened considerably. In addition to the study of CHD, there has been a more intensive focus on how patients perceive and cope with cardiac illnesses such as heart valve defects, congenital heart disease, and cardiac arrhythmias. Rapid technological progress in diagnosis and therapy has led to the emergence of psychocardiology as a new field; studies have investigated the psychological processes of coping with interventions like bypass grafting, heart transplantation, angioplasties, and the fitting of cardiac pacemakers or implantable cardioverter defibrillators. The scientific disciplines that contribute to psychocardiological research are numerous and include epidemiology, health systems analysis, medicine, psychology, rehabilitation science, public health, and sociology. Thus, psychocardiology is not a new research field, but rather a bringing together of widely disparate areas of knowledge. The term *psychocardiology* is analogous to those describing other interdisciplinary research fields that have developed over the past 30 years, such as psychonephrology, psycho-oncology, neuropsychology, and psychoendocrinology, among others. Given the great importance of social variables in the development of CHD, a more accurate term would be *social psychocardiology* or *biopsychosocial cardiology*. However, these terms are not generally accepted. Other terms like *behavioral cardiology* or *cardiac psychology* are also common.

PSYCHOCARDIOLOGY STATUS CONFERENCE

In 1998, in response to these challenges, we organized the Psychocardiology Status Conference, which was held in Germany and was attended by 32 scientists from five countries. Our main goal was to review the existing literature systematically and document the results in such a way as to foster open scientific discussion on every issue (see Appendix 1).

Method

We divided the broad field of psychocardiology into precisely demarcated areas, which we then delegated to the respective specialists. Fourteen systematic reviews were produced, and 10 of these are included as chapters in this volume.[1] Each of the reviews was distilled from systematic and comprehensive literature searches in international databases (Medline, PsycINFO, PSYNDEX, Cochrane Library). Predetermined methodological criteria (based on those of evidence-based medicine) were used: All of the existent literature was systematized, evaluated in terms of methodological soundness,

---

[1] Because of length considerations, the following papers could not be included in this volume: "The Influence of Partnership on the Development and Course of Coronary Artery Disease (Sexuality, Communication, Social Support, Risk Behavior)," by G. Titscher and C. Schöppl; "The Significance of Anger and Anger Expression in the Etiology of Coronary Disease," by P. Hank and O. Mittag; "The Concepts of Vital Exhaustion, Anxiety and Depression, Helplessness, and Despair Before the Outbreak of Coronary Artery Disease," by K. H. Ladwig, N. Errazzo, and R. Rugulies; and "Women and Coronary Diseases: Gender-Specific Factors in Etiology," by H. Weidemann, K. Meyer, and T. Fischer.

and presented in a form designed to permit critical review by other scientists at any time.

The draft reviews were debated in detail by all 32 scientists involved in the conference, thus ensuring high quality standards. Discussions took place at eight meetings, each lasting 2 or 3 days, between 1998 and 2002. The reviews were reworked many times before being approved by consensus. It is our hope that the final reviews will serve as authoritative sources for the formulation of guidelines by scientific societies and institutions like the World Health Organization.

High-quality medical protocols today cost many thousands of dollars, and most independent research funds are restricted by their constitutions from funding this type of work. Fortunately, the Boehringer Ingelheim Foundation made it possible for the project team of the Psychocardiology Status Conference to work with great thoroughness over the course of 4 years. Other financial help came from the German Research Foundation, the Senckenbergische Foundation, the German Society for Cardiac Rehabilitation and Prevention, and the Werner Reimers Foundation.

The present volume aims to integrate the extensive scientific discourse on psychological considerations in CHD. It is our hope that research teams worldwide will be encouraged to pursue the path our contributors have shown in their syntheses of the literature on topics in need of additional investigation. Systematic reviews are urgently needed of conceptual models of the etiology of cardiovascular diseases, including the impact of psychological factors on pathobiology and pathophysiology; psychological aspects of and interventions to promote risk-reducing nutrition; the psychological aspects of cardiac interventions in children; experiences of and ways of coping with cardiac interventions (including bypass grafting, heart valve surgery, heart transplantation, cardiac pacemakers, and defibrillators); and the psychological aspects of heart defects and cardiac arrhythmias. Such proposals can be submitted to the editors of the present volume and will be evaluated by internationally recognized experts. It is our hope that this volume will provoke further studies that will help to refine our knowledge base.

Findings of the Conference

The present volume clearly represents remarkable scientific progress. Its authors have facilitated the systematic evaluation of scientific dialogue and thus have permitted fruitful discussion of controversial issues. Our focus on methodological issues in comparing studies will help researchers compare these data with any given specialty area and will facilitate a comprehensive approach.

The systematic reviews in this volume took a great deal of time to compile (from 1998 to 2002); the necessary transformation and translation, as well as the production of the book, required many additional months. In the meantime, many new scientific publications have appeared, and the findings of several important studies, including the Sertraline AntiDepressant Heart Attack Randomized Trial (SADHART), INTERHEART, and Enhancing Recovery in Coronary Heart Disease (ENRICHD) studies, could not be reviewed in this book. The results described in these chapters have long-term relevance, however, because they are based on a substantial number of high-quality studies. Only a large number of empirical publications that challenged these findings would necessitate revision of the chapters' conclusions.

Readers should also remember that in everyday clinical practice, knowledge is applied through the unique experience and personality of the clinician. The specific nature of the relationship between patient and clinician lays the foundation on which knowledge can be applied. In empirical research, it is easy to overlook such fundamental realms of experience as existential threat, death, loss, and helplessness and hopelessness and the psychic processes involved. The biographical framing and rooting of human experience similarly create an individual psychological makeup that manifests itself in interpersonal relations. As researchers, we know that studies of high scientific quality (with randomized and controlled selection of patients and manualized psychological intervention) are those that create precise and reliable results. However, we also recognize that these standards are often not helpful for clinical practice, because no psychotherapist would ever be willing to perform a clinical intervention under precisely these conditions, following a manual to the letter. Selected and randomized participants from multicenter studies are relatively rare in clinical samples and rehabilitation centers. The majority of patients have unique characteristics, such as multimorbidity, that prevents the direct transfer of clinical trial results to clinical practice. It is thus important to emphasize that clinical psychology is the use of precise and comprehensive scientific knowledge by a well-educated and experienced psychotherapist in an appropriate institutional context. This requires the constant adaptation and translation of scientific knowledge to clinical work (see section 2.7 in chap. 2).

One of the most voluminous and costly psychotherapeutic investigations, the ENRICHD study, has shown the kinds of methodological difficulties that can arise in a multicenter randomized controlled study. Randomizing patients in such a study is difficult, because they must provide informed consent to participate in a randomized study; as a result, they are immediately aware of the aims of the study. The participants in the ENRICHD study received extensive background information about the study, and the control group was not comparable with the usual standard care patients. The ENRICHD study found that the spontaneous rate of remission of depression was significantly higher than would be expected on the basis of results from recent studies. Although placebo groups are impossible in psychological intervention studies, in principle an attention placebo group should be included so that the influence of social attention on patients can be evaluated. Participating in a study can influence outcome variables, so it is necessary to control the effects of social attention, because this can be seen as a kind of social support. In addition to the intervention and control groups, an attention placebo group is needed to control these effects. Usually, the randomized members of the attention placebo group are told that someone will come and talk with them about the cardiac intervention. The person then comes, listens actively, and talks in a nondirective way, focusing on family, job, interests, or any other areas the patients relate to. Furthermore, the manualization of the intervention, although methodologically necessary, is not only difficult but also somewhat unwieldy. In the

context of the ENRICHD study, it is justifiable to doubt whether depression therapy following that of Aaron T. Beck, which was developed for depressive patients without comorbidity, could be considered adequate following a heart attack. Anxiety and depression shortly after a heart attack are sometimes symptoms of an adjustment disorder and may require alternative concepts of psychotherapy.

Finally, one obstacle seems nearly insurmountable in intervention studies. The extraordinary success of medically based therapy for CHD has resulted in a consistently lower mortality rate for patients; after a heart attack, a patient has a significantly raised risk of mortality in the first 6 to 10 months, but after that period, the mortality rate drops to 2% to 3%. To influence this remaining variance of 2% with a specific psychological intervention is not only extremely difficult but also requires large study samples and long-term follow-up.

Not only in studies of psychological interventions, but also in somatic and technical intervention studies (e.g., of the use of cardioverter defibrillators), mortality rates are declining in control groups. We could thus conclude that participation in a study has favorable health effects (i.e., lowered mortality). This demonstrates that future studies will need to be conceived with extraordinary care. ENRICHD has—quite unfoundedly in our opinion—created discouragement and disappointment among researchers and clinically active psychocardiologists because hard endpoints like mortality were not significantly changed in the intervention group compared with the controls. Such a reaction is not legitimate from the scientific point of view. Studies on the importance of cholesterol, for example, were controversial for a long time, and for a long time millions of research dollars were unable to shed light on the issue. From a scientific point of view, we have learned numerous lessons from ENRICHD and should be grateful for that.

A crucial question we now face is whether it makes sense to perform further large-scale, costly studies to study the effects of psychotherapy on mortality in cardiac patients. To date, psychotherapy studies have not been carried out with the goal of investigating the effects on mortality. It may be wise to aim research efforts at those effects only when preliminary studies have examined intervention techniques and proved that the intended psychological parameters can be effectively changed.

FUTURE STEPS IN INTERVENTION RESEARCH

As a first step, future psychotherapeutic intervention studies should focus on different types of interventions for various subgroups of cardiac patients. It is important that these interventions be easily integrated into health care systems and that they be acceptable to both patients and medical staff. It is also critical to have specific interventions for clearly defined variables. Without a clear and specific indication for psychotherapy, and without taking into consideration the specific characteristics of subgroups, psychological interventions are not promising.

As a second step, future research should assess whether psychological interventions are effective: Can they change psychological risk factors, health-related lifestyles, emotions, mood, and cognitions, and do these effects persist over time? It is important that psychological interventions primarily seek to change psychological variables and that outcomes be stable over time. Finally, the third step for future studies is to evaluate whether the modified psychological variables have any effects on morbidity and mortality.

OVERVIEW OF THE BOOK

This book contains 10 chapters, each of which reviews the highest quality literature relevant to its topic. Because of space limitations, we have created a Web site (http://www.apa.org/books/resources/jordan/) to accompany this book. It provides short summaries and information concerning the methodological quality of the publications and on additional studies that had to be excluded from the present volume as well as supplementary material supporting study results. The Web site material is referred to at appropriate points throughout the book.

Chapter 1, "Sociological Aspects of the Development and Course of Coronary Heart Disease: Social Inequality and Chronic Emotional Distress in the Workplace," focuses on two selected sociological aspects of CHD: the social inequality in the risk of CHD in modern Western societies and the impact of chronic emotional distress in the workplace on the disease. Both subjects are key issues in medical sociological research, and an impressive volume of theoretical articles and empirical research has been published on both.

Today there is conclusive empirical evidence that at least since the 1970s, in most Western societies, CHD is disproportionately prevalent in persons of low socioeconomic status (SES). In addition to this finding, several studies have shown that social inequality in CHD is not apparent only in comparisons of individuals with the lowest and highest SES; a continuous inverse association between SES and risk of CHD has been observed.

Emotional distress in the workplace has long been suspected as an etiological factor for the development of CHD. Current research in this field is dominated by two theoretical models: the demand–control model and the effort–reward imbalance model. These models assume, on the basis of sociological and stress research theories, that certain sets of conditions in the workplace increase the risk for CHD. The theoretical assumptions of both models give rise to specific hypotheses that can be tested in empirical studies. Chapter 1 presents and discusses the results of these studies.

Chapter 2, "Psychodynamic Hypotheses on the Etiology, Course, and Psychotherapy of Coronary Heart Disease: 100 Years of Psychoanalytic Research," provides a systematic review of all publications in English, German, and French that have reported psychodynamic research on patients with CHD. Until now, no systematic review of this area of research has been published. The chapter evaluates the contribution of psychodynamic research to a scientific understanding of the etiology and course of disease and reviews the most important theoretical models focusing on the etiology of the disease and the associated emotional disturbances. It also reviews experiences with psychodynamic interventions and the important question of how best to handle transference and countertransference in the psychotherapeutic relationship.

Chapter 3, "Smoking Cessation in Patients With Coronary Heart Disease: Risk Reduction and an Evaluation of the Efficacy of Interventions," summarizes the effects of smoking on cardiovascular morbidity and mortality and the benefits of refraining from smoking after a cardiac event. The chapter also provides a meta-analysis of 21 randomized controlled trials on smoking cessation in patients with cardiovascular disorders. Together, these studies showed an effect of smoking cessation intervention on abstinence. The chapter describes and evaluates interventions to promote smoking cessation for their appropriateness and contraindication in patients with cardiovascular disorders. This systematic review is useful for clinicians and researchers in secondary prevention of cardiovascular disorders.

Chapter 4, "Psychosocial Interventions to Influence Physical Inactivity as a Risk Factor: Theoretical Models and Practical Evidence," deals with a significant psychosocial risk factor: physical inactivity. The negative effects of a sedentary lifestyle on cardiovascular health have been well documented. Numerous empirical results have demonstrated the benefits of regular physical activity in primary and secondary prevention as well as in the rehabilitation of severe cardiac diseases. Despite the benefits of exercise, few people start an exercise program, and most of those who do fail to adhere to it. The vast majority of the population is completely inactive. Interventions to reduce inactivity and foster the initiation and maintenance of regular exercise (e.g., three times a week for about 30 minutes at moderate intensity) are necessary for both individual and public health promotion. In the long run, such interventions are more cost effective than any medical or pharmacological intervention. The chapter raises the question of how to motivate and foster commitment to regular physical exercise in individuals at coronary risk. Answers are provided in a systematic narrative and meta-analytic review of available empirical results. The chapter deals primarily with the process of motivation and adherence; the physiological and psychological effects of regular physical exercising are discussed

only briefly, because these effects are well documented in the scientific literature and in the recommendations of various health organizations.

Chapter 5, "Anxiety and Depression in Patients With Coronary Heart Disease," is a systematic review of prospective studies of anxiety or depression or both (including self-ratings of depressed mood without a categorical diagnosis of depression) in patients with documented or suspected CHD. Cross-sectional prevalence and correlation studies are included. Given the large number of studies covered, the authors have ranked the qualification of each study using a scale they developed based on sample size, validity and reliability of the instruments, and the completeness of the reporting of results (e.g., significance levels, effect sizes, multivariate analyses). This review of more than 500 publications establishes that depression develops in a significant number of cases after myocardial infarction (with a prevalence of 30% to 45%) and is a strong predictor of the course of disease. The findings regarding anxiety are more ambiguous. (A meta-analysis based on this chapter was published by Barth, Schumacher, & Herrmann-Lingen [2004] in *Psychosomatic Medicine*.)

Chapter 6, "Type A Behavior and Hostility as Independent Risk Factors for Coronary Heart Disease," presents a meta-analysis of all existing high-quality studies on this topic. The database for Type A behavior is excellent. The most compelling design using "hard" criteria and healthy persons (with a combined N of only 1,110), however, revealed an insignificant population effect size. Studies with the hard criterion and CHD patients showed a trend toward a negative association between Type A behavior and subsequent CHD events. Therefore, it would be inadvisable to initiate any intervention to alter Type A behavior. Taking into consideration all studies on Type A personality, no significant association with CHD can be observed. It may thus be concluded that Type A behavior is not an independent risk factor for CHD.

The database for hostility and CHD is much smaller than that for Type A behavior. About 15,000 persons in 10 prospective studies were analyzed. This effect size is significant ($p = .022$; the correlation was very low), but the practical meaning for diagnosis and treatment is questionable.

Chapter 7, "Chest Pain, Angina Pectoris, Panic Disorder, and Syndrome X," gives an excellent review of these clinical phenomena. Chest pain is an epidemiologically important symptom that has a lifetime prevalence of 25% to 33% and represents the most common symptom in outpatient practice. Depending on the population investigated, however, only 20% to 30% of people with episodes of chest pain were found to have cardiac pathology. The remaining episodes were classified as esophageal or chest wall pathology or as psychological disturbances, including anxiety, panic disorder, somatization, or depression. Because of the life-threatening potential of cardiac symptoms, pathology must be excluded first.

As efforts to better define syndrome X have increased, several important examinations of the vascular microenvironment and the physiology of flow regulation have been published. Explanations of interindividual and intraindividual differences in perceptions of angina pectoris have included, on the one hand, vascular abnormalities such as microvascular angina pectoris, receptor regulation problems in vascular relaxation, and elevated levels of nitric oxide and other local hormones and, on the other hand, psychological processes such as pain generation and transmission, symptom perception, and central processing of enteroceptive, situational, or emotional cognition regarding angina pectoris. Chapter 7 provides a thorough meta-analysis of the literature on noncoronary angina pectoris, including cardiac syndrome X and microvascular angina pectoris, and defines the borders of other patho-anatomical or pathopsychological processes involved, especially depression with recurrent pain episodes.

Chapter 8, "Psychosocial Aspects of Coronary Catheterization, Angiography, and Angioplasty," reviews the literature in this dominant area of cardiology. These procedures are the most frequent in cardiology worldwide, yet from a methodological point of view, related psychosocial studies are of lesser quality. The chapter highlights the results of studies on coping with the procedures, quality of life following a procedure, interventions that pre-

pare patients for a procedure, and comparisons of the efficacy of angioplasty with bypass surgery and pharmacological treatment.

This review shows that thorough preparation of patients before they undergo a cardiac procedure reduces anxiety, improves coping, and promotes lifestyle changes. Both patients and their partners require personalized and comprehensive information about the procedure itself and about the possible risks. Preparation should also include information about sensory and pain reactions and their significance. During the procedure, particularly in the first minutes, most patients find it helpful to be able to communicate with staff, who should encourage patients to ask questions and report their sensory experiences.

Chapter 9, "Psychological Interventions for Coronary Heart Disease: Stress Management, Relaxation, and Ornish Groups," deals with one of the foremost and current scientific topics in psychocardiology: controlled interventions to influence health behavior, emotional status, and coping processes. This review focuses on the question of whether the addition of psychological therapy to the usual cardiac care can have a positive impact on the morbidity and mortality of cardiac patients following a first event. Numerous large, well-controlled trials and meta-analyses of outcomes were available to help answer the question. These studies do not lead to simple, categorical conclusions because of continuous improvements in the quality of medical care and methodological problems of the studies. In light of current discussion about the SADHART and ENRICHD large-scale intervention studies, the clinical practice recommendations of this chapter are very important. Particularly relevant issues in psychological interventions with cardiac patients include the need to offer gender-specific treatments, to ensure that only distressed patients are treated and that treatment continues until distress is reduced, and to conduct further research on the best timing for identifying distress and offering treatment.

Chapter 10, "Cardiac Rehabilitation From a Health Systems Analysis Perspective," gives a systematic overview of programs and guidelines for cardiac rehabilitation. Currently, cardiac rehabilitation is offered as a more or less integral part of comprehensive cardiac care in all developed countries. Initially, cardiac rehabilitation was considered suitable predominantly for (male) patients recovering from uncomplicated myocardial infarction. After strict immobilization for a minimum of 6 weeks, these patients were in poor physical and psychological condition on discharge from the hospital. Thus, early rehabilitation programs were focused on physical exercise to restore patients' cardiopulmonary capacity and on psychosocial support to restore their self-esteem and facilitate coping with the chronic heart disease and its serious somatic, social, and psychological consequences.

In the past 20 years, the aims, assumptions, and components of cardiac rehabilitation programs have changed fundamentally as a result of the changing characteristics of cardiac patients, the immense advances in knowledge about CHD, and the changing spectrum of medical and surgical therapies for cardiac illnesses. A wider range of patients are eligible for rehabilitation programs because of the increasing variety of diagnostic groups (e.g., patients recovering from various medical interventions such as revascularization procedures or heart valve surgery, patients with stable angina pectoris or heart failure). Another contributing factor is increased participation by older adults and the advent of programs tailored to patients with severe types of CHD.

Currently, however, beyond official guidelines and statements, the details of how cardiac rehabilitation is implemented in different countries remain a mystery. How are cardiac rehabilitation services organized? Who participates in the programs, and what are the rates of referral or utilization? How long do the programs last? Which professionals are responsible for specific interventions, and which components of rehabilitation (e.g., training, medical advice, education, counseling, behavioral interventions) are included in the programs? This chapter represents the first attempt to collect and systematize the available international data about cardiac rehabilitation delivery in developed countries, including the United States, Great Britain, and Germany.

CONCLUSION

As a result of our experience as editors of this book, we have come to the conclusion that the sheer volume of material and the contradictory nature of the findings from psychosocial research constitute the principal reasons for the relative lack of attention to psychosocial factors in standard prevention, treatment, and rehabilitation practices. Transferring knowledge across disciplines is another challenge. Medicine and the social sciences differ widely in approach and research strategies. Interdisciplinary dialogue is difficult, and moreover, there are few opportunities for the exchange of views to take place. We hope this will change.

Participants in the Conference

Bernhard Badura, Bielefeld, Germany

Benjamin Bardé, Frankfurt am Main, Germany

Jürgen Barth, Freiburg, Germany

Jürgen Bengel, Freiburg, Germany

Klaus Bös, Karlsruhe, Germany

Hans-Günther Budde, Bad Münster am Stein, Germany

Ullrich Buss, Göttingen, Germany

Franziska Einsle, Dresden, Germany

Gesine Grande, Leipzig, Germany

Petra Hank, Trier, Germany

Christoph Herrmann-Lingen, Marburg, Germany

Jochen Jordan, Frankfurt am Main, Germany

Martina Kanning, Stuttgart, Germany

Volker Kollenbaum, Kiel, Germany

Volker Köllner, Blieskastel, Germany

Karl-Heinz Ladwig, München, Germany

Kurt Laederach-Hofmann, Bern, Switzerland

Wolfgang Langosch, Bad Krozingen, Germany

Claudia Lazanowski, Frankfurt am Main, Germany

Wolfgang Linden, Vancouver, Canada

Nadine Messerli-Buergy, Bern, Switzerland

Katharina Meyer, Bollien, Switzerland

Oskar Mittag, Luebeck, Germany

Michael Myrtek, Freiburg, Germany

Karl Heinz Rüddel, Bad Kreuznach, Germany

Reiner Rugulies, Copenhagen, Denmark

Hartmut Schächinger, Trier, Germany

Wolfgang Schlicht, Stuttgart, Germany

Johannes Siegrist, Düsseldorf, Germany

Georg Titscher, Vienna, Austria

Hermann Weidemann, Bad Krozingen, Germany

Andreas Michael Zeiher, Frankfurt am Main, Germany

SOCIOLOGICAL ASPECTS OF THE DEVELOPMENT AND COURSE OF CORONARY HEART DISEASE: SOCIAL INEQUALITY AND CHRONIC EMOTIONAL DISTRESS IN THE WORKPLACE

Reiner Rugulies and Johannes Siegrist

1.1. INTRODUCTION

This chapter focuses on two sociological aspects of coronary heart disease (CHD): social inequality in the risk of coronary heart disease in modern Western societies and the impact on the disease of chronic emotional distress in the workplace. Both subjects are key issues in medical sociological research, and an impressive volume of theoretical articles and empirical research has been published for both. Other topics in medical sociology that are relevant to CHD—for example, findings on protective factors and resources (e.g., social network and social support) and sociocultural stability and social demands outside the workplace (e.g., personal relationships, family, neighborhood, critical life events)—are not addressed or are only briefly touched on in this chapter. Two considerations led us to focus only on social inequalities and emotional distress in the workplace: (a) the relatively good scientific evidence in these two areas, and therefore the high relevance of the results for medicine and health policy, and (b) our specific expertise in these two areas.

The literature review on which this chapter is based was originally conducted in the context of the Psychocardiology Status Conference. Between 1998 and 2002, the members of this panel wrote comprehensive reviews of psychosocial aspects of CHD and met several times a year to discuss and peer review their work (Jordan, Bardé, & Zeiher, 2001). Our review (Rugulies & Siegrist, 2002) was based on literature published through 1999. For

this chapter, we updated our findings to include articles published through May 2003.

The chapter has the following structure:

- Section 1.2 discusses methods and problems in medical sociology and social epidemiology, especially measurement issues, types of study design, and considerations for statistical analysis.
- Section 1.3 reviews selected studies on social inequality in the risk of CHD.
- Section 1.4 analyzes the impact of chronic emotional distress in the workplace on the development and course of CHD. The section discusses in detail the theoretical assumptions and the empirical evidence for the demand–control model and the effort–reward imbalance (ERI) model, the two dominating models in this field.
- Section 1.5 summarizes the main findings of the review and gives suggestions for future research.

1.2. MEDICAL SOCIOLOGY AND SOCIAL EPIDEMIOLOGY

Medical sociology uses the terms, methods, empirical knowledge, and theories of general sociology to analyze phenomena related to health and illness. Research interests are as diverse as the social aspects of help seeking and coping with diseases, the social roles of physicians and patients, the sociology of physician–patient relationships, the structure and development of the health care system, and social influences on health and illness; the latter line of research is also called *social epidemiology* (J. Siegrist, 1995). Social epidemiological research is an important part of medical sociology, especially when hypotheses are explicitly derived from sociological theories. Because this chapter is about a social epidemiological issue—the contribution of socioeconomic status and chronic emotional distress in the workplace to the risk of CHD—we will start with a brief discussion of the content and methods of social epidemiological research.

1.2.1. Content of Social Epidemiological Research

Social epidemiology investigates the social distribution and the social determinants of health and illness in a population. It had its beginning in the middle of the 19th century, and early scholars include Rudolf Virchow (1821–1902), who reported on the social causes of the typhus epidemic in Upper Silesia (R. Taylor & Rieger, 1985; Virchow, 1849/1968), and Friedrich Engels (1820–1895), who described the condition of the working class in England and its effects on health (T. M. Brown & Fee, 2003; F. Engels, 1845/1987, 1845/2003).

Quantitative methods to determine the distribution and causes of disease also arose in the middle of the 19th century. Pioneering statistician and epidemiologist William Farr (1807–1883) began collecting and analyzing statistical information on mortality in the 1830s at the British Registrar General of Birth, Deaths, and Marriages. His work led him to the conclusion that social living conditions heavily influence mortality (Hamlin, 1995; Susser & Adelstein, 1975). In France, Émile Durkheim (1858–1917) investigated the social determinants of suicide by preparing meticulous tables on the frequency of suicide among Catholics and Protestants (Durkheim, 1897/1951).

Despite this long tradition, social epidemiology still struggles for recognition by general epidemiology. For example, in most epidemiological textbooks, social epidemiology is only briefly covered (Krieger, 1994). However, the recent publication of the first textbook on social epidemiology (Berkman & Kawachi, 2000) and the growing number of publications on the social determinants of health in recent years (Kaplan & Lynch, 1997) indicate that social epidemiology is becoming a more established field of research.

1.2.2. Methods and Challenges in Social Epidemiological Research

Like epidemiology in general, social epidemiology places strong emphasis on biostatistics and quantitative methods. The main focus is on comparing the incidence and prevalence of morbidity and mortality among different groups. These groups are defined by their *exposure status*, or whether they have been exposed or not to specific factors that might have an impact on health.

1.2.2.1. Measuring the constructs. Social epidemiology faces a special challenge in that an exposure of interest usually is not a physical entity (like cholesterol or blood pressure) but a latent construct. Latent constructs cannot be directly observed but rather are inferred using scientific methods (J. Siegrist, 1995). Therefore, there is a heightened risk that the measurement of the exposure of interest is unreliable or invalid. For example, the socioeconomic status of an individual is usually measured using variables such as education, income, or occupational status. Although studies that have used these indicators have found a clear association with health outcomes (see section 1.3), these variables are nevertheless rather crude indicators for such a complex construct as socioeconomic status. One can assume that relying on these imperfect variables will result in a certain amount of misclassification. This misclassification, when it is unspecific, leads to a bias toward the null and therefore to an underestimation of the true effect (K. Rothman & Greenland, 1998).

An invalid measurement of an exposure can lead to a misinterpretation of the study's results. For example, a questionnaire that intends to measure objective problems in the work environment may in fact measure the mood of the respondents. When an association between high scores on the questionnaire and a health outcome is found, the researchers would then draw the conclusion that problems at work cause poor health when in fact, negative mood is the cause of the health problems.

An alternative to using questionnaires is to assess distress by job title. Usually, on the basis of previous large-scale representative surveys, researchers assign a specific score for distress to every person with the same job title, thus ruling out bias due to subjective factors. This method has been used in several studies from Sweden, which has a comprehensive classification system for job titles and associated exposure to psychosocial factors (J. V. Johnson, Hall, & Theorell, 1989; J. V. Johnson, Stewart, Hall, Fredlund, & Theorell, 1996). The disadvantage of this method is that differences in the work environment within an occupational group are not taken into account.

A third method for measuring occupational distress is workplace observations. The exposure is measured for the individual not by self-report, but objectively. Some recent social epidemiological studies using this method have yielded interesting results (Bosma et al., 1997; Greiner, Krause, Ragland, & Fisher, 1998). However, workplace observations are time consuming and expensive and therefore difficult to conduct, especially among large study populations.

Measurement problems are not limited to the assessment of exposure; they can also have an effect on the assessment of endpoints. For example, it is possible that people with high levels of neuroticism experience both more emotional distress and non-CHD-related chest pain that might be mistaken for angina pectoris symptoms (Serlie, Erdman, Passchier, Trijsburg, & ten Cate, 1995). In such a case, exposure and mistakes in the measurement of the endpoint are systematically associated with each other, and the relative risk (RR) is overestimated. Therefore, results from studies that use angina pectoris as an endpoint should be viewed with caution.

1.2.2.2. Study designs. Like epidemiology in general, social epidemiology is based mainly on observational—meaning nonexperimental—studies. The methodological gold standard is therefore not the double blind randomized controlled clinical trial but rather the prospective cohort study. In a cohort study, a number of subjects (the cohort) are followed for a certain amount of time. The predictors

(e.g., distress in the workplace) are assessed at the beginning of the study. The incidence rates of new clinical endpoints during follow-up are then compared for the exposed subjects (e.g., those with distress in the workplace) and the nonexposed subjects (e.g., those without distress in the workplace) by calculating a ratio. Depending on the type of data and the method of analysis used, this ratio can have different names, but *relative risk* (RR) is probably the most widely used, and we will use it in this chapter. Other terms are *incidence density ratios* (when length of exposure for study participants [*person time*] is taken into account), *cumulative incidence ratios* (when person time is not taken into account), and *hazard ratios* (when the analysis is based on a Cox proportional hazard model).

Among observational studies, cohort studies are the most powerful for investigating the causal relationship between a predictor and an endpoint, because by design, the presence of the predictor is established before the incidence of the disease. Therefore, reverse causation (i.e., that the endpoint has caused the occurrence of the predictor) can be ruled out. However, cohort studies usually require large resources and are often difficult to conduct, especially if the disease under study is relatively rare. Even if the disease is frequent, like CHD, it is usually necessary to follow up on thousands of subjects over several years to get enough incidences for statistical analyses.

Alternatives to cohort studies are *case–control studies*, which need substantially fewer resources and are therefore very popular in epidemiology. In these studies, individuals with a specific disease (the cases) are compared with individuals without this disease (the controls) to find out if the predictor of interest is more frequent in one or the other group. The RR in case–control studies is calculated using so-called *odds ratios*, a term that originated with racetrack betting. An odds ratio compares the chances of being exposed to the predictor among the cases with the chances of being exposed among the controls.

The main challenge in case–control studies is to find appropriate controls. Failure to ensure the appropriateness of controls can heavily bias study results. For example, a comparison of heart disease patients from California (a region with very low smoking rates) with healthy controls from China (a region with very high smoking rates) would probably find higher odds for smoking in the controls, which would lead to the conclusion that smoking protects from CHD.

Another challenge for case–control studies is that exposure is assessed after the occurrence of the disease. For example, it is possible that subjects with heart disease report more emotional stressors at the workplace than controls because they are motivated to find an explanation for their illness. In such a case, emotional stressors would not be the cause of increased CHD rates, but CHD would be the cause of an increased reporting of emotional stressors.

Special types of case–control studies can address some of the challenges. In *nested case–control studies,* a specific population is monitored for a specific time (e.g., all nurses in a hospital for 1 year). When a person develops the disease of interest, one or more control subjects are randomly matched from the population under study. This means that cases and controls contribute an identical amount of person time, and therefore the odds ratios can be interpreted like incidence density ratios. In a *case–cohort study*, cases and controls are also selected from a predefined cohort. However, person time is not taken into account, which means that the odds ratios should be interpreted as cumulative incidence ratios (Pearce, 1993; Rodrigues & Kirkwood, 1990). Nested case–control studies and case–cohort studies can have almost the same high quality as prospective cohort studies, especially when the exposure is determined not by self-report in retrospect but by objective measures (e.g., job titles).

Another type of study, the *cross-sectional study*, investigates associations between exposure and endpoint at the same time in a specific population. In social epidemiology, the usefulness of these studies is limited, because they do not establish the time sequence between exposure on one hand and morbidity and mortality on the other and therefore do not allow causal inference. However, cross-sectional studies are sometimes useful to compare the prevalence of risk factors (e.g., hypertension or high cholesterol) in exposed and nonexposed groups.

Ecological studies have a long tradition in social epidemiology, starting with Durkheim's research on suicide (Durkheim, 1897/1951). These studies measure exposure and endpoint not on the individual level but on the group level (e.g., correlations between hours of sunshine in specific regions and local rates of melanoma). A few years ago, findings from ecological studies on the association between level of income inequality and mortality rates caused a controversial debate in social epidemiology (Lynch, Davey Smith, Kaplan, & House, 2000; Lynch, Due, Muntaner, & Davey Smith, 2000; Marmot & Wilkinson, 2001; Muntaner & Lynch, 1999; Muntaner, Lynch, & Oates, 1999; Wilkinson, 1996, 1999, 2000).

Intervention studies are rare in social epidemiology, not surprising given the challenges and difficulties in influencing the social environment, which is very different from administering drugs and placebos in randomized controlled trials in clinical epidemiology. Nevertheless, intervention studies are important, and at least a few examples from workplace intervention studies have targeted hazardous psychosocial exposure (see section 1.4).

1.2.2.3. Statistical adjustment and overadjustment.

A crucial issue in epidemiology is ensuring that an association between a predictor and an outcome is not biased by confounding. A *confounder* is a factor associated with the risk factor that independently affects the likelihood of the outcome. For example, suppose one finds an increased risk of myocardial infarction among people who drink coffee compared with coffee abstainers. Suppose also that coffee drinkers are more likely to be smokers than non–coffee drinkers. In this case, it is not clear if the higher risk of myocardial infarction among coffee drinkers is due to their coffee consumption or to their higher smoking rates.

The problem of confounding is usually addressed by multivariate analyses, which allow one to adjust for possible confounding effects and to calculate an RR that is independent of the confounder. Multivariate analysis is a powerful tool for controlling confounders and is a standard procedure in epidemiology. However, there are two major limitations. First, one obviously can control only for variables that have been measured in the study. Second, one must conceptually clarify whether a variable is a confounder or a step in the causal pathway. For example, studies that investigate the impact of psychosocial stressors in the workplace on the risk of myocardial infarction usually control for high blood pressure. This is the correct procedure if one wants to isolate the effects of psychosocial stressors, which are independent from blood pressure. However, there is evidence that psychosocial stressors in the workplace are a cause of high blood pressure, which then subsequently increases the risk of myocardial infarction (Schnall, Belkić, Landsbergis, & Baker, 2000; Schnall, Schwartz, Landsbergis, Warren, & Pickering, 1998). In this case, blood pressure is not a confounder but rather an intermediate step in the causal pathway between psychosocial workplace stressors and myocardial infarction. Adjusting for blood pressure in multivariate analyses would therefore lead to an underestimation of the effects of psychosocial workplace stressors on myocardial infarction.

Adjusting for confounding becomes even more difficult when the causal chain includes several intermediate steps in which both biomedical and additional psychosocial factors are involved. For example, adverse social living conditions might cause negative emotions, which might cause physiological changes (e.g., a rise in cholesterol level or blood pressure), which might finally result in a specific disease. Such complex hierarchical steps cannot be appropriately analyzed with regression models. The addition of other statistical approaches, such as structural equation modeling (Ullman, 1996), could provide a better understanding of the associations between the variables; however, epidemiologists rarely use these approaches (for exceptions, see Knesebeck, 1998; J. Siegrist & Matschinger, 1989).

1.3. SOCIAL INEQUALITY IN THE RISK OF CORONARY HEART DISEASE

Social inequalities in health are a core subject in both medical sociology and social epidemiology.

Following the tradition of sociologist Max Weber (1864–1920), most scholars in medical sociology and social epidemiology assume that societies are hierarchically organized and that they consist of different social groups. These social groups differentiate themselves from one another by identifying common characteristics, such as education, assets, or values, that determine group members' "life chances" and success in the marketplace (Abel, 1991; Lynch & Kaplan, 2000; Weber, 1922/1968). Empirical research usually differentiates social groups by relatively simple and quantifiable characteristics, such as years of education and highest degree, amount of income, and type of occupation. The resulting social hierarchy is usually labeled *socioeconomic status*, although the terms *social class*, *social stratum*, and *socioeconomic position* are also in use.

Researchers have shown that low socioeconomic status is a strong determinant of poor health. This association is ubiquitous in space, persistent in time, and pervasive across diverse health outcomes. In a brilliant review, Antonovsky (1967) tracked anecdotal evidence of a shorter life expectancy for people of lower socioeconomic status as early as the 12th century. Another major breakthrough in research on social inequality and health, the Black Report, was published in 1980. This report, which was named after Sir Douglas Black, the chair of a research commission on social class and health, was the first major study showing that strikingly higher morbidity and mortality rates for people of lower socioeconomic status also exist in modern societies (in this case Great Britain during the 1970s). Inspired by this pioneer work, research on social inequalities in health has increased exponentially in Western Europe and North America (Kaplan & Lynch, 1997). The findings from these research activities show conclusively that marked social inequalities in health exist in all nations. Whether the indicator is education, income, or occupational status, men, women, and children of lower socioeconomic status are always at substantially higher risk of developing illnesses, becoming disabled, and dying prematurely (European Science Foundation, 2000; Lynch & Kaplan, 2000; Mackenbach et al., 1997; Rugulies, Aust, & Syme,

2004; Syme & Balfour, 1998). One of the most fascinating epidemiological findings has been the discovery of a gradient relationship between socioeconomic status and health (Adler et al., 1994; Evans, Barer, & Marmor, 1994; Marmot, 1994; McDonough, Duncan, Williams, & House, 1997; Syme, 1996). The importance of the topic of social inequalities in health is reflected in a research initiative by the European Science Foundation on Social Variations in Health Expectancy in Europe (for a detailed description, see European Science Foundation, 2000, and the Web site http://www.uni-duesseldorf.de/health).

There are very few diseases for which the association between low socioeconomic status and increased risk of poor health is absent or even reversed; the most notable is breast cancer, which is found more often in women of higher socioeconomic status. It has been speculated that this exception is caused by the later average age of first full-term pregnancy in women with higher education and income (Kelsey & Bernstein, 1996). Many scientists have considered (and many among the general public still consider) CHD to be another exception—in other words, people of higher socioeconomic status were believed to have a higher risk for CHD. There is indeed some evidence, mainly from the United States and Great Britain, that at the beginning of the 20th century, men (but not women) of higher socioeconomic status were more likely to develop CHD (Kaplan & Keil, 1993). Since the second half of the 20th century, however, this association has reversed, and today CHD is much more prevalent in both men and women of lower socioeconomic status in North America and Western Europe, as shown in several comprehensive reviews (e.g., Gonzáles, Artalejo, & del Rey Calero, 1998; Kaplan & Keil, 1993; Marmot, 1994). Gonzáles et al. (1998), for example, conducted an analysis on all cohort and case–control studies on social inequality in CHD published between 1960 and 1993. In the studies from the 1960s, persons performing manual occupations and persons with low education levels had a lower CHD risk than persons performing nonmanual occupations and persons with college educations. The studies from the 1970s, 1980s, and 1990s, how-

ever, showed a substantially higher risk for CHD among persons working in manual occupations and with low levels of education. This change over time was statistically significant ($\beta = .033$, $p = .02$) and was independent of sample size, endpoint (mortality: *yes* or *no*), and location of the study (within or outside the United States).

Socioeconomic status not only is associated with a higher risk of CHD but also has a negative impact on the clinical course of manifested CHD. Coronary patients of low socioeconomic status have significantly higher mortality risk than coronary patients of high socioeconomic status (Ruberman, Weinblatt, Goldberg, & Chaudhary, 1984; Weinblatt et al., 1978; R. B. Williams et al., 1992).

The following sections present in more detail two of the most important research projects on social inequalities in the development of CHD. The first is a comprehensive review of the European Union Working Group on Socioeconomic Inequalities in Health, and the second describes two large-scale prospective cohort studies on occupational status and CHD among British civil servants.

1.3.1. Results From the European Union Working Group on Socioeconomic Inequalities in Health

Under the direction of social epidemiologists Johan P. Mackenbach and Anton E. Kunst from the Netherlands, numerous studies and reviews on social inequalities in health and mortality have been published in recent years (Kunst et al., 1999; Kunst, Groenhof, Mackenbach, & European Union Working Group on Socioeconomic Inequalities in Health, 1998; Mackenbach et al., 1997). Figure 1.1 shows findings on socioeconomic status and mortality due to coronary heart disease for men 30 to 44 years old in Finland, Sweden, Norway, England and Wales, Italy, and the United States (Kunst et al., 1999). All results are based on prospective cohort studies and on a representative sample of the male working population followed over several years. Socioeconomic status was determined by occupational status. Persons not belonging to the workforce (e.g., because of early retirement, disability, or unemployment) were excluded from the analyses. The analyses compared the CHD mortal-

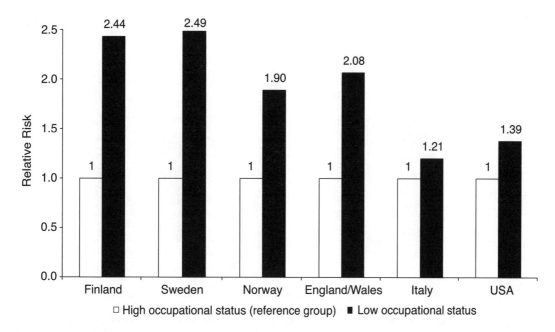

FIGURE 1.1. Relative risk for coronary heart disease mortality in men (ages 30–44) with high and low occupational status in different cohort studies. Data from "Occupational Class and Ischemic Heart Disease Mortality in the United States and 11 European Countries," by A. E. Kunst et al., 1999, *American Journal of Public Health, 89*, p. 51. Copyright 1999 by the American Public Health Association. Reprinted with permission.

ity rates for persons of low socioeconomic status (manual occupations) with those of persons of high socioeconomic status (nonmanual occupations, including employers) and showed an increased risk of dying from CHD for people of low socioeconomic status. Similar results were found for other age groups, although the social inequalities for those groups were less pronounced than for the 30 to 44 age group.

1.3.2. The Whitehall Studies

Although there is a consensus among researchers that risk of CHD is higher among people of low socioeconomic status, the causes for this finding are heatedly debated. Some researchers have pointed to the higher prevalence of problematic health behaviors among people of low socioeconomic status (especially smoking) as well as material deprivation as the causes for social inequalities in health, whereas other researchers have emphasized the importance of psychosocial stressors (Lynch, Davey Smith, et al., 2000; Macleod & Davey Smith, 2003;

Marmot & Wilkinson, 2001; Rugulies, 1998; J. Siegrist, 1996b). To investigate this issue empirically, large-scale prospective cohort studies are required that measure not only socioeconomic status and CHD but also health behaviors and potential psychosocial stressors. Among the best studies using such a research design have been the Whitehall studies (Marmot et al., 1991; Marmot, Ryff, Bumpass, Shipley, & Marks, 1997; Marmot, Shipley, & Rose, 1984). These prospective studies on 17,530 male civil servants (Whitehall I, completed in the 1980s) and 10,308 male and female civil servants (Whitehall II, ongoing) in London have measured not only socioeconomic status and health outcomes but also potential mediating factors. Figure 1.2 shows results from Whitehall I for death due to coronary heart disease. The left side of the figure illustrates the age-adjusted mortality rates in relation to occupational class (Marmot et al., 1984). There is a clear gradient, with the lowest mortality rate in the highest occupational class and the highest mortality rate in the lowest class. The

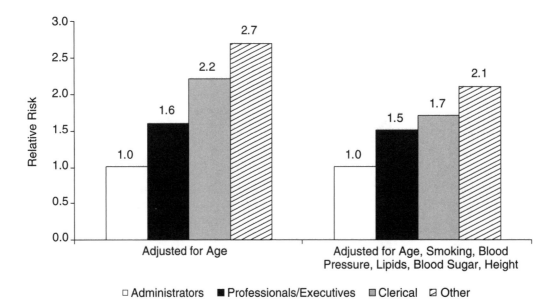

FIGURE 1.2. Relative risk for coronary heart disease mortality in male British civil servants. Data from M. G. Marmot et al., "Inequalities in Death—Specific Explanation of a General Pattern?" 1984, *Lancet, 1*, p. 1005. Copyright 1984 by Elsevier. Reprinted with permission.

right side of the figure shows what happens when the coronary risk factors are controlled for, including smoking, blood pressure, cholesterol, blood sugar, and height (as a proxy measure for deprivation in childhood). The gradient becomes somewhat smaller, indicating that these risk factors indeed explain part of the association between socioeconomic status and coronary mortality. However, although reduced, the gradient is still clearly visible, so there must be other powerful, as yet unknown factors that contribute to the higher coronary heart disease risk in persons of lower socioeconomic status.

The currently ongoing Whitehall II study has replicated the social gradient for men and identified in women the same association between low occupational status and increased risk of CHD (Marmot, Bosma, Hemingway, Brunner, & Stansfeld, 1997; Marmot et al., 1991). Similar results were found in a female-only case–control study in Sweden. As in Whitehall II, the social gradient remained after adjusting for biomedical risk factors (height, menopause, hypertension, smoking, physical activity, obesity, and lipids). For instance, women of the lowest occupational status group had 3.9 times (unadjusted; 2.6 times adjusted) the risk of CHD of

women of the highest occupational status (Wamala, Mittleman, Horsten, Schenck-Gustafsson, & Orth-Gomér, 2000).

1.3.3. Current Explanations for the Social Gradient in Coronary Heart Disease

Five explanations have been developed to explain the association between socioeconomic status and CHD. The relative contribution of and interaction among these explanations have been topics of intensified recent research.

1. *Social selection.* This approach maintains that ill health causes low socioeconomic status rather than the other way around. Social "downward mobility" in terms of disability and early retirement is considered a consequence of suffering from severe social selection. Several prospective studies tested this argument. Findings indicate that only a small proportion of the variance of the social gradient of CHD (usually 1% to 2%) is explained by social selection (Marmot & Feeney, 1996). Furthermore, this hypothesis cannot explain the robust association of education, an intraindividually stable trait, with CHD that leaves those with lower education at substantially higher risk.

2. *Health care inequalities.* This approach maintains that therapeutic and preventative progress in cardiology more often reaches higher socioeconomic status groups and that these differences may account for a substantial part of the social gradient. In fact, there is some evidence that this phenomenon may explain about 10% to 15% of the CHD variance by socioeconomic status (Mackenbach, Stronks, & Kunst, 1989). However, indicators of frequency of health care utilization and treatment procedures in cardiology do not show a social gradient, at least not in European countries.

3. *Prenatal development and early development.* Recent birth cohort studies have cast new light on the significance of maternal health during pregnancy, and particularly on mothers' health-related behaviors and their impact on fetal metabolism and subsequent birth weight. Metabolic dysregulation during pregnancy has been associated with increased metabolic and cardiovascular risk in middle adulthood (Barker, 1994). The quality of the social relationship between parents and children has also been shown to be an important determinant of differential susceptibility to illness later in life. Adverse socialization may lead to poor education and restricted occupational opportunities, which in turn elevate the risk of chronic disease (Blane, Brunner, & Wilkinson, 1996). Future research results will demonstrate the impact of these conditions on social variations in morbidity and mortality. These conditions may account for up to one third of the total variance observed between different social groups.

4. *Health-damaging behaviors in early and middle adulthood.* There is now convincing evidence of a social gradient in health-damaging behaviors, in particular cigarette smoking, unhealthy diet, weight gain, lack of physical exercise, and alcohol consumption. Health-adverse behavior is the most important explanatory factor for the social gradient in CHD. This conclusion is supported by analyses of socially differential reduction in CHD incidence (Keil & Hense, 1996; Mielck, 2000). Yet a significant proportion of the social gradient of CHD remains unexplained

after adjusting for health-related behaviors in multivariate statistical analysis (Marmot & Feeney, 1996). Moreover, the higher prevalence of health-adverse behaviors among people of lower socioeconomic status needs to be explained. In this perspective, the fifth explanatory approach is of particular importance.

5. *Exposure to an adverse material and psychosocial environment in adulthood.* The lower one's socioeconomic status, the higher one's exposure to adverse physical, chemical, and psychosocial stressors in occupational life and in everyday life. Direct effects (e.g., noise and hypertension, chronic distress and elevated fibrinogen and lipid concentrations) and indirect effects (e.g., increased cigarette consumption) on cardiovascular risk are topics of intense scientific analysis. Available results indicate that both material and psychosocial stressors follow an inverse social gradient and that these stressors contribute to the explanation of social differentials in CHD (Marmot & Wilkinson, 1999). Occupational stressors are of particular importance in this context, as will be shown later in this chapter, due to the long duration of exposure and the high intensity of distinct physical and psychosocial stressors in occupational life.

Although the role of genetic influences on CHD may be relevant for individual risk prediction, these factors may be less important in a population health perspective. For instance, the rapid change in CHD incidence during the past few decades cannot be substantially attributed to genetic influences; genetic factors would require a much longer time period to produce a comparable level of change. In terms of research methodology, it is therefore important to analyze the interactions of the five explanatory approaches developed so far and to combine prospective cohort studies with experimental and interventional approaches. Moreover, multilevel analysis might be appropriate because some of the determinants mentioned are located at an aggregate rather than an individual level of data collection (e.g., income distribution, regional disparity, business cycle). Research so far has focused heavily on risk factors but has neglected the role of protective conditions at both the biomedical and psychosocial levels. A more balanced analysis of risk and protective factors thus is needed.

This brief review indicates that further progress in explaining the social gradient of CHD is critically dependent on intensified transdisciplinary research and innovative study designs. The following section discusses only the fifth of the explanatory approaches, with a focus on the psychosocial stressors in occupational life that vary according to socioeconomic status and thus might contribute to an explanation of the social gradient in CHD. This in-depth analysis provides evidence-based information as a basis for specific recommendations for clinical medicine and for public health policy.

1.4. CHRONIC DISTRESS IN OCCUPATIONAL LIFE AND CORONARY HEART DISEASE

The inverse association between socioeconomic status and CHD must be considered a clear indication of the important role of social change in explaining variations in disease patterns over time. Some decades ago, CHD was considered a disease of civilization that resulted from a wealthy lifestyle, including a diet rich in cholesterol and calories, lack of physical activity, and smoking. Therefore, CHD was considered a typical upper class disease with a high prevalence among managers. More recently, this pattern has changed dramatically in developed countries and is changing rapidly in developing countries as well. Health-adverse behaviors are now recognized as more prevalent in individuals of lower socioeconomic status, and they contribute to a less favorable risk profile for cardiovascular and metabolic diseases.

Taking into account these developments, a robust inverse social gradient of CHD persists after adjustment for healthy lifestyle among both men and women (Marmot et al., 1984, 1991; Wamala et al., 2000). This observation points to the importance of psychosocial determinants of CHD. There is also evidence that the social gradient has increased in the recent past and that this increase accompanies a growing burden of socioeconomic and psychosocial stress. At the same time, scientific

progress in the area of stress research has cast light on the pathophysiological processes triggered by exposure to chronic psychosocial stressors that are of relevance to CHD (S. Cohen & Herbert, 1996; Manuck, 1994; Manuck, Marsland, Kaplan, & Williams, 1995; Sapolsky, 1995). In this section, we focus on adverse psychosocial work environment conditions, perhaps the most important source of exposure to a stressful environment in adult life.

There are several ways to investigate associations between job characteristics and risk of CHD. One approach is to compare statistics about CHD incidence in different occupational groups. Tüchsen recently published a gender-stratified list of occupations that were found to be associated with an increased risk of CHD in at least two independent epidemiological studies; 19 occupations for men and 6 for women were identified (Steenland et al., 2000). The best and most impressive epidemiological data were collected for inner-city bus drivers. Several reviews have shown that this occupational group has an increased risk for cardiovascular disease (CVD) in general and CHD and hypertension in particular (e.g., Aust, 1999; Belkić et al., 1994; Winkleby, Ragland, Fisher, & Syme, 1988). In 28 of 32 studies, professional bus drivers showed adverse outcomes with regard to blood pressure, ventricular arrhythmia, myocardial infarction, and other forms of ischemic heart disease (Aust, 1999; Belkić et al., 1994).

Another approach is to identify specific factors within an occupational group that are associated with an increased risk of CHD. For example, a study from Kornitzer and colleagues followed CHD incidence among employees of a private bank and a semipublic bank in Belgium (Kornitzer, Dramaix, & Gheyssens, 1979; Kornitzer, Kittel, Dramaix, & de Backer, 1982). The authors noted that the employees in the private bank were under intense pressure because of frequent workplace changes and the dynamic and aggressive style of the company. In the semipublic bank, pressure on the employees was considerably lower. After the 10-year follow-up period, the researchers found a doubled incidence of CHD in the private bank, even after taking other coronary risk factors into account.

The third, and in our opinion most promising, approach is to build hypotheses about working conditions that increase risk of CHD that are based on theoretical models. Such an approach is in accordance with the principle of falsification introduced by Popper (1966) and adopted by many epidemiologists (Weed, 1986). This principle requires that a researcher start with general sentences (theories) from which specific sentences (hypotheses) can be deducted. The specific sentences must be formulated in a way that they can be proved wrong by empirical research. If the hypotheses are not proved wrong, the theory is viewed as corroborated. If empirical research produces results that are not in accordance with the hypotheses, both the hypotheses and the theory are rejected (falsified). However, because epidemiological studies are complex and because measurement errors and major differences in the sociodemographic and sociocultural composition of samples are always possible, social epidemiological researchers usually have to view the evidence from several studies before deciding whether to accept or reject hypotheses and theories.

At the current stage of research, two theoretical models have evolved to explain associations between workplace factors and CHD in accordance with the principle of falsification: the demand–control model and the ERI model. Both models describe, on the basis of sociological theories and stress theory, specific psychosocial work environments that might be hazardous to coronary health. The hypotheses of both models have been tested in several prospective cohort studies. Hypotheses have also been generated for other theoretical models, such as the person–environment fit model (Caplan & Van Harrison, 1993) and action regulation theory (Hacker, 1994; Landsbergis, Theorell, Schwartz, Greiner, & Krause, 2000), but these hypotheses have not yet been tested in prospective cohort studies.

1.4.1. The Demand–Control Model

1.4.1.1. Theoretical assumptions and methods.
The demand–control model was developed in the 1970s by U.S. sociologist Robert A. Karasek (1979)

and subsequently tested, in close cooperation with the Swedish cardiologist and epidemiologist Töres Theorell, in several epidemiological studies (Karasek & Theorell, 1990; Theorell & Karasek, 1996). The model assumes that the interaction of psychological demands and job control (*decision latitude*) is crucial for understanding psychological workload. High psychological demands consist, for example, of time pressure, high work intensity, or tasks that require a great amount of concentration. Job control involves the ability to make decisions during the work process (*decision authority*) and to acquire and use new personal skills (*skill utilization*). According to the model, the combination of low demands and high control and of low demands and low control do not affect physical and psychosocial health. The combination of high demands and high control is viewed as positive, because it motivates and helps the individual acquire new skills and experience success (Theorell & Karasek, 1996).

The critical combination is high demands and low control, which is called *job strain*. This combination triggers anxiety, worry, and exhaustion, which subsequently reduce the ability of the person to learn and to develop new skills. According to the model, chronic exposure to this negative state leads to psychophysiological changes that increase the risk of CHD.

J. V. Johnson and Hall (1988) suggested expanding the demand–control model by including social support in the workplace; they hypothesized that the combination of high psychological demands, low control, and lack of social support (called *iso-strain*) might be even more hazardous to coronary health. Several empirical studies on the iso-strain concept have been conducted, and we include a discussion of the results in this section.

1.4.1.1.1. Measurement of job strain. Job strain has been measured by job titles, by specific questionnaires, and by workplace observations. One of the most widely used instruments is the Job Content Questionnaire, developed by Karasek. This questionnaire includes, among others, scales to measure psychological demands and job control at the workplace. An evaluation of the Job Content Questionnaire has shown that its psychometric properties are satisfactory (Karasek et al., 1998).

1.4.1.1.2. Literature search and selection of studies. As pointed out earlier in this chapter, the best study designs for social epidemiological research are prospective cohort studies, nested case–control studies, and case–cohort studies. We included all studies on the demand–control model with these designs in the review, and we also present findings from one intervention study.

We conducted the initial literature search in January 2000. The most important sources for references were the reviews "Job Strain and Cardiovascular Disease" (Schnall, Landsbergis, & Baker, 1994) and "The Workplace and Cardiovascular Disease" (Schnall, Belkić, Landsbergis, & Baker, 2000). In addition, we searched the Web site of the Center for Social Epidemiology (http://www.workhealth.org). Finally, we conducted a Medline search with the key words *demand control model* and *job strain*. The Medline search resulted in 998 hits covering a time span from 1966 to December 1999. When we combined the findings with the key word *coronary*, 96 hits remained. Those 96 articles included 14 studies that were cohort studies, nested case–control studies, or case–cohort studies (Table 1.1). For this chapter, we updated the literature search in May 2003 and identified two more articles (Kivimäki et al., 2002; Kuper & Marmot, 2003), also included in Table 1.1 (the article by Kuper & Marmot did not add a new cohort study but provided further analysis of Bosma, Peter, Siegrist, & Marmot, 1998, which was already included in the review).

1.4.1.2. Results. The following sections show the results of the review on job strain and CHD.

1.4.1.2.1. Job strain and the development and course of coronary heart disease. Job strain (high demands and low control in the workplace) or iso-strain (high demands and low control and low social support in the workplace) predicted the development of CHD or CVD in 6 of 14 studies. The following RRs were found: 4.95 (Haan, 1988), 4.0 (Karasek, Baker, Marxer, Ahlbom, & Theorell, 1981), 2.22 (Kivimäki et al., 2002), 1.92 (J. V. Johnson et al., 1989), and 1.38 (Kuper & Marmot, 2003). One study (Alfredsson, Spetz, & Theorell, 1985) used standardized mortality ratios and found

ratios of 118 for men and 164 for women, which were significantly higher than the expected value of 100.

In five studies, job strain was partially associated with CHD. LaCroix and Haynes (1984) found a significant association between job strain and CHD in women (RR = 2.9) but not in men. Alterman, Shekelle, Vernon, and Burau (1994) found that the increased risk for job strain was of only borderline significance. Low job control, however, was a significant predictor of an increased risk for CHD (RR = 1.32). Three other studies also found significant relative risks for low job control of 2.38 (Bosma et al., 1998), 1.83 (J. V. Johnson et al., 1996), and 1.41 (Steenland, Johnson, & Nowlin, 1997).

Especially interesting is the study by Johnson et al. (1996), because it used a large survey of 12,517 employed Swedish men. On the basis of job titles, psychological demands, job control, social support, and iso-strain were calculated for each subject. Because the survey also included information about subjects' job titles for the past 25 years, the authors created a job exposure matrix that included not only current but also past exposure to iso-strain. The analyses showed that 14 years after the survey, 521 men had died of CVD. The authors randomly matched five control subjects to each case. Subjects with low job control experienced 1.60 to 1.83 times the risk of dying from CVD. The combination of low job control and low social support at the workplace resulted in 2.62 times the risk (J. V. Johnson et al., 1996).

Three studies could not find any harmful effect of either job strain or its subcomponents that was of statistical significance. Hall, Johnson, and Tsou (1993) found that low job control tended to increase the risk in the expected direction (RR = 1.28), but Reed, LaCroix, Karasek, Miller, and MacLean (1989) found a trend toward a protecting effect of job strain. Suadicani, Hein, and Gyntelberg (1993) also did not have significant findings.

Only two studies investigated the impact of job strain on the course of CHD (see Table 1.1). Theorell, Perski, Orth-Gomér, Hamsten, and de Faire (1991) examined 79 men of relatively young age (≤45 years) who had recently suffered a

TABLE 1.1

Studies on the Impact of Job Strain on Coronary Heart Disease and Cardiovascular Disease

Study citation	Population and outcome measured	Main results	Level of significance	Factors controlled for
		Etiological studies		
Alfredsson, Spetz, & Theorell, 1985	958,096 male and female Stockholm residents with a 1-year follow-up Outcome: Hospitalization for MI	Hectic and monotonous work: SMR = 118 (men) SMR = 164 (women)	Significant[a] (men) Significant (women)	Age, risk factors, physical workload
Alterman, Shekelle, Vernon, & Burau, 1994	1,683 men in the United States with a 25-year follow-up Outcome: CHD mortality	Job strain: RR = 1.40 Low job control: RR = 1.32	Job strain: Borderline significant[b] Low job control: Significant	Age, risk factors, education
Bosma, Peter, Siegrist, & Marmot, 1998	10,308 men and women in the United Kingdom with a 5-year follow-up Outcome: CHD incidence	Job strain: Not significant Low job control: RR = 2.38 Note: Same study population as in Kuper & Marmot (2003)	Low job control: Significant	Age, gender, risk factors, effort–reward imbalance
Haan, 1988	902 men and women in Finland with a 10-year follow-up Outcome: CHD incidence	Job strain: RR = 4.95	Significant	Age, risk factors
Hall, Johnson, & Tsou, 1993	5,921 women in Sweden with a 9-year follow-up Outcome: CVD mortality	Job strain: Not significant Low job control: RR = 1.28	Low job control: Borderline significant	Age
C. C. Johnson, Hunter, Amos, Elder, & Berenson, 1989	7,219 men in Sweden with a 9-year follow-up Outcome: CVD mortality	Isostrain (all workers): RR = 1.92 Isostrain (blue collar workers): RR = 2.58 Isostrain (white collar workers): RR = 1.31	All workers: Significant Blue collar workers: Significant White collar workers: Not significant[c]	Age
J. V. Johnson, Stewart, Hall, Fredlund, & Theorell, 1996	12,517 men in Sweden with a 14-year follow-up Outcome: CVD mortality	Isostrain: Not significant Low job control: RR = 1.83 Low job control and low social support: RR = 2.62	Low job control: Significant Low job control and low social support: Significant	Age, risk factors, education, socioeconomic status
Karasek, Baker, Marxer, Ahlbom, & Theorell, 1981	1,461 men in Sweden with a 9-year follow-up Outcome: CVD mortality	Job strain: RR = 4.0 Low job control: RR = 1.5	Job strain: Significant Low job control: Not significant	Age, risk factors, CHD at baseline, education
Kivimäki et al., 2002	812 men and women in Finland with a 25-year follow-up Outcome: CHD mortality	Job strain: RR = 2.22	Significant	Age, gender, risk factors, occupational group

(continued)

TABLE 1.1 (Continued)

Studies on the Impact of Job Strain on Coronary Heart Disease and Cardiovascular Disease

Study citation	Population and outcome measured	Main results	Level of significance	Factors controlled for
Kuper & Marmot, 2003	10,308 men and women in the United Kingdom with an 11-year follow-up Outcome: All CHD incidence; fatal CHD and nonfatal MI	Job strain (all CHD incidence): RR = 1.38 Job strain (fatal CHD and nonfatal MI): RR = 1.16 *Note:* Same study population as in Bosma et al. (1998)	All CHD incidence: Significant Fatal CHD and nonfatal MI: Not significant	Age, gender, risk factors, occupational grade
LaCroix & Haynes, 1984	911 men and women in the United States with a 10-year follow-up Outcome: CHD incidence	Job strain (women): RR = 2.9 Job strain (men): Not significant	Women: Significant	Age, risk factors
Reed, LaCroix, Karasek, Miller, & MacLean, 1989	8,006 men of Japanese descent on Hawaii with an 18-year follow-up Outcome: CHD incidence	Job strain: Not significant Low job control: Not significant	Not significant	Age, risk factors
Steenland, Johnson, & Nowlin, 1997	3,575 men in the United States with a 14-year follow-up Outcome: CHD incidence	Job strain: RR = 1.08 Low job control: RR = 1.41	Job strain: Not significant Low job control: Significant	Age, risk factors, education
Suadicani, Hein, & Gyntelberg, 1993	1,638 men in Denmark with a 4-year follow-up Outcome: CHD incidence	Job strain: Not significant	Not significant	Age, risk factors, socioeconomic status
Prognostic studies				
Hlatky et al., 1995	922 men and women in the United States with advanced coronary atherosclerosis with a 5-year follow-up Outcome: CHD mortality and MI	Job strain: RR = 0.96	Not significant	Age, severity of CHD
Theorell, Perski, Orth-Gomér, Hamsten, & de Faire, 1991	79 men in Sweden who had returned to work after first MI with a 5-year follow-up Outcome: Fatal reinfarction	Subjects with fatal reinfarction during follow-up had rated their workplace as more stressful ($p = .02$)	Significant	Age, risk factors, severity of CHD

Note. MI = myocardial infarction; SMR = standardized mortality ratio; CHD = coronary heart disease; RR = relative risk; CVD = cardiovascular disease.
[a]$p \leq .05$ or lower interval limit ≥ 1, or both. [b]$p = .06–.09$ or lower interval limit < 1 but $\geq .90$, or both.
[c]$p \geq .10$ or lower interval limit $< .90$, or both.

myocardial infarction (MI). The subjects were asked to rate the level of psychological demand and job control at their workplaces. All men returned to their workplaces after their recovery. After 5 years, 13 men had died from a second MI, 17 had either survived a second MI or had undergone coronary bypass surgery, and 49 had not experienced a new coronary event. Analyses showed that subjects who later died had rated their workplaces as more stressful than subjects who did not experience a later event. This difference remained after adjusting for cholesterol level, fibrinogen level, blood pressure, extent of atherosclerosis, Type A behavior, and education.

In the second study, 922 men and women with CHD (documented by angiograms and with stenosis of ≥75%) were followed for 4 years (Hlatky et al., 1995). No association between job strain and course of CHD was found. However, this study had several methodological problems: Only a few subjects were of low socioeconomic status, it was not documented how many subjects had given up their jobs because of the disease, and the analyses were not stratified by gender.

1.4.1.2.2. An intervention study on the demand–control model. As pointed out earlier, it is difficult to conduct intervention studies of high methodological quality in the context of social epidemiology. Among the best intervention studies conducted with regard to the demand–control model is a study by Orth-Gomér, Eriksson, Moser, Theorell, and Fredlund (1994) of male and female public employees in Sweden. This study followed 94 employees in the intervention sample and 35 in the nonrandomized control group. The intervention consisted of meetings to inform employees about the association between work environment and stress reaction and of stress management classes. Participants also organized focus groups to identify stressful working conditions and to develop ideas for improvement.

The evaluation of the program after 8 months of intervention showed that participants in the intervention group reported an increase in job control and an improvement in their relations with their supervisors. There were no changes in the control group. On the biomedical level, researchers found a 6% reduction in the apolipoprotein B–apolipoprotein AI ratio, which was statistically significant. However, the clinical consequences of a 6% reduction in this measure are unclear.

1.4.1.3. Summary of research on the demand–control model. In 6 of 14 prospective studies with initially healthy subjects, job strain or isostrain significantly increased the risk of CVD. In 2 other studies, the associations were of borderline signifi-

cance or were found only in women but not in men. Three other studies found that low job control, but not job strain, had a significant impact. In 1 study, low job control was of borderline significance. In 2 studies, job strain, iso-strain, and low job control did not have a harmful impact on cardiovascular health.

The demand–control model has also been tested with regard to other health outcomes, especially musculoskeletal disorders (Bongers, de Winter, Kompier, & Hildebrandt, 1993; Bongers, Kremer, & ter Laak, 2002). Most of these studies are cross-sectional in design and thus do not allow causal inference. However, this limitation does not apply to a recent prospective study from the United States on the impact of job strain on all-cause mortality. This study used a job exposure matrix to assess the experience of job strain throughout subjects' occupational careers and analyzed mortality after 5 and 10 years. Although job strain was not a significant predictor for mortality, subjects with low job control showed a significantly increased 1.43 higher risk of mortality (Amick et al., 2002).

1.4.2. The Effort–Reward Imbalance Model

1.4.2.1. Theoretical assumptions. The ERI model was developed in the late 1980s in Germany and has since been tested in several international studies. It assumes that people expend effort at work as part of a socially organized exchange process to which society at large contributes in terms of rewards. Rewards are distributed via three transmitter systems: money; esteem; and career opportunities, including job security.

The ERI model postulates that lack of reciprocity between "costs" and "gains" (i.e., when high effort is compensated by low rewards) produces emotional distress that can lead to the arousal of the autonomic nervous system and associated strain reactions (J. Siegrist, 1996a, 1996b; J. Siegrist et al., 2004). For instance, having a demanding but unstable job or achieving at a high level without being offered promotion prospects are examples of high cost–low gain conditions at work. According to the ERI model, people experience low reciprocity under three conditions:

1. Lack of alternative choices in the labor market may prevent people from leaving even unfavorable jobs because the anticipated costs of change outweigh the costs of accepting inadequate benefits ("a bad job is better than no job").
2. People may accept unfair job arrangements for a certain period of their occupational trajectory for strategic reasons, perhaps to improve chances for career promotion and related rewards at a later stage.
3. A specific personal pattern of coping with demands and of eliciting rewards that is characterized by overcommitment may prevent people from accurately assessing cost–gain relations. *Overcommitment* is a set of attitudes, behaviors, and emotions reflecting excessive striving in combination with a strong desire for approval and esteem. People who exhibit overcommitment expend effort beyond levels usually considered appropriate in relation to gain.

ERI therefore may involve extrinsic as well as intrinsic motivation. The presence of both components is considered especially hazardous to coronary health (for a more detailed description, see J. Siegrist et al., 2004).

1.4.2.1.1. Measuring effort–reward imbalance. The extrinsic and intrinsic components of the ERI model are measured with separate standardized questionnaires that are then combined in statistical models (J. Siegrist, 1996a; J. Siegrist et al., 2004). Historically, two different versions of statistical testing have been developed. The first version, called the *weak test*, assumes that at least one component of effort (extrinsic or intrinsic) and at least one component of low reward have to be present in a person to increase his or her risk of CHD. Both the early studies on the ERI model, which used the original questionnaire, and studies that used proxy variables to measure ERI (because the original questionnaire was not available) used this "weak" version.

The second version of statistical testing, which is the currently used approach, constitutes a *strong test* of the model by building two scores. One score

expresses the relation between extrinsic effort and reward, with a value greater than 1.0 indicating a health-hazardous mismatch between high efforts and low rewards. The other score is a sum score for overcommitment. The upper tertile of this score indicates a level of overcommitment that is thought to be too high in intrinsic effort and in the need for esteem (J. Siegrist et al., 2004).

1.4.2.1.2. Literature search and selection of studies. The literature search for studies of the impact of ERI on the development and course of CHD followed the same logic as that described for the demand–control model and was restricted to studies with a prospective, nested case–control, or case–cohort design. In addition, we present findings from an intervention study.

The most important sources for references were the reviews by Aust (1999), J. Siegrist (1996b), and Schnall et al. (2000). We conducted a Medline search with the key words *effort–reward imbalance* and *Gratifikationskrisen* covering a time span from 1966 to December 1999 that resulted in 17 hits. Of these, we identified three prospective studies on ERI and two prospective studies on restenosis after angioplasty (percutaneous transluminal coronary angioplasty) and on the progression of atherosclerosis of the carotid artery. For this chapter, we updated the literature search in May 2003 and identified two more articles (Table 1.2). (The article by Kuper, Singh-Manoux, Siegrist, & Marmot, 2002, did not add a new cohort study but provided further analysis of Bosma et al., 1998).

1.4.2.2. Results. The following sections show the results of the review on effort–reward imbalance and CHD.

1.4.2.2.1. Effort–reward imbalance and the development and course of coronary heart disease. In the Marburg Industrial Worker Study, J. Siegrist and colleagues followed 416 male blue collar steelworkers over a period of 6 1/2 years. Twenty-one of the subjects experienced a myocardial infarction during the follow-up period (J. Siegrist, Peter, Junge, & Cremer, 1990). Among these 21 subjects, 38.0% had shown the combination of high effort and low reward at baseline, compared with only 7.4% of subjects who did not develop an MI. When

TABLE 1.2

Studies on the Impact of Effort–Reward Imbalance on Coronary Heart Disease
and Cardiovascular Disease

Study citation	Population and outcome measured	Main results	Level of significance	Factors controlled for
Etiological studies				
Bosma, Peter, Siegrist, & Marmot, 1998	10,308 men and women in the United Kingdom with a 5-year follow-up Outcome: CHD incidence	ERI: RR = 2.15 *Note:* Same study population as in Kuper et al. (2002)	Significant[a]	Age, gender, risk factors, job control
Kivimäki et al., 2002	812 men and women in Finland with a 25-year follow-up Outcome: CHD mortality	ERI: RR = 2.42	Significant	Age, gender, risk factors, occupational group
Kuper, Singh-Manoux, Siegrist, & Marmot, 2002	10,308 men and women in the United Kingdom with an 11-year follow-up Outcome: All CHD incidence and fatal CHD and nonfatal MI	ERI (all CHD incidence): RR = 1.26 ERI (fatal CHD and nonfatal MI): RR = 1.21 *Note:* Same study population as in Bosma et al. (1998)	All CHD incidence: Significant Fatal CHD and nonfatal MI: Not significant[b]	Age, gender, risk factors, occupational grade
Lynch, Krause, Kaplan, Tuomilehto, & Salonen, 1997	2,297 men in Finland with an 8-year follow-up Outcome: MI	ERI: RR = 1.57 *Note:* When adjusted separately for behavioral and biological risk factors and without psychological problems, the relative risk was significant (RR = 2.30 and RR = 1.94, respectively)	Not significant	Age, behavioral and biological risk factors, and psychological problems
Lynch, Krause, Kaplan, Salonen, & Salonen, 1997	940 men in Finland with a 4-year follow-up Outcome: Progression of atherosclerosis of the carotids	Height of atherosclerotic plaques increased more in subjects with effort–reward imbalance (0.32 vs. 0.27. $p = .04$)	Significant	Age, risk factors
J. Siegrist, Peter, Junge, & Cremer, 1990	416 men in Germany with a 6.5-year follow-up Outcome: MI	ERI: 3.42 (regression coefficient)	Significant	Age, risk factors
Prognostic studies				
Joksimovic et al., 1999	106 men in Germany after angioplasty with a 1-year follow-up Outcome: Restenosis	Work-related overcommitment: RR = 2.86	Significant	Age, risk factors

Note. CHD = coronary heart disease; ERI = effort–reward imbalance; RR = relative risk; MI = myocardial infarction.
[a]$p \leq .05$ or lower interval limit ≥ 1, or both. [b]$p \geq .10$ or lower interval limit $< .90$, or both.

adjusted for age, body mass index, systolic blood pressure, and low-density lipoprotein cholesterol levels, the regression coefficient for ERI was 3.42 (SE = 0.83) and highly significant ($p < .001$). However, both the study population and the numbers of subjects were very small, and therefore the effects are unstable. For example, the regression coefficient expressed as a multivariate odds ratio would be 30.57, with very wide confidence intervals ranging from 5.05 to 155.52. Therefore, in additional analysis, the case definition was broadened to include subjects with subclinical signs of CHD as defined by electrocardiogram changes. Subjects with ERI had 6.15 times the risk of CHD, a significant effect (95% CI = 2.01–18.82) after adjustment for age, weight, and blood pressure (J. Siegrist, 1996b, pp. 219–220).

In the British Whitehall II study, Bosma et al. (1998) analyzed the impact of ERI on the incidence of angina pectoris and doctor-diagnosed CHD in 10,308 men and women after a 5-year follow-up. Because the ERI questionnaire was not used at baseline, proxy measures were built from other items. Subjects with ERI were 3.1 times more likely to develop CHD. After statistical adjustment for occupational status, negative affectivity, coronary risk factors, and job control, there was still 2.15 times the risk. This study showed for the first time that high ERI and low job control increased the risk of CHD independently from each other.

Kuper et al. (2002) recently ran a new analysis on the Whitehall cohort. Their analyses differed in some important areas from those of Bosma et al. (1998). Kuper et al. used more items to build proxy measures for ERI and validated them against the original items from the ERI questionnaire that was used in later phases of the Whitehall study. As with the original instrument, they calculated a ratio between effort and reward. Their analyses also covered a longer follow-up period (11 years) and measured incidence of CHD, fatal CHD, and nonfatal myocardial infarction separately. Kuper et al. found that high ERI increased the risk of CHD 1.26 times, which was significant ($p < .001$). A significant linear trend of $p = .008$ was also discovered. For the outcome of fatal CHD and nonfatal myocardial in-

farction, the relative risk for the fourth quartile was 1.21, which was not significant, and there was no significant linear trend.

The Finnish Kuopio Study used high demands and low psychosocial resources in the workplace and low income as measures for ERI (Lynch, Krause, Kaplan, Tuomilehto, & Salonen, 1997). ERI significantly increased the risk of myocardial infarction, even when adjusted for behavioral risk factors (smoking and alcohol consumption, RR = 2.30) and biological risk factors (blood pressure, cholesterol, and other biomarkers, RR = 1.94). The association only became insignificant (RR = 1.57) when the adjustments were made simultaneously for behavioral and biological risk factors and also for psychological problems (depression and hopelessness). Further analyses from this study showed that individuals with ERI had greater progression of carotid atherosclerosis at a 4-year follow-up (Lynch, Krause, Kaplan, Salonen, & Salonen, 1997).

Another study from Finland (Kivimäki et al., 2002) analyzed proxy measures for ERI obtained in a survey from 1973 and linked them to the national mortality register. ERI was calculated as the ratio between efforts and rewards and was categorized into tertiles. The follow-up period was 25 years. Compared with the most favorable tertile, subjects in the second tertile had 1.91 times and subjects in the third tertile 2.42 times the risk of CHD mortality after adjustment for occupational group and behavioral and biological risk factors.

The impact of ERI on the course of CHD has been investigated in one study so far. In this study, 106 men with coronary heart disease filled out the ERI questionnaire on the evening before they underwent angioplasty. A control angiogram 6 months later showed that men with high levels of overcommitment were 2.9 times more likely to show a restenosis of the dilated artery (Joksimović et al., 1999).

1.4.2.2.2. An intervention study on the effort–reward imbalance model. One intervention study has addressed the ERI model. It was a so-called feasibility study that investigated how the assumptions of the model could be translated into workplace health promotion (Aust, 1999; Aust, Peter, & Siegrist, 1997). In a public transit company in a major city in the western part of Germany, 54 bus drivers participated in a controlled nonrandomized trial. The 12-week intervention program was aimed at both the individual level (e.g., information about the hazardous effects of distress on health, reflection on one's attitude toward stress in the workplace, relaxation techniques) and the interpersonal level (e.g., training in social competence and conflict management, group discussions with supervisors). At the end of the program, subjects in the intervention group showed a significant decrease in work-related overcommitment, and there was no change in the control group. Another measurement 3 months after the course showed that these changes had remained stable (Aust et al., 1997). In addition, the researchers conducted a comprehensive analysis of problems in the organization and developed solutions that they presented to employers and employees of the company (Aust, 1999).

1.4.2.3. Summary of research on the effort–reward imbalance model. Although the ERI model has been used in only a few prospective studies to date, the results are relatively consistent and indicate that the mismatch between high efforts and low rewards increases the risk of CHD. However, before reaching a final conclusion, it seems advisable to wait for the results of current ongoing large-scale prospective studies on ERI and CHD. Other studies have shown associations between ERI and other health outcomes, such as gastrointestinal and musculoskeletal disorders, psychological problems (especially depression), and poor subjective health (Joksimović, Starke, Knesebeck, & Siegrist, 2002; Peter, Geissler, & Siegrist, 1998; Rugulies & Krause, 2000; Stansfeld, Bosma, Hemingway, & Marmot, 1998; Stansfeld, Fuhrer, Shipley, & Marmot, 1999; Tsutsumi, Kayaba, Theorell, & Siegrist, 2001).

1.5. CONCLUSION

We have shown in this chapter that there is clear and compelling evidence of a higher risk of CHD in people of lower socioeconomic status. There is also some evidence that exposure to adverse psychosocial working conditions increases the risk of CHD. However, the results on work environment factors are not yet as coherent and strong as those for socioeconomic status, so further research is needed in this area. It is especially important to conduct more prospective studies that measure psychosocial working conditions, not only at baseline but also at several times during the course of the study, so that changes in exposure over time can be assessed.

Both the demand–control model and the ERI model are focused on few but central psychosocial workplace factors. The parsimonious nature of the models is one of their strengths and an important reason for their attractiveness. However, there may be other psychosocial working conditions not included in these two models that are relevant to coronary heart disease. For example, emotional demands have been discussed recently in the literature as an important psychosocial workplace factor, especially among hospital workers and other employees in the service sector (de Jonge, Mulder, & Nijhuis, 1999). Other workplace factors that are currently being tested are the predictability and the meaningfulness of work (Kristensen, 2001; Nielsen, Kristensen, & Smith-Hansen, 2002; Nielsen et al., 2004).

1.5.1. Chronic Distress and Social Inequality in the Risk of Coronary Heart Disease

A very important and currently controversial issue in social epidemiology is whether the increased risk of CHD among people of lower socioeconomic status can be explained at least partly by differences in exposure to psychosocial workplace factors. Some researchers have argued that exposure to adverse psychosocial working conditions might be a causal step in the pathway between socioeconomic status and CHD, but other researchers have stressed that socioeconomic status and adverse psychosocial workplace factors might be merely correlated and that the causal impact of psychosocial working conditions on health remains to be proved (Lynch, Davey Smith, et al., 2000; Macleod & Davey Smith,

2003; Marmot & Wilkinson, 2001; Singh-Manoux, 2003). Empirically, only a few findings are available that address this issue, and their interpretation is difficult. In the Whitehall II study, statistical adjustment for psychosocial working conditions made the social gradient in CHD disappear (Marmot, Bosma, et al., 1997). This can be interpreted as a mediating effect of psychosocial workplace conditions (Syme & Balfour, 1997). However, researchers who are skeptical about psychosocial explanations have argued that this finding may show that psychosocial working conditions, and especially low job control, are more or less proxy measures for socioeconomic status (Davey Smith, 1997). To make things even more difficult, a Swedish case–control study on women with coronary heart disease showed that even after adjusting for psychosocial workplace factors, the social gradient was still largely intact (Wamala et al., 2000). Clearly, more and better research is needed on this important issue.

1.5.2. Sociological Aspects of Other Psychosocial Factors

Socioeconomic status and distress in the workplace are associated with several other psychosocial factors discussed as predictors for CHD. The very first study on Type A behavior (M. Friedman & Rosenman, 1959) was in fact inspired by a previous study on the impact of occupational stress on cardiovascular risk factors in tax accountants (M. Friedman, Rosenman, & Carroll, 1958). Regarding hostility, the most popular psychosocial explanation for CHD in the 1990s, studies from the United States, Great Britain, and Germany demonstrated that levels of hostility are higher in people of low socioeconomic status (Barefoot, Peterson, Dahlstrom, & Siegler, 1991; Marmot et al., 1991; Mittag, Peschel, & Chrosziewski, 1997; Scherwitz, Perkins, Chesney, & Hughes, 1991). These findings indicate that it is important to investigate psychological factors in a broader sociological context. As Myrtek shows in chapter 6 in this volume, Type A behavior was predictive of CHD in the Western Collaborative Group study (Rosenman et al., 1975) but failed to predict CHD in later studies (Ragland & Brand, 1988a, 1988b; Shekelle, Hulley, et al.,

1985), so it can no longer be regarded as important in CHD. For hostility the evidence is mixed, and the overall effect sizes are relatively small. Although admittedly speculative, we wonder if research on Type A behavior and hostility would be more successful if these two factors were viewed as psychological reactions, patterned and influenced by a larger sociological context, instead of isolated personality aspects.

The most convincing evidence of the impact of a psychological factor on coronary heart disease currently exists for clinical depression and depressive mood. A recent meta-analysis of 13 prospective studies with subjects showing no sign of CHD at baseline found that depression led to 1.64 times the risk of CHD, a significant result ($p < .001$; Rugulies, 2002). The sensitivity analysis revealed that the effect was strongest for clinical depression, which resulted in 2.69 times the risk. Subjects with depressed mood had 1.49 times the risk, which was still statistically significant ($p < .002$). Studies of the impact of depression on the course of CHD have shown even greater effect sizes (Frasure-Smith, Lespérance, & Talajic, 1995a; Ladwig, Kieser, Konig, Breithardt, & Borggrefe, 1991; Lespérance, Frasure-Smith, Juneau, & Théroux, 2000). From a sociological point of view, there is evidence for a higher incidence and prevalence of depression in people of low socioeconomic status and in persons who have experienced chronic distress (G. W. Brown & Harris, 1978, 1989; Kaplan, Roberts, Camacho, & Coyne, 1987; J. M. Murphy et al., 1991; Stansfeld, Head, & Marmot, 1998). It has also been shown recently that both low control in the workplace and ERI increase the risk of depression (Stansfeld et al., 1999), suggesting that negative emotions, such as depression, might be an intermediate step in the causal pathway between psychosocial workplace factors and CHD.

These examples show that factors on the macrosocial level (socioeconomic status), the mesosocial level (experience of distress, especially in the workplace), and the personal level (e.g., depression and hostility) are not independent phenomena. Psychocardiology (or, more precisely, sociopsychocardiology) should therefore not limit itself to the identification of isolated social and psychological predictors of CHD. Instead, a broader and transdisciplinary framework is needed to investigate the complex interplay of social living conditions, psychological states, and physiological processes in the epidemiology of health and illness in general and of coronary heart disease specifically (Rugulies et al., 2004). Transdisciplinary research is certainly not easy, but we believe it is the best way to improve our knowledge about the determinants of coronary heart disease and to find strategies to reduce CHD morbidity and mortality.

CHAPTER 2

PSYCHODYNAMIC HYPOTHESES ON THE ETIOLOGY, COURSE, AND PSYCHOTHERAPY OF CORONARY HEART DISEASE: 100 YEARS OF PSYCHOANALYTIC RESEARCH

Jochen Jordan and Benjamin Bardé

2.1. INTRODUCTION

This chapter reviews psychodynamic contributions to the literature on psychological factors in coronary heart disease (CHD) published in English, German, and French since 1920 (not included are publications dealing with coping processes during the course of the disease).[1] After this introduction, section 2.2 describes the strategies we used in the systematic literature search of scientific databases, section 2.3 reviews the history of research on CHD, section 2.4 examines research on triggers of the onset of heart attacks, and section 2.5 reviews the literature concerning the development and therapy of posttraumatic stress disorder (PTSD) after myocardial infarction (MI). The concluding section reports on how psychodynamic knowledge can contribute to the psychotherapy of patients with CHD.

A systematic review of the psychodynamic literature involves three special difficulties: (a) limitations in search processes, (b) problems in identifying specifically psychodynamic contributions, and (c) the methodological quality of the publications. First, the literature search process is limited by the fact that psychodynamic articles encounter difficulties in being accepted by mainstream scientific journals; for example, psychodynamic articles are usually much longer than permitted. In addition, their methodological standards often are not accepted by the scientific community, which prefers short empirical papers. Thus, for decades psycho-

analytical publications have appeared in specialized journals or in books, many of which are not integrated systematically into scientific databases, and we cannot be sure that our search identified all applicable publications. Furthermore, psychoanalytic authors prefer to publish in their own language (particularly German, French, Spanish, and Italian). Thus, this review may exclude important publications in languages other than those included (English, German, and some in French).

The second problem is identifying specifically psychodynamic articles from among the large number of publications. Many abstracts mentioned a conceptualization that suggests a psychodynamic orientation, but intensive study of the article revealed that it could not be classified as psychodynamic. Concepts like denial, defense mechanisms, intrapsychic conflict, and dynamic therapy suggest psychodynamic thinking, but these concepts are also used in other theoretical contexts.

We included a publication in this review if it referred to essential characteristics of psychodynamic ways of thinking reflected in at least one of the following five concepts and statements:

1. It clearly distinguished between conscious and unconscious processes and formulated corresponding hypotheses.
2. It referred to a psychodynamic conflict model.
3. It described defense mechanisms according to inner psychodynamic processes.

---

[1] Note that quotations throughout from German and French sources have been translated into English by the authors.

4. It referred to the phenomena of psychodynamic transference and countertransference.
5. It provided a psychodynamic description of intrapsychic processes.

Finally, psychodynamic work opens a window on unconscious emotional processes and contributes in this way to an understanding of the psychosocial aspects of CHD. Therefore, we decided to include articles without regard to their methodological quality. This decision was based on the assumption that psychodynamic knowledge is one type of expert knowledge even if the sample size is small (N = 1–100) and even when basic methodological standards are neglected (e.g., sample description, selection mechanisms, description of the psychological interventions). No systematic review has previously been published on the psychodynamic literature, and we hope that this chapter will inspire further development of research in this field.

2.2. SYSTEMATIC LITERATURE SEARCH

For the literature search, we used the PSYNDEX, PsycINFO, and Medline databases. We did not specify limits concerning the publication date. The search terms we used were *heart attack, myocard*, coronar*, koronar*,* and *cardiovasc*,* in combination with *psychoanal*, tiefenpsy*, psychodyn*, psycholog*,* and *psychosom*.* We did a supplementary search using the key words *psychother*, group*, gruppe*, psycholog*,* and *psychosoc*.*

We also searched articles in such journals as *Group Analysis, Gruppentherapie, Gruppenanalyse, Psychotherapie und Gruppendynamik, International Journal of Group Psychotherapy,* and many others. Beyond journal articles, our search included reference books and textbooks (e.g., *Psychosomatic Diagnosis,* Dunbar, 1943, and *Emotions and Bodily Changes,* Dunbar, 1954; *Psychosomatic Medicine: A Clinical Study of Psychophysiologic Reactions,* Weiss & English, 1957; *Psychology of the 20th Century,* Balmer et al., 1976–1981; *Heart and Mind,* Allan & Scheidt, 1996; *Psychosomatic Medicine,* Uexküll, 2002). In all articles and chapters, we analyzed the reference lists, and we found many new publica-

tions in this way. We also systematically searched the holdings of the German Library in Frankfurt am Main and the world's largest collection of psychoanalytical journals, magazines, and books at the Sigmund Freud Institute in Frankfurt am Main.

This process enabled us to identify more than 700 publications in international scientific journals and books, each of which we analyzed word for word. In the end, we included 233 publications in this review.

2.3. PSYCHODYNAMIC RESEARCH ON CORONARY HEART DISEASE

For hundreds of years, people have intuitively known that the emotions and heart functioning are interrelated. Colloquial speech in nearly every language worldwide reflects this knowledge in metaphors and idioms. Numerous examples demonstrate the common knowledge and everyday experience of psychological influences on the etiology and mortality of heart disease (see, e.g., http://www.whonamedit.com/doctor.cfm/84.html). In such folk usage, only a limited spectrum of emotions appear systematically: the loss of loved ones, depression, serious disappointment, stress, hostility, and every type of anger.

Until the end of the 19th century, the interaction between emotional and somatic factors in heart functioning did not have to be proved; it was evident. "Modern" medicine increasingly became a natural science (sometimes, especially with cardiology, it is called an "engineering science"). Subsequently, the correlation between emotional and social factors had to be proved by empirical and experimental studies using rigorous methodology (known as *evidence-based medicine*). Systematic research in this area began in 1925, but the development of research instruments took a long time. In the classic textbook *Psychosomatic Medicine* (Weiss & English, 1957), the authors described the research up to 1957 as unsatisfactory. They asserted that there was still no sufficient empirical base proving that psychological factors influence the etiology of CHD. Although Weiss and English (1957) considered this hypothesis plausible, they rated the evidence base as low. They also argued, however, that the scientific knowledge base provided evidence that following the onset of CHD, the course of the disease is influenced by psychological factors (coping processes as well as mortality).

2.3.1. The Prescientific Phase of Psychocardiology

A systematic literature search is impossible for publications before 1930, because scientific databases do not thoroughly inventory the work of this period. Consequently, we identified these early sources using the original reference lists of publications of this time period. This effort was not only extremely time consuming but also faulty and often incomplete. Medical publications on psychosomatic issues published before 1930 reflect many methodologies and include empirically based observations, literary and philosophical treatises, reports on everyday psychological experience, and educational essays (texts that sought to educate the public). Many publications could be classified as "expert descriptions": Well-known specialists would give a talk on their personal experiences and subsequently publish a report (e.g., Braun, 1920, 1932; Fahrenkamp, 1941). Publication titles are often imprecise; sometimes only after reading the whole work did we realize that the content was not related to the title. (Interesting from a historical perspective are the following publications, which we will not review in this chapter: Braun, 1920, 1932; Deutsch & Kauf, 1923; J. C. Edwards & White, 1934; Eichenberger, 1929; Fahrenkamp, 1929, 1941; Heyer, 1925; Katzenelbogen, 1932; Kilgore, 1929; Klemperer, 1929; MacWilliam, 1923; H. E. Richardson, 1933; W. H. V. Wyss, 1924, 1927, 1931.)

Researchers in this period dealt extensively with the question of how psychological events are relevant to CHD. Authors asked which concrete psychophysiological interactions exist between emotional conditions and heart circulation functions. A first review of psychosomatic models of etiopathological processes was presented in 1954 by Flanders Dunbar in her book *Emotions and Bodily Changes—A Survey of Literature on Psychosomatic Interrelationships 1910–1953*. The chapter entitled

"Cardiovascular System" contains a brilliant review of the scientific work from this time. We could not find much of this work in the databases we searched, so the essay is a treasure trove of literature from the initial phase of psychosomatic research.

2.3.2. The Beginning of Systematic Scientific Research

The beginning of systematic scientific research can be dated from 1925. Two groups were foremost in collecting data systematically, one in the Menninger Clinic (Houston, Texas) and the other in New York at the Presbyterian Hospital.

One of the first systematic psychodynamic attempts was to formulate specific conflict constellations that characterize the personality of people suffering from CHD. Menninger and Menninger (1936), on the basis of three short case reports, formulated a psychodynamic hypothesis—that aggressive tendencies lead to CHD—with great caution: "Our data are entirely insufficient to prove anything clinical. They only suggest that these psychological factors are sometimes of importance in the development of cardiopathology" (p. 21). Menninger and Menninger included a note that mentioned a discussion of their hypothesis among their circle of colleagues at the Psychoanalytical Society in Chicago, among them Franz Alexander and Thomas French. They reported that discussions were intense and that a number of case and treatment reports were shared that supported their hypothesis. This note shows that their colleagues were intensely interested in the topic of CHD.

Menninger and Menninger (1936) proposed that, particularly in men, CHD is the result of repressed strong aggressive tendencies. The core conflict is centered in a negative oedipal scene:

> Characteristically they [the aggressive tendencies] appear in a man who was strongly attached emotionally to his father and often more or less definitely hostile to his mother. The conscious affection for the father completely obliterated the deeply buried hostilities for him. If, then, the father has heart

disease or symptoms of heart disease, it is very typical for the patient to include these symptoms in his identification with the father but carry out the inexpressible patricidal impulses reflexively by unconscious focal suicide. It has been suggested . . . that this identification is not with the father so much as with the father's preferred love objects, i.e., his wife, the patient's mother, and that in this sense the heart disease is at the same time symbolic of the "broken-hearted-ness" of disappointment. (p. 20)

In conclusion, Menninger and Menninger (1936) stated that the aggressive tendencies seemed to be the most important factor in the development of CHD in men. The authors expressed the desire to engage in further research in cooperation with cardiologists. From a historical perspective, it is interesting that Menninger and Menninger summarized an article by a cardiologist, L. A. Conner, who in 1930 published a paper describing the psychological burden on patients with coronary diseases:

[Conner] listed the common (superficial) *psychogenic precipitating traumas* as: (1) the thoughtless statement of some physicians; (2) the knowledge of heart disease and/or sudden death in the family or friends; (3) the occurrence of some sudden symptom such as pain, which focuses attention on the heart; and (4) profound emotional disturbance as in "shell shock." He stated very definitely that treatment belongs essentially to the realm of psychotherapy. (quoted in Menninger & Menninger, 1936, p. 11)[2]

This quotation shows that the traumatic impact of an MI and the need for psychotherapeutic interventions have long been recognized.

2.3.3. Flanders Dunbar and Her Work Group

In the history of psychosomatic medicine, the work of Flanders Dunbar and her group at the New York Presbyterian Hospital is a milestone. Their publications concerning CHD have been those most often cited in the past 50 years, and they continue to be cited even today. They were the first researchers to systematically examine large samples of patients and controls (i.e., persons with injuries or organic diseases; Dunbar, Wolfe, Tauber, & Brush, 1939). They developed a system for documenting specific variables (described later in this section). In numerous articles and books, they portrayed patients with CHD and their psychosomatic backgrounds, compared them with other clinical groups and controls, and illustrated their etiology in short case reports.

Extensive experience with numerous clinical groups characterizes the empirical studies and publications of Dunbar's work group. Their work was based on a long-term study (14 years) with several comparison and control groups. Dunbar regarded psychotherapeutic interventions using psychodynamic education as an essential component of inpatient medicine. In one article (Dunbar, Wolfe, & Rioch, 1936), she wrote, "The time should not be too long delayed when psychiatrists are required on all our medical and surgical wards, and in all our general and special clinics" (p. 679). Dunbar and her colleagues described the emotional factors in the course of disease as occupying three dimensions, including the etiology of disease, the consequences of experiencing and coping with medical treatments, and the interaction between medical factors and the personality of the patient (Dunbar et al., 1936; see also Dunbar, 1936, 1939, 1940, 1942; Dunbar et al., 1939).

Much research of the time on cardiovascular disease shared some difficulties. The obvious clinical evidence of emotional factors in the course of the disease often could not be differentiated from medical factors, because the diagnostic technology was limited. The differential diagnosis between

---

[2] Menninger and Menninger (1936) did not cite the article correctly, and we could not find the original.

functional disturbances and organic illnesses was difficult to separate. In many studies, the patients examined were described as "cardiac patients," but the case reports showed that various cardiac symptoms were combined and not differentiated, including functional psychosomatic troubles, high blood pressure, respiratory troubles, mitral stenosis, aortic insufficiency, MI, and myocarditis.

Nevertheless, in her prominent textbook *Psychosomatic Diagnosis,* Dunbar (1943) differentiated various subgroups of cardiac patients very precisely and tried to work out specific psychological characteristics. Four chapters concerned cardiac diseases: (a) "Hypertensive Cardiovascular Disease," (b) "Coronary Insufficiency and Occlusion," (c) "Anginal Syndrome," and (d) "Cardiac Arrhythmias." A footnote at the end of the chapter "Coronary Insufficiency and Occlusion" showed her intensive effort to differentiate subgroups: "Note: The coronary occlusion patient with preexisting hypertension or anginal symptoms usually diverges from this profile (Coronary occlusion, JJ/BB) in the directions indicated in the two respective profiles, especially in categories 4, 5, 6, and 10" (p. 310).

The studies by Dunbar and her coworkers are cited in nearly every scientific publication concerning psychosomatic aspects of cardiac diseases. However, they are often reported unsystematically and in a very short and unrepresentative way. For this reason, we summarize their findings in this section (but we highly recommend that readers examine this important work firsthand). All quotations in this section, unless otherwise specified, are from *Psychosomatic Diagnosis* (Dunbar, 1943).

Part 1 of *Psychosomatic Diagnosis* described the "Nature and Magnitude of the Problem," and Part 2 describes the "Onset of Symptoms." Part 3, entitled "Predisposition to Illness," listed the following factors to be evaluated:

- *Heredity:* "Cardiovascular disease in parents and siblings about average for the groups studied (42 per cent). . . . Exposure to cardiovascular disease or to sudden death in about 90 per cent of the cases" (p. 309).
- *Constitution:* Age, sex, and marital status.

- *Previous health:* "These patients consistently neglected their health, principally through lack of sleep, working long hours, taking no vacation or recreation, going contrary to doctor's orders, excessive use of tobacco and coffee, consolation in food, either forbidden or thought to be harmful" (p. 306).
- *Previous injury.*
- *Early influences and traumatic experiences:*

  In brief then, all patients with coronary occlusion . . . had been exposed to cardiovascular disease in some dramatic way. . . . There was also a relatively frequent *history of severe shock* [italics added] as a result of death of a person to whom they were closely bound emotionally, usually by cardiovascular disease or occasionally by accident. . . . Even more prominent than these factors, however, was the excessively strenuous work history; the patients worked long hours without vacations under considerable stress and strain. There was regularly a sudden reverse just after achieving the goal for which they had been working. *A sudden traumatic "ruin"* [italics added] was regularly reported by these patients and rarely by patients in the group with fracture. (p. 300)

- *Salient information about personality history:* Vocation and education, income and occupation, general behavior, social behavior, sexual behavior, attitude toward parents.
- *General behavior:*

  In terms of general adjustment the major difficulties of these patients with coronary occlusion seemed to fall in the spheres of family and of sex. They had unusually stable work records, most of them with histories of beginning at the bottom and working up to the top. (p. 302)

- *Social behavior:* "These patients were always well liked and sociable except that they tended to have difficulties with their superiors and to keep others at a distance" (p. 302).

- *Sexual behavior:*

  Although sex had always been important to them (and their impulse had been stimulated early), very few had made what they regarded as a satisfactory sexual adjustment. Half had not bothered to secure adequate contraceptive advice and continued to practice withdrawal although they disliked it. The women in the group were frigid, and the majority of the men had frigid wives, or suffered from premature ejaculation, or both. (p. 303)

- *Characteristic behavior patterns:* "As has been noted, traumatic events of considerable seriousness, deaths in the family, financial disaster, or the sudden ruin of ambitious plans were prominent in the histories of all the coronary patients . . ." (p. 304). The discussion of characteristic behavior patterns includes the following list:

  Compulsively consistent action. Tendency to work long hours and not take vacations. Tendency to seize authority; dislike of sharing responsibility. Conversation an instrument of domination and aggression. Tendency to attach emotions to ideas and goals. Articulate about feelings. Living for future. (p. 309)

- *Neurotic traits, early and present:* "Few early neurotic traits, tendency to brood and keep their troubles to themselves. In later life inner tension and a tendency to depression which is rarely admitted to others, together with compulsive asceticism and drive to work" (p. 309).
- *Addictions and interests.*
- *Life situation immediately prior to the onset:*

  The situation prior to the onset of the illness in these patients was always an acute one, although preceded by a long period of overexertion and worry with

inadequate rest. The major emotional factor was usually a disappointment in relation to vocational life. (p. 307)

- *Reaction to illness:* "When ill these patients attempt to deny the fact. If activity is curtailed they become depressed and lonely" (p. 307).

The following summarizes Dunbar's argument in Part 4, "Dynamic Formulation": "The focal conflict was peculiarly repressed in patients with coronary disease" (p. 307). Despite trouble with authority, she noted that it had been observed that these patients try to outdo and seek appreciation from their superiors and strive to be as good as their "fathers." They tend to favor the leading role in relationships to others. Dunbar formulated that these patients must be rulers of men. The particularity of the patients' illness is their identification with the father. Dunbar stated further that

  the identification with the father is of special interest in view of the nature of the patients' illness. Although the cardiovascular disease to which these patients were exposed occurred most frequently in the mothers, sudden death, including cardiovascular and other accidents, occurred primarily in the males of the family, and it was with the male that the identification together with the domination pattern was established. A large number of these patients had a dual psychosomatic conditioning: exposure to cardiovascular disease in the mother including early focusing of attention on the heart, to which was added the shock of sudden death in a male relative. (pp. 307–308)

According to Dunbar, the mothers are the caretakers of the family regardless of their ability to satisfy the required needs. They remain the ones usually maintaining contact within the family. Mothers were never reported as being the dominant person in the family.

The sections that follow Part 4 describe forms and expressions of inner conflicts ("degree and nature of somatic expression of conflicts") and, finally, psychotherapeutic implications. Prominent is the psychoeconomic function of work, which Dunbar described as a defense mechanism against inner poverty and uncertainty. Consumption of tobacco and coffee were mentioned as functioning to increase fitness for work and concentration. The intensity of the inner conflicts can be estimated directly from the intensity of the abuse of professional work, which many did without consideration of their own health and without vacation or sufficient breaks. The more difficult their (inner and outer) situation became, the more they worked. They would prefer to die sooner than fail. Dunbar saw in this constellation a suicidal component and a connection to depression after the onset of illness. In her opinion, patients were extremely restrained in expressing emotional conditions and in verbalizing difficulties.

The section of *Psychosomatic Diagnosis* discussing the psychotherapeutic treatability of patients with CHD is of historical interest; in the ensuing decades, psychoanalytic experts tended to be much more pessimistic than Dunbar. Dunbar began the section on psychodynamic treatment with a critical presentation of the doctor–patient relationship that was similar to those of many later experts: The treating doctor feels a strong tendency to correct risky behavior, which Dunbar called "unhygienic habits" and which is currently called "coronary-prone behavior," but very often the doctor fails to inspire any change in patient behavior. Dunbar pointed out that many patients who are seemingly cooperative in the beginning are subsequently unwilling to change their behavior; seeming to be cooperative is a subtle way of showing their resistance to medical authority. Dunbar understood the difficulties patients encountered in enacting lifestyle changes as being the result of unconscious self-destructive tendencies and repressed depression. Dunbar emphasized that without psychotherapeutic help in overcoming inner conflicts and finding new solutions, long-term changes in risk behaviors are not possible; this conclusion is still ignored today. The following rarely cited passage highlighted the opportunities and challenges inherent in psychotherapy with patients with CHD:

The coronary patient is a particularly satisfying person with whom to work therapeutically. His life-long habit of working things out for himself makes it easy to enlist his interest and cooperation. His interest in ideas and concepts makes it relatively easy for him to understand what the physician has in mind, and the traumatic effect of the illness itself, usually reinforced by a preceding traumatic emotional situation, creates a disequilibrium in his own inner adjustment which makes it relatively easy to relieve his life-long repression and inhibitions. The danger relative to this latter point is the intensity of the emotions repressed, hence the physician must proceed cautiously in order not to place an undue strain on an already damaged heart. In our series, however, there were few patients in whom therapy was contraindicated for this reason, and in none of the cases in which therapy was attempted were the results anything but favorable. (pp. 320–321)

Dunbar pointed out that the psychotherapist must pay particular attention when patients seem to be cheerful, cite little trouble, speak easily about their own illness, and tell light-hearted jokes. Dunbar found these phenomena to be part of a special type of countertransference that is dangerous and prognostically unfavorable: "In our series the patients who were the 'best sports' about their illness were the ones that died" (p. 321). Other technical difficulties in treatment Dunbar cited relate to sexual problems and conflicts with partners; she cited the need for help that is carefully supporting and encouraging (see p. 321).

The research of Flanders Dunbar and her colleagues not only was impressively systematic but also resulted in the formulation of many concepts and hypotheses that were cited and replicated in the decades that followed. Their work provided the foundation for much psychosomatic research. For example, the conceptualization of Type A behavior by Friedman and Rosenman (1959) reflects

Dunbar's work. It is unfortunate that later psychodynamic studies did not replicate Dunbar and her colleagues' research; for example, it would have been useful to validate Dunbar's results in samples with different sociodemographic characteristics.

A fundamental dilemma in psychodynamic research and theoretical models in general is found in Dunbar's formulation of a specific conflict in CHD. The careful formulation of the etiological hypothesis and the similarity between the coronary patients and the controls leads to only one conclusion: In the end, a specific conflict does not exist. We have summarized Dunbar's work extensively because her formulations show how much inner effort—one could say against the empirical evidence—she needed to expend in formulating a specific psychosomatic hypothesis for the etiology of CHD. Her hypothesis has resonated strongly in the literature, however; many publications have emphasized the psychodynamic conflict as she described it.

Arlow (1945), who also worked at the New York Presbyterian Hospital, integrated the work of Dunbar's group with that of Menninger and Menninger (1936) and hypothesized that inner insecurity and a sense of weakness play an important role in the psychodynamics of CHD patients. He analyzed 13 patients using a psychiatric interview and the Rorschach test. He observed the following:

> These patients with coronary occlusion represent a specific type of character development. They make a spurious and only partial identification with the father. The image of the father is exaggerated out of all proportion by the childhood anxiety. The identification is made less out of admiration and more out of fear. The identification, however, is not complete and thoroughgoing. Above all, in the deeper layers of the patient's personality, it is unconvincing. The patient feels much like a youngster who is masquerading successfully in his father's clothes, and who is frightened lest at any moment he be caught exposed and punished. In order to make this masquerade seem more convincing, the patient pursues his usurped role all the more aggressively. To a certain extent the disguise deceives the patient himself, but this is never completely so—his deep seated lack of conviction accounts for both the compulsive competitiveness and the traumatic effect of the experience of failure. Inwardly convinced that he is a sham, the patient cannot accept success. This inner insecurity and sense of weakness which the patient fears to face, and which he seeks to deny, remain unaffected by realistic achievements. For this reason he needs ever more successes to alleviate his own doubts.
>
> It is not simply the experience of failure which proves so traumatic to the coronary patient. What disturbed these patients most was to fail under circumstances which convinced both the outer world and themselves that they were not as good as they had thought. Such failures have the significance of an unmasking. When the façade of feigned omnipotence is ripped away, the patient is forced to face his inner sense of weakness and fear. These are the very feelings which the patient tried to exclude from consciousness by compulsive aggression. (p. 201)

The failure of not convincing the outer world and themselves that they were as good as they had thought themselves to be disturbed them more than the experience of failure per se. When the mask is dropped, the patient is faced with his inner sense of weakness and fear; these remain persistent in consciousness.

This passage provided the first characterization of the psychodynamic function of professional work. The author was highly restrained concerning the causal etiological hypothesis, but he excluded 2 of the 14 patients because the interview and test were "unproductive," and he excluded 2 other patients because they did not match his psychodynamic hypothesis. This strategy was used in many other psychoanalytic publications over the years, resulting in a long-lasting scientific legacy of homogeneity of patient groups and reduced differentiation in research. Scientific progress would have been better supported by the development of alternative hypotheses, which researchers might have considered had they not excluded patients in this way.

Numerous empirical studies on psychosomatic aspects of the etiology and course of CHD in the next 40 years were based on the hypotheses of Dunbar's work group. An excellent review by Mordkoff and Parsons (1967) showed that the results of these studies were contradictory; some controlled studies could not confirm the hypotheses (Miles, Waldfogel, Barrabee, & Cobb, 1954; C. K. Miller, 1965; O'Connell & Lundy, 1961; Storment, 1951), whereas others can be seen as a confirmation (Cleveland & Johnson, 1962). Mordkoff and Parsons interpreted the inconsistency in the results as being a consequence of the general nature of statements concerning substantially different emotional conditions and the lack of operationalization of different life experience areas. Further sources of inconsistency in the results are the use of different assessment instruments and study samples that are not comparable. Mordkoff and Parsons concluded that many studies did not control for important variables such as age, gender, socioeconomic status, race, and personality factors. They also asserted that sociodemographic differences likely produced more variation in results than differences between patients with CHD and other clinical subgroups.

Weiss, Dlin, Rollin, Fischer, and Bepler (1957) systematically examined Dunbar's hypotheses and found that a specific personality among CHD patients does not exist. Moreover, they stated that evidence of psychopathology among the samples could not be identified. On a historical note, Weiss et al. observed that only 39% of Miles et al.'s (1954) sample were Jewish, compared with 59% of Dunbar's; they hypothesized that this difference produced the inconsistencies between the studies.

2.3.4. Other Studies From the United States

In the years after 1950, studies placed increasing emphasis on the psychosocial aspects of CHD (primarily stress, especially workplace stress, and heart disease, as well as social inequality). Friedman and Rosenman (1959) formulated their thesis of specific risk-increasing behavior in the *Journal of the American Medical Association* (*JAMA*). Many psychodynamically oriented authors tried within the following 20 years to understand and interpret so-called "Type A" behavior.

From a psychodynamic point of view, some impressive articles were developed based on the Middlesex County Study (Bahnson & Wardwell, 1962; Wardwell, Bahnson, & Caron, 1963). This study, which began in 1957, was one of the most important foundations for examination of the social and psychological factors causing CHD. In Middlesex County (Connecticut), researchers followed all White men who had heart attacks for a period of 1 year. Thirty-five men were still living 1 year after the MI; 3 were excluded for different reasons, resulting in a sample of 32. A control group of 32 comparable (matched on some sociodemographic data) White men with serious illnesses was chosen; the difficulties encountered in composing this control group were discussed critically and in detail in the publication. Questionnaires and interviews were completed for both groups by qualified academic and additionally trained professional interviewers. In addition to describing specific aspects of both groups, the researchers formulated a subtly differentiated description of the men's specific defense mechanisms, including reaction formation, rationalization, intellectualization, and denial. They also mentioned further variables that later researchers also found to be frequent in patients with CHD:

- the high importance of and dissatisfaction with work;
- increased stress levels;
- unstable self-esteem;
- compulsive character;
- tendency to somatize inner conflicts;
- acting-out behavior with authority figures;
- hyperactivity as a reaction formation against fear; and
- reactions to trouble (anger) that include tension, confusion, and aggression.

Wardwell et al. (1963) described the man who shows a greater probability of having an MI as urban, middle class, Protestant, and of northwest European descent. This man grew up in a cultural environment

> which is repressive and demanding on the individual but which lacks the supportive authoritarian character of the rural or old-world community. He tends to govern his behavior through internalised societal controls and ethical standards . . . , a characteristic which may be interpreted as an alternative to a simpler, but probably more gratifying, affectional involvement with other persons. His resulting anxiety and tenseness are barely concealed by such psychological defensive mechanisms as denial and reaction formation that permit him to function adequately in society. We hypothesise that the fundamental psychological problems of the male most likely to suffer a myocardial infarction center around unsatisfactory identification, unstable self-image, and ambivalence with regard to authority. (p. 165)

With regard to the etiological and genetic hypotheses, the authors spoke cautiously, calling for future studies; they suspected that the essential etiological mechanism is the chronic repression of anger impulses, which produces a chronic psychophysiological tension.

Bahnson and Wardwell (1962) also provided an interesting examination of parental identification styles, citing the results of Arlow (1945). After comparing an MI group with a control group, they described two important subgroups with respect to their dominant parental identification styles: a mother-centered group, which they called "self-centered-regressive," and a father-centered group, which they called "socio-centric, striving, controlled." They described the self-centered-regressive patients as follows:

> The mother-oriented coronary patients, who were younger and more passive, appeared to have low ego strength and little internalization of the masculine values usual in the United States. They had fathers without heart conditions and mothers who died relatively young. They came from, and themselves stayed within, lower socio-economic and occupational levels. They married wives older than themselves, of higher socio-economic status . . . and with more education than themselves. Apparently they carried over to their choice of wives their basic dependency on their mothers. They had lower self-acceptance than the other coronary subgroups, showed dependency by tending to turn to others for help when in trouble, stated that they often daydreamed, and were less compulsive and concerned over "face." They also expressed passivity through stating that they often "sat and did nothing" and through their lack of interest in and commitment to their work. (p. 844)

Work pressure and exhaustion was reported by these patients, although their contribution in the workforce and social life was minimal. They reported as well a general dissatisfaction with their life along with depressive moods and inability to relax, which characterized their marginal neurotic adjustment. Bahnson and Wardwell (1962) went on to describe the psychodynamic constellations of the three types of identification (with the parents) within the coronary sample. They showed that a psychodynamic investigation could have a controlled and intelligent study design and that a precise hypothesis can lead to new and creative results.

2.3.5. Work Group From the Netherlands

Psychodynamic research concerning CHD has been carried out in the Netherlands since 1947. Groen (1951, 1964) and coworkers studied not only specific personality traits, sociological factors, and unconscious phenomena with different psychosomatic illnesses but also psychophysiological mechanisms (Groen, Welner, & Ishay, 1970). Bastiaans (1968, 1969, 1982) studied specific mechanisms for coping with aggression and anger in the context of psychosomatic diseases. This work group established an interdisciplinary cooperation and a long tradition of research on psychocardiology that continues to the present in Maastricht. The work group under Groen published a first article, "Acute Myocardial Infarction: A Psychosomatic Study" (Groen et al., 1965) on 30 men in 1965 that was never translated into English, but the many group members published results in international journals in subsequent years (Groen, 1951; Heijningen & Treurniet, 1966; Pelser, 1967, 1988; Valk & Groen, 1967; van Heijningen, 1960).

In this section we review in detail the work of this group, with special attention to the psychological (dys)function of work characteristic of people with CHD: Individuals with CHD work much harder and more intensely than other people. Work often is the only really important activity in their lives. They have a strong sense of responsibility and are ready to drastically curtail other aspects of life (e.g., family time, social contacts) to increase time for work.

Groen and coworkers (Groen, 1951; Groen et al., 1970) were the first to use the term *workaholic* in a scientific discussion of CHD, and their publications addressed how to interpret this specific work behavior psychodynamically. The authors were very creative and formulated different arguments that are compatible only to a certain degree, but all authors identified a fundamental etiological function of work as providing a means of coping with aggressive impulses. They described varying biographical structures as leading to this aggression, but all identified an unstable personality structure. These patients' urge for autonomy, success, and dominance characterizes their feelings and behavior in stable life phases, but underlying unconscious wishes for loving care, security, passivity, and regression (and corresponding fears) break through in periods of psychological crisis. These crises of destabilization can be triggered by overloaded, stressful, and demanding situations; failure to succeed; or provoking remarks by other people. The narcissistic destabilization resulting from such

stressful circumstances can provoke aggressive explosive reactions even in men who were "innocent" and inhibited before. Uncontrolled aggressive outbursts often are followed by feelings of guilt, which may then activate "masochistic" mechanisms and lead to dangerous physiological states that can trigger a heart attack.

Some authors identified an early separation crisis (e.g., Bowlby, 1958) as the cause of these mechanisms. During childhood, these patients experienced a lack of loving care, warmth, and security. They had to work hard and had little time to play with other children. As a reaction formation, they developed the ideal of early separation and autonomy, together with a strong competitiveness and drive for success; they developed "compulsive striving characters." Heijningen and Treurniet (1966) described the psychodynamic and defense mechanisms concisely, and they pointed to an excessive defense against passive desires. Valk and Groen and others (Trijsburg, Bal, Parsowa, Erdman, & Duivenvoorden, 1989; Trijsburg, Erdman, Duivenvoorden, Thiel, & Verhage, 1987; Valk & Groen, 1967) analyzed the object relationship of patients with CHD to their fathers and developed an interesting multigenerational perspective on their incapacity to handle oedipal conflicts; the following passage provides a characteristic description of the core conflict: "When I am big and when I can make big products and great streams immediately, nothing can happen to me, everyone will love me" (Bastiaans, 1968, p. 206).

Bastiaans (1968) summarized the psychodynamic reflections of this work group as follows:

> It may be stated that the essence of coronary neurosis is given in the patient's inability to deal effectively with his narcissism and his strivings for competition and rivalry. Particularly the oedipal competition is seldom coped with in a flexible way. Although in their later psychic development, potential CHD patients seem to develop well in many aspects of their personality organization, they regress too easily to the infantile ideal of omnipotence as

presented in early security, establishing magical thinking and clinging to the phallic-aggressive position. When stress increases and when the phallic position does not guarantee security and admiration sufficiently, regression proceeds in the direction of compulsive anal behavior, marked by moral masochism and unhappiness. As soon as this position in its turn does not guarantee security and satisfaction, the above-mentioned psychosomatic paralysis may start abruptly. Myocardial infarction usually occurs in those moments when narcissistic injury and frustration in job activity coincide with frustration in a libidinal relationship with partner, children or friends. (p. 207)

Groen's work group clearly formulated in various publications the similarity in personality traits of MI patients and normal and successful men from Western industrial nations. They identified a slightly intensified version of a common behavior pattern: strong competitiveness and drive to succeed. Furthermore, they described a probable conflict background that deals mostly with external recognition of a failed endeavor. Hahn, Nüssel, and Stiehler (1966) summarized the conflict of this group as follows:

> The usual reaction in such conflict situations for infarct patients is not an immediate or aggressive statement. Apparently it is an overly calm and optimistic behavior pattern, and with that the flowing of inner tensions is introjected. Infarct patients compensate for their failures in general with more work and cope in this way with their conflicts. (p. 243)

The length and continuity of this Dutch research effort are scientifically and historically remarkable; in these areas, scientists have worked continuously since 1947 on psychosocial studies dealing with CHD. Their interdisciplinary cooperation, multimethod research designs, and comprehensive academic thinking have produced meaningful results that have been recognized worldwide, especially their descriptions and evaluations of the concepts of *vital exhaustion* (Appels, Kop, Meesters, Markusse, Golombeck, & Falger, 1994; Appels, Bär, Bär, Bruggeman, & de Baets, 2000; Appels, Siegrist, & De Vos, 1997; Kop, Appels, Mendes de Leon, & Baer, 1996; Kop, Hamulyak, Pernot, & Appels, 1998; Mendes de Leon, Kop, de Swart, Bar, & Appels, 1996) and *distressed personality* (Denollet, 1998a, 2000).

2.3.6. Marseilles Work Group and Other French Researchers

Our literature searches of French authors and work groups encountered a series of difficulties. First of all, we were uncertain whether all relevant French publications were recorded in international databases; for this reason and because we had limited time to research in France, we may have missed some publications. To be as thorough as possible given these constraints, we used the reference lists of some of the publications we identified as a further source of citations. The review in this chapter of French scientific work is best considered a selection, therefore, and may not represent the totality of papers. We review in this section the most important work we identified.

The work group led by Andre Jouve at the Center for the Prevention of Cardiovascular Diseases at the Cantini Hospital in Marseilles is, in our estimation, the most meaningful research from France. Between 1960 and 1985, this group published a series of works dealing with psychosocial aspects of CHD (Bernet, Drivet-Perrin, Blanc, Ebagosti, & Jouve, 1982; Jouve & Dongier, 1962; Jouve, Dongier, & Delaage, 1960; Jouve, Dongier, Delaage, & Mayaud, 1961; Jouve & Ebagosti, 1985; Jouve, Sommer, Avierinos, & Fondarai, 1973; Jouve, Sommer, Gerard, Casanova, & Malfroy, 1962; Jouve & Torresani, 1961). Jouve's coauthors were also involved in other research and cooperated with many other French research centers (e.g., that of Pierre Pichot in Paris) and collaborated in a multicenter prospective study of 2,147 people and their partners in Paris (Pichot), Brussels

(Denolin), and Gent (Pannier; see Pichot, de Bonis, & Somogyi, 1977).

Jouve and his coworkers used questionnaires to evaluate aspects of patients' personality typology (particularly the Type A concept). Many of their publications did not have a psychodynamic orientation, and these will not be discussed in this chapter. One investigation (Jouve et al., 1960), however, tested a psychodynamic hypothesis: They examined 109 cardiac patients and a control group of 100 persons. Following the character neurosis concept of Wilhelm Reich (1925, 1949), they examined a set of personality characteristics they called "obsessive character." The authors concluded that a compulsive structured personality occurred more frequently in the patients than in the controls; 73% of the MI patients, compared with 40% of the control group, showed these characteristics. These authors emphasized that a basic characteristic of infarct patients is a specific reaction to stressful situations, and they hypothesized that a better knowledge of the mechanisms of this reaction could lead to meaningful implications for prevention and therapy.

Two other French publications were of interest. In the first, de Dowiakowski and Luminet (1969) selectively reviewed the literature and discussed previous findings. They also described a publication by Vauthier (1966) reflecting the dominant French psychosomatic school (e.g., *pensée operatoire*; Marty & de M'Uzan, 1962) that we could not obtain. de Dowiakowski and Luminet listed Vauthier's results concerning psychodynamic factors in male MI patients:

- Patients show a dysfunctioning ego ideal: Strictly forbidden aspects are very dominant in the personality structure.
- The desire to be loved (fundamental but rarely verbalized) expresses itself in quixotic overactivity.
- A very rigid self-concept causes compulsive efforts to fulfill unattainable goals.
- An archaic and intense aggressiveness expresses itself through intense activity and causes inhibited behavior that has oral and anal characteristics.

- Overactivity functions to dominate dangerous feelings of passivity and can be seen as a defense against passive wishes. Feelings of addiction are intense but intolerable.
- The personality is characterized by a deficiency of regressive abilities. If regression takes place, it leads to two destructive archaic reactions: depression and psychosis. Somatic complications appear as an absurd concealment.
- The trigger of a coronary event can be found in the situational context of personal defeat.

In their clinical investigation, de Dowiakowski and Luminet (1969) interviewed 32 men who experienced an MI before the age of 46 but had no previous history of high blood pressure (the authors mentioned but did not describe in detail a control group of 16 men). Following Arlow's (1945) hypothesis, the authors evaluated the object relationships of the patients with their fathers. The authors stated that the men in their study surpassed by about 50% their fathers' professional qualifications (they provided no operationalization for how they measured this variable) and were well entrenched at the hierarchical level. More than 50% (19 of 32) of the men had dominating, castrating fathers, as described by Arlow; 7 of the 32 subjects had "ideal fathers" who enabled mature oedipal development; and 6 of the 32 men had "absent fathers" who prevented mature oedipal development. They described these object relationships in three case reports, which they compared with the controls. The authors concluded that the men in the study had attained a broken and insufficient oedipal identification (pseudo-identificational object relationship to castrating and dominating fathers). The psychoeconomic activity of professional work (i.e., the emotional occupation of work) had a pseudo-oedipal meaning and was compensatory, and the heart attack was triggered by a failure of this dysfunctional identification.

The second French publication of interest is an article by Lesage-Desrousseaux (1981). This author, a student of J. Lacan, characterized the communication cardiologists use with patients in a unique way, as resembling that of an engineer (i.e., the heart is an engine, pumping blood and repairable like the motor of a car; p. 366). Lesage-

Desrousseaux, who had much experience in the medical field, described patients' fear of death and emphasized an unconscious role of cardiologists as stabilizers of patients' narcissistic grandiose fantasies of becoming immortal. It is remarkable that in an otherwise brilliantly written essay, the reference list mentions no other authors besides Freud and Lacan.

2.3.7. German Work Groups

As we pointed out at the beginning of this chapter, there is a long tradition of psychocardiology research in Germany. In this section we describe some important publications from the work groups of Peter Hahn (Heidelberg) and Emma Moersch (Sigmund Freud Institute, Frankfurt am Main) and summarize the work of several other researchers. Finally, we briefly present the results of investigations with projective tests, which include articles in both German and other languages.

2.3.7.1. Work group of Peter Hahn. In Heidelberg, Germany, Hahn and his colleagues have worked systematically in the field of psychocardiology and have included psychodynamic hypotheses in their empirical work. Hahn's holistic perspective integrates somatic, sociological, and psychodynamic aspects. Hahn has argued that a psychological specificity—that is, that all patients with CHD have at least one characteristic psychological pattern that they share with all others—is not probable. Instead, he has argued, the psychosomatic specificity concept connected with the work of Franz Alexander (e.g., Alexander, 1950; Alexander & French, 1948) should be renewed as a replacement for all linear causality models, including the materialistic model (i.e., somatic processes cause psychological processes) and the spiritual model (i.e., psychological processes cause somatic processes), and integrated holistic concepts should be developed. Following the *Gestaltkreis* concept of Victor von Weizsäcker (1950), Hahn formulated the "cybernetic principle," which integrates somatic and psychological phenomena in an interdependent process model.

Hahn developed an Infarct Profile consisting of a patient's risk personality, situational analysis, and infarct personality. *Risk personality* encompasses both a personality analysis and all medically meaningful risk factors, including behaviors and constitutional and genetic factors, that are relevant to the etiology of the infarct (Christian, 1966, p. 103). *Situational analysis* is an analysis of the conditions surrounding the MI, including special somatic or psychosocial stressors that could be linked to the onset of the MI. The *infarct personality* includes the somatic and psychosocial condition of the patient both before and after the infarct.

The Infarct Profile is suitable both for critically evaluating existing case reports and gathering data for case studies. For individual patients, the Infarct Profile can inform differential diagnoses and psychosomatic and somatopsychological therapy. This very promising concept established a basis for further research, and it is disappointing that it has not received further attention in subsequent psychodynamic investigations. Hahn himself ceased work in this field after some years (Hahn, 1968a, 1968b, 1969, 1971, 1987, 1988; Hahn & Hüllemann, 1972; Hahn & Kämmerer, 1985).

Hahn's Infarct Profile may be useful not only in single case studies but also in longitudinal studies of risk personality and infarct personality and cross-sectional studies of the situational analysis, potentially contributing to the formulation of a multifactorial pathogenic model. Hahn concluded that it was no longer plausible to formulate a concept implying a nosological category *myocardial infarction*. More plausible is the concept of a myocardial ischemia syndrome, which would allow one to differently characterize cases with varying pathophysiological clinical symptomatology.

Another meaningful implication of the Infarct Profile is that interpretations of cardiovascular pathophysiological mechanisms should be carried out only for groups with similar risk patterns. Hahn's concept explains the large variance in study results over the years and contributes to a clear categorization of specified subgroups and the formulation of new hypotheses for further studies. Such studies would strongly support the development of specific therapeutic strategies.

Although Hahn repeatedly described his skepticism about the classic "specificity concept" (i.e., classification of the whole group of patients with CHD), at the end of his book (Hahn, 1971) he formulated a psychodynamic hypothesis:

> Summarizing the findings concerning obsessional personality traits and extraversion, one is able to formulate a psychodynamic etiological hypothesis that explains the manifestation of extraversion and that explains the margin of deviation after the infarct clearly. The personality structure foundation of the described obsessive personality segment . . . is connected substantially with the introjections of morally demanding instances, leading to a reevaluation of the superego compared to the ego. (p. 86)

On the surface, the patient with an obsessive character seems well behaved and reality oriented, but on the inside he or she contains latent aggressive impulses that underlie defense mechanisms. These latent aggressive adjustments to the demands of the social environment create additional extraversion. A latent aggressive person is forced to invest more energy in social adjustment than fully identified persons with a deep experience of trusting and is constantly on the lookout for unexpected or hostile reactions from his or her surroundings: He or she must try to do nothing wrong and to anticipate friendly and hostile impulses in order to protect an unstable self-esteem. The projection of hostile impulses onto others is fostered by the person's own aggressiveness. Thus, self-esteem is always dependent on the reactions of the situational social environment, which means that self-esteem is always in danger of destabilization. Additionally, these dependencies explain the underlying compensated depressive feelings.

Hahn hypothesized that to counteract feelings of dependency (through the superego), aggressive impulses arise that interfere with social adjustment processes, and various defense mechanisms are activated to control aggressive impulses and hostility. Each process of consciousness interferes with the individual's perception of his or her own aggressive impulses and inner tensions. Therefore, passive and regressive impulses, as well as psychodynamic therapy, could cause feelings of danger, increased tension and anxiety, and a sense that relief is out of reach (Hahn, 1971, pp. 86–87; see also Condrau & Gassmann, 1989; Fassbender, Cziepluch, & Nippe, 1984). From this hypothesis, Hahn derived a set of implications for psychotherapeutic treatment, which we describe in section 2.6.2.3. Because we consider Hahn's concept very innovative, in the following paragraphs we present part of one of his case reports in detail (see Hahn, 1971).

The *risk personality* analysis of this patient included examination of his CHD history, which indicated a hereditary pattern (heart disease–related death of his father). The patient's constitution was described as strong and muscular. There was no indication that an atherosclerotic process existed before the infarction. Blood pressure was moderately elevated. The patient did not exercise, was 30 kg overweight, and abused nicotine (40 to 60 cigarettes per day). In his younger days, the patient had been an award-winning athlete; he had had to give up sports because of a meniscus injury. As for coexisting illnesses, the patient had diabetes mellitus, complained of fatigue and pectanginous symptoms, and had recurring ulcus duodeni.

The *situational analysis* highlighted a background of psychological and social conflicts. This patient's extraversion was not as pronounced as his compulsive traits, which were evident in his behavior in work situations. The patient's wife had been under medical treatment for 14 years for nervous heart complaints (cardiac neurosis), causing stress for the patient. The patient had taken over part of his father's business 3 years before his first MI; 2 years later, his father died suddenly of an MI, and the patient took over the entire administration of the business. He was overtaxed by this role and frequently obliged to make important decisions. He used the word *Männle* (the diminutive form of *man* in German) to describe his feelings about his role. He became increasingly dependent on his mother. He experienced further psychological strain while under treatment for ulcus duodeni when the fraudulent activity of a customer necessitated legal action and threatened the patient's business with bankruptcy. Furthermore, the diagnosis of diabetes mellitus substantially disconcerted him. Immediately before the MI, the patient was attacked by a drunken worker and had to defend himself physically, and he had also had angina pectoris symptoms; nevertheless, he continued to go to work.

The analysis of the *infarct personality* indicated that after the MI, the patient lost weight, and his cholesterol level decreased into the normal range. He increased his level of physical activity. His blood pressure normalized, and because of the shock of the infarct he gave up smoking cigarettes. Hahn's psychodynamic characterization of the patient described his personality structure as fixed in his psychosexual development in a negative oedipal constellation. The patient had been his father's favorite because of his athletic abilities. The father was described as a strict and dominating instructor and boss. The patient had been unable to live up to his father's ideal; thus, after the sudden death of his father, the patient's deficits in self-esteem and leadership broke through and led to an identity crisis. His lack of preparation for this paternal authority loss prompted a regressive dependence on his mother, who he hoped would take over the authority of the father. This conflict, Hahn suggested, resulted in psychological suffering and pressure, triggering depressive symptoms. This interpretation fit the self-verbalization of the patient, who said to himself in critical situations, "*Männle, do it already!*"

2.3.7.2. Work Group of Emma Moersch. One of the last psychodynamic investigations was published in 1980. A work group at the Sigmund Freud Institute in Frankfurt examined 100 patients, using a retrospective interview, shortly after they had experienced an MI. The study design was simple; no hypothesis and no specific questions were formulated, and data were collected using exclusively unstructured interviews (i.e., no questionnaires). Nonetheless, an entire issue of the journal *Psyche—Journal of Psychoanalysis and Its Applications* was devoted to publication of the results (Moersch et al., 1980). The authors described their method, following that of Malan (1962), as the "workshop method," and they concluded that MI patients show a wide range of substantial defects in ego

structure that can be explained as maladaptive processes of separation and individuation as well as defects in the development of the ego and the self.

Kerz-Rühling (1980) summarized the conflict structure as follows: "Due to their familial experience of missing care and emotional security . . . many interviewed patients intensively try to avoid social situations in which they feel dependent or which could cause disappointment in others" (p. 549). She concluded that for these patients, "all psychological conflicts are significant (and dangerous) and able to destabilize the narcissistic balance, causing, for example, shame and disappointment on the job as well as in the family" (p. 545). This study focused not on finding a typical personality profile or specific behavior pattern, but on identifying typical conflict constellations. Kerz-Rühling described four typical psychodynamic conflict constellations:

1. Failure to achieve the ambition of attaining security and acknowledgment was connected with failure in power and rivalry situations:

   The life history of all patients from this group show that these people, since childhood, have strived to compensate for the lack of security and care, disappointment, and shame (feelings of weakness, inferiority and dependency). However, the compensatory efforts to achieve social success and material wealth never really provide safety, and relatively slight malfunctioning can destabilize self-confidence and feelings of independence. (p. 547)

2. A second area of conflict involved object loss or the fantasy of possible object loss (p. 548). The retreat or loss of a dominated object "reactivates infantile disappointment with the primary objects, which were not mastered by the patient" (p. 549). Experienced loss and separation not only reactivate unconscious early problems of dependency, but also trigger "hate" toward the current disappointing object (p. 549). Simultaneously, the aggressive fantasies are accompanied by fear of being punished by illness or

death (p. 550). This psychodynamic constellation had previously been described by Menninger and Menninger (1936) and others.

3. Because of strict impulses of the superego, unconscious feelings of guilt arose when desired emotional ("libidinal") impulses were fulfilled (p. 550): "In 13 cases the onset of illness was during vacation. A third of the interviewed patients suffered the MI during weekends or on work holidays" (p. 552). Kerz-Rühling interpreted this as a psychodynamically meaningful situation involving temptation and failure.

4. Another group of patients experienced feelings of disappointment about a deficiency of satisfaction concerning oral impulses (from primary objects and later partners) as well as feelings of envy toward people "who got more" (p. 551). Following the Netherlands work group (see Section 2.3.5), Kerz-Rühling concluded that these patients compensated for traumatic experiences in childhood and the resulting aggressive impulses by working hard and being socially successful. Satisfactory experiences, which were deeply missed for so many years, reactivate the unconscious basic traumatic complex. This hypothetical reconstruction led this author to the conclusion that an intensive mobilization of internal conflicts can trigger an MI in some cases (she offered no hypothesis that could explain this process psychophysiologically).

The results of this investigation should be treated with caution, as acknowledged by Kerz-Rühling (1980a) herself:

> The heterogeneity of conflict constellations permits neither the acceptance of a conflict specificity for infarct patients compared with other psychosomatics, nor does it permit one to reliably postulate a significant difference in this population, because one can assume that these constellations are ubiquitous. What we can maintain with some security, however, is that infarct patients experience stressful, life-threatening events immediately before the infarct occurs that lead to a revival of unconscious infantile conflicts. (p. 554)

2.3.7.3. Other researchers. Condrau and Gassman (1989) presented detailed case studies of three MI patients and concluded that the personality structure of these patients exhibited all of the characteristics that also had been described by Bloch and Bersier (1979). They concluded that coronary patients most frequently show obsessive–compulsive behavior patterns and additionally a narcissistic fragility, and they listed the following characteristics as typical in these patients:

> enormous effort at work, a predilection for taking responsibility, exaggerated perfectionism, anticipation of criticism, pedantry, a love of order, strong impulses toward self-control and control of others, suppression of feelings (in particular anxiety), a tendency to rationalize, difficulty expressing aggressiveness other than through impulsive and explosive attacks, an intense struggle for professional success, feelings of omnipotence and invulnerability, denial of personal limitations, ruthlessness, absence of self-criticism, fragility in the face of failure, a great desire to be needed and loved and esteemed, addiction to success, extremely poor fantasies and dreams . . . , unfulfilling lives outside professional activity, unusual hyperactivity, inability to relax and rest, apparently exemplary social adjustment despite existing discontent, unsatisfactory sex life, general inability to enjoy oneself. (p. 86)

2.3.8. Research Using Projective Testing

Several studies used projective tests (e.g., Rorschach test, Thematic Apperception Test [TAT]; see Aronow, 1999; Cramer, 2000; H. A. Murray, 1953; Rorschach, 1951; Sargent & Hirsch, 1954) in addition to questionnaires. As far as we know, Arlow (1945) was the first to report on the application of such a procedure (Rorschach test). Two studies emphasized the infantile traumatizations and unstable object relationships of cardiac infarct patients (Remer, 1972; Revers, Revers, & Widauer, 1978). It is impossible to summarize the results of such studies in detail; suffice it to say that there are numerous inconsistencies in their results. Investigations with projective tests continue to be published, however (Bonami & Rime, 1972; J. M. J. Bruce & Thomas, 1953; Cleveland & Johnson, 1962; Defourny, Hubin, & Luminet, 1976; Defourny, Timsit, & Dongier, 1972; Frankignoul & Melon, 1971; Karstens, Köhle, & Weidlich, 1970; Keltikangas-Järvinen, 1992; Kemple, 1945; Melon, 1971; Melon, Dongier, & Bourdouxhe, 1971; T. Q. Miller, Smith, Turner, Guijarro, & Hallet, 1996; Schilling, 1980; Siltanen et al., 1975; Stoiberer, 1984).

2.4. RESEARCH ON TRIGGER SITUATIONS

Although CHD is initially caused by (usually undetected) plaque deposits that accumulate over years, the question of what conditions trigger an MI has stimulated great interest. If such a significant event occurs at some point during an unnoticeable process, the question of what triggers it is important. Patients' lay theories often include psychological or physical stress as a probable explanation. "Life event research" provides a pragmatic research-oriented perspective on such lay theories. It suggests that generally stressful events of varying intensity have a causal relationship to the origin of physical and psychological illnesses (Rahe, 1990, 1994; Rahe & Arthur, 1978). The literature on life event research will not be presented in this section because of its size and complexity and its incompatibility with the central focus on psychodynamic research.

From a psychodynamic point of view, the examination of trigger events is important because temptation and disappointment situations can often be identified as the starting point for the development of symptomatic and pathological processes (see, e.g., Fenichel, 1977). The question of under what circumstances and in which situations a heart attack happens at a particular time is important from a scientific (cardiological, physiological, and psychological) perspective and must be considered if the situational analysis can be expected to provide conclusions about relevant etiological factors of the heart attack event. Analysis of the trigger event must enable one to identify central psychological contexts that are causally relevant.

Authors interested in the psychodynamic aspects of CHD often consider the trigger event to be a symbolic conversion of a neurotic symptom (e.g., "language of the organs" [symptoms and diseases as a way to communicate unconscious conflicts, wishes, or "forbidden" impulses], expressive event) and the trigger situation as containing the whole of the psychogenesis of the heart attack. Epidemiological lines of research focusing on temporal factors (e.g., times of day, days of week, special events such as birthdays and holidays, seasons), relationship factors immediately preceding physical stress, and life events such as wars and natural disasters are not clearly relevant to psychodynamic issues. Of interest is an autobiographical publication by one of the best-known psychosomatic researchers, George Engel. Engel lost his identical twin to a heart attack and himself suffered a heart attack 1 year later. He subsequently reported on how he dealt with it emotionally (G. L. Engel, 1975, 2001; Wise, 2001).

2.4.1. Psychodynamic Hypotheses Regarding Trigger Situations

2.4.1.1. Psychological conflicts and trauma as triggers: Retrospective cross-sectional studies. In this section we briefly review the findings and conclusions of cross-sectional studies that involve psychodynamic constellations. The time between trigger and MI identified in these studies varies widely, ranging from hours to weeks.

Dunbar (1943) concluded that a heart attack generally follows a psychodynamically important situation in which the authority of the patient is threatened by his or her environment and the patient feels humiliated and insulted: "The coronary accident in these patients is precipitated by an apparently irreparable mutilation of their picture of themselves through external threats to their authoritative role" (p. 336). Their biographies are often characterized by striking traumatic events: "There was also a relatively frequent history of severe shock as a result of death of a person to whom they were closely bound emotionally" (p. 301). Failures are experienced as catastrophic–traumatic psychological stress: "There was regularly a sudden reverse just after achieving the goal for which they had been working. A sudden traumatic 'ruin' was regularly reported by these patients" (p. 301). In her view, the typical situation experienced shortly before the occurrence of the infarct is a failure, mistake, or disappointment in relation to vocational life:

> The situation prior to the onset of the illness in these patients was always an acute one, although preceded by a long period of overexertion and worry with inadequate rest. The major emotional factor was usually a disappointment in relation to vocational life. (p. 307)

Dunbar's hypothesis that trigger situations involve loss, insult, lack of recognition, and failure was subsequently taken up by other authors (Applebaum et al., 1955; Bastiaans, 1968; de Dowiakowski & Luminet, 1969; Dreyfuss, 1953; Hahn et al., 1966; Hauss, 1954; Kapp, 1954; Luminet, 1969; Paterson, 1939; Pelser, 1967; Valk & Groen, 1967; Vauthier, 1966; P. D. White, 1951).

2.4.1.2. Triggers of illness identified after the onset of CHD.
There are only a few clinical reports in the literature on the psychotherapeutic treatment of patients who have had heart attacks. Often they provide hypotheses about the trigger situations that can be formulated if the patient receives treatment relatively soon after the infarct.

Bardé and Kutter (1996) reported on a psychotherapeutic session that took place during inpatient treatment in a cardiac rehabilitation clinic (p. 92). The circumstances in which the patient, a freelance electrician (in Germany), found himself just before his heart attack were marked by a complete loss of control. He had received an order to install television cable connections in several houses on the same street. He could not get the connections to work, causing a high degree of physical strain because of the need to move between various floors

and the basement to check why the connections did not work. After several failed attempts, he contacted the postal technicians, who ascertained that they had installed the wrong central connections and informed him that their workers were busy elsewhere and would not be able to rectify the error for a week. The patient felt intense disgust about the sluggishness and "parasitic nature" of the "government apparatus," whose members lived at the expense of the people who "did the real work."

This patient experienced the situation as a failure and spent several days extremely annoyed about the incident. On the weekend, he mowed the lawn, drank a bottle of beer, smoked a cigarette, and collapsed on his freshly mowed lawn.

Later in the rehabilitation clinic he saw his heart attack as a "deliverance" that allowed him to rest at last. He had lived much of his life with an "apocalyptic outlook" and often wandered through the nearby woods after a frustrating day of work with the feeling that it was all meaningless and that there was no real future for him. These existential states were related to his early childhood experiences in bunkers that provided protection from bomb attacks. In the clinic he could for the first time sleep, relax, and experience a feeling of essential safety. This patient had had heart complaints for over 10 years before his MI; his doctor had drawn his attention to the imminent danger and had advised him to adopt a healthier lifestyle.

Bardé (1997) provided another account of a patient, who received 63 hours of intensive psychodynamic psychotherapy, in which the trigger situation was very telling. The patient, also German, was in politics, and one evening the members of his party dismissed him as a candidate for an upcoming election. The patient was surprised by the dismissal, and he suffered a heart attack at 3 o'clock the following morning. This extremely stressful situation, which for this patient meant existential failure and coming undone, evoked other psychologically stressful situations that, as became apparent during the course of his treatment, were related to early traumatic events. From a psychodynamic point of view, the loss of a prominent position of power in his party was paramount to the ruin of a grandiose narcissistic fantasy that held for him a twofold purpose: On one hand, it served the purpose of diverting his immense aggressiveness, fed by a basic disturbance, that exhibited itself as social and political hostility (e.g., hatred of foreigners). On the other hand, it was meant to compensate for his immense narcissistic lack of self-worth in the sense that he could create for himself the feeling that "they" (i.e., the nation) were "someone" again through his distinguished leadership position and his identification with the ideology of his party. Both functions, which from a psychodynamic point of view had the purpose of stabilizing a fragile and threatened self, were rendered ineffective with his dismissal.

Similarly, a case report by Marshall (1965) described a heart attack as a deliverance from the patient's unbearable and unresolved oedipal conflict. The patient was looking for a figurative ideal, caring father in the person of his boss, who nevertheless disappointed him. He looked for a "better father" in another firm and distinguished himself through exceptional achievement, substantiated by an increase in profits. However, in this job too he failed to receive the recognition of the ideal father on whom he had intrapsychically fixated. According to Marshall's case description, the psychological state of the patient could be characterized directly by a twofold disappointment and failure reaction in the context of a highly charged, near-limitless eagerness to perform and sacrifice himself with the purpose of attaining recognition, attention, and love. The patient dissociated himself from his first boss–father out of disappointment, hoping to get, from his second boss–father, all the masculine love and recognition that, in his opinion, his first supervisor had purposefully failed to provide. However, the patient's second boss also disappointed his need for love and recognition. When it became apparent that the patient had to leave this man as well, he collapsed with a heart attack brought about by a state of hopelessness and depressive exhaustion. Remarkably, after the heart attack the patient told Marshall of a depressive deliverance fantasy: The heart attack, and ultimately the heart failure, would make it possible for the patient to unite with his dead mother in his grave and in this way attain eternal rest.

A few years later Dreyfuss, Dasberg, and Assael (1969) devised a similar hypothesis. In their opinion, the situation in which the patient's heart attack occurred can be related to an unconscious suicide fantasy: The depressive patient used the heart attack to be delivered from the anguish of vain efforts to fulfill his never-ending longing for love, recognition, attention, and appreciation by his limitless eagerness to perform and sacrifice himself. The deliverance through heart failure allowed the patient the opportunity to rest and relax that he was denied in the state of "living" (see also the discussion of the Sisyphus syndrome in Wolf, 1967).

A case report by Stephanos (1982c) described the psychological state of a female MI patient who was 36 years old and the mother of three children and who received inpatient analytical psychotherapeutic treatment for 3 months (a model at the University of Ulm, Germany). Stephanos (1982c) related the story of this hard-working farmer's wife. He observed, "Her physical appearance is tough, muscular and broad-shouldered and she appears aged beyond her years and worn out" (p. 216). Her father died of a heart attack when she was 2, and her depressive and highly stressed mother had raised five children by herself on a farm: "As a result, the patient experienced a lack of emotional affection and basic security, which resulted in a latent depressive disposition" (p. 219).

At the age of 23 she was abandoned by her great love, a man from her town whom she had wanted to marry. This abandonment left her with long-lasting depression, which she tried to compensate for with hard work. At the age of 26, while suffering from depression, she met her future husband, a foreman bricklayer from a neighboring town with an established fortune; she took over management of his parents' farm. During her third pregnancy she experienced a crisis during which she felt as if she were a failure, as well as weak, helpless, and despairing.

A year before the heart attack, she seemed to herself "useless to the family, sometimes even superfluous. She was plagued by feelings of inferiority" (Stephanos, 1982c, p. 220). She could not talk to her husband about her difficulties. After quoting the patient—"Sometimes I had the feeling that I had become unable to cope with the task of raising the children"—Stephanos concluded "that in the last months before the heart attack, she had fallen into a state of increasing resignation, characterized by depression and dangerous isolation" (p. 221). One of the crises leading up to the heart attack was the departure of her 9-year-old son for travel abroad with her older sister: "'I could only agree to the journey with a heavy heart.' In the evening after the departure she suffered the attack with dizziness and a sensation of deafness" (p. 222). An additional separation experience troubling her at that time was the entrance of her youngest son into kindergarten.

She related the specific sequence of events surrounding the infarct to a nurse: She had attended a church wedding that day, and as she got out of the car and saw the wedding couple, she experienced sharp pains in her chest. A short time later, while in the church, the pains became more intense. The next morning she was admitted to inpatient treatment for a heart attack. "When I see a wedding couple," she admitted to the nurse, "I cannot help but think of my boyfriend. It was the most wonderful time of my life" (Stephanos, 1982c, p. 222).

In Stephanos's (1982c) opinion, the situation in which the heart attack occurred involved a psychological conflict that was central to her life. From the point of view of psychodynamic drive theory, the patient began "splitting off the world of drives," most recently after the separation from her "great love" (p. 228). She then compensated for the resulting "basic lack of security" by showing "great enthusiasm for her work," through which she obtained a "pseudoindependence" from her environment. In this way she constructed her own world consisting of work, which satisfied her narcissistic potency, but subject to the splitting off of her drives (p. 228). Her great love for the man "in whom she believed she perceived her forgotten dreams" awoke within her the childhood wish for love and security, which she then tried to realize by proxy with a man whom she did not love and whom she had married in a civil, rather than religious, ceremony. In this way she developed a defense against the failure in the development of her

passionate and sensual being through excessive work in "close partnership with her husband" and satisfaction by proxy in the "sensuous emotional exchange with her children" (p. 228).

Her urge-blocking conflict was triggered by the fact that her children were becoming independent, which became apparent through her son's journey abroad with his aunt; her increasing awareness of rejection by her husband, whom she had married for "reasons of convenience" (Stephanos, 1982c, p. 220); and conflicts with her parents-in-law. "In this way, we determined that in the last months before the heart attack she had fallen into a state of increasing resignation, characterized by depression and dangerous isolation" (p. 221). In this state she confronted the church wedding scenario that caused her "artificial state of existence" (p. 228) to disintegrate and the loss of her essential dreams. At this moment in the church, the heart attack set in. Stephanos implicitly hinted at the hypothesis that the infarct was triggered, in the context of a state of total exhaustion, by the fact that suppressed emotions belonging to split-off drives were activated and "somatized" (Stephanos, 1982a, 1982b).

2.4.1.3. Triggers of illness in patients during the course of psychotherapy.
Chessick (1977, 1987a, 1987b) provided a case study of a patient who suffered a heart attack during the course of a 6-year-long psychodynamic therapy. The sudden death of the patient's father triggered an existential crisis that brought on both depression and the development of homicidal tendencies toward his analyst (Chessick), who, in his eyes, had rejected him. It was at this point that the heart attack occurred.

Chessick described the psychodynamic constellation present shortly before his patient's heart attack. The patient suffered, according to Chessick, from a pronounced narcissistic personality disorder and was strongly dependent on self–object relationships to stabilize and integrate his personality and his feeling of identity. Chessick referred to Condon (1987), who had also emphasized the presence of a pronounced narcissistic personality disorder in heart attack patients. Before the heart attack, Chessick's patient had experienced a series of heavy setbacks: His father had died, his beloved daughter had left home to pursue her studies, his wife had been on the brink of divorcing him, and he perceived that Chessick had rejected his wishes (transference) to find in the therapist a sympathetic, warm-hearted (primary) object.

After the death of his father, the patient wanted to reduce the frequency of his sessions from twice a week to once a week because he could not anticipate an improvement in his condition through treatment. Chessick encouraged the patient to continue treatment but agreed to once-weekly sessions. Chessick described the patient's psychological state as characterized by his basic conflict: He had an intense wish for "intimacy" and "need for merger" that at the time he felt he was being denied in all of his social relationships, including that with his analyst. This basic conflict led to an existential helplessness and (one can infer) to despair and exhaustion in view of the hopelessness of his situation that "endangered the very cohesion of his nuclear self."

In the following paragraphs we summarize Chessick (1987b) at length because his is one of only two reports describing the situation shortly *before* the occurrence of a heart attack:

> The patient seemed to be fighting off his disappointed archaic longings for intimacy by classical paranoid dynamics, projection of oral sadistic rage, and withdrawal, out of his fear of being overwhelmed and fragmented by the need for merger stirred up by the death of his father, all of which occurred against the background of his wife's coldness. Another reason for his rage may have been the intuitive recognition that further discussion about his past and present experiences with his mother endangered the very cohesion of his nuclear self, because he felt helpless to deal with his archaic needs.
>
> He went off for a week's vacation and returned with fleeting but intense fantasy of shooting me, when I opened the office door. He related this to his own fear of being too attached to me and having to adjust to seeing me half

of the time he was seeing me before. He, superficially as usual, seemed relatively comfortable and was busy adjusting his life to find various ways of pleasing and soothing himself. (p. 139)

Chessick (1987b) continued,

> About 6 weeks after he returned from the week of vacation, he called me from a hospital and told me that he thought he was having a heart attack. . . . I telephoned him in the hospital several times to see how he was doing. I also repeatedly attempted to contact the internist, but he never returned my calls. According to the patient, the angiography was said to show severe triple coronary artery disease. (p. 139)

Noteworthy are the events that ensued: The patient ended his treatment with Chessick; he felt that the heart attack had resulted in the relief for which he had fought for so long. He was pampered by nurses and his wife, whom he had before perceived as a cold and rejecting person. His wife had suddenly transformed into a warm-hearted, sympathetic, and caring human being who never left his side.

Chessick (1987b) described his problems with countertransference; the transference of the patient's "depleted empty self " was to him a serious narcissistic injury, because the patient did not progress toward the expected psychoanalytic cure:

> I believe the most dangerous aspect of countertransference in the treatment of such a case is the injury to the therapist's narcissism when he recognizes that a case that appears amenable to intensive psychotherapy has reached a rock bottom, unalterable core of the depleted empty self; the time lag that occurs between reaching this point and the filtering of this information through the therapist's countertransference-based need to see the patient progress and recover is a delay which . . . is exceedingly dangerous. It is most important in intensive psychotherapy . . . to keep a

sharp lookout for signs that the patient has gone as far as he or she can go, and to relinquish and modify treatment goals on the basis of this material in spite of ostensive superficial professed motivation of the patient toward achieving structural change and analytical cure. (p. 142)

Chessick's (1987b) report contains indirect self-critical clues that he had blocked the way for himself to manage the dynamic developing in the patient's transference through his identification with the ideal of what constitutes psychoanalysis. He speculated that this countertransference may have set off the patient's "overwhelming rage that he somatized in the coronary artery disease" (p. 141).

It remains unclear what Chessick meant by "somatized" in this context; he may have meant either the emotional equivalent or the accompanying psychophysiological preparatory reactions. It should also be noted that on the one hand, Chessick talked of chronic intrapsychological conflict, which on the other hand became a *reconstellation* (a repetitive circular unconscious pattern) in the context of the therapy. The therapist seemed unable to deal with and classify these and, looking back, to feel guilty about his lack of empathy. Accordingly, the patient's inability to solve his internal conflict seemed to result in an interpersonal blockage that took the form of a reversed dissolution within the partnership: First, the patient experienced his spouse as cold and inapproachable; then, following the heart attack, he experienced the therapist as cold and inapproachable and his wife as loving and caring. According to Balint (1973), one could infer that it was difficult to integrate the patient's "basic fault" into an empathic therapeutic relationship. One suspects that it may have been precisely the analyst's resistance to the countertransference (Racker, 1978) that had set off considerable destructive consequences (aggression, hate) in the patient that were no longer resolvable within the context of the treatment.

Rust (1990) reported on the intensive psychotherapy treatment (72 hours), using primarily *katathym-imaginative techniques* (guided affective imagery; see Leuner, 1955, 1994), of a 58-year-old patient. The patient suffered a heart attack after the 31st treatment session. Rust reconstructed this treatment according to psychodynamic points of view. The patient sought psychotherapeutic treatment about 10 months before the infarct because he was experiencing extreme internal tension and unrest, a lack of motivation, reduced performance ability, a general down-in-the-dumps feeling, and an inability to cope with his work (p. 258). His wife had left him unexpectedly a year before because she felt neglected as a result of his heavy workload.

From a psychodynamic point of view, this loss reflected earlier severe losses. His father, a dedicated member of Hitler's Nationalist Socialist Party, was killed in the final year of World War II during a bombing raid. His mother, who was a political fanatic and a very strict person, had committed suicide in 1945 after the Americans invaded. The patient, who had received a privileged education, was thus orphaned and was raised by an uncle. His depressive symptoms began at that time, but he had a strong urge to control and felt that he had to "stand on his own" in life.

Rust (1990) described (as did Hahn) a compulsive personality that purposefully resisted and blocked from consciousness the underlying depressive experiences involving a complex of extreme loss and deficiency experiences:

> The patient's compulsive structure seemed to be at the forefront at first, with a controlled and orderly bearing and a vague, indicative manner of speaking. Reaction formation, rationalization, intellectualization, and emotional isolation, as well as denial, seemed to keep his depressive and aggressive emotions under control. He seemed to want to tie up his experiences of loss in physical symptoms and replace his grief by deficit in performance. (p. 259)

From a treatment point of view, Rust (1990) adopted a strategy of circumventing the compulsive character resistance of the patient, which was the result of a "rigid, strong superego," by the application of katathym-imaginative psychotherapy. He hoped to uncover the resisted depressive core and thereby resolve the patient's symptoms (physical ailments, poor work performance). Rust believed that the introduction of a regressive process may have, if not set off the infarct event, at least favored it. In an induced daydream in the 31st session, the patient imagined looking at a house from the outside and discovering a crack in the exterior wall: "I am sitting here in anxious distress, and I am staring at the wall" (p. 258). A week later the patient suffered an MI. In his analysis of the treatment, Rust went as far as to assert that "a chronological correlation appeared between the regressive process and the infarction." He interpreted this correlation as causal (p. 260).

Rust (1990) continued his psychotherapeutic work with the patient after the infarct with the intention of making it possible for him to gain access to his emotional experiences not only of peril, loss, and grief, but also of aggression, and to overcome his compulsive resistance. As a result, according to Rust, the patient "regained his ability to work by the 72nd session." As proof of the success of the treatment, he presented the second daydream, in which the patient again described the house of the 31st session:

> "It is the same house as before, but there is no crack in the exterior wall; it has probably been repaired in the meantime. I do not want to remain sitting on the bench—I want to see the house from the inside." He is then able to walk through all the rooms in the house, linger in the living room, get himself some milk out of the refrigerator in the kitchen and lie down to rest in the bedroom. (p. 262)

In his "critical reflection" Rust (1990) analyzed the trigger situation of the infarct event. Like Chessick, he emphasized the dissolution of a narcissistic self–object relationship that was meant to compensate for an unstable and flimsy self-discipline. The compulsive structure, based on the superego pa-

thology, was related to a severe emotional disturbance (an "alexithymia" and a *pensée operatoire*). Rust explained the emotional disturbance as consisting of the fact that the emotional agitation set off by the treatment could not be symbolized in controlled emotions: "The infarct event can be understood as the expression of a deep need combined with the enormous force of primal aggression which found its expression in this situation in turning against its own person" (p. 263).

Rust (1990) asked himself afterward how a patient whom he was treating could suddenly suffer a heart attack. He raised the notion of a "distortion of the countertransference": "In cases of pronounced superego pathology and early object-relational disorders, one has to have prepared oneself for a long-term contortion of the countertransference" (p. 263). Rust speculated that because the patient's compulsive structure made him appear well adjusted, Rust was tempted to assume that the proper working conditions for psychotherapeutic treatment were available. He was unable, however, to find direct access to the emotional experience of the patient in the transference relationship and thus could not deal with this constructively, so the patient had to "somatize" his impaired emotional self in the form of the infarct:

> The apparent positive transference relationship must have been affected in the background by the weak ability to form relationships and primal aggression. In this internal state the patient must have had no other way of dealing with the situation than with a most severe, existentially threatening somatic reaction. (p. 263)

In this reconstruction of Rust's account, the infarct is interpreted as an expressive event and is in theory compared to a neurotic syndrome or a tic (Brody, 1968, formulated a similar interpretation).

2.4.1.4. Hahn's conceptualization of the infarct trigger. Hahn (1971) attempted to describe the situations in which a heart attack occurs systematically on a clinical and empirical basis. (His concept of the Infarct Profile and the results of his research were summarized in Section 2.3.7.1). Hahn applied his Infarct Profile (consisting of the risk personality, the situation analysis, and the infarct personality) to an examination of 50 heart attack patients and concluded that the trigger situations of the infarct events were complex and that psychological strain by itself played a relatively minimal role in his group of patients. At the same time, cases of exclusively physical strain were just as rare. Instead, most patients experienced mixed psychological and physical strain. Accordingly, Hahn concluded, trigger situations are neither typical nor specific, but rather complex:

> Trigger situations are distributed over a broad spectrum from inconspicuous situations (occurring during or after rest and stress) and postprandial events to dramatic events involving unusual physical and psychological strain. The significance of the trigger situation in relation to the premorbid personality can hold clues, in some instances, to the seriousness of the basic ailment. (p. 26)

2.4.2. Summary of Psychodynamic Research on Trigger Situations

Numerous epidemiological investigations have addressed the question of whether specific circumstances influence the occurrence of a cardiac event. Our brief review indicates that the data are variable and often contradictory, indicating that trigger situations are complex. As in so many cases, the approach of identifying common patterns is not justified by the data. Just as in the physiological realm (e.g., circulatory conditions, electrical instability, vagal tonus, hormonal and metabolic imbalances, physical and psychological stress), different trigger clusters exist that combine different psychosocial variables (e.g., psychophysiological reagibility, age, sex, social status, vocational status, preparedness to sacrifice oneself). The search for unimodal distributions in the case of such a complex event as MI holds little promise from a methodological point of view.

The question that now remains is whether the study of psychological aspects of trigger situations can increase our understanding of coronary heart disease. The search for typical or specific relationships (e.g., points in time, such as day of the week or time of day) should be replaced by a search that is led by hypotheses and builds on existing etiological knowledge. More rigorous scientific approaches are needed to identify specific and distinct subgroups. For instance, study of heart attacks that occurred during a relaxation period requires a different theoretical framework than the study of infarcts in the context of intense emotional agitation. Research led by psychological hypotheses and etiology must begin with knowledge about the various pathomechanisms (e.g., psychoimmunological processes, electrical instability, variation in heart rate, hyperregulation) as the starting point in the study of trigger situations.

2.5. ACUTE MYOCARDIAL INFARCTION AS A TRAUMATIC EVENT

Acute myocardial infarction (AMI) is an extremely dangerous occurrence that leads to death within 28 days in about 50% of cases. Gradual change in the capillary system (the development of congestion and stenosis through deposits) remains undetected over a long period until the symptoms of cardiac angina pectoris occur or AMI sets in. AMI is experienced most often as a completely unexpected occurrence, but it is the final stage of a process that stretches over years and even decades.

The characteristics of an AMI vary. A few patients do not notice the infarction at all (silent heart attack), and it is later discovered by chance. Others, however, suffer extreme physical symptoms at the time of the attack, experience fear of death, and occasionally collapse into unconsciousness. The AMI is, if the patient survives, the start of a long succession of medical procedures: emergency transport, emergency treatment, intensive care, diagnosis and therapy (angiography, percutaneous transluminal coronary angioplasty [PTCA], bypass surgery, pharmacological therapy), transfer to a rehabilitation facility, transfer to a long-term outpatient treatment program, and eventually reestablishment of a normal life incorporating the necessary lifestyle changes.

From a psychosomatic point of view, AMI is an important biographical interruption with considerable psychological consequences. Conscious thoughts about death arise in the person's mind (sometimes for the first time), and constant fear of death or signs of its denial occur in most patients. For many, new questions arise and come to the fore; for some, so do serious emotional disturbances and emotional disorders that may be intense enough to qualify as a stress disorder.

This section deals with PTSD after a heart attack. First, we will examine when and to what extent one can say that PTSD occurs after a heart attack, according to the criteria specified in several more recent editions of the *Diagnostic and Statistical Manual of Mental Disorders* (3rd ed. [*DSM–III*]; American Psychiatric Association, 1980; 4th ed. [*DSM–IV*]; American Psychiatric Association, 1994). We will describe the typical symptoms and prevalence of stress disorder after an AMI as reflected in the literature. In conclusion, we will examine the implications for psychotherapeutic treatment.

The American Psychiatric Association incorporated the category of acute and posttraumatic stress disorder into the *DSM–III* (American Psychiatric Association, 1980) classification in 1980. The criteria for the diagnosis of a life-threatening disease were added in 1994 to the *DSM–IV* (American Psychiatric Association, 1994). The occurrence criterion for PTSD is formulated differently, and more restrictively, in the *International Classification of Diseases* (ICD; World Health Organization, 1991) than in the *DSM–III* or *DSM–IV:* According to the ICD, an AMI is not an occurrence criterion for PTSD. Consequently, the scientific literature on the topic refers exclusively to the *DSM–III* and *DSM–IV.*

Research has established that patients' subjective perceptions and appraisals (and therefore biographical factors and factors determined by personality) play a key role in cases of severe traumatization and, therefore, that trauma is not just an "objective" event with a linear dosage–effect relationship. It has long been recognized that an AMI can be a trau-

matic experience (Allan & Scheidt, 1996, 1998; Alonzo, 1999, 2000; Alonzo & Reynolds, 1998; Cameron, 1989; Jordan, Bardé, Stirn, & Girth, 1997; Kazemier, 1982; Klasmeier, 1991; Köhle & Gaus, 1986; Köhle, Gaus, & Wallace, 1996; Lachauer, 1984; Strasser, 1982). Researchers have hypothesized that the heart attack is an extraordinary life event that requires the person affected to reorient him- or herself and that can trigger many psychological, psychosomatic, and emotional disturbances. The crisis may be so serious that it causes severe shock to the personality in its biographical construction, in its previous nature and dynamics, and even in its formerly valid subjective sense of reality, just as do other types of trauma. A traumatic crisis can take on an existential character to the extent that it renders inoperative the requisite beliefs of belonging to the everyday world—that is, social cooperation, physical autonomy, and continuity (W. Fischer, 1984; Gerhardt, 1984).

2.5.1. Psychological Symptoms of a Traumatic Reaction

Many clinically relevant symptoms appearing with the onset of PTSD are not listed in the *DSM* criteria B through F. Some others are not listed because they are accompanying rather than major symptoms; somatization disorders, affective disorders (especially depression, fear, and compulsive behavior), fatalism, intentionally unhealthy lifestyles, and substance abuse are examples of common complaints resulting from a psychological trauma (and also an AMI). They are not classified separately and so are lost to clinical documentation, leading to difficulty in documenting changes in the intensity of PTSD over the course of disease. PTSD thus is an "on–off diagnosis"; either it exists or it does not, and classification of severity is difficult.

2.5.2. Clinical Diagnosis of Posttraumtic Stress Disorder Following a Heart Attack

In the daily clinical routine, PTSD is seldom diagnosed after a heart attack because patients rarely exhibit behavior problems and because the relevant diagnosis requires both time and the attention of qualified experts with substantial knowledge and experience. Kutz, Garb, and David (1988) published a comprehensive report on four cases involving posttraumatic disorder after heart attack and outlined their psychotherapeutic treatment; this is the only publication we identified that documents the therapeutic treatment in detail. Their psychiatric work in Israel involved standard procedures for examining patients for possible stress disorders (e.g., war experiences, combat stress reaction). In the course of this routine practice, their attention was quickly drawn to the fact that many people who had had a heart attack had developed the same disorders.

The first patient was a 40-year-old man who was sent by his general practitioner for psychiatric consultation because he had demonstrated a complete personality transformation 4 months after his heart attack and, despite good angiographic measurements, was not recovering. The second patient also was a 40-year-old man who had had a heart attack only 7 days previously and who was being treated pharmacologically and had a cardioversion in the intensive care unit for life-threatening arrhythmia. Although he appeared afraid, passive, and apparently unemotional but was noticeably depressed (he had been highly sedated), he became openly fearful after being transferred to the regular ward and lay motionless on his bed, often for hours on end, interacting very little with his environment. He clung stubbornly to his oxygen mask, although it had been disconnected. He complained of chest pains. The third patient, a 55-year-old man, was referred for consultation because he had developed a cough that was unresponsive to treatment and that had raised the suspicions of the cardiologist that he was "attention seeking." The fourth patient, a 61-year-old man who had been a Holocaust victim, was transferred because of evident nervousness, depression, and an increasing use of angina medication.

These four patients were referred for psychiatric consultation for different reasons, and none of the referrals mentioned symptoms of PTSD. Only the psychiatric examination showed that the symptoms were signs of a stress disorder. Kutz et al. (1988) described each patient's stress disorder symptoms, which varied widely.

The first patient had displayed unusual behavior in the intensive care unit. He had had strong emotional reactions, including fear, confusion, and agitation. He had required high doses of sedatives during the entire intensive care stay. Later he appeared calm, brooding, and detached but suffered from sleeplessness and would not let his wife leave his side. At home, his reclusiveness continued and increased; he experienced unanticipated fits of anger. His strength did not return, he continued to complain of chest pains and shortness of breath, and he suffered increasingly from sleeplessness.

The second patient displayed oversensitivity to noise and such a severe attention deficit that he was unable to follow the psychiatrist's questions. Additionally, he suffered from a sleep disorder (difficulty getting to sleep and staying asleep) and from nightmares (of carrying heavy loads and of choking to death) that woke him up every time he had them.

The third patient, after intensive exploration, reported deep-rooted feelings of helplessness, abandonment, and rejection. He too suffered from sleeplessness, concentration deficit, and severe irritability. His wife and children described his restlessness, irritability, and uncontrollable fits of rage, as well as low noise tolerance and nightmares from which he would wake up screaming.

The fourth patient suffered openly, was emotionally unstable, and was prone to crying and feeling helpless. He, too, suffered from nightmares, loss of appetite, and intense fits of fear about having another heart attack.

Thus, different clinical symptoms can indicate underlying PTSD, but clinical staff and cardiologists usually take little notice of these silent and unspecific symptoms. Great clinical experience on the part of psychiatrists and psychologists is needed to identify and treat the specific behavior as a sign of PTSD, and the inclusion of colleagues is helpful.

2.5.3. Literature Review on Trauma Disorders and Acute Myocardial Infarction

We conducted a review of the literature published through August 2003 by searching PSYNDEX, PsycINFO, and Medline using the terms *coronar* and (a) *traumatic near1 stress*, (b) *PTSD*, or (c) *emotional*

TABLE 2.1

Overview of the Literature Reviewed

Type of publication	Citations
Systematic review	S. S. Pedersen, 2001
Original empirical works	P. Bennett & Brooke, 1999; P. Bennett, Conway, Clatworthy, Brooke, & Owen, 2001; Doerfler, Pbert, & DeCosimo, 1994; Hackett, Cassem, & Wishnie, 1968; Kutz, Shabtai, Solomon, Neumann, & David, 1994; Kutz et al., 1988; Neumann, 1991; Shemesh et al., 2002; van Driel & Op den Velde, 1995
Case studies	Bardé, 1997; Hamner, 1994; Kutz et al., 1988; Menninger & Menninger, 1936; Ohlmeier, 1989
Publications about theoretical and clinical aspects of trauma following a heart attack	Allan & Scheidt, 1996, 1998; Alonzo, 1999, 2000; Alonzo & Reynolds, 1998; Cameron, 1989; Jordan et al., 1997; Kazemier, 1982; Klasmeier, 1991; Köhle & Gaus, 1986; Köhle et al., 1996; Lachauer, 1984; Strasser, 1982
References in *Dissertation Abstracts International*	Devaul, 2000; Lukach, 1996; McPherson, 1999; R. N. Thompson, 1999

near1 distress. We also used other search terms (e.g., *myocard* near1 infarc** or *AMI*), but these did not supply any additional hits. Furthermore, we did a manual search of the indexes of manuals and textbooks.[3] The 32 publications listed in Table 2.1 comprise the literature on the subject of acute posttraumatic stress disorder following a heart infarction. In addition, two studies not included in this review mentioned aspects of acute suicidal tendencies after a heart attack (and other serious illnesses; Kishi, Robinson, & Kosier, 2001; Kishi, Robinson, Kosier, & James, 2002).

Although it may seem unusual, we decided to include case reports and theoretically or clinically oriented publications describing traumatic reac-

tions after a heart attack. This type of publication not only contains valuable expert knowledge but also makes sense in view of the current state of scientific research. This strategy allowed us to include the work of Kutz et al. (1988) described in the preceding section and the experience of researchers who are also involved in clinical work (e.g., Allan & Scheidt, 1996, 1998; Klasmeier, 1991; Köhle et al., 1996; Köhle & Gaus, 1986).

The 32 studies vary with regard to the following:

- sample size (Ns = 21 to 102), quality of the sample description , selection criteria, and analysis of dropout rates;
- delay between infarct and examination, ranging from immediately after intensive care treatment (usually a few days after the event) to 96 months later; and
- instruments used to assess the symptoms of PTSD—many had obvious weaknesses and recorded only selected aspects of PTSD (e.g., the Impact of Event Scale; Horowitz, Wilner, & Alvarez, 1979).

The articles selected show a prevalence of PTSD of between 5% and 25%, or an estimated mean prevalence of 11% to 12%, for the first 6 months. For periods longer than 6 months, the data are insufficient and contradictory; however, we speculate that the rate of spontaneous remission is low.

2.5.4. Implications for the Psychotherapeutic Treatment of Trauma in Acute Myocardial Infarction Patients

Many different intervention techniques have been applied in psychotherapy for posttraumatic stress disorder, including those founded on or derived from psychodynamic, behavioral, cognitive–behavioral, and neurobiological concepts and models (Flatten et al., 2004, pp. 60 ff). Among others, specific therapeutic techniques include imagina-

---

[3] We did not include research that dealt with the related construct of adjustment disorder (searching on the term *emotional near1 distress*). Also not included were works dealing with the question of whether PTSD has effects on the cardiovascular system. Among the works found in our search were publications on the issue of dealing with the psychological (traumatic) experience of defibrillator use, cardiac arrest, heart transplants, and bypass surgery. We excluded these works from our examination, as well as those examining the consequences of severe stress (especially participation in a war) for the subsequent development of heart disease and works that compared persons who had previously experienced PTSD with those who had not.

tion, cognitive–behavioral restructuring, exposition strategies, eye movement desensitization and reprocessing, and procedures relating to activation through physical and artistic expression, as well as psychopharmaceutical treatment.

Central to psychodynamic therapy are procedures to revive traumatic experiences that have been suppressed or split off leading to the traumatic syndrome (e.g., intrusion, dissociation, apathy, heightened sensitivity, somatization). These experiences are revived through transference with the aim of helping the client process and ultimately integrate the surprising and overwhelming traumatic events through symbolization, typification, and normalization in a therapeutic dialogue (Horowitz, 1974; Lindy, 1993, 1996). This therapeutic procedure usually includes three components: (a) stabilization, (b) trauma processing in the narrower sense, and (c) rehabilitation or reintegration of the traumatic destructivity. The basic therapeutic attitude is availability, presence, and authenticity in the recognition and treatment of the trauma and the existential topic of life and death. For this reason, the treating psychotherapist must have personally come to terms with the existential dimension of being and must have integrated this in the form of a basic competence in his or her own personal existence.

There is a great shortage of research on the evaluation of the various PTSD treatment procedures. Future research is needed to clarify to what extent the many trauma therapeutic procedures developed in the past few decades are effective both generally and specifically in regard to specific patient groups. It might be necessary to develop further specific intervention procedures.

No empirical intervention study has focused on PTSD following infarction. A pivotal problem in the treatment of PTSD in heart attack patients is the specific transference they exhibit: They often adopt a distanced approach, appear inconspicuous in the everyday activity of the clinic, and tend to avoid close contact with medical personnel. Such patients avoid topics and feelings related to the heart attack in conversation; they express themselves in a superficial fashion (common in people who have been traumatized; G. Fischer & Riedesser, 1998).

Thus, they risk remaining unnoticed by the doctors treating them in intensive care units and rehabilitation clinics as well as during long-term care. Many seemingly unaffected patients do not seek psychotherapeutic help of their own volition, so their symptoms remain unnoticed. Normally, friends or family members such as a spouse notice the changes and take the initiative in seeking help. Many patients and practitioners assume that the symptoms of PTSD will go away by themselves in time. This assumption is wrong: A large body of evidence indicates that after different traumas (such as cancer, accident, or MI), one cannot expect a spontaneous remission of PTSD after 6 months (Alter et al., 1996; Andrykowski, Cordova, McGrath, Sloan, & Kenady, 2000; Cordova et al., 1995; Hamner, 1994; Kessler, Sonnega, Bromet, Hughes, & Nelson, 1995; Pelcovitz et al., 1996; Shalev, Schreiber, Galai, & Melmed, 1993; Tjemsland, Soreide, & Malt, 1996).

In psychotherapeutic treatment, it is first necessary to consider the specific transference for heart attack patients and to accurately monitor any countertransference. Therapists should not encourage trivializing or marginalizing, even if patients utter this wish unconsciously or "present" it as a means of dealing with the trauma. Dunbar (1943) pointed out that trauma can be treated effectively, but she noted that good-humored patients dealing with their illness in a lighthearted or contemptuous way are in danger. Therapists should emphasize the gravity of the situation and initiate discussion about the patient's grief over the loss of invincibility and confidence. A crucial but perhaps unconscious issue in the lives of patients is the constant fear of death and the need to cope with this fear (Allan & Scheidt, 1996; Klasmeier, 1991). Many do not speak even to their partners about this fear or merely discuss it in a jovial, playfully defensive way. It is essential that cardiac patients have a place where they can discuss this fear earnestly. The uncertainty of their continued existence—the ever-present threat of suffering a renewed and possibly deadly reinfarction—is the existential theme in their lives.

The basic therapeutic attitude can be described as follows: to be personally available for the patient's existential cares while not losing sight of the reality of the next steps in life and to allow the patient to express his or her fear of death and yet develop worthwhile and satisfying perspectives on life. Therapists must avoid merging with the patient and be alert to the unconscious countertransference of distancing themselves too much (J. P. Wilson & Lindy, 1994). From the practical perspective of behavioral therapy, it is necessary to systematically break down the avoidance behavior that usually develops and to involve the family in an active supporting role. Patients should learn that they can extend their radius of activity and that they do not have to stay close to a doctor permanently. They should further understand that they can assess and make use of their physical potential and that, in fact, they should use and improve this within the framework of secondary prevention.

It is advisable to discuss the causes of the heart attack with the patient in detail and to do so repeatedly. Additionally, the therapist should explore the patient's own lay theory about the heart attack, because each patient gives it a specific meaning that varies according to his or her background and biographical structure and development (including such relevant structures as punishment, humiliation, moratorium, salvation, or liberation; *moratorium* is the idea of providing a "time out" in the sense that a disease provides time to think about principal questions of life; see Erikson, 1959). The patient's analysis of the cause and attribution of meaning often leads him or her to a deeper sense of understanding and more effective coping strategies, because the patient frequently unconsciously relates the trauma of the heart attack to other, previous traumatic experiences. Exploration of these personal attributions of meaning encourages the patient's gradual readjustment and helps him or her to endure and integrate the permanent uncertainty and fear of death. Moreover, personal attributions of meaning help patients mitigate risk factors through adjustments in lifestyle. Lifestyle changes are most effectively encouraged not by wagging a threatening finger, but by helping patients deal with their grief, work through anxiety and depression, gain new perspectives, and identify resources. The duration of such treatment can be

gauged from clinical experience; the literature cites 3 to 25 sessions.

For many patients, the involvement of the spouse or partner is very important. Empirical findings show that the quality of the partnership influences the way the patient copes with the illness. Research has also shown that many partners also suffer from the consequences of the heart attack and may develop diverse functional, psychosomatic, and emotional disorders during the 18 months following the event (Titscher & Schöppl, 2000). The partner may find it difficult to talk about his or her feelings and fears about the illness because he or she is afraid of troubling the patient. The wife of one patient said the following in the context of psychotherapeutic treatment: "You cannot imagine how difficult it is to live with a man for 10 years who fears that he might die any day and who on top of this mentions it at least once a week" (personal communication by a patient, July 2002).

2.5.5. Summary of Acute Myocardial Infarction as a Traumatic Event

A heart attack is a life-threatening event. It triggers fears and far-reaching demands for change in everyday life. Patients' psychological reactions vary greatly and are dependent on many factors. Most patients survive the ordeal without noteworthy psychological effects. Perhaps 20% to 40% of patients, however, show various psychological disturbances (many of them probably adjustment disorders), and a stress disorder is diagnosed in about 11%. Psychological adjustment has long- and short-term consequences for psychological health, compliance with treatment, quality of life, and prognosis. Which variables predict who will experience a stress disorder is still unknown; factors mentioned include age, sex, seriousness of the heart attack, duration of treatment in the intensive care unit, and ethnic and social characteristics (P. Bennett, Owen, Koutsakis, & Bisson, 2002). An as yet unanswered question is whether people who have suffered posttraumatic stress disorder earlier in life are more susceptible to renewed PTSD following an AMI.

The prevalence of PTSD in cases of serious (non-illness-related) trauma (e.g., experiencing a natural catastrophe or being tortured, taken hostage, or kidnapped) is about 35%. The prevalence of PTSD with many illnesses (e.g., cancer, transplants, heart attacks) is therefore comparatively low, at approximately 11%. Many explanations have been offered for this apparent discrepancy. The most common is that a grave and life-threatening illness is a very probable event that can be expected in the normal course of life. People are usually able to deny the threat of becoming seriously ill ("it will happen to others, not me"). The problem for patients following a heart attack is "informational trauma" (B. L. Green, Lindy, & Grace, 1994; Shalev et al., 1993), which occurs when they are informed that death has become imminent and that they also must face other difficult events and consequences. Their trust in their own capability and invincibility is shaken (G. Fischer & Riedesser, 1998).

Identifying the specific subgroup of patients with stress disorder is highly relevant both for research and for clinical treatment for a number of reasons:

- Failure to recognize stress disorder results in high costs and later illnesses (Solomon & Davidson, 1997).

- Patients with stress disorder are less compliant with treatment regimens (Shemesh et al., 2002), and their prognosis is often worse.

- Stress-disordered patients need trauma-specific psychological interventions.

Related research in psychotraumatology shows that the symptoms of stress disorder tend to become chronic if left untreated (this was confirmed in a case study by P. Bennett et al., 2002). If the disorder persists untreated after 12 months, there is little possibility of a spontaneous remission (Maercker & Ehlert, 2001).

2.6. PSYCHODYNAMIC TREATMENT REPORTS

The psychodynamic publications we found on the treatment of coronary patients are listed in Table W2.1 (see the accompanying Web site: http// www.apa.org/books/resources/jordan/) by date of

publication and study methodology. We found seven systematic empirical studies, 15 case studies from outpatient and inpatient settings, 24 expert reports with and without clinical implementation reports, and several unsystematic reviews.

2.6.1. Systematic Empirical Studies

In this section we review the publications we identified that describe specific and methodologically controlled interventions. Comparison of these intervention studies is problematic for several reasons:

- Sample sizes ($N = 31$ to $N = 106$, average 56) were too small in some cases to validly compare the different treatment groups or treatment and control groups.

- Different treatment characteristics and doses were applied in various settings. For example, five interventions were for outpatients and two were for inpatients. Four studies had a treatment dosage of 10 to 15 sessions (of 60 to 75 minutes each); one appeared to involve (the details were not clear) six 2-hour sessions, and another involved about 50 outpatient sessions, an extremely high dosage (again, the details were not clear).

- The descriptions of the interventions are, in most cases, very brief. The qualifications of the intervening staff are generally insufficiently specified, and the clinical quality of the interventions is unclear. Therefore, replication studies are not possible for most of these studies.

A fundamental deficiency in the design of almost all the studies is that they lacked a so-called attention-placebo group (only one study had such a control group; Ebert & Moehler, 1997). A control group receiving "standard care" is inappropriate in psychological studies, because this care and attention may have important effects. A classical (no-treatment) control group or attention-placebo control group is better able to control for a generalized social effect. Four of the seven studies had a control group; the other three did not need a control group because they tested present-course details and not outcome variables.

The goals of the studies varied widely. Four studies tested exclusively psychological or psychometric areas (e.g., quality of life, depression, coping). One study measured psychophysiological parameters, and only one study measured cardiac endpoints in addition to psychological parameters (Rogner, Bartram, Hardinghaus, Lehr, & Wirth, 1994).

We assessed the quality of the interventions, following Herrmann-Lingen and Buss (chap. 5, this volume), and Jordan and Lazanowski (chap. 8, this volume), according to the following criteria: A treatment was classified as being of high quality when it included at least four of the following six points:

1. Qualified staff administered the intervention, or qualified materials (e.g., videos, brochures) were used.
2. The intervention was clearly and thoroughly described.
3. The groups were randomly selected.
4. There was a control group and/or an attention-placebo group.
5. There were 15 or more persons in each treatment group.
6. Results demonstrate differential outcomes.

We assigned points to indicate the quality of the intervention as described in Exhibit 2.1. In addition, Table W2.1 incorporates these seven studies (see accompanying Web site). The following paragraphs provide short descriptions of the studies.

Rogner et al. (1994) reported on two studies. The first involved 67 heart attack patients in an inpatient rehabilitation clinic; it attempted to validate the hypothesis of depressive-style coping (patients after a heart attack often show depressive symptoms in the 1st month). The second, a controlled study, involved 81 cardiac patients also in an inpatient rehabilitation clinic. This study tested a 15-session group therapy treatment program using "indirect-suggestive" techniques for cardiac rehabilitation. The group therapy included two parts: (a) "hypnotherapeutic dialogue to promote the recovery of the depressive type" and (b) a mental relaxation program intended to help patients use relaxation in everyday life and to reduce their fear of experiencing another heart attack. The authors collected pretest and posttest data as well as data

on other dimensions that Dunbar (1943) found to be cardiopathologically relevant (e.g., fear, depression, willingness to wear oneself out, and aggression, as well as personality dimensions), using a questionnaire, and they compared the results with those of a randomized control group taking part in a rehabilitation program. The authors concluded, "Participation in group therapy can reduce the depressive tendencies of patients recovering from illnesses" (Rogner et al., 1994).

Altmann-Herz, Reindell, Petzold, and Ferner (1983) described an outpatient treatment program. They differentiated (without using a randomized and controlled design) between two groups: the sociable group and the impulsive–regressive group; the latter comprised two subgroups, the impulsive–aggressive subgroup and the regressive–apprehensive subgroup. The groups differed regarding achievement orientation, tendency toward social withdrawal, conservative attitudes, and psychophysiological state. Impulsive–regressive patients suffered more, were less achievement oriented, were more introverted, were more dependent, and in general were more psychosomatically disturbed in comparison with sociable patients. For impulsive–aggressive patients, the authors recommended coronary sports groups to allow them to work out their aggressions, increase their social competence, and prepare for group therapy. For regressive–apprehensive patients, who have both a high degree of suffering and high ideals, they recommended individual therapy. For sociable patients, who generally had a functioning defense system, they recommended support therapy (autogenic training combined with group therapy).

Stern and colleagues (Stern, Gorman, & Kaslow, 1983; Stern, Plionis, & Kaslow, 1984) described a methodologically rigorous study involving three randomized groups that showed the positive effects of the psychodynamic interventions. Unfortunately, both intervention groups also took part in fitness training outside of the study, which may have influenced the results.

In another well-designed study, Ebert and Moehler (1997) used a control group and an attention-placebo group and showed that social integration clearly improved as a result of the inter-

EXHIBIT 2.1

Classification of the Quality of Treatment Studies

Study characteristic	Points assigned			
	1	2	3	4
Relevant *n*	<30	30–99	100–499	≥500
a. Quality of instruments used	Ad hoc instruments or single items	Unknown instruments	Well-established instruments *or* interviews	Well-established instruments *and* interviews
b. Quality of intervention (list in section 2.6.1)	1 point was assigned for one of the six criteria met from the list in section 2.6.1	2 points were assigned, if two or three of the six criteria met from the list in section 2.6.1	3 points were assigned, if four or more of the six criteria met from the list in section 2.6.1	(No studies were assigned 4 points)
c. Results criteria reported	Only mean value	*M* + *SD* or percentage	*M* + *SD* and percentage	

Methodological Score = (a + b + c) / 3

Quality	No. of studies
Very well qualified (>8 points)	1
Very qualified (>6 to ≤8 points)	2
Partially qualified (>4 to ≤6 points)	2
Not qualified (≤4 points)	2

Quality of the study = sample size points × methodological score

vention. We ranked the quality of this study as low, however, because the data for the two control and one intervention groups (*N* = 32) involved too few recipients (i.e., fewer than 15 persons per group). Nevertheless, the results of this study are impressive.

A study by Kavanagh, Shephard, Pandit, and Doney (1970) compared a standard intervention to promote movement and fitness with a nonstationary hypnotherapeutic intervention. They were unable to carry out the study as designed because patients would not accept being randomized to control and treatment groups. The system for assessing cardiologic parameters was explained, but no description was provided of the method they used to assess patients' psychological characteristics. The empirical significance of this study is thus limited.

Taken together, these studies show that participating patients complied very well with treatment regimens and achieved positive psychological changes. Only one of these studies is less than 20

years old (Rogner et al., 1994). The studies were not able to overcome the methodological problems that frequently plague intervention studies, such as problems with forming control and attention-placebo groups. In addition, they were unable to sufficiently control for confounding influences on cardiological health; cardiac patients naturally desire to change their way of life, for example by intensifying their level of physical activity. Also, it is difficult to describe an operationalized psychodynamic therapy in sufficient detail to serve as a manual. In summary, the research to date remains unsatisfactory but indicates that further research is justified.

2.6.2. Case Reports

The following section describes case reports of psychodynamic treatments (outpatient and inpatient).

2.6.2.1. Outpatient treatment. On the basis of our literature search, we found only two publications that described ambulatory psychotherapeutic treatments with patients who began their treatment before their heart attack and suffered from an MI during this period (Chessick, 1977, 1987a, 1987b; Rust, 1990). Three publications reported ambulatory treatments with patients soon after they experienced a heart attack (Bardé, 1997; Marshall 1965; Nuland, 1968).

2.6.2.1.1. Treatment begun before a heart attack. We found two single case reports in the literature, by Chessick (1977, 1987a, 1987b) and Rust (1990), on psychodynamic-oriented treatment that started before the patients had a heart attack (these reports are also described in section 2.4.1.3). These authors had treated their patients for several years before the patients' heart attacks and reflected on the question of how to understand the infarct in the context of therapy. We strongly recommend reading the original works, which we summarize only briefly here.

Both case studies described the narcissistic and compulsive character styles of the patients, which were supposed to explain their deep-set traumatic and depressive experiences. The authors described the patients' conflict constellations and personal configurations as Dunbar had earlier, as being specific to coronary patients. Both authors reported on their own difficulties as psychotherapists. They tended to use treatment methods involving warm and intensive contact with the traumatically depressive complex of the patient, which was inevitably set free during treatment. The authors reported a feeling of failure in their therapeutic ethos, because they worried that they did not provide comfort to their patients. The weak point of both studies was based on a grave misunderstanding: Because a heart attack happened during the course of psychotherapy, the authors seemed to say, they must have failed or made a professional error. They seemed to expect that no patient should suffer a heart attack while undergoing psychotherapeutic treatment, especially when the therapy has been carried out by experienced trained professionals. The reasons for this expectation are not explicit and, moreover, could not be plausible. This hypothesis may have led to both authors' conviction that some unconscious countertransferences could have caused the illnesses.

2.6.2.1.2. Treatment begun after a heart attack. Three publications reported on psychodynamic treatment begun after the patient had experienced a heart attack. Marshall (1965) provided at least 120 hours of psychoanalysis to a 43-year-old patient who had had a heart attack a year after he finished his first psychoanalysis, which had lasted 4 years. Marshall reported on the positive effects of the analytical method of interpretation. This method concentrated on the deep-seated problems of destructive aggressiveness and death fantasies (murder or suicide). He explained that intensive transference is a burden and that the analyst has to confront the patient's position on death, destruction, hopelessness, and helplessness.

Nuland (1968) briefly described four cases involving hypnotherapy, and Garma (1969) described some ideas regarding psychosomatic illness. These publications describe concepts that now are outdated, and we will not discuss them further.

Bardé (1997) described a patient for whom he had provided psychodynamic treatment in the intensive care unit following a heart attack and continuing after discharge outside the clinic (totaling approximately 50 hours, one session per week). He found that because of the specific transference constellation that led to the reconstruction of his traumatic structures, this patient was psychodynamically dependent in terms of character defense. Regarding the treatment methods, Bardé described the difficulties with aggressive hostility; murder and suicidal fantasies played a major role, and Bardé made it clear that fragile self-integration, extreme self-pity, and resulting aggression in therapy sessions must be given priority.

2.6.2.2. Inpatient treatment. Inpatient psychological rehabilitation does not exist in many countries; however, it is common in Germany (see Grande & Badura, chap. 10, this volume). There are few studies in which intensive arguments about institutional conditions do not take place, and therefore discussions primarily concern technical modifications. A great deal of importance is given to the interpersonal relationships among staff members and to institutional resistance to the concept of somatic determination. Articles in this area typically discuss considerations for involving the family in treatment and the specific needs of subgroups of patients.

The first publications on inpatient psychotherapy date back to 1963 (Hattingberg, 1967, 1968; Hattingberg & Mensen, 1963). Hattingberg and his colleagues reported on the risk personality of heart attack patients based on his experiences with a total of 2,500 workers in group therapy (7 hours a week over 6 weeks) in a rehabilitation clinic. They found that through the resistance of love and passive wishes and through a very strong relationship with a father figure, certain patients had a tendency to seek authority in order to be led; this finding demonstrates how important it is to go beyond psychotherapeutic doctrinal attitudes to promote a transference relationship that can better address the fears induced by the illness. Hattingberg found that there is no single category of "heart attack patient" and named four subgroups: the melancholic, the sanguine, the choleric, and the heart-fear types. He concluded that not only pathophysiology but also differences in personal characteristics that qualify as "borderline neurosis" (i.e., neuroses that are almost outside the margin of neurosis) should be taken into consideration in rehabilitation.

Concerning stationary rehabilitation (from the Heart Center in Rotenburg an der Fulda, Germany), Siepmann (1980) reported on individual discussion therapy with heart patients. He believed that heart attack patients in general have basic depressive problems: They feel worthless and have to compensate for this (i.e., by having a Type A personality). In early childhood, such patients were disappointed in their passive wishes and their wish to be taken care of, and in reaction to this they developed an impulsive character defense. The heart attack shatters this resistance, and patients become helpless and weak (through the physical illness, the repressed past returns). What they have sought to avoid in their lives actually happens. Siepmann felt that Rogerian psychotherapy was the appropriate method to address both the current situation following a heart attack and the patient's underlying personality issues.

Siepmann (1980) reviewed many common psychodynamic concepts and described the traditional rehabilitation programs that stressed mainly physical exercise and education. He concluded that most of these methods were unhelpful in addressing patients' personality issues and in this sense were contraindicated. He argued that the intensity of physical exercise and therapy and the emphasis on ergometer training outcome measures strengthens the pre-CHD etiological relevant psychological behavior patterns of the patients (i.e., high achievement). He therefore recommended that exploration of regressive feelings and the heretofore ignored impulses should be encouraged.

Roettger (1982) reported from a rehabilitation center about a stationary program for creative therapy. He identified three groups and described their characteristics using case examples. The first group consisted of patients who were not willing to take part in psychotherapeutic work and received no treatment. The second group comprised patients who received information regarding risk-related behaviors. The third and smallest group underwent intensive psychotherapeutic sessions during which they examined their feelings and social relationships. The psychological intervention (gestalt therapy) was poorly explained and not reproducible.

A case report from Stephanos (1982b) is remarkable not only because it is the only treatment report from a female patient but also because the treatment setting was unusual. Stephanos treated a woman with coronary illness using an integrated internistic psychosomatic model in a clinic in Ulm over an exceptionally long period (3 months). This model involved an integrative in-patient unit in which internal medicine and psychosomatic medicine worked together equally. The basic thesis of the report was that psychoanalytic therapy is helpful for inpatients because psychotherapy can positively influence feelings and conditions and in this way trigger the course of the illness (Stephanos, 1982c, p. 211). Stephanos described his methods as follows:

> The art of the psychoanalyst is to put himself in the place of his patient, to feel the crisis and complexity of the inner dramatic feelings. He can then, throughout the treatment, help his pa-

tient achieve better insight into the reasons for this crisis. The patient can then slowly but surely find solutions for his problems, objectively related. The healing process starts here.
(p. 216)

Stephanos showed that sometimes the MI reactivates a traumatic unconscious experience and that psychodynamic therapy shortly after an MI is integrated into the patient's ability to cope with the illness.

Ettin, Vaughan, and Fiedler (1987) presented a detailed and plausible program for stress management in 12 sessions. They described every session thematically and discussed the relationship between psychoeducational and psychodynamic elements of group leadership.

Ohlmeier (1989) provided five sessions of psychotherapy to an inpatient group in Germany. Although seven reports of this program were published (Köhle, Gaus, Karstens, & Ohlmeier, 1972; Ohlmeier, 1980, 1982, 1985, 1989, 1999; Ohlmeier, Karstens, & Köhle, 1973), none clearly described the setting and the institutional organization. In addition, Ohlmeier did not describe his intervention technique in sufficient detail. Ohlmeier interpreted the fact that the technique led to a point that the group therapist was no longer of importance and felt shut out of the group in connection with the background of the subordinately unconscious father conflict.

Kutter (1997) reported (without providing details) on the treatment of several inpatient groups in a rehabilitation clinic. He characterized his intervention methods as interactional psychodynamic. As in other studies, this author encountered difficulties in convincing patients to participate. He worked with relatively small groups (3 to 5 persons) over 12 sessions lasting 1.5 hours each. This is a relatively high therapy dosage (in comparison with other studies, surely the highest dosage in the limited area of a rehabilitation clinic). Kutter's conclusions concerning the role of the group leader are surprising; although he was a very experienced group therapist and supervisor, he emphasized that no classical interpretation technique should be

used, that the group therapist should not be distanced or strict, and that the basic rules of psychoanalysis should not be used. Interesting is a brief discussion of the use of an item from a coping questionnaire to initiate a group discussion that had good results; one could interpret this as an alternative treatment method for dealing with group situations (e.g., long silences).

Bardé and Kutter (1996) reported on the inpatient treatment of a self-employed electrician as part of a pilot project in a rehabilitation clinic for coronary illnesses. Because the length of stay was short, seven sessions were held in one phase, during which the patient was highly sensitive. He had worn himself out over decades, and after his heart attack he could sleep as much as he needed. In this relaxation phase, the patient gladly accepted the offer of counseling, and the theme of the counseling was the patient's immense annoyance and hatred of the illness situation, connected with loss of control.

Lesage-Desrousseaux (1981) reported on an open inpatient discussion group with heart attack patients. The group met once a week for 20 one-hour sessions; 9 patients and the author, a staff nurse, took part. Following this Lacan-oriented therapy, the nurse concluded that these patients were not psychoanalytically treatable. She asserted that because their traumas were triggered by their illness, there was no "symbolic order" to use in analyzing an unconscious wish (*le désir*). According to her, the patients found themselves in a "mirror-stage" in which they as "subjects" could not speak because they were beyond language (*parole*). The main priority for these patients was to address their need for help and attention from someone who could directly and practically take care of their needs (p. 370). She especially emphasized the death threat felt by patients and described a specific dynamic of transference and countertransference between patients and cardiologists characterized by a medical-model machine–engineer discourse: The patient is being threatened by death, is helpless and desperate, and feels needy, and the cardiologist responds with an omnipotence fantasy in which, through the use of technology, the patient can ward off death and be reborn, a kind of reincarnation (*re-naissance*,

p. 373). This unconscious agreement between doctor and patient constitutes an "iatrogenic pathology" (p. 376) established on a narcissistic level (the mirror stage) that definitely allows access to the patient. Patients join with their doctors in an "engineering discourse," which means that even in the future, they will not be able to speak for or express themselves.

Mittag and Ohm (1987) described psychodynamic psychotherapy focused on a group model in an inpatient rehabilitation center. Psychodynamic psychotherapy usually is not appropriate for short inpatient stays because patients need more time to achieve depth in their internal processes. Therefore, they use an adapted method they called "theme-centralized interaction" but stressed that it is important for the group leader to have good psychological insight in order to understand and guide the group process.

Mittag and Ohm (1987) explained the contents of the four group sessions and used case reports to illustrate. In the first session, the group explored the patients' status following the heart attack, appropriate expectations for rehabilitation, and the psychological intervention methods to be used in the group. The second session was devoted to exploration of Type A behavior (e.g., controlling ambitions) and internal and external stress factors. In the third session, group leaders discussed strategies for dealing with pressure, providing concrete examples. In the fourth and final session, leaders helped patients prepare to return to their families and jobs (see also Esser, 1987).

Mittag and Ohm (1987) described how dealing with difficult patients (e.g., those showing resistance, trivialization, or lack of concrete insight) caused personal problems for them as therapists (see Ohm, 1987, and Hübel & Kauderer-Hübel, 1987, for relaxation and hypnosis techniques and D. Lehr, 1996, for hypnotherapy techniques). In their conclusion the authors called for more attention throughout the clinic to the psychological side of the illness and for more peace and quiet in the rehabilitation center.

2.6.2.3. Poststationary setting. In some countries, after the acute cardiological treatment, an in-patient rehabilitation follows. *Poststationary therapy* is the outpatient psychotherapy that follows acute or rehabilitative therapy. There are few publications describing poststationary psychological rehabilitation. In an early intervention study by Adsett and Bruhn (1968), which can be considered classic and is often quoted, the psychodynamic orientation remains unclear. The authors developed a therapeutic treatment that offers interesting possibilities but unfortunately has not been copied or systematically researched. They led groups for couples, treating ill men and their wives in separate groups for approximately 10 sessions. The authors described the group process and main themes in more detail than is usual in the literature. They observed that the sick men participated more fully in the group process than their wives, who were reserved and did not work together as a group. The patient group developed a warm, trusting climate and talked about their feelings of shame, dependency, and inferiority. One point stood out in particular: The men did not want to go into depth about their relationships with their partners because they were scared of their partners' dominance and control. In the wives' group, themes of guilt (regarding the husband's heart attack), worries about the course of the illness, and overprotectiveness played a major role.

Adsett and Bruhn (1968) named their intervention model after Piers (Piers & Singer, 1953); it involves a "circular model of psychodynamic interaction with alternating periods of activity and reaction" (Adsett & Bruhn, 1968, p. 583). They identified a vicious circle in their therapeutic experiences that patients must work on: Aggressive impulses cause feelings of guilt and fear, which are followed by the fear of being passively dependent. The feeling of being dependent is shameful, and this shame causes negative aggression, once again setting off the vicious circle. According to the authors, psychotherapeutic interventions must be adapted to the various medical treatment phases. Individual treatment in the acute phase can help prepare patients for the group therapy treatment, and long-term effects are best achieved in a setting that enables further treatment immediately following the first rehabilitation stage.

Hahn (1968a) was the first author to describe group therapy using the psychodynamic model. His description is remarkably applicable to the problems of psychodynamic psychotherapy in the present-day medical milieu. He noted that it was very difficult to motivate coronary patients to take part in long-term group therapy. A considerable change in motivation was achieved only after the settings had been rearranged; the group therapy was placed just after the heparin therapy, meaning that the patients had to travel only once for both treatments. Hahn describes the therapy he conducted with two groups of 13 members each that were merged after a lengthy period. His publications differ from a lot of other psychodynamic publications in that he presents very careful descriptions of the randomized samples and specific medical data of the treated patients (Deter, Hahn, & Petzold, 1987; Hahn, 1968a, 1968b, 1969, 1988; Hahn & Hüllemann, 1972).

Titscher and Göbel-Bohrn (1988) described an outpatient group therapy intervention conducted over 15 sessions. Their work shows how important it is to integrate such interventions into cardiological care and how influential such interventions can be on the progression of the disease. The first author was a cardiologist with additional psychotherapy qualifications, and the intervention was described as being a regular part of treatment and not as a secondary effort. The authors described the treatment to potential participants not as group therapy, but as a "discussion group" for exchanging views and experiences. This approach resulted in 33 of 40 patients accepting the offer, but the dropout rate reached 50% over the course of therapy, a clear indication of how difficult it is to obtain patient participation. The authors found that a strict analytical group therapy intervention technique was not appropriate and that the information approach worked much better when the leader integrated his psychodynamic understanding of the events. The authors provided a brief description of the developing group process; they reported that the participants had a strong fixation on the male group leader (there was a female coleader) and did not have much contact among themselves. In their description, the idealization of the father figure

(especially the authority of the doctors) stands out, but this seems a reflection not of the persons involved but rather of the system and institution.

2.6.3. Expert Reports

In this section we describe publications by authors who have had long clinical experience in the psychotherapeutic treatment of coronary patients, regardless of whether they provide detailed case reports. Such perspectives are of great importance for clinical work.

One publication that is remarkable from a clinical point of view is that of Freund (1987). It is very detailed and draws on the author's long years of experience with techniques and problems in group therapy treatment of coronary patients in a rehabilitation clinic. Because it is a unique work, we provide a more detailed summary. Drawing on Milton H. Erickson's psychodynamic hypnotherapy (see Erickson, Rossi, & Rossi, 1976), Freund considered it unwise to break patients' resistance, because the resistance of coronary patients holds productive life energy with which, paradoxically, they connect with themselves therapeutically. Attempting to break the patient's resistance may make it stronger and could lead to an extremely aversive reaction (e.g., continuing smoking, no changes in lifestyle, noncompliance), which has often been reported in the literature:

> Denying the illness means that the patient wants to be everything else, just not ill. And this fear of illness is the energy that helps him recover. . . . I have learned that it expends my own energy to consider the patient's resistance as senseless. I had to stop myself from trying to do anything about this denying resistance. It is not the patient who resists the illness, but the therapist who shows resistance against what the patient feels. (p. 89)

Freund believed that a heart attack patient is the opposite of the "classic psychotherapy patient" and that therefore "classic psychotherapy treatment" methods will fail. He emphasized that the heart attack patient has a psychological problem that has been induced through unconscious physical events.

The patient tries to attach some kind of significance to the noncontrollable physical developments, and trying to get this explanation under control plays a central strategic role. The usual psychotherapy schools, with their special professionalization, do not take into account the special physical themes. Freund observed, "I rather think you can be more helpful to the heart attack patient if you do the opposite of what you learned to be correct. This is the basic experience: to accept the paradox as a method" (p. 89).

In a sensitive way, Freund (1987) developed strategies based on his observations of typical psychological features in the population of heart attack patients. He thus developed a specific concept of psychotherapeutic resistance analysis: that patient resistance should not be broken (as conceptualized in psychotherapeutic norms) but rather the opposite—that the strength of resistance should be used in healing.

Klasmeier (1991), a clinical psychologist, reported on her experiences in a rehabilitation clinic. She described her discoveries regarding unconscious institutional defense mechanisms in interactions between medical personnel and patients. First, she emphasized a conflict in interdisciplinary cooperation between cardiology and psychology: Medical diagnostics and therapy assist in patients' striving for omnipotence, expressed through power, influence, control, and security. Psychological treatment must work on these personality traits, and this is difficult to do if the traits are reinforced by cardiologists (p. 278). A special transference–countertransference constellation is found within the staff: Cardiologists represent optimistic and active coping (striving for omnipotence), and psychotherapists are responsible for the corresponding defended feelings of fear, helplessness and hopelessness, despair, and so forth:

> From the beginning the psychotherapist in the cardiac rehabilitation clinic is confronted with patients' inferiority complexes and compensatory omnipotence fantasies. Again and again, the psychotherapist reaches, in different ways, the boundaries of his or her psychotherapeutic influences. (p. 280)

Klasmeier (1991) warned about transferring the medical model to psychotherapeutic work. Because such an implementation can involve only imposing highly structured learning programs for changing the standard risk factors, patients' feelings of desertion, destruction, and especially fear are neglected. The difficulties Klasmeier encountered in addressing these experiences, which for her was the central goal of psychotherapeutic work connected to specific treatment methods, are similar to those described by Chessick (1977, 1987a, 1987b) and Marshall (1965). One problem is that psychotherapists start to reject, hate, and distance themselves from patients, because therapists feel that patients are inferior and nothing can be done for them. Many patients with CHD will configure the psychotherapeutic relationship according to their lifestyle (achievement oriented, readiness to achieve), which means that they try to be good patients, and they manage the therapeutic relationship on the principle "through performance to love" (p. 282).

Therapists often feel inadequate, helpless, and powerless, and Klasmeier (1991) pointed out that they may tend to reactively devalue the patient and draw back from him or her in a typical countertransference constellation. She asserted that the therapist must understand this feeling of countertransference as a reflection of the patient's inner psychological state and use this in the therapeutic work. She provided some case examples from individual and group therapy discussions.

Klasmeier (1991) addressed the finding often reported in the literature that cardiac patients experience explosive outbreaks of aggression and strong feelings of anger. She interpreted the explosiveness and patients' violent, aggressive, rationalized, trivial, devaluing, intellectual, omnipotent, and disowning expressions as a reflection of their trial in coming to terms with their fears of destruction, disownment, and possible death:

> Especially in group therapy, I have often witnessed how vague feelings of "not being understood" set off dissatisfaction and anger in the patient, made worse by a "conspiracy" among each other. These reactions can lead the

therapist to feel betrayed and destroyed. (p. 283)

A crucial and stressful problem for the therapist is to allow these situations to unfold, understand them, and try to reframe them for patients in such a way that they can be discussed. Klasmeier observed,

> I noticed how hard I was trying to find an answer, how hard I tried to offer them something, to give them hope. Their increasing contempt made me feel faint and incompetent. With this contempt and devaluation, the patients defended themselves against the helplessness of being left alone. . . . When I was able to talk about how lonely and abandoned they must feel because of their illness . . . the atmosphere in the group changed from contemptuousness to a mood of dismay and sadness. This showed me that the patients felt accepted and understood. The feeling of human destiny and suffering, which we all felt, became clear, and I as the therapist no longer shut myself out of it. (p. 284)

Klasmeier's work provides an example of how the analysis of countertransference can help therapists in their work with coronary patients. She also demonstrated the importance of (unconscious) institutional conditions and medical staff interactions.

Allan and Scheidt (1996, 1998) reported in two publications about their experiences and conclusions from outpatient group therapy with cardiac patients. Allan was a registered doctor of clinical psychology, and Scheidt was a cardiologist at the New York Presbyterian Hospital; the articles were published by both, but Allan led the group alone. For 15 years, Allan offered half-open outpatient groups (i.e., groups in which membership is open to new patients as old patients leave the group, in contrast with closed groups, in which all members begin and end treatment together) for cardiac patients. Allan used multimethod (psychodynamic and what he termed "eclecticistic") techniques oriented toward interventions for changing Type A behavior (Recurrent Coronary Prevention Project).

His major focus was on working with anger and anger modulation.

In the section on group atmosphere, Allan and Scheidt (1998) posited that each session should be lively and educational and have a liberal atmosphere. Every individual should have enough time to get involved, which should motivate participants to come to the next session. The therapist must ensure that interactions within the group do not become excessively aggressive; the authors noted that outbreaks of anger can be important but that they should not get out of hand. Allen coped with outbreaks of aggression by suggesting to the person that they talk one on one about this topic and that afterward, when things had cooled down, they discuss it in the group. The authors considered it fundamental to remind the patients that anger is bad for heart illnesses and that patients should ask themselves if getting angry is worth risking their health (see L. H. Powell, 1996).

Allan and Scheidt (1996) included a section on countertransference. They believed that fear of death, a subject of great significance for patients who have survived sudden death, is involved in a fundamental countertransference therapists experience in work with this group. They emphasized that such an experience can cause a posttraumatic stress reaction and that the therapist must acknowledge patients' fear of death in order to motivate patients to change their way of life.

The second fundamental countertransference they identified is connected to anger. It is essential that the therapist be able to cope with anger and aggression. The most important technical advice is that therapists never allow themselves to get involved in angry or aggressive discussions (see Powell, 1996, p. 313). The authors explicitly recommended remaining silent as being very helpful. Therapists must be able to lead feelings of anger into a productive dialogue and prevent these feelings from taking an excessively affective form. This report describes many typical problematic relationship constellations frequently encountered in heart patient groups; unfortunately, experiences with typical psychodynamic conflict–defense configurations have received sparse empirical and theoretical analysis.

Jordan et al. (1997) reached similar conclusions in an analysis of prevailing institutional conditions involved with PTCA. These findings paralleled, without being influenced by, those of Allan and Scheidt (1996, 1998), which were published contemporaneously, and Klasmeier (1991), who published in German. On the basis of clinical experience, scientific research, and theory, Jordan et al. described how patients are influenced by the technical possibilities of medical diagnostics and therapy in the given institution, their past experiences, their subjective theory about their illness, and their psychological processes. Medical procedures and staff cause a lasting somatic fixation because patients' fears and feelings of uncertainty are defended through optimistic attitudes about the power and effectiveness of technology.

Technical improvements and the joining of diagnostics (angiography) and therapy (PTCA) into a single procedure creates a dense situation from the psychological point of view: Positive dilatation results lead to a trivialization or minimization of the severity of the underlying illness (CHD). Most patients do not dwell on the facts that the intervention only relieves the symptoms, that the reason for the illness (atherosclerosis) is not treated, and that a relapse or shortened life expectancy can be warded off only by changing one's habits and not by undergoing the PTCA. The "rapid recovery" possible with the aid of technical advances may lead patients to dismiss their fear of death. This trivialization causes the patient to place responsibility for his or her recovery elsewhere (e.g., "I do not have to do anything but take my pills"; "I just have to find a good cardiologist who will do everything for me"). Such a reaction may lead patients to do less to reduce risks.

This is how patients conjure wonderful feelings, fantasies about miracles, unrealistic beliefs in technology, and minimizing cognitions (e.g., "It was only a short stenosis"; "Only about 80% of the artery was blocked"). Patients are discharged quickly and almost immediately resume everyday life. If they have a restenosis, the intervention can be done again. Subjectively, this results in an unrealistic feeling of being healthy, especially in patients who had no MI before and no cardiac symptoms after the intervention.

Like Klasmeier (1991), Bastiaans (1968, 1982) published articles about psychotherapeutic intervention techniques with patients who have had traumatic conflicts and experiences. Drawing from his personal experience treating these patients and supervising treatment teams, he described a frequent countertransference whereby psychotherapists and doctors, in response to specific personality and defense mechanisms of patients, feel pressure to become overactive. In response to patients' inability to relax and wait, professionals may find themselves feeling that they have to do everything immediately for the patient.

M. Barth and Sender (1991) described an individual case using the biographical reconstruction method ("objective hermeneutics," in accordance with Oevermann, Allert, Konau, & Krambeck, 1979). We present this work because it concentrated on specific institutional setting conditions that decisively moderated the course of treatment and results, although the article gave higher priority to the inpatient rehabilitation routine than the patient's biographical background and current situation. The patient had the conflicts and personality characteristics that, since Dunbar, have been regularly described as being typical for coronary patients. He had a narcissistic and disturbed way of dealing with aggression as well as extreme conflicts with authoritative persons at work. This cycle produced a chronic stress situation noticeably connected with his cardiovascular illnesses. The patient was treated in an inpatient rehabilitation center, which acted as an artificial benign climate, for the purpose of reducing only risk factors. This strategy succeeded in reducing the patient's stress indicators; thus, according to the official definition, this heart patient was rehabilitated and returned to normal working life. The authors speculated that when the patient went back to work he would probably have another heart attack if he did not take part in outpatient psychotherapeutic treatment to enable him to find ways of coping with his conflicts with authority and aggression.

Hummel (1992) developed an illness- and body-oriented psychological conceptualization for heart patients in his book *Heart Language: A Psychoanalysis of the Heart*. This book was based on his long experience providing psychodynamic treatment to heart attack patients (and cardiac sport groups). A doctor and psychotherapist, Hummel sharply criticized both professions. Hummel saw the main task of psychotherapeutic care of these patients as helping them use symbolic–psychological language. He gave reasons for the extensive definition nomenclature from Jacques Lacan and ultimately arrived at simple autogenic training.

Cunningham, Strassberg, and Roback (1978) reported on 11 emotionally important factors in group therapy. These factors refer to Yalom's work (Yalom, 1975) and are specifically adapted for cardiac rehabilitation.

Poettgen (1981) described an intervention combining supportive discussions with psychodynamic psychotherapy. Psychodramatic role-playing was sometimes used in dealing with conflictual situations, and this process was then later discussed in the group.

Garamoni and Schwartz (1986) focused on treatment for coronary patients with Type A behavior patterns or obsessive structures. The authors argued for an integration of cognitive–behavioral therapy and psychodynamic approaches, which they saw as complementary, as a way of enhancing treatment. In this type of patient, therapy typically focuses on conflicts produced by the fear of losing control. Psychodynamic-oriented approaches offer the possibility of concentrating on the internal control mechanism with the goal of "feelings management." Behavioral approaches, conversely, address the external control conditions and therefore focus on "situational management." A characteristic aspect of the transference relationship is that patients judge positive reinforcement for compliance as a criticism of their earlier way of life or as an exhortation to make bigger efforts to modify their Type A behavior. Consequently, the patient, who at first idealizes the therapist, comes to see him or her as threatening. If the therapist ignores these transference and resistance phenomena, therapy may develop into a tug-of-war over control, further provoking Type A behavior patterns.

Singer (1987) reported about experiences in group treatment of patients and their partners after a heart attack. This treatment addressed the patients' Type A behavior, especially the mechanisms of denial and rationalization. The author described the infarct as being a traumatic experience, and the outpatient group therapy was intended to help patients come to terms with their emotional experience. In this hospital, every patient received information sheets and was told about the group and about its goals and benefits. Individual discussions were held with the patient and his or her partner before they took part in the group (a nurse coordinated and was coleader of the group). Singer noted his surprise at how reserved patients were with their partners, and he wondered what kind of psychological stress brought on such reactions. He sensitively and differentially described the emotional problems, inner conflicts, and defense mechanisms of these patients and their families.

2.6.4. Summary of Psychodynamic Treatment Reports

Our review of the literature on the psychodynamic treatment of patients with CHD sheds light on the controversial question of whether this treatment is beneficial. The skepticism often expressed by researchers and psychotherapists (see, e.g., Gildea, 1949; Herzog, 1984; Herzog, König, Maas, & Neufert, 1982; Moersch et al., 1980) can be relativized or even partly repudiated; the publications reviewed in this chapter clearly show that some groups of coronary patients can be successfully treated. The case reports show that patients experience and psychologically process a heart attack in different ways depending on differences in their fantasies and the contexts of the infarct: The patient may experience the heart attack as a relief and liberation from unending continuous stress; alternatively, he or she may experience the infarct as a total narcissistic defeat ("castration") or as a traumatic trigger of powerful and unexpected feelings about disappointments. Together, these publications show how informative and worthwhile work with coronary patients is. The intervention methods described in the literature were helpful for the patients, and positive treatment effects were achieved. These findings legitimize further studies.

The weak point of the case reports is their almost complete lack of connection: They neither work with each other nor stand alone. The case reports do not permit comparative analysis, but they do provide a picture of psychoanalytical scientific history; through these studies, research in the area of psychoanalytical knowledge of coronary illnesses has become less important. In the future, psychoanalytic methods can be used to inform studies that build on one another, are built on current knowledge about CHD, and are connected to operationalized hypotheses that allow replication.

The few existing intervention studies on the effects of psychodynamic treatment for CHD patients are outdated and have significant shortcomings. The lack of detail in the descriptions of treatment protocols is an important flaw in the scientific literature in this area; without detailed descriptions, it is not possible to do similar studies.

2.7. CRITICAL REMARKS ON THE PSYCHODYNAMIC LITERATURE ON CORONARY HEART DISEASE

Since about 1936, researchers have written about psychodynamic hypotheses regarding CHD. After a creative and original first phase of research, various groups published systematic psychodynamic research results, primarily from 1940 until 1970. Thereafter, little research was conducted, and since 1980 almost none at all has been done. The last psychodynamic publication was an unsystematic review by O'Neill (2000) of the psychodynamic treatment of patients with CHD in a book on psychodynamic perspectives on health and sickness in general.

Between 1940 and 1970, systematic work was done in many different places in the world, and the formulation of theoretical models on the etiology of CHD was influenced by psychodynamic findings and hypotheses. Various theoretical concepts on the psychological specificity of illnesses dominated the scientific discussion. Our review shows that models concerning CHD, as would be expected, were adapted to the prevailing psychodynamic theory development of the time. During the first phase, existing knowledge was described from the perspective of drive theory. In the next phase, ego-psychological reflections were based on the current thinking in terms of object relations and later narcissism theory. After a specific coronary-prone personality was formulated, theoretical concepts were

developed that focused on specific conflicts behind coronary-prone behavior.

In all of these phases of psychodynamic research, researchers used an implicit hypothesis: that etiological knowledge could be gained using retrospective studies with small samples. As evidenced by concepts concerning psychological specificity, researchers additionally assumed that specific intrapsychological conflicts, which they evaluated in investigations and in the course of psychotherapy with infarct patients, provided evidence relevant to all patients with this illness. They often minimized the problem of generalizability (Jordan, 1999). Very few psychodynamic researchers reflected on this question systematically, as Flanders Dunbar did. She examined large samples of patients with different diseases using the same categorization, and she also included control groups. In addition, almost all psychodynamic publications (exceptions include Dunbar, 1943; Hahn, 1971; and Wardwell et al., 1963) have been weak in their postulating argumentation and have lacked provable empirical evidence. Psychodynamic authors typically postulated that there is a connection between the occurrence of specific conflicts (which are evaluated after the onset of disease) and the etiology of CHD, but they did not consider the possible and appropriate psychosomatic mechanisms.

The psychodynamic study by Moersch et al. (1980) is paradigmatic for the deficiencies that can be found in most psychodynamic publications of the last six decades. This study, and the literature in general, show at least four limitations:

1. *Lack of attention to previously published research.* The authors of a majority of psychodynamic publications failed to review and incorporate the existing research literature (including the psychodynamic, as well as psychological, sociological, and epidemiological, empirical literatures). For example, Moersch et al. (1980) should have reviewed the systematic study designs of Dunbar (1943) and Hahn (1971) and undertaken a replication of the results with their own sample. Instead, their analysis was laid out as if there had never been any research conducted on

cardiac infarct patients, and their study design and presentation of results thus are difficult to interpret in the context of existing psychodynamic knowledge.

2. *Lack of detail in the description of samples.* Psychodynamic researchers frequently failed to describe in sufficient detail how they selected patients for their treatment and control samples, as well as the selection effects and dropout rates. Also missing from their descriptions were sociodemographic characteristics and relevant medical data of their intervention samples.

3. *Exclusion of subgroups from analyses.* Many publications excluded patients who did not fit the main line of interpretation from further evaluation and presentation. Few authors explicitly recognized that they had done this (e.g., Arlow, 1945). Moersch et al. (1980) also paid little attention to subgroups; for example, despite calls in the literature for a gender-specific point of view, they did not report separately on the women they examined. The literature as a whole omitted analysis of subgroups such as social class, age, and ethnic origin.

4. *Lack of systematic analysis of results on the background of literature.* The insufficiency in differential evaluation and presentation also applies to the systematic analysis of results. Most investigations evaluated only a small selection of existing psychodynamic hypotheses, and this led to a reduced analysis of their own empirical data. For example, Moersch et al. (1980) concentrated mainly on "classic" psychodynamic topics. Other aspects described in previous literature (e.g., relationship with the father, psychoeconomic function of work, trigger situations, narcissistic deficits, depression, obsessive–compulsive characteristics) are ignored in favor of one main thesis. The existing empirical material of many studies would have enabled the authors to analyze more than one variable. However, this often was not done, because their interest was to specifically concentrate on one question, and existing literature was not used to formulate different questions for the same material. This makes comparison difficult and also hinders scientific progress.

These criticisms of psychodynamic research are not an argument for disregarding this research or excluding psychodynamic thinking from the scientific discourse. As we sought to show in this chapter, a scientifically important corpus of hypotheses can be derived from these publications. However, the critical, comprehensive, and systematic conduct and description of investigations is a basic prerequisite for further research. Thus, we hope that our chapter will contribute to the development of higher methodological standards in psychodynamic research.

The psychodynamic literature can be meaningful in two different regards. First, it can inform clinical work by providing a cognitive structure that is helpful to the process of psychotherapy. Second, psychodynamic research contributes additional interpretations of empirical findings and thus produces new hypotheses for future research. Despite the methodological deficits, psychodynamic publications have shown many points of agreement and overlapping hypotheses, including striving, depression, the role of anxiety, narcissistic imbalance, vital exhaustion, denial, and many others. In the following paragraphs we review some of these themes in further detail.

At the beginning of psychodynamic research (drive theory), the early childhood relationship models were the reference for dynamic hypotheses. Therefore, male infarct patients were seen as having, for different reasons, an incomplete or conflictual identification pattern connected to their fathers that led to a set of risk-increasing behaviors. Many different attachment patterns were cited as playing a role in the various intrapsychic conflicts, including a high ego-ideal conception, anxiety, mood, disturbed self-regulation, or a permanent inner drive to stabilize narcissistic needs. Because of their father relationships, these patients developed fragile behavior patterns that led to a chronic imbalance in regard to narcissistic regulation. Their characteristics included chronic overexertion, abnormal ambition, a high validation of professional work, and ambitious behavior in all areas of life.

Authors who have discussed the psychodynamic role of the workplace have cited different motivations as contributing to the fact that the patients chronically abused professional work, from the psychoeconomic point of view, in order to compensate for and hide deficiencies. From this followed highly ambitious striving, an ambivalent or disturbed relationship to authorities, and an irrational loss of energy. Chronic exertion (vital exhaustion) emerged, as well as behaviors intended to increase productivity (e.g., smoking, caffeine abuse, lack of activity, bad nutrition), leading in consequence to CHD. Substantial disappointments ("catastrophic ruin"; Dunbar, 1943) and feelings of deep personal defeat were cited as leading to an infarct, especially if the heart was already unstable and damaged.

Psychodynamic hypotheses regarding the psychoeconomic abuse or (dys)function of work are consistent with the sociological research (e.g., exertion model, demand–control model, gratification–crisis model) and with social–psychological concepts (e.g., Type A behavior, distressed personality, vital exhaustion, depression). These connections point to future perspectives for psychodynamic studies.

Frequently CHD patients are described as having personalities that are impaired because of early disturbances in their development of primary narcissistic self-regulation. Therefore, these patients are impaired by a deficit that makes them extremely vulnerable but that also helps them develop specific compensatory patterns and defense mechanisms. Nearly every publication or case report has emphasized patients' extraordinary overvaluation of striving behavior that seeks to guarantee present and future success and produces a chronic narcissistic gratification (de Dowiakowski & Luminet, 1969; Defontaine-Catteau, Pedinielle, & Bertagne, 1992; Luminet, 1969). Thus, through striving, patients raise their basal low narcissistic level of self-regulation.

These publications described a specific pattern of object relations that also has the function of stabilizing weakened narcissistic self-regulation. These patterns involve self–object relationships: The other person has a mirror-image function; by providing constant appreciation and uninterrupted presence, the other guarantees a basic existential acknowledgment and security. This pattern explains a phenomenon that is repeatedly described in studies as typical for infarct patients: These patients often are easily offended, and experiences of separation, loss, and failure become catastrophic, life-threatening, and total-ruin experiences. They react to such situations with either rage and explosive aggression or depression and vital exhaustion. Coronary events are connected both with a more or less explicitly deficient expression of aggression that they are unable to symbolize and with emotional experiences of depression and exhaustion. Dreyfuss et al. (1969) even went so far as to presume that depression and even a latent suicidal tendency are an etiological component of the development of a heart attack. These publications commonly make reference to social–psychological studies (on, e.g., hostility, anger-in and anger-out, Type A and Type D behavior).

Case studies describe how conditions of aggressive (destructive) and depressive experiences caused by relevant narcissistic losses and shame can be warded off and brought back under control through different compulsive defense mechanisms. The most common compulsive mechanism is highly ambitious and narcissistically charged work-related behavior. There is evidence of a cyclic recurring process: Narcissistic deregulation (loss, failure, mortification, anger, or depression) leads to a compulsive defense mechanism through increased productivity. Such a maladaptive cycle is then repeated over decades, leading to typical lifestyle risk factors. In consequence, a coronary event occurs when the ego is weakened and can no longer defend and control the narcissistic crises.

On the basis of that theoretical background, authors have formulated models explaining specific trigger situations. Psychodynamically oriented authors have described the potential traumatic causes of an infarct, concluding that narcissistic imbalances, depression, and other affects immediately before or after the infarction can be reconstructed from biographical information.

2.7.1. Construct of Depression
Since 1925, the literature repeatedly has claimed a correlation between clinically relevant signs of depression and the course of CHD. It seems certain

that depression is a predictive variable for the development and progress of CHD (see Herrmann-Lingen & Buss, chap. 5, this volume; see also Ladwig, Erazo, & Rugulies, 2003; Wulsin & Singal, 2003). Taking a historical view, it is interesting that many clinically oriented authors who were very observant described and reflected this correlation at a time when empirical data were not available, and the first systematic studies of psychosocial factors in CHD attributed importance to the dimension of depression (Arlow, 1945; Menninger & Menninger, 1936; H. Williams, 1950). The close relationship between compulsive symptoms and depression, which is very important in psychodynamic considerations, was not described until many years later, but Dunbar (1936) emphasized compulsive perfectionism in cardiac patients early on. Menninger and Menninger (1936), as well as Hübschmann (1966), Seemann (1964), and Aresin (1960), also referred to the significance of obsessive characteristics in connection with depression.

As far as we know, Hahn (1971) provided the most detailed reconstruction of the psychodynamic problem of depression:

> A further possible interpretation is a psychoetiological understanding of compulsive behavior. The specific defense of conflict perceptions by obsessive mechanisms assumes a previous and processed compensated depression. . . . The obsessive mechanisms therefore serve as a psychological defense against earlier unsolved underlying depressive ambivalence conflicts. In contrast to the neurotic development, these defense mechanisms are fixed attitudes (integrated in the personality structure) which are experienced only in their appearing consequences and not during psychological conflict situations. This denial of the inner reality causes a reinforced orientation on the perceptible outside reality and actually enables a healthy adjustment for a long period. (p. 79)

Hahn believed that a basic depressive conflict underlies a defense by compulsive mechanisms. In accordance with the analytical mode of thinking at that time, the obsessive structures serve to prevent a regression to an "oral fixation." Intensive stressors or psychological destabilization lead to decreasing defense mechanisms, which cause depressive symptoms. The depression defense is psychogenetically connected with the father image: The father, as an unreachable model, forms part of the ego ideal. The individual feels that he or she can never surpass the father, but he or she would like one day at least to be praised and accepted by him.

In this context, Hahn (1971) interpreted the enormous motivation of CHD patients to work hard and their tendency to easily be offended at work. Hahn pointed out that underlying depression makes it enormously difficult to find a psychotherapeutic path with these patients, because the depression must be constantly defended and minimized. Many psychodynamically oriented authors came to similar conclusions (Appels, 1979; Chessick, 1977, 1987a, 1987b; Dreyfuss, 1953; Dreyfuss et al., 1969; Dreyfuss, Shanan, & Sharon, 1966; Faller, 1989; Klasmeier, 1991; Rogner et al., 1994; Stephanos, 1982a, 1982b; H. Williams, 1950).

An important difficulty in the literature concerning depression and CHD is the differing and contradictory uses of the term *depression*. For example, some authors speak of a "depressive conflict," a "vital depression," or a "depressive feeling" to refer to both a clinical diagnosis of depression and symptoms or feelings of mourning and self-doubt. The "defense of depression" is discussed again and again but is never comprehensively explained.

2.7.2. Construct of Denial

Numerous psychodynamic publications emphasized the importance of depressive symptoms after the outbreak of CHD. These publications gave special attention to the acute phase and drew a connection between the constructs of depression and denial. Köhle et al. (1996) concluded that about 58% of their sample of acute-phase coronary patients showed depressive symptoms (see also Herrmann-Lingen & Buss, chap. 5, this volume).

They saw these symptoms as understandable and appropriate reactions to the illness and the blow to patients' self-confidence.

Psychodynamic authors, more than authors with other theoretical orientations, interpret depression after the infarct not only as a normative coping mechanism but also as a consequence of psychological processes already in place at the onset of the infarct. Patients' personality styles make it difficult for them to accept the loss of confidence in their bodily functions that results from the MI. The reality of the illness confirms their unconscious conflictual uncertainty and lack of self-confidence. According to this hypothesis, any illness can trigger the mobilization of deep repressed unconscious conflicts, but patients with coronary heart disease experience these psychological disturbances more acutely because of the severity of the illness and the vulnerability of their backgrounds. The threatening life event (infarction) brings to the fore topics such as loss of autonomy, professional degradation and financial problems, loss of status, and requirements for lifestyle changes, all of which cause a deep mourning process that can produce an intensive defense over years.

In some publications, the phenomenon of denial has been discussed in the context of the psychotherapeutic treatment of depression. Early psychodynamic research explored the phenomenon of denial and its development in the course of CHD. Hackett and Cassem were among the first to examine under what circumstances denial has a protective (adaptive) or a maladaptive and dangerous function in CHD (Cassem & Hackett, 1971; Froese, Hackett, Cassem, & Silverberg, 1974; Froese, Vasquez, Cassem, & Hackett, 1974; Hackett & Cassem, 1970, 1974; Hackett, Cassem, & Wishnie, 1968; Stern, Caplan, & Cassem, 1987; Wishnie, Hackett, & Cassem, 1971).

In recent decades, many authors have emphasized the importance of denial in the course of disease (Breitkopf, 1983; Cameron, 1989; Dimsdale & Hackett, 1982; Esteve, Valdez, Riesco, & Jodar, 1992; Fassbender et al., 1984; Janne, Reynaert, & Cassiers, 1990; Soloff, 1978; Trijsburg, 1989; Valk & Groen, 1967), but they have used the term in various ways. Furthermore, some authors have used the term but have not connected it with psychodynamic thinking; thus, denial has been mostly described as a mechanism to avoid the experience of depression and anxiety. Often *denial* is used imprecisely to describe other defense mechanisms such as minimizing, intellectualization, and splitting.

Early in this recent period, Breitkopf (1983) pointed out that the term *denial* describes an unconscious phenomenon that is very difficult to study because it is not directly detectable or measurable. Identification of denial is always embedded in social interactions; because denial is an intrapsychic and unconscious process, an observer is required to state that someone is in denial. Therefore, the perspective of the person who is in denial is very important to obtain. For example, a physician or researcher may state in a specific situation that a patient is in denial because the patient does not show the feelings the physician or researcher views as adequate. Thus, researchers frequently interpret an absence of anxiety as denial, without further description of the construct or the symptom. Esteve et al. (1992) found denial processes in only 20% to 22% of the examined cases. Examination of denial processes can also lead to prognostic hypotheses; Trijsburg et al. (1987) found that men who showed symptoms of denial at the time of their infarction complained of more somatic symptoms 6 months after the first examination.

Chapter 3

SMOKING CESSATION IN PATIENTS WITH CORONARY HEART DISEASE: RISK REDUCTION AND AN EVALUATION OF THE EFFICACY OF INTERVENTIONS

Jürgen Barth and Jürgen Bengel

3.1. INTRODUCTION

In this chapter, we examine, evaluate, and integrate primary studies on interventions to promote smoking cessation in patients with coronary heart disease (CHD). The aim of this chapter is not to formulate guidelines, which would require consensual decisions from professional associations (see, e.g., U.S. Department of Health and Human Services, 2000). We also have avoided evaluating interventions from a health care economic perspective, which would require a thorough cost–benefit analysis (see, e.g., Barendregt, Bonneux, & Maas, 1997; Lightwood & Glantz, 1997).

We examined primary studies for answers to the following four questions:

1. What is the influence of smoking as a risk factor for CHD? Which specific diseases show a high incidence, and which treatment approaches are most frequently indicated?
2. What is the effect on morbidity and mortality of abstinence from tobacco use after a cardiac event?
3. Which methods for promoting smoking cessation have been proved effective?
4. What percentage of patients stop smoking after a cardiac event? Is it necessary to offer additional specific interventions to encourage patients with CHD to stop smoking, or is the standard care enough? Is it possible to transfer successful smoking cessation strategies from patients without somatic illnesses to CHD patients?

3.2. METHOD

We used both key words and free text in the literature search for this review. We searched three databases: PSYNDEX, PsycINFO, and Medline (it was not financially viable to use the Embase database). We also performed a free text search in the Cochrane Library's CCTR database in April of 2000 (a detailed description of the literature search is found in Appendix W3A on the accompanying Web site; see http://www.apa.org/books/resources/jordan/). The key word search mainly identified studies on the effect on cardiac patients of smoking cessation, whereas the free text search mainly brought up publications with an epidemiological emphasis and unspecified intervention methods for cardiac patients. We limited the search to works published between 1985 and 2000. We identified older studies with the help of available reviews and bibliographies from newer publications and more recent studies by publishing alerts in relevant journals.

3.2.1. Selection of Relevant Studies

To answer our two epidemiological questions (Questions 1 and 2), we chose studies with the following characteristics: They had a prospective design, assessed smoking status at the beginning of the survey, and recorded relevant endpoints (e.g., morbidity and mortality from CHD). For Question 1, we used studies with large samples (>1,000 for each group). For Question 2, we also included studies with smaller samples. To answer Question 3, we chose reviews from the Cochrane

Library that analyzed the effect on abstinence from tobacco use of a specific intervention and that provided a sufficient base of empirical data (>5 randomized controlled trials) to evaluate the intervention. To answer Question 4, we chose randomized intervention studies that differentiated at least one intervention group and one control group (or an intervention group with an alternative treatment method) and that assessed efficacy in an appropriate follow-up period (>6 months).[1] We also examined studies with a pre–post design when they contributed to an understanding of the process of smoking cessation or the influence of moderators (see also chap. 6, this volume). Studies that were excluded are listed in Appendix W3B on the Web site (compare Tables W3B.1 and W3B.2).

We chose 26 of the studies we identified through our search to answer the epidemiological questions (some of the studies were by the same groups of authors). We based our assessment of the efficacy of measures to promote smoking cessation (Question 3) on nine reviews from the Cochrane Library. We used 22 studies for the meta-analysis of the efficacy of measures to promote smoking cessation among patients with CHD (Question 4).

3.2.2. Independent Variables

Epidemiological studies reported both bivariate correlations between smoking and morbidity and mortality and adjusted correlations that controled for other risk factors. Because no adjusted analyses with control variables for all studies had previously been performed (e.g., age, gender, other risk factors), we calculated bivariate correlations for this chapter. If the study specified whether a subject had never smoked, was a former smoker, or was a current smoker, we compared the never-smoked group with the current-smoker group (implying a tendency to overrate the effect of smoking on CHD). Studies that distinguished only between smokers and nonsmokers usually assigned former smokers to the nonsmoker group (implying a conservative assessment of the effect of smoking on CHD). Some epidemiological studies used the

number of cigarettes smoked per day as a criterion to differentiate the effect of smoking on CHD using subgroup analysis (e.g., of low, medium, and high consumption). The present review uses only a dichotomized analysis—smokers versus nonsmokers. We assessed the efficacy of smoking cessation methods by comparing the "best possible" intervention (related to the hypothesis of the authors) with the normal intervention ("standard care").

3.2.3. Dependent Variables

We analyzed the dependent variables of morbidity and mortality for the first two epidemiological questions. Data were available both for general morbidity and mortality and for cardiac events or procedures (e.g., myocardial infarction [MI], coronary artery bypass grafting [CABG]) and cardiac causes of death (e.g., deadly MI).

The dependent variable for intervention studies was patient abstinence from nicotine use. Follow-up periods were heterogeneous, and data recording methods varied among the studies. Both self-reports and medical tests (i.e., objective self-reports) were used. However, the validity of participant self-reports is debatable. D. K. Wilson, Wallston, King, Smith, and Heim (1993) examined the validity of self-reported smoking in comparison to medical methods of analysis and concluded that they deviated by approximately 5% (this study did not include an intervention).

Social desirability biases have been found to be stronger in intervention studies, and smoking rates were lower, if persons were interviewed by the researcher. A meta-analysis by Tang, Law, and Wald (1994) of the effect of nicotine replacement products showed that self-reports made at home provided more valid data than personal interviews with participants. Socially validated reports were occasionally sought by asking the patients' partners about patients' tobacco use, but the partners of many participants who classified themselves as smokers declared them to be abstinent. Methods of assessing current smoking status are included in the presentation of studies in Appendix W3C

---

[1] Hedbäck and Perk (1987) is an exception. Although no randomized allocation was made, we included the study because of the long follow-up period (5 years).

(see Web site). We assumed that no systematic biases occurred that would lead to an overrating of abstinence among the intervention groups.

Because of insufficient reliability and validity, we did not analyze the number of cigarettes consumed as a dependent variable, primarily because the main goal of smoking cessation interventions is abstinence, not reduction in consumption. We also did not assess the cost-effectiveness or efficacy of treatments or analyze treatment and secondary costs (see Lightwood & Glantz, 1997).

3.2.4. Data Entry

We used Review Manager 4.1 (Cochrane Collaboration, 2004) for data entry and literature management.

3.2.4.1. Evaluation.

Only values from four-way tables or bivariate correlation values can be used for epidemiological studies. If values were specified as relative risk or odds ratio (OR), we recalculated them as absolute values (e.g., number of persons per group). This is only an estimate, but it enabled us to consider a greater number of primary studies. We did not include correlation values that were adjusted by further variables (e.g., age, gender) because they are estimation models, and real case numbers are needed for data entry.

We used two models of calculation to interpret the findings of the intervention studies. For a conservative estimate, we calculated the proportion of abstinent persons ("intention to treat") who left the original sample, regardless of how many persons were reached by follow-up (see section 3.5.2). The term *intention to treat* predicts inclusion of all randomized subjects in the analysis. We rated patients without recorded data at the last measurement point as smokers in both the intervention and control groups. For an optimistic estimate, we restricted the calculation to people who were reached at follow-up, and we calculated ORs from the remaining sample (see section 3.5.1). As a rule, this model leads to higher abstinence rates than the conservative model. It is also reasonable to assume that if the sample is not biased, the ORs calculated using the optimistic model will coincide with those calculated using the conservative model. If the re-

port did not provide the number of participants before the intervention, only optimistic estimates could be calculated. We decided not to use an extremely conservative estimate, which would assume that people in the intervention group who were not contacted had relapsed and that people who stayed in the control group remained nonsmokers. If the number of smokers after the intervention was higher than at the beginning of the data collection, we counted smokers as such only if they were smokers right from the start.

3.2.4.2. Presentation of statistical parameters.

The influence of smoking as a risk factor for the occurrence of CHD is presented using ORs. A number greater than 1.00 indicates that there is a higher risk for those who smoke than for those who do not. ORs for the mortality of CHD and general mortality are presented in the same manner. Values greater than 1.00 indicate a greater mortality of smokers. Intervention effects are also presented as ORs. Values greater than 1.00 indicate that the newly implemented intervention led to a larger reduction in the number of smokers within the experimental group compared with standard care.

We calculated confidence intervals (CIs) of 95% for all ORs in the tables, and we also calculated the number needed to treat (NNT) with CIs. We calculated chi-square values to check the homogeneity of the findings for all pooled effect sizes. Significant results ($p < .05$) indicate heterogeneous effects in the primary studies. We did not perform a homogeneity test for the epidemiological questions, because even small differences would lead to statistically significant nonhomogeneity.

3.2.4.3. Weighting and order of studies.

For the epidemiological questions, we weighted the studies according to the number of people examined. This is a sufficient criterion for weighting because the studies are of uniformly good quality. We arranged the studies in ascending order according to the period of follow-up, with no relation to their content.

Sample characteristics, lengths of follow-up, and data collection methods were very heterogeneous across intervention studies. As with the epidemiological studies, we weighted them using sample size and ranked the results in ascending order by quality of study in order to check whether studies of lower quality showed different effects than studies of higher quality.

We evaluated the quality of intervention studies according to their methodological characteristics. We considered and coded the following five criteria:

1. *Sample.* Relevant to sample quality were the description of the data collection methods and the institution where the study took place and the description of the selection criteria, including period of data collection, patient characteristics, and institutional characteristics. We coded as follows: No information available = 0; information available but descriptive features missing = 1; good description provided of sample acquisition and of persons in the sample = 2. We also examined the representativeness of the sample relating to the question. We coded as follows: No information available or strong selection apparent = 0; some information available but differences apparent compared with the initial sample = 1; sample consistent with CHD patients to be examined and only small selection effects apparent = 2.

2. *Randomization.* We examined whether the randomization controlled for clinical parameters and sociodemographic variables (coded as 0 = no and 2 = yes). We also examined whether the randomization was made externally. If a third, uninvolved person performed the randomization, this feature was coded as 2. If persons who were involved in the study performed the randomization, it was coded as 1. Randomization by the experimenter or therapist was coded as 0.

3. *Bias effects.* We examined evidence of selection bias (i.e., systematic differences between the experimental group and the control group before the intervention), coded as follows: No differences apparent = 2; small differences apparent = 1; large differences apparent, or not screened = 0. We also examined evidence of dropout bias (i.e., systematic differences between the experimental and control groups in

the number of people remaining at follow-up), coded as follows: No difference in number reached at follow-up = 2, members of experimental and control groups reached at follow-up different on sociodemographic variables = 1, large reduction in experimental and control groups or wide differences among group members reached at follow-up = 0.

4. *Data collection of dependent variables.* We coded data collection methods as follows: Blinding of the interviewer = 2,[2] anonymous self-report via questionnaire = 1, and personal interview with the experimenter = 0. We coded validation of a self-report of smoking status with the help of a test result as no = 0 and yes = 2.

5. *Standardization of intervention.* We examined whether study reports specified the selection and training of those performing the intervention. We coded as follows: Manual was included and training took place = 2; manual was included or therapeutic steps were clearly described = 1; neither condition met = 0. We also examined adherence to the therapist's instructions (i.e., whether the successful realization of the planned procedure and quality control were recorded). We coded as follows: Standardized external control = 2, occasional control or therapist's self-reports = 1, no control = 0. We did not consider the length of the follow-up period for the evaluation of primary studies, because the follow-up period was most often 12 months.

Using the codes we assigned the quality criteria, we calculated a total value (minimum = 0, maximum = 20) that we used to rank the studies (see section 3.5 and Table 3.1).

3.3. SMOKING AS A RISK FACTOR FOR CORONARY HEART DISEASE

In Germany, according to surveys by the German Health Authority (*Bundesgesundheitsamt*) in 1998, approximately 37% of men and 28% of women between 18 and 80 years of age smoke (Junge & Nagel, 1998). Smoking in patients with CHD is

---

[2] If a validation of the self-report was made, it was coded as 2, because blinding of the interviewer was not necessary.

TABLE 3.1

Quality Assessment of the 22 Primary Studies Used in the Meta-Analysis

Study citation	Sample	Randomization	Bias effects	Data collection of dependent variables	Standardization of intervention	Total quality
B. Linden, 1995	2 (1, 1)	0 (0, 0)	0 (0, 0)	0 (0, 0)	2 (1, 1)	4
Burt et al., 1974	3 (1, 2)	2 (0, 2)	0 (0, 0)	0 (0, 0)	0 (0, 0)	5
Erdman & Duivenvoorden, 1983	3 (2, 1)	0 (0, 0)	1 (1, 0)	1 (1, 0)	0 (0, 0)	5
Mitsibounas, Tsouna-Hadjis, Rotas, & Sideris, 1992	1 (1, 0)	0 (0, 0)	3 (1, 2)	0 (0, 0)	1 (1, 0)	5
C. B. Taylor, Houston-Miller, Haskell, & DeBusk, 1988	4 (2, 2)	0 (0, 0)	0 (0, 0)	0 (0, 0)	2 (2, 0)	6
Hedbäck & Perk, 1987	4 (2, 2)	0 (0, 0)	2 (2, 0)	0 (0, 0)	1 (1, 0)	7
Lisspers et al., 1999	3 (2, 1)	0 (0, 0)	2 (2, 0)	1 (1, 0)	1 (1, 0)	7
Marra, Paolillo, Spadaccini, & Angelino, 1985	3 (2, 1)	0 (0, 0)	3 (2, 1)	0 (0, 0)	1 (1, 0)	7
Engblom, Rönnemaa, Hämäläinen, & Kallio, 1992	4 (2, 2)	0 (0, 0)	2 (2, 0)	1 (1, 0)	1 (1, 0)	8
Carlsson, Lindberg, Westin, & Israelsson, 1997	4 (2, 2)	0 (0, 0)	4 (2, 2)	1 (1, 0)	0 (0, 0)	9
Fridlund, Högstedt, Lidell, & Larsson, 1991	4 (2, 2)	1 (1, 0)	2 (1, 1)	1 (1, 0)	1 (1, 0)	9
van Elderen-van Kemenade, Maes, & van den Broek, 1994	4 (2, 2)	0 (0, 0)	3 (2, 1)	0 (0, 0)	2 (2, 0)	9
Heller, Knapp, Valenti, & Dobson, 1993	4 (2, 2)	2 (1, 1)	2 (2, 0)	0 (0, 0)	2 (1, 1)	10
Sivarajan et al., 1983	2 (1, 1)	0 (0, 0)	4 (2, 2)	1 (1, 0)	3 (2, 1)	10
van Elderen, Maes, Seegers, Kragten, & Relik-van Wely, 1994	4 (2, 2)	0 (0, 0)	3 (2, 1)	1 (1, 0)	2 (2, 0)	10
Allen, 1996	4 (2, 2)	2 (0, 2)	3 (1, 2)	1 (1, 0)	1 (1, 0)	11
Campbell, Ritchie, et al., 1998; Campbell, Thain, Deans, Ritchie, & Rawles, 1998	3 (2, 1)	4 (2, 2)	4 (2, 2)	1 (1, 0)	0 (0, 0)	12
Dornelas, Sampson, Gray, Waters, & Thompson, 2000	4 (2, 2)	2 (0, 2)	2 (2, 0)	4 (2, 2)	1 (1, 0)	13
Rigotti, McKool, & Shiffmann, 1994	2 (1, 1)	0 (0, 0)	4 (2, 2)	4 (2, 2)	3 (2, 1)	13
J. K. Ockene et al., 1992; Rosal et al., 1998	3 (2, 1)	0 (0, 0)	3 (2, 1)	4 (2, 2)	4 (2, 2)	14
C. B. Taylor, Houston-Miller, Killen, & DeBusk, 1990	4 (2, 2)	2 (0, 2)	2 (2, 0)	4 (2, 2)	3 (2, 1)	15
DeBusk et al., 1994	4 (2, 2)	4 (2, 2)	2 (1, 1)	4 (2, 2)	2 (2, 0)	16

Note. Codes are defined in section 3.2.4.3. Each criterion was coded for two aspects; these are listed in parentheses.

well documented. For this chapter, we selected only prospective studies that examined smoking as a predisposing factor for morbidity and mortality in CHD. Considering the abundance of findings, this review is not complete, but it is an acceptable sampling, considering the homogenous data and the broader emphasis of this review.

3.3.1. Morbidity

On the basis of 10 epidemiological studies on smoking, the mean OR was 2.62 (CI 2.06–3.32) for suffering an MI and 2.07 (CI 1.24–3.47) for CHD as a whole (see Table 3.2). There were heterogeneous effects of smoking on morbidity from MI, $\chi^2(6, N = 263{,}672) = 49.44$, $p < .00001$, and from CHD as a whole, $\chi^2(3, N = 21{,}403) = 22.47$, $p < .00001$. These heterogeneous findings are mainly ascribable to methodological variations: The studies analyzed varied greatly in both size and length of follow-up. As expected, the study with the longest follow-up period (Jacobs et al., 1999) found the lowest influence of smoking on CHD. Studies with shorter follow-up periods found substantially stronger effects.

TABLE 3.2

Smoking as a Risk Factor for Morbidity From Myocardial Infarction and Other Cardiovascular Disorders

Study citation	Follow-up period (years)	Smokers experiencing morbidity		Nonsmokers experiencing morbidity		Weight (%)	Odds ratio	95% confidence interval
		n	N	n	N			
Myocardial infarction (MI)[a]								
Shaper et al., 1985	4	108	3,185	18	1,819	9.9	3.51	2.13, 5.80
Willett et al., 1987	6	150	39,801	92	79,603	14.7	3.27	2.52, 4.24
Nyboe, Jensen, Appleyard, & Schnorr, 1991	6.5	277	7,790	83	4,406	14.9	1.92	1.50, 2.46
Keil et al., 1998	8	52	345	40	709	11.2	2.97	1.92, 4.58
Prescott, Hippe, Schnorr, Hein, & Vestbo, 1998	12	1,282	14,951	481	9,712	17.1	1.80	1.62, 2.01
Njølstad, Arnesen, & Lund-Larsen, 1996	12	428	5,998	170	5,845	16.1	2.57	2.14, 3.08
Kawachi et al., 1994	12	416	38,845	166	50,663	16.1	3.29	2.75, 3.94
Total for MI (random effects model)		2,713	110,915	1,050	152,757	100.0	2.62	2.06, 3.32
Unspecified cardiovascular disorders[b]								
D. G. Cook, Shaper, Pocock, & Kussick, 1986	6	189	3,185	30	1,819	30.7	3.76	2.55, 5.55
Tunstall-Pedoe, Woodward, Tavendale, A'Brook, & McCluskey, 1997; Woodward, Moohan, & Tunstall-Pedoe, 1999	7	77	1,808	95	3,941	32.9	1.80	1.33, 2.45
Jacobs et al., 1999	25	1,228	7,829	327	2,821	36.4	1.42	1.25, 1.62
Total for unspecified disorders (random effects model)		1,494	12,822	452	8,581	100.0	2.07	1.24, 3.47

Note. Odds ratio > 1 means a higher risk for smokers. Studies are listed in order of increasing follow-up period. [a]$\chi^2(6, N = 263,672) = 49.44$, $p < .00001$; $z = 7.89$, $p = .00001$. [b]$\chi^2(2, N = 21,403) = 22.47$, $p < .00001$; $z = 2.76$, $p = .006$.

3.3.2. Mortality

Table 3.3 shows the influence of smoking on mortality from CHD. The mean OR of 2.20 (CI 1.83–2.63) indicates a higher risk for smokers of dying from CHD. This finding was uniformly confirmed in several studies. The reported effects are not homogenous, $\chi^2(8, N = 741,372) = 91.57$, $p < .00001$; as expected, studies with a longer follow-up period reported a smaller influence. Smoking also has an influence on total mortality, although we did not include such studies in the meta-analysis for this chapter (see K. Wilson, Gibson, Willan, & Cook, 2000). Tobacco use increases the incidence of MI and is associated with earlier death from CHD; whether it increases the need for additional bypass

operations and angioplasties has not yet been examined.

Besides such direct influences of smoking on the risk of CHD, we also believe there are synergistic effects—that is, that risk factors act not only in an additive manner but also in a multiplicative manner. A prospective study from Finland, for example, showed a multiplicative connection between the risk factor of smoking and increased levels of serum cholesterol. Jousilahti, Vartiainen, Korhonen, Puska, and Tuomilehto (1999) examined the effects of smoking, increased cholesterol level, and increased blood pressure on about 8,000 men and about 8,000 women. They dichotomized these factors using the criteria of presence of or death

TABLE 3.3

Smoking as a Risk Factor for Mortality From Coronary Heart Disease

Study citation	Follow-up period (years)	Smokers who died		Nonsmokers who died		Weight (%)	Odds ratio	95% confidence interval
		n	*N*	*n*	*N*			
Willett et al., 1987	6	39	39,801	26	79,603	7.0	3.00	1.83, 4.93
Cullen, Schulte, & Assmann, 1997	7	62	7,374	15	3,482	6.0	1.96	1.11, 3.45
Kuller et al., 1991	10.5	3,444	133,117	2,973	228,545	14.3	2.02	1.92, 2.12
Kawachi et al., 1993	12	284	35,217	131	50,427	12.1	3.12	2.54, 3.84
Kawachi et al., 1994	12	121	38,724	49	50,633	9.7	3.24	2.32, 4.51
Tverdal, Thelle, Stensvold, Leren, & Bjartveit, 1993	13	1,270	23,456	381	19,838	13.6	2.92	2.60, 3.28
Luoto, Prättälä, Uutela, & Puska, 1998	13	306	3,738	696	15,236	13.3	1.86	1.62, 2.14
Fulton & Shekelle, 1997	25	176	956	81	575	10.6	1.38	1.03, 1.83
Jacobs et al., 1999	25	1,214	7,829	307	2,821	13.4	1.50	1.32, 1.72
Total (random effects model)		6,916	290,212	4,659	451,160	100.0	2.20	1.83, 2.63

Note. Odds ratio > 1 means a higher risk for smokers. Studies are listed in order of increasing follow-up period. $\chi^2(8, N = 741,372) = 91.57, p < .00001; z = 8.46, p < .00001$.

from a coronary disease. Compared with men with none of the three risk factors, men with all three risk factors had relative risks of 11.8 of dying from a coronary disease and 7.3 of developing CHD. For women, the relative risks of dying from coronary disease were 9.6 and of developing CHD, 8.6. These findings indicate that tobacco use has a higher influence on the risk of MI in men than in women.

Prescott, Hippe, Schnohr, Hein, and Vestbo (1998) reported different findings in a sample of 11,000 people. They found a relative risk of MI of 2.24 for women and a relative risk of coronary disease or death from a cardiac infarct of 1.43 for men. Luoto, Prättälä, Uutela, and Puska (1998) reported similar results in their Finnish study; the OR for dying of coronary disease was 2.9 (CI 1.9–4.5) for women and 1.9 (CI 1.5–2.5) for men. A final conclusion regarding a gender-specific effect on the manifestation of CHD is not yet possible.

Besides one's own tobacco use, passive smoking is also important in the development of CHD. A re-

view by He et al. (1999) that controlled for other risk factors found a mean relative risk of 1.26 (CI 1.16–1.38). Their review also highlights the influence of the duration and intensity of passive smoking on the probability of CHD, demonstrating that for a smoker who is trying to stop, having a partner who smokes not only causes motivational problems, but also represents a direct risk factor for CHD.

3.4. EFFECT OF ABSTINENCE ON MORBIDITY AND MORTALITY

The findings described in Section 3.3 suggest that smoking is associated with increased morbidity and mortality from CHD. We next examined whether abstinence from tobacco use would have a positive influence on patients already suffering from CHD. This section focuses on a secondary prevention question: Does abstinence from tobacco use have any influence on relapse and mortality among premorbid smokers with existing coronary disease?

3.4.1. Influence on Morbidity

A review by Burling, Singleton, and Bigelow (1984) reported heterogeneous findings regarding the importance of abstinence from tobacco use after a cardiac infarct in slowing the further development of CHD. The available studies consistently found an increased risk of falling ill again or of an early death for patients who continued to smoke. However, the ORs are inconsistent, ranging from 1.33 to 2.55 for a CHD relapse. Jost (1994) mentioned several studies in his review that provide evidence that smoking increases the risk of relapse. However, we could not compare these studies with others because Jost examined only prevalences. According to Jost, abstinence from tobacco use led to a reduction in mortality of 25% to 60%. He specified changes in morbidity ranging from a reduction of 60% and an increase of 280%, with a weighted mean of about −30%.

We aggregated 11 primary studies that show that abstinence from tobacco use is associated with lower morbidity for patients with MI (OR = 0.62, CI 0.46–0.83, equivalent to a relative risk reduction of 18%; see Table 3.4). However, the primary studies found heterogeneous results regarding the efficacy of abstinence from tobacco use, $\chi^2(10, N = 6,602) = 23.46$, $p < .01$. We discarded publication bias as an explanation because verification of the funnel plot showed no unexpected findings. The heterogeneity of the findings is in fact from the Coronary Artery Surgery Study (Hermanson, Omenn, Kronmal, & Gersh, 1988); in that study, several continuing smokers died during the follow-up period of 6 years (see Table 3.4). No MI was registered in their sample during the follow-up period. We found homogeneous effects ($p > .65$) when we excluded this study from the meta-analysis. The OR of 0.62 indicates that continuing smokers have 1.2 times the risk of relapse after an MI.

We found no effect on relapse of either percutaneous transluminal coronary angioplasty (PTCA; OR = 0.80, CI 0.37–1.71) or CABG (OR = 0.95, CI 0.68–1.34). These findings should be interpreted carefully, because only a few primary studies (two for PTCA and one for CABG) were available and because of the high CI.

Taken together, these findings point to a protective influence of smoking cessation on cardiac health of patients with CHD (especially MI), although the intensity of the influence varies. For PTCA and CABG, other factors than cardiac disease were also decisive in the results. Because MI is a clearly measurable variable, we expected to find that smoking has a direct influence on relapse, and this expectation was confirmed.

3.4.2. Influence on Mortality

Table 3.5 summarizes findings regarding the influence of abstinence from tobacco use on mortality from CHD (it does not consider effects on total mortality). We observed a preventative effect of abstinence from smoking on mortality from CHD (OR = 0.66, CI 0.54–0.80, corresponding to a relative risk reduction of 24%). We used a funnel plot to verify whether the effect was stable or whether the selection of publications was jointly responsible for the stability (see Appendix W3D on the Web site). The absence of small studies to the right of the centerline led us to assume that studies with small samples were not published. The three studies with larger samples in Table 3.5 found an OR ranging from 0.65 to 0.85, resulting in a mean OR of 0.73 (CI 0.61–0.88). This value is realistic, because we have to assume that there was a selection bias in the publication of findings, even though they suggest a statistical homogeneity, $\chi^2(6, N = 8,109) = 9.42$, $p = .15$.

To summarize, abstinence from tobacco use improves the mortality of patients with CHD (see also Critchley & Capewell, 2003). The effect on coronary heart morbidity is similar for a reinfarct. That there is not enough evidence of a protective influence of smoking cessation on a relapse for patients with CABG and PTCA can be ascribed to the small number of primary studies.

3.5. EFFICACY OF SMOKING CESSATION INTERVENTIONS FOR PATIENTS WITH CORONARY HEART DISEASE

The proportion of former smokers in epidemiological studies increased with the increasing age of the population (Junge & Nagel, 1998). The wish and need for behavioral change seemed to be especially high in persons over 40 years of age (the smoking

TABLE 3.4

Influence on Morbidity of Abstinence From Tobacco Use After a Cardiac Event

Study citation	Persons experiencing morbidity who abstained from tobacco use after cardiac event		Persons experiencing morbidity who continued smoking after cardiac event		Weight (%)	Odds ratio	95% confidence interval
	n	*N*	*n*	*N*			
Myocardial infarction[a]							
Aberg et al., 1983	104	542	127	441	16.1	0.59	0.44, 0.79
Galan, Deligonul, Kern, Chaitman, & Vandormael, 1988	2	76	3	84	2.2	0.73	0.12, 4.49
Hasdai, Garratt, Grill, Lerman, & Holmes, 1997	9	435	22	734	8.0	0.68	0.31, 1.50
Hermanson, Omenn, Kronmal, & Gersh, 1988	46	759	43	1,039	13.7	1.49	0.98, 2.29
Rivers, White, Cross, Williams, & Morris, 1990	8	156	7	35	5.2	0.22	0.07, 0.64
Ronnevik, Gundersen, & Abrahamsen, 1985	44	551	45	368	13.4	0.62	0.40, 0.97
Sato et al., 1992	0	59	2	28	0.9	0.09	0.00, 1.92
Sparrow, Dawber, & Colton, 1978	8	56	26	139	7.1	0.72	0.31, 1.71
Ulvenstam, Aberg, Pennert, Vedin, & Wedel, 1985	77	296	83	232	14.7	0.63	0.43, 0.92
Voors et al., 1996	11	72	28	95	8.1	0.43	0.20, 0.94
Wilhelmsson, Vedin, Elmfeldt, Tibblin, & Wilhelmsen, 1975	20	231	31	174	10.6	0.44	0.24, 0.80
Total for MI (random effects model)	329	3,233	417	3,369	100.0	0.62	0.46, 0.83
Percutaneous transluminary coronary angioplasty[b]							
Galan et al., 1988	29	76	46	84	43.3	0.51	0.27, 0.96
Hasdai et al., 1997	108	435	167	734	56.7	1.12	0.85, 1.48
Total for PTCA (random effects model)	137	511	213	818	100.0	0.80	0.37, 1.71
Coronary artery bypass grafting[c]							
Hasdai et al., 1997	62	435	109	734	100.00	0.95	0.68, 1.34

Note. Odds ratio < 1 corresponds to a lower risk for former smokers in comparison to continuing smokers. Studies are listed in alphabetical order.

[a]$\chi^2(10, N = 6,602) = 23.46, p = .0092; z = -3.23, p = .001.$ [b]$\chi^2(1, N = 1,329) = 5.02, p = .025; z = -0.58, p = .6.$
[c]$\chi^2(0, N = 1,169) = 0.00, p < .00001; z = -0.28, p = .8.$

cessation rate for both women and men is over 40%). For women, the percentage of abstinent persons in higher age groups remained relatively constant (maximum of about 50% between 70 and 80 years), whereas for men the percentage of former smokers continued to rise with age (maximum of about 80% between 70 and 80 years). Experts estimated that 90% to 95% of former smokers stopped smoking without either obtaining professional help or resorting to abstinence support measures (Carey,

Snel, Carey, & Richards, 1989; Fiore, Novotny, Pierce, Giovino, & Davis, 1990).

Epidemiological studies on patients with coronary disease have varied widely in the percentage of smokers. Smoking prevalence was very dependent on cultural habits, characteristics of the patients treated (e.g., social class, age), treatment provided (PTCA, CABG), and year of survey.

In the following tables, we address the results of the meta-analysis regarding the efficacy of

TABLE 3.5

Influence on Mortality of Abstinence From Tobacco Use After a Cardiac Event

Study citation	Persons who abstained from tobacco use after cardiac event who died		Persons who continued smoking after cardiac event who died		Weight (%)	Odds ratio	95% confidence interval (random)
	n	*N*	*n*	*N*			
Aberg et al., 1983	80	542	94	441	19.7	0.64	0.46, 0.89
Cavender, Rogers, Fisher, Gershi, & Coggin, 1992; Vlietstra, Kronmal, Oberman, Frye, & Killip, 1986	164	1,490	341	2,675	30.8	0.85	0.69, 1.03
Hermanson et al., 1988	121	759	229	1,039	26.5	0.67	0.53, 0.86
Mulcahy, Hickey, Graham, & MacAirt, 1977	11	89	17	59	4.7	0.35	0.15, 0.81
Salonen, 1980	24	221	53	302	10.7	0.57	0.34, 0.96
Sato et al., 1992	5	59	6	28	2.2	0.34	0.09, 1.23
Wilhelmsson et al., 1975	11	231	17	174	5.4	0.46	0.21, 1.01
Total	416	3,391	757	4,718	100.0	0.66	0.54, 0.80

Note. Odds ratio < 1 corresponds to a lower risk for former smokers compared to continuing smokers. Studies are listed in alphabetical order. $\chi^2(6, N = 8,109) = 9.42$, $p = .15$; $z = -4.24$, $p = .00002$.

interventions in stopping patients with coronary heart diseases from smoking. We distinguish between an analysis for people with follow-up information (optimistic estimation) and an analysis according to the "intention to treat" method (conservative estimation).

3.5.1. Optimistic Estimate of Intervention Efficacy

The overview in Table 3.6 shows the effects of the primary studies we assessed that evaluated specific and nonspecific interventions aimed at stopping cardiac patients from smoking. Integrating the 19 primary studies shows that the interventions were successful at stopping people from smoking (OR = 2.25, CI 1.57–3.03). Although the majority of primary studies did not show a significant intervention effect, aggregating the studies produced evidence for the efficacy of smoking cessation interventions. The efficacy of the individual studies is heterogeneous; the test for homogeneity indicates statistically relevant differences among the studies, $\chi^2(18, N = 2,027) = 34.29$, $p < .05$. However, studies with extremely high effects (OR > 20) may also

be responsible for that heterogeneity (Erdman & Duivenvoorden, 1983; Lisspers et al., 1999; Mitsibounas, Tsouna-Hadjis, Rotas, & Sideris, 1992). If we exclude those primary studies from the analysis, we achieve a homogeneous effect, $\chi^2(15, N = 1,946) = 23.14$, $p > .05$.

The funnel plot (see Figure WD3.8 in Appendix W3D on the Web site) shows a relatively uniform sample size for most studies. As expected, the effects of those studies scatter around the mean OR. Because we found no indication of a publication bias in this diagram, we did not perform a statistical verification of possible biases. If we limit the analysis to studies with high internal validity and therefore high quality, we can exclude eight studies with a value of 7 or less (Burt et al., 1974; Erdman & Duivenvoorden, 1983; Hedbäck & Perk, 1987; Lisspers et al., 1999; Marra, Paolillo, Spadaccini, & Angelino, 1985; Mitsibounas et al., 1992; C. B. Taylor, Houston-Miller, Haskell, & DeBusk, 1988; see Tables 3.1 and 3.6). With this quality restraint we obtained a homogeneous odds ratio of 1.95 (CI 1.44–2.64), $\chi^2(11, N = 1,297) = 15.04$, $p > .20$. We can therefore maintain that in-

TABLE 3.6

Efficacy of Interventions in Promoting Abstinence From Tobacco Use in Patients With Coronary Heart Disease: Optimistic Estimate

Study citation	Members of intervention group who remained abstinent at last point of measurement		Members of control group who remained abstinent at last point of measurement		Weight (%)	Odds ratio	95% confidence interval
	n	*N*	*n*	*N*			
Erdman & Duivenvoorden, 1983	9	18	0	15	0.9	31.00	1.61, 596.04
Mitsibounas et al., 1992	13	18	2	18	2.3	20.80	3.45, 125.30
Burt et al., 1974	79	125	27	98	8.7	4.52	2.55, 8.01
C. B. Taylor et al., 1988	29	42	16	26	5.1	1.39	0.50, 3.89
Hedbäck & Perk, 1987	41	104	25	108	8.5	2.16	1.19, 3.92
Lisspers et al., 1999	5	7	0	5	0.8	24.20	0.93, 629.35
Marra et al., 1985	56	74	47	72	7.3	1.65	0.81, 3.40
Engblom et al., 1992	11	25	4	20	3.5	3.14	.081, 12.13
Carlsson et al., 1997	16	32	9	35	5.1	2.89	1.03, 8.07
van Elderen-van Kemenade, Maes, & van den Broek, 1994	9	15	6	16	3.2	2.50	0.59, 10.62
Heller et al., 1993	34	52	34	64	7.0	1.67	0.78, 3.54
Sivarajan et al., 1983	13	27	14	37	5.2	1.53	0.56, 4.17
van Elderen, Maes, Seegers, et al., 1994	40	64	32	64	7.5	1.67	0.82, 3.37
Allen, 1996	9	14	6	11	2.7	1.50	0.30, 7.53
Campbell, Ritchie, et al., 1998	1	102	11	98	1.8	0.08	0.01, 0.62
Dornelas et al., 2000	28	40	16	40	5.7	3.50	1.39, 8.84
J. K. Ockene et al., 1992; Rosal et al., 1998	47	82	37	78	8.2	1.49	0.80, 2.78
C. B. Taylor et al., 1990	51	72	26	58	7.3	2.99	1.45, 6.17
DeBusk et al., 1994	92	131	64	120	9.3	2.06	1.23, 3.47
Total (random effects model)	583	1,044	376	983	100.0	2.25	1.67, 3.03

Note. Odds ratio > 1 corresponds to higher benefit to the intervention group compared to the control group. Studies are listed in order of increasing quality. $\chi^2(18, N = 2,027) = 34.23, p = .012; z = 5.36, p < .00001$.

terventions lead to a higher abstinence from tobacco use. We found the real effect in an OR of between 1.4 and 2.6. After conversion into the clinically important statistic NNT, we obtained a value of 7 (CI 4–11).

3.5.2. Conservative Estimate of Intervention Efficacy

The conservative model includes only nine primary studies, because most studies did not indicate the base rate of smokers at the beginning of the study or provided no data for the remaining people at the time of follow-up. The mean OR was 1.81 (CI 1.15–2.83). We found a trend showing that the

higher the quality of the study, the lower its efficacy (see Table 3.7). Overall we found heterogeneous effects, $\chi^2(8, N = 835) = 16.17, p < .05$.

The funnel plot in Appendix W3D (see the Web site) shows the relatively heterogeneous effects in primary studies. The missing accumulation of studies around the mean odds ratio is remarkable. Instead, we observed a wide scattering of those effects with relatively uniform sample sizes. If we also limit the studies to those with a quality index of over 7 for a conservative estimate of efficacy, the OR decreases to 1.35 (CI 0.89–1.86; this estimate excludes Hedbäck & Perk, 1987; B. Linden, 1995; and Mitsibounas et al., 1992; see Table 3.1). The

TABLE 3.7

Efficacy of Interventions in Promoting Abstinence From Tobacco Use in Patients With Coronary Heart Disease: Conservative Estimate

Study citation	Members of intervention group who remained abstinent at last point of measurement		Members of control group who remained abstinent at last point of measurement		Weight (%)	Odds ratio	95% confidence interval
	n	*N*	*n*	*N*			
B. Linden, 1995	4	5	3	8	2.6	6.67	0.49, 91.33
Mitsibounas et al., 1992	12	18	2	20	5.1	18.00	3.10, 104.54
Hedbäck & Perk, 1987	41	59	25	60	14.3	3.19	1.50, 6.79
Carlsson et al., 1997	16	40	9	38	11.2	2.15	0.81, 5.72
Fridlund et al., 1991	19	30	16	27	10.2	1.19	0.41, 3.46
Sivarajan et al., 1983	13	39	14	37	11.7	0.82	0.32, 2.10
Dornelas et al., 2000	28	54	16	46	13.5	2.02	0.90, 4.53
Rigotti et al., 1994	19	44	19	43	13.0	0.96	0.41, 2.24
Rosal et al., 1998; Ockene et al., 1992	47	135	37	132	18.3	1.37	0.82, 2.30
Total (random effects model)	199	424	141	411	100.0	1.81	1.15, 2.83

Note. Odds ratio > 1 corresponds to higher benefit to the intervention group compared with the control group. Studies are listed in order of increasing quality. $\chi^2(8, N = 835) = 16.17$, $p = .04$; $z = 2.59$, $p = .01$.

effect is then no longer statistically significant. This finding corresponds to an NNT of 14, with a lower confidence interval of 6 (because of the statistically nonsignificant OR, this value has no upper limit).

3.6. AVAILABLE META-ANALYSES AND THEIR FINDINGS FOR CORONARY HEART DISEASE

According to Fiore et al. (1990), it is possible to differentiate between professional external interventions (i.e., offerings from the health care system) and self-management attempts (i.e., smoking cessation with no help from the professional health care system). In this section, we discuss the findings of reviews concerning the efficacy of professional methods in smoking cessation (for an overview, see Lancaster, Stead, Silagy, & Sowden, 2000). We then present studies by method used to treat people with CHD. It is impossible to arrange the studies by intervention strategy without blurring, because most studies used several interven-

tion components. We also analyze side effects that might be caused by medications and by nicotine replacement therapy in patients with CHD.

3.6.1. Medical Advice

Advice from a doctor is frequently used to wean patients from smoking. *Medical advice* is commonly defined as a verbal instruction from a doctor indicating that the patient should stop smoking. The advice may include information regarding the damaging consequences of smoking, but it does not have to. It is possible to differentiate minimal, complete, and intensive interventions. A minimal intervention normally includes advice (with or without provision of a leaflet) within a single consultation lasting less than 20 minutes. A complete intervention includes a maximum of one follow-up visit. An intensive intervention consists of a doctor giving advice within a longer consultation, providing further resources besides a leaflet (e.g., demonstration of exhaled carbon monoxide or pulmonary function test, self-help manuals) and more than one follow-up visit.

Silagy (1998) presented a meta-analysis on the effect of medical advice on smoking cessation; 31 studies met the inclusion criteria (two treatment groups and a randomized allocation of participants). The author compared the efficacy of medical advice in promoting abstinence from tobacco use in a treatment group (at the last measurement point) after a minimal intervention with the control group who did not receive a doctor's advice (OR = 1.69, CI 1.45–1.98). Additional support, such as patient leaflets, had no additive effect (OR = 1.88, CI 1.63–2.18) compared with the intervention without additional support (OR = 2.00, CI 1.60–2.49).

Although medical advice had no effect on abstinence in people without a specific risk profile (OR = 1.20, CI 0.97–1.47), there is evidence of a positive effect on abstinence from smoking among people with an increased risk for developing a disease (OR = 1.82, CI 1.44–2.29). Even after only one session, this group was more successful at smoking cessation than the control group (OR = 1.66, CI 1.41–1.95). For temporary interventions lasting several sessions, compared with control groups, we found an OR of 2.54 (CI 2.02–3.19). However, it is questionable to conclude that the rate of abstinence from smoking increases with the number of sessions offered; intensive sessions with follow-up interviews had an OR of 1.6 (CI 1.10–2.33) compared with minimal interventions, contradicting that conclusion. There was no positive effect of medical advice on the 20-year mortality rate (OR = 0.87, CI 0.75–1.02); however, only one study examined this question (see Silagy, 1998).

Thus, for smoking cessation, medical advice had a positive effect, especially for patients at risk, compared with a control group. Therefore, this intervention should be provided during the treatment of patients after a cardiac event, because it has been shown to be effective on physically ill patients. The findings regarding the efficacy of additional contacts for abstinence from tobacco use are inconsistent, and we cannot assume that they have an additive effect.

No randomized study has exclusively analyzed the efficacy of medical advice for patients with CHD. Nevertheless, a doctor's advice is often the starting point for a comprehensive intervention (see Rigotti & Pasternak, 1996). In their nonrandomized study with patients who had experienced a cardiac event, R. R. Scott, Mayer, Denier, Dawson, and Lamparski (1990) reported a rate of abstinence from smoking of about 30% after 12 months.

3.6.2. Intervention by Nurses

We examined both nurse's advice and other supportive strategies as part of interventions by nurses to promote smoking cessation. *Nurse's advice* is defined as a verbal instruction from a nurse to a patient to stop smoking, regardless of whether the nurse provides information about the damaging consequences of smoking. Nursing interventions can also be categorized as low or high intensity. A low-intensity intervention comprises advice (with or without provision of a leaflet) within a consultation of a maximum of 10 minutes, plus a maximum of one follow-up visit. A high-intensity intervention includes contacts of more than 10 minutes using further materials and strategies (e.g., manuals) in addition to leaflets and more than one follow-up visit (see Rice & Stead, 1999).

In eight studies, interventions by nurses, regardless of their intensity, were effective in promoting smoking cessation (OR = 1.43, CI 1.24–1.66; Allen, 1996; Burt et al., 1974; Campbell, Ritchie, et al., 1998; Campbell, Thain, Deans, Ritchie, & Rawles, 1998; Carlsson, Lindberg, Westin, & Israelsson, 1997; DeBusk et al., 1994; Fridlund, Hogstedt, Lidell, & Larsson, 1991; Rigotti, McKool, & Shiffmann, 1994; C. B. Taylor, Houston-Miller, Killen, & DeBusk, 1990). The interventions were most effective for patients with CHD (as an element of multimodal interventions, OR = 2.14, CI 1.39–3.31) and inpatients (OR = 1.68, CI 1.26–2.24), although no positive effects could be found for patients with other somatic illnesses (OR = 1.20, CI 0.92–1.56; see Rice & Stead, 1999). Including current studies and reanalyzing the data for CHD patients resulted in a higher OR of 3.01 (CI 2.04–4.43) for an optimistic estimate (see Table 3.8). Only three studies provided data for a conservative estimate; we found a reduced OR of 1.31 (CI 0.76–2.27).

TABLE 3.8

Categorization of Studies by Intervention Type and Calculation Model

Study citation	Intervention by nurses	Self-help	Behavioral therapy group	Telephone counseling	Physical exercise
Campbell, Ritchie, et al., 1998; Campbell, Thain, et al., 1998	F	F		F	
Burt et al., 1974	F				
B. Linden, 1994		ITT			
Erdman & Duivenvoorden, 1983			F		F
C. B. Taylor et al., 1988					F
Hedbäck & Perk, 1987					ITT, F
Lisspers et al., 1999			F		
Marra et al., 1985					F
Engblom et al., 1992			F		F
Carlsson et al., 1997	ITT, F		ITT, F		ITT, F
Fridlund et al., 1991	ITT				
van Elderen-van Kemenade, Maes, & van den Broek, 1994			F	F	
Heller et al., 1993		F	F		
Sivarajan et al., 1983			ITT, F		ITT, F
van Elderen, Maes, Seegers, et al., 1994			F		
Allen, 1996	F	F			
Dornelas et al., 2000				ITT, F	
Rigotti et al., 1994	ITT		ITT		
J. K. Ockene et al., 1992; Rosal et al., 1998			ITT, F	ITT, F	
C. B. Taylor et al., 1990	F	F	F	F	
DeBusk et al., 1994	F	F		F	
Odds ratio, conservative estimate	1.31 (CI 0.76–2.27) 3 studies	6.67 (CI 0.49–91.33) 1 study	1.26 (CI 0.87–1.83) 4 studies	1.54 (CI 0.99–2.38) 2 studies	1.84 (CI 0.82–4.10) 3 studies
Odds ratio, optimistic estimate	3.01 (CI 2.04–4.33) 6 studies	2.25 (CI 1.54–3.28) 5 studies	2.07 (CI 1.52–2.81) 10 studies	2.35 (CI 1.63–3.38) 6 studies	2.04 (CI 1.44–2.88) 7 studies

Note. Mitsibounas et al. (1992) is not listed because it was the only study we located of a psychodynamic intervention. F = follow-up (used in the optimistic estimate); ITT = intention to treat (used in the conservative estimate; predicts inclusion of all randomized subjects in the analysis); CI = confidence interval.

3.6.3. Self-Help

We defined *self-help* as any material or program meant to support an individual's attempts to stop smoking without the help of health care experts, counselors, or group interventions. Self-help includes written materials, audio and video recordings, computer programs, and telephone hotlines. The target groups for these interventions may be smokers in general or specific populations of smokers (e.g., certain age groups, students). Some self-help materials have been tailored to individual smoking habits. We did not include the provision of brief leaflets about the health risks of smoking as a self-help intervention.

We defined *self-help offers* as those interventions with minimal face-to-face contact with the sole purpose of describing self-help programs. If such contact included a discussion of the program content, we called it "brief counseling with additional self-help offers." Recurrent additional counseling meetings were not considered self-help offers (see Lancaster & Stead, 1999b).

According to the findings of a meta-analysis by Lancaster and Stead (1999b), self-help offers had no positive effect on abstinence from smoking. Use of both a telephone hotline (one primary study, OR = 1.67, CI 1.11–2.52) and individually tailored therapy materials promoted smoking cessation (OR = 1.41, CI 1.14–1.75).

Six studies on patients with CHD explicitly used self-help programs or guided patients to apply self-help strategies (Allen, 1996; Campbell, Ritchie, et al., 1998; Campbell, Thain, et al., 1998; DeBusk et al., 1994; Heller, Knapp, Valenti, & Dobson, 1993; B. Linden, 1995; C. B. Taylor et al., 1990). Using the conservative model, we found no significant effect in the qualitatively inferior study by B. Linden (OR = 6.67, CI 0.49–91.33). We could perform an optimistic estimate using only the remaining studies with better methodology. We found that the effect of self-help offers on abstinence from smoking was OR = 2.25 (CI 1.54–3.28). The question as to whether specific self-help measures can be recommended for smokers with CHD cannot be answered on the basis of these findings.

3.6.4. Behavioral Therapy Groups

Behavioral therapy groups include all interventions aimed at changing behavior and lasting at least two sessions. In addition to concrete cognitive–behavioral therapy, we also included measures providing information, placement, advice, and encouragement. Common methods in the behavioral therapy approach included training of patients, self-monitoring, reinforcement plans, social competency training, cognitive restructuring, and relaxation exercises. Consistent with Stead and Lancaster (1998), we did not count group interventions, nicotine replacement therapy, aversive methods, acupuncture, and hypnotherapy as behavioral therapy interventions. Group therapies based on behavioral therapy principles (Stead & Lancaster, 1998) were more effective than self-help group offers (OR = 2.10, CI 1.64–2.70), but for abstinence from smoking, group therapy was not superior to individual therapy (Lancaster & Stead, 1999a).

Twelve studies described treatment of patients with CHD in group therapy based on behavior therapy concepts. Most used a mixed intervention system, including telephone contact, written media, and other techniques, but in these 12 studies, group therapy formed a substantial part of the intervention (Carlsson et al., 1997; Engblom, Rönnemaa, Hämäläinen, & Kallio, 1992; Erdman & Duivenvoorden, 1983; Heller et al., 1993; Lisspers et al., 1999; J. K. Ockene et al., 1992; Rigotti et al., 1994; Rosal et al., 1998; Sivarajan et al., 1983; C. B. Taylor et al., 1990; van Elderen-van Kemenade, Maes, & van den Broek, 1994; van Elderen, Maes, Seegers, et al., 1994).

For the meta-analysis, we used the conservative method to evaluate four studies and found no statistically significant effects for group therapy interventions on smoking cessation (OR = 1.26, CI 0.87–1.83). We found behavior therapy group offers to be effective only using the optimistic model (OR = 2.07, CI 1.52–2.81). The heterogeneous findings on the efficacy of interventions are consistent with the clinical perspective on the applicability of such treatment for outpatient settings; J. K. Ockene et al. (1992) found that although patients were motivated to reduce smoking, only a few were willing to participate in group treatment over a long period if telephone counseling dates were offered as an alternative. The participants had been preselected by proximity of residence (less than 25 miles from the clinic), but compliance was still low, and consequently the group treatment was soon cancelled. Thus, in addition to efficacy, the practicality of and evidence for compliance with behavior therapy groups in outpatient settings must be examined further.

3.6.5. Telephone Counseling

Telephone counseling is effective at stopping people from smoking, but the effect is lower than for intensive measures with more frequent and regular contacts (Fiore, Jorenby, & Baker, 1997). J. K. Ockene et al. (1992) showed that telephone counseling helped participants with cardiac disease in a smoking cessation program who were attending a clinic for a physical examination to "bond" effectively with the clinic. Although only half of the 80% of participants who made an outpatient appointment actually kept it, 90% were willing to contact the counseling team by telephone. The framework of the study was to call every patient after 1 and 3 weeks. Those who still abstained from tobacco use received a further call after 3 months, whereas those who had relapsed received a call after both 2 and 4 months. The authors specified that every patient had approximately 90 minutes of contact with the intervention team, which is a relatively low therapy dose. The whole intervention achieved a positive effect (OR = 1.41 for 12 months). This intervention was also superior over the long term to advice not to smoke (see Rosal et al., 1998). However, at 5-year follow-up, the additive effects of telephone counseling were relatively small and constituted only a trend (49% vs. 40% abstinence rate).

Six studies examined the efficacy of additional telephone contacts on patients with CHD (Campbell, Ritchie, et al., 1998; Campbell, Thain, et al., 1998; DeBusk et al., 1994; Dornelas, Sampson, Gray, Waters, & Thompson, 2000; J. K. Ockene et al., 1992; C. B. Taylor et al., 1990; van Elderen-van Kemenade, Maes, & van den Broek, 1994). In the optimistic model, telephone aftercare offers were helpful for patients with CHD (OR = 2.35, CI 1.63–3.38). Even with the conservative model, we found an almost statistically significant effect for telephone aftercare (OR = 1.54; CI 0.99–2.38). In these studies, telephone aftercare always built on the success achieved with an inpatient or outpatient pretreatment; intervention exclusively by telephone would probably not be effective.

3.6.6. Physical Exercise

Physical exercise programs are an important element of cardiac rehabilitation, and many intervention studies included them to modify risk factors. There is no systematic review available of the significance of such programs in smoking cessation. The studies we present in this section offered programs of physical exercise, but in addition they offered educational or therapeutic choices.

We located seven relevant studies (Carlsson et al., 1997; Engblom et al., 1992; Erdman & Duivenvoorden, 1983; Hedbäck & Perk, 1987; Marra et al., 1985; Sivarajan et al., 1983; C. B. Taylor et al., 1988); we used four of these to calculate a conservative estimate of the efficacy of physical exer-

cise in promoting abstinence from smoking. The findings do not confirm the efficacy of physical exercise programs for smoking cessation using the conservative model (OR = 1.84, CI 0.82–4.10). We obtained a similar effect with the optimistic model (OR = 2.04, CI 1.44–2.88), but the effect is statistically significant because of the higher number of primary studies.

3.6.7. Nicotine Replacement

Nicotine previously obtained through smoking is substituted by chewing gum, patches, nose spray, or inhalers containing nicotine. Nicotine replacement therapy may also be supplemented by personal support for the smoker. Routine personal support is commonly considered an additional low-intensity support. A support is considered high intensity if the duration of the first consultation exceeds 30 minutes or if more than two additional consultations are given (see Silagy, Mant, Fowler, & Lancaster, 1999; Silagy, Mant, Fowler, & Lodge, 1994).

For heavy smokers (>15 cigarettes a day), a combination of nicotine replacement (chewing gum, patches) and behavior therapy clearly enhanced abstinence results (Fiore, Smith, Jorenby, & Baker, 1994). The meta-analysis by Fiore and colleagues of 17 studies showed that after 6 months, 22% of people in the intervention group (patches) were still abstinent (CI 19.7–23.9), compared with only 9% of people without that help (CI 7.8–11.0), corresponding to an OR of 2.6 (CI 2.2–3.0) for immediate success and 3.0 (CI 2.4–3.7) over a period of 6 months. A meta-analysis by Silagy et al. (1999) resulted in an OR of 1.63 (CI 1.48–1.78) for nicotine chewing gum, an OR of 1.77 (CI 1.58–1.97) for nicotine patches, and the highest efficacy for nose spray (OR = 2.27, CI 1.61–3.20), compared with results for placebos. Increasing the dose of the nicotine patches (4 mg vs. 2 mg) had a positive influence on smoking cessation for heavy smokers (OR = 2.67, CI 1.69–4.22).

Tang et al. (1994) specified an efficacy of 9% (CI 6%–13%) over 12 months. Po (1993) indicated an OR of 3.10 (CI 2.65–3.62) for a short period and 2.26 (CI 1.80–2.86) for a 12-month period. From this meta-analysis, we can conclude that the probability of lasting 1 year without smoking is doubled by using nicotine patches and other substitutes (Richmond, 1997). Nicotine chewing gum or patches are used, among other reasons, to reduce withdrawal symptoms. Patten and Martin (1996) provided a skeptical evaluation of the coherence between withdrawal symptoms and a higher probability of relapse in their review. One of the reasons the authors provided for the heterogeneous findings was problems in recording withdrawal symptoms; different assumptions were made for the corresponding criteria and the exact moment of recording. Reducing tobacco consumption gradually had no advantages compared with stopping abruptly (Silagy et al., 1999).

No randomized controlled studies have analyzed long-term abstinence from smoking using nicotine surrogates among patients with CHD. In an observation study on patients with risk factors for cardiac diseases, Basler, Brinkmeier, Buser, and Gluth (1992) achieved an abstinence rate of over 50% for a period of 1 year. The intervention used both group therapy methods and nicotine surrogates (chewing gum). Unlike other studies, this one did not involve people with acute cardiac events.

We also examined short-term abstinence for patients with CHD, covering periods from 2 to 24 weeks. In their randomized study, Tverdal, Thelle, Stensvold, Leren, and Bjartveit (1993) treated patients with patches containing either 14 milligrams or 21 milligrams of nicotine. They achieved an abstinence rate of 27% (14 of 52 subjects) after 2 weeks for the experimental group, whereas the control group achieved an abstinence rate of only 13% (7 of 54 subjects). The dosage was dependent on cigarette consumption, with higher dosages given to those who smoked more than 20 cigarettes a day. Patients in a study by the Working Group for the Study of Transdermal Nicotine in Patients With Coronary Artery Disease (Working Group, 1994) had the chance to increase the dose from 14 milligrams to 21 milligrams per day after 1 week, either by choice or because of a relapse. The control group had an abstinence rate of 21% (17 of 79 subjects) after 5 weeks, whereas the treatment group had an abstinence rate of 36% (28 of 77 subjects). Besides providing an educational interven-

tion, Joseph et al. (1996) also used nicotine patches to treat veterans with CHD who were discovered through a detailed medical history. Over 10 weeks, people received a dose of 21 milligrams per day for 6 weeks, then 14 milligrams per day for 2 weeks, and finally 7 milligrams per day for the last 2 weeks. After 14 weeks, 21% of former smokers in the treatment group and 9% in the control group were still not smoking. For the longest follow-up (24 weeks), abstinence from smoking decreased in the treatment group to 14% and increased in the control group to 11%. The meta-analysis showed that treatment with nicotine replacement therapy is more effective than treatment with a placebo (OR = 1.63, CI 1.12–2.37).

Some findings of individual case reports and clinical tests have reported negative effects of nicotine replacement on cardiovascular parameters or incidents. In their review, Benowitz and Gourlay (1997) listed 11 patients who experienced incidents during treatment. We summarize two of the cases as examples (see also Dacosta et al., 1993). Besides frequent side effects such as skin irritation and sleep disorders with high nicotine doses of 44 milligrams per day, P. A. Frederickson et al. (1995) reported a nonlethal myocardial infarction in one patient. It occurred in the 5th treatment week, 2 days after the dose was reduced from 44 mg to 22 mg per day. The patient received cardiac care during the study duration of 3 months and experienced no further complications. Ottervanger, Festen, de Vries, and Stricker (1995) also reported a myocardial infarction in a 39-year-old patient using nicotine patches. This patient's history did not indicate any organic cardiac abnormalities. His symptoms had been examined 2 years previously because of chest pains, and he consumed 50 to 100 cigarettes a day. Nicotine was replaced via a 21-milligram patch, and the cardiac event happened on the 20th day of treatment. After inpatient treatment, the patient had left-ventricular restricted blood flow. His performance and cardiac parameters were not limited in the long term.

The question of the causal influence of nicotine replacement therapy on cardiac death cannot be answered with these case descriptions. We found no systematic correlations (e.g., day of treatment, previous diseases). Furthermore, the documentation is not always sufficient for a comprehensive analysis. For example, smoking status during replacement therapy is documented only for some patients. We therefore examined and evaluated the following cardiac parameters in clinical and observation studies:

- *Influence of nicotine replacement on heart rate.* Keeley et al. (1996) showed that compared with a placebo spray, the administration of nicotine with a spray did not lead to a short-term change in heart rates. In this intraindividual design, the largest increase in heart rate was observed after inhaling cigarettes. Tzivoni et al. (1998) also reported no mean change in heart rate for people using nicotine patches. The findings of Tanus-Santos et al. (2001) for smokers with and without hypertension were similar. The findings of the Working Group (1994) suggested an increase in heart rate for the placebo group compared with the treatment group.
- *Influence of nicotine replacement on blood pressure.* Keeley et al. (1996) found no direct effect of nicotine sprays on blood pressure. Tzivoni et al. (1998) also found no significant change in blood pressure in subjects treated with nicotine patches (similar findings were reported by the Working Group, 1994). Smokers with hypertension also showed no short-term change in blood pressure after applying a nicotine patch (Tanus-Santos et al., 2001). However, nonhypertensive control group members showed a short-term increase in blood pressure independently of their smoking status.
- *Influence of nicotine replacement on other cardiac parameters.* Tzivoni et al. (1998) found no evidence of increased ischemic episodes or more frequent arrhythmia in patients under stress who were treated with nicotine patches compared with placebo, nor was the maximum cardiac capacity influenced by the treatment. The Working Group (1994) analyzed angina pectoris symptoms and found no differences between the treatment and placebo control groups. Furthermore, that study could not find any sys-

tematic differences for the parameters of tachycardia, arrhythmia, or ST-segment depression in the electrocardiogram.

- *Other side effects of nicotine replacement.* The studies we selected searched for other possible side effects of nicotine replacement therapy. Data were recorded with both the patients and the testing doctor blind, although we emphasize that it is difficult to achieve complete blinding, especially for nicotine replacement therapy with patches, because the size of the patches, and therefore of skin irritations, varies according to the dose. Patches caused skin irritation in about 20% to 30% of patients, whereas placebo patches caused irritation in only about half that number (Lewis, Piasecki, Fiore, Anderson, & Baker; 1998; Working Group, 1994). To try and maintain the blinding, patients were instructed to place the patch in a different place every day to avoid skin irritation (see Joseph et al., 1996).

Contrary to expectations, the Working Group (1994) study resulted in a substantially higher dropout rate in the placebo group. Beside medical indications (e.g., side effects), this result is possibly ascribable to the patients' desire for treatment, which would necessitate deblinding. Also contrary to their hypothesis, the Working Group reported greater weight gain among the treatment group than the placebo group.

Thus, there are single case reports of manifest coronary events while using nicotine replacements. It should not be concluded, however, that nicotine replacement for patients with CHD is problematic in general (see Arnaot, 1995). A doctor should always perform a continuous observation, and there should be no additional consumption of cigarettes during the replacement period (for a case description, see Dacosta et al., 1993). Any potential complications should receive immediate attention.

The consumption of cigarettes during the treatment is a problem in nicotine replacement. Abstinence rates of 10% to 20% suggest that most people continue smoking, and even many patients with CHD do not take the recommendation to stop smoking seriously. The small alterations in cardiological parameters with nicotine replacement suggest that the side effects are due to the consumption of cigarettes rather than to the treatment (see Benowitz & Gourlay, 1997).

According to the American College of Cardiology and American Heart Association (2002) guidelines, replacement therapy should not take place during the phase immediately after an MI or cardiac event (see also Lewis et al., 1998). An exception is when the patient suffers intense withdrawal symptoms (see Spinler et al., 2001). Relatively small sample size is a problem in studies that examine side effects. Because of the infrequency of cardiovascular changes (only about 10% to 20% of people report side effects), large samples are necessary to perform a detailed analysis of side effects, and studies to date have not achieved sufficient sample sizes. Larger scale application tests are also required. In addition, an integrative evaluation of the efficacy (i.e., abstinence from tobacco use and subsequent lower morbidity and mortality; see section 3.4) and possible long-term costs (i.e., because of higher morbidity due to treatment) of nicotine replacement remains to be done.

3.6.8. Psychopharmacological Treatment

We examined studies evaluating two types of medication for their effect on withdrawal from smoking: anxiolytics and antidepressants. Anxiolytics are not as effective for smoking cessation as antidepressants (see Hughes, Stead, & Lancaster, 1999), which several studies have proved to be effective in promoting smoking cessation. Hughes, Stead, and Lancaster (2002) examined five substance groups, two of which proved to be effective. Nortriptyline was tested in four studies and was superior to a placebo treatment (with or without nicotine replacement; OR = 2.77, CI 1.73–4.44). In seven comparison studies, the atypical antidepressant bupropion was effective in treating smokers; significantly more people in the treatment group were still not smoking after 6 to 12 months (OR = 2.54, CI 1.90–3.41). Selective serotonin reuptake inhibitors, the monoamine oxidase inhibitors, and serotonin–noradrenaline reuptake inhibitors did

not prove effective in placebo-controlled studies (Hughes et al., 2002).

The side effects of nicotine replacement in combination with bupropion and nortriptyline have been comprehensively analyzed in case studies (Lineberry, Peters, & Bostwick, 2001; Pederson, Kuntz, & Garbe, 2001) and clinical studies. Because of its side effects profile, particularly cardiac side effects such as arrhythmia and hypertension, the U.S. Department of Health and Human Services classified nortriptyline as a second-choice drug (U.S. Department of Health and Human Services, 2000). Its use on patients with CHD disease is therefore not recommended. T. L. Wenger, Cohn, and Bustrack (1983) reported finding only small changes in the electrocardiograms of depressive patients treated with bupropion compared with amitriptyline (see also T. L. Wenger & Stern, 1983). In their analysis comparing nortriptyline and bupropion, Kiev et al. (1994) concluded that treatment with bupropion had substantially less influence on cardiac parameters and that it can therefore be used by patients with CHD.

Roose et al. (1987) conducted studies on depressive patients with cardiac disease, analyzing the effect of imipramine and bupropion on cardiac insufficiency. The authors found no clinically relevant changes in the 10 people tested using either substance. A second study included patients with cardiac insufficiencies, atrioventricular block, and arrhythmias (Roose et al., 1991). Although they found statistically significant increases in blood pressure for all 35 participants (mean changes ranged from 1 to 5 mmHg), the authors interpreted this result as not clinically relevant. Of more concern was the number of patients who had to stop using the medication because of complications; four had to stop because of cardiac problems (mainly hypertension), although three of these had a complete remission of the symptoms after a short time. For this reason, the U.S. Department of Health and Human Services (2000) suggested that the blood pressure of patients treated with bupropion be monitored.

Case reports forced the manufacturer of bupropion to give warnings about the risk of epileptic seizures (rate of 1 per 1,000 applications). The antidepressant dose of 450 milligrams used in Roose et al.'s (1987, 1991) studies was higher than that used in clinical studies for withdrawal from smoking; most used 300 milligrams as the highest dose (see Jorenby et al., 1999), which is the maximum dose recommended by the manufacturer for smoking cessation. The question of whether using bupropion leads to augmented suicidal thoughts and acts is still being examined (see Poethko-Müller, 2002). Because of current uncertainty about side effects, bupropion should not be used until after the appraisal is done and recommendations made to ensure that patients are not endangered needlessly.

3.6.9. Other Methods and Intervention Principles

3.6.9.1. Hypnosis. Abbot, Stead, White, Barnes, and Ernst (1998) showed no systematic effects in their review of the efficacy of hypnotherapy in smoking cessation; studies by Holroyd (1991) likewise showed no effect. Mittag and Ohm (1992) performed hypnosis as part of inpatient treatment of cardiac patients. The 22 participants suffered from CHD or arterial occlusive disease and were all smokers averaging 40 cigarettes per day before the heart attack. A maximum of 10 sessions took place with each patient, with an average duration of 15 to 20 minutes. During the trance, the patients received suggestions intended to strengthen their willpower or were encouraged to use self-praise about their achievements in giving up smoking. The intervention was very effective in the short term (success rate about 80%), but at 12 months only 8 patients remained abstinent from smoking, and 4 continued to smoke. A conservative estimate is that 50% of those treated with hypnosis successfully gave up smoking. However, comprehensive studies are required before conclusions can be drawn about the efficacy of this method.

3.6.9.2. Contract management. D. K. Wilson, Wallston, and King (1990) analyzed the effect of designing a behavior contract for people with cardiac complaints. The contract, to last a predetermined period of between 1 and 12 weeks, was made during a counseling interview. Achieved goals were rewarded with previously defined reinforcers. The wording of the contract was varied experimentally; some referred to the reward alone, and others also included reference to loss of that reward. There was no significant main effect of this experimental variation. However, there were significant interaction effects between the wish to give up smoking and self-efficacy expectations. Highly motivated people benefited more from a contract with a reward alone, whereas people with low motivation benefited more from a contract providing both reward and loss. People with high self-efficacy also profited more from a contract with both gain and loss. There are no randomized controlled studies of the efficacy of behavior contracts. However, because the method is also important for goal definition, the question regarding efficacy is secondary.

3.6.9.3. Aversive methods. Aversive methods for smoking cessation are based on assumptions from learning theories. Examples of aversive methods include fast puffing (noninhalation) culminating in the use of electric shocks and imaginative methods, where smoking is associated with negative images. Because of the wide range of interventions that are labeled as aversive treatment methods and the comparatively small samples (Hajek & Stead, 1997), the efficacy of the individual methods cannot be described. Fast smoking was effective compared with an attentiveness placebo group (OR = 2.08, CI 1.39–3.12). Other aversive methods analyzed to date have shown no positive effect on abstinence from smoking (OR = 1.19, CI 0.77–1.88).

The important factor in smoking cessation is the strength of the aversion. The more aversive a method is, the more effective it is in promoting abstinence from smoking (OR = 1.66, CI 1.00–2.78). However, statistical relevance was only just reached. There have been no controlled studies of the use of this smoking cessation method with patients with CHD, perhaps because a short-term (involuntary) abstinence from smoking is already achieved by the cardiac event, and this method would therefore be used at the wrong moment.

3.6.9.4. Confrontation with the negative consequences of smoking.

Confrontational media and fear-inducing messages (see J. Barth & Bengel, 1997) are a part of health education about the harmful consequences of smoking for CHD patients (Trost, 1995; see the theoretical review by J. Barth & Bengel, 2000). In a study by R. R. Scott et al. (1990), participants were confronted with information about the carbon monoxide concentration of their exhalation and its consequences. This intervention had no effect on abstinence from smoking. The authors explained this finding by noting the relatively long elapsed time of 6 years between the first heart attack and the intervention.

3.6.9.5. Acupuncture.

Acupuncture is defined as treatment with needle stings on the surface of certain body regions, known as acupuncture points. Acupuncture points are found on the ear, the face, and the upper body. Normally the needles are kept in position for between 15 and 20 minutes. Electroacupuncture stimulates the acupuncture points with electricity. As an alternative or in addition to the traditional use of needles, manufactured "permanent" needles may be used that are normally fixed in the ear for a few days with the help of a medical patch. The patients are instructed to press on the needle if they feel withdrawal symptoms. As an alternative to needles, it is also possible to fix small grains on the ear with the help of patches or to introduce surgical stitches into the earlobe and knot them with a pearl (see A. R. White, Rampes, & Ernst, 1999).

Controlled studies have provided no proof of the efficacy of acupuncture on smoking cessation (see White et al., 1999). A study of the efficacy of acupuncture in treating CHD (Baillie, Mattick, Hall, & Webster, 1994) was also unable to show an effect.

3.6.9.6. Psychodynamic interventions.

Psychodynamic interventions play a subordinate part in smoking cessation, and so far there are no meta-analyses available regarding their efficacy. To date, one randomized controlled study described patients with CHD treated in group therapy. Mitsibounas et al. (1992) reported very good results using both the conservative (OR = 18, CI 3.10–104.54) and the optimistic models (OR =

20.80, CI 3.45–125.30). However, this study was of low methodological quality (e.g., a heavy selection bias), and therefore its generalizability is considerably limited.

3.7. SUMMARY AND DISCUSSION OF FINDINGS

A heart attack is associated with substantial psychological burdens (e.g., fear, worries about the future) and with intense physical symptoms, such as pain. For these reasons, heart attacks often have consequences for withdrawal from smoking. The cardiac event may motivate not only changes in health behavior, but also modification of underlying attitudes and behavior patterns. Studies have shown that people in control groups (who receive standard treatment) also make considerable changes to their way of life and tobacco use. In control groups, rates of abstinence in the primary studies ranged between 35% and 45% over about 12 months. Thus, interventions for cessation of smoking address only about 60% of patients, who a priori have rather low motivation to change their smoking behavior. Hence, even elaborate interventions achieved an increase in abstinence rates of only 45% to 55%. However, compared with studies on the general population, this rate is very high. Without a cardiac event, most intervention studies achieve an abstinence rate of only 10% to 20%.

Most people who experience a heart attack are over 40 years old, and many may already have tried to stop smoking in the past. This previous experience has two main consequences. On the one hand, these people have already been through the withdrawal phase and know the negative experiences associated with it. On the other hand, those particular experiences can influence current expectations for success, so a new attempt to give up smoking should involve an intensive analysis of former strategies.

Depression is connected with unfavorable coping strategies, and patients may increase their tobacco consumption to regulate their emotions (see Herrmann-Lingen & Buss, 2002; chap. 5, this volume). For patients who have had a heart attack, Wray, Herzog, Willis, and Wallace (1998) showed that continuing smokers were more depressed compared with nonsmokers or successfully abstinent people (bivariate results). However, they included no psychosocial dimensions in their integrative regression model of predictors of smoking cessation. Huijbrechts et al. (1996) also described increased depression and increased state anxiety for continuing smokers compared with abstainers. The explanation may be that continuing smokers were regulating their emotions by consuming tobacco, but the study description is insufficient to evaluate whether this was the case. Current epidemiological studies have found an independent correlation between tobacco consumption and increased suicidal thoughts and actions (see M. Miller, Hemenway, Bell, Yore, & Amoroso, 2000). Further research on the correlation between depressive disorders and CHD is essential (see Heßlinger et al., 2002).

The severity of CHD (e.g., the number of affected vessels) has not consistently shown an effect on abstinence from tobacco use. Some studies have found such a correlation (e.g., J. K. Ockene et al., 1992), but others have not (e.g., K. A. Perkins, 1988). In an observational study with patients who had had heart attacks, Havik and Maeland (1988) showed that the severity of the disease decreased the risk for a relapse among smokers who abstained from tobacco use.

People who suffer a cardiac event may differ in specific ways from the general population. Wray and colleagues (1998) reported on the influence of education on the probability of smoking cessation after a heart attack. Although the attack itself had a significant influence, the victim's education also had an interactive effect. They found an OR of 1.44 for smoking cessation among heart attack patients with more education compared with those with less education. There is also evidence of better study compliance in patients with more education. In Coronary Artery Smoking Intervention Study (CASIS; Rosal et al., 1998), ability to reach the patient at follow-up correlated with more education; it is unknown if those not reached by follow-up had a higher relapse rate.

Some interventions addressed aspects of the social environment (e.g., partner, work) as well as individual parameters (e.g., disposition to change) in

promoting smoking cessation (see the overview by Fuchs & Schwarzer, 1997; Schwarzer, 1996). A person's social environment is important for both initiating and changing a risk behavior. Carey et al. (1989) found a positive effect of social support in their review of the abstinence rates of people who stopped smoking without an intervention. They speculated that it may be easier to cope with withdrawal when social support is available. The partner's support is especially important during both the intention-building and the withdrawal phases. The term *social support* is therefore slightly inappropriate; the social control exercised by the partner is also important. Havik and Maeland (1988) showed that heart attack patients with more conflictual partnerships relapsed earlier after a phase of abstinence from tobacco.

The transtheoretical model of change has also been used to promote smoking cessation. Prochaska and DiClemente (1986) described the stages in building intentions to change and in operationalizing health behavior changes. These stages include precontemplation, contemplation, preparation, action, and maintenance. Implicit in this model is that a change of attitude is a process. Rumpf, Meyer, Hapke, Dilling, and John (1998) conducted a cross-sectional analysis of these phases with smokers in a German city. Most people were in the phase of precontemplation (76%) or contemplation (17%). Only 6% of current smokers were in the preparation phase. According to this study, the motivational disposition of the general population for a change in tobacco consumption is low. Therefore, besides abstinence from smoking, interventions could also have the objective of developing patients' motivation to contemplate changing their tobacco consumption.

Phase-specific intervention techniques have been developed, but most studies have observed only the process of behavior modification. The stages of change model was used descriptively in the CASIS study (J. K. Ockene et al., 1992; Rosal et al., 1998), but they differentiated only the phases of precontemplation, contemplation, and disposition to change. Kristeller, Rossi, Ockene, Goldberg, and Prochaska (1992) found no differences between the cognitive and behavioral smoking cessation strategies used by patients with CHD and the general population (e.g., stimulus control, increased health awareness). Furthermore, the CASIS study (Rosal et al., 1998) showed that people not reached at follow-up were more often in the stage of contemplation and less often in the stage of action. The effectiveness of stage-related interventions has recently been discussed critically (see Riemsma, Pattenden, Bridle, Sowden, & Mather, 2003).

As we discussed in section 3.6, measures for smoking cessation appear to be effective if one uses the optimistic model to estimate their effects. However, if the conservative model is used and limited to studies of high quality, no statistically significant effect is shown. Which of these results is the more accurate? The answer may lie between the optimistic and conservative estimates. Successful cessation of smoking leads to an improvement of clinical parameters (morbidity and mortality). The success of an intervention is unpredictable in individual cases; only about 1 in 10 patients benefits from a comprehensive intervention. Nevertheless, it should be standard procedure for doctors, psychologists, nurses, and other information distributors working in cardiac rehabilitation to discuss the risk factor of smoking and to recommend a smoking withdrawal measure to reduce the risk of cardiac disease.

Trost (1995) interviewed former smokers with cardiac problems about their withdrawal strategies. Seventy-five percent used candies, chocolate, or similar substitutes. Nine percent used nicotine replacement patches or chewing gum. Available studies used mainly structured interventions administered by professionals (e.g., doctors, nurses)

while also encouraging patients' potential for self-help and providing additional self-help materials.

However, cardiological rehabilitation mostly uses multimodal interventions that combine several of the strategies mentioned in section 3.6 (Allen, 1996; Burt et al., 1974; DeBusk et al., 1994; Erdman & Duivenvoorden, 1983; Fridlund et al., 1991; Hedbäck & Perk, 1987; Lisspers et al., 1999; J. K. Ockene et al., 1992; Rigotti et al., 1994; Rosal et al., 1998; Sivarajan et al., 1983; C. B. Taylor et al., 1990). The results are inconclusive as to whether the choice and use of specific strategies is important and whether causation, or only a correlation, exists between dose and effect. The use of nicotine replacement has proved to be effective both for the general population and for patients with CHD, but a conclusive evaluation of the effects and side effects of therapy with bupropion has yet to be conducted.

There are convincing meta-analyses that show the efficacy of measures to promote smoking cessation. This chapter considered only efficacy studies, but proof of the practicability and applicability in everyday clinical life (effectiveness) is also important. The studies that used carefully selected populations generated interesting results, but their generalizability is limited. A loss approaching 50% from the population of potential study participants who satisfy the inclusion criteria is problematic; some studies do not even describe their selection criteria. The question arises as to how the other half of the patients can be treated or which interventions are indicated for patients with multiple morbidities.

CHAPTER 4

PSYCHOSOCIAL INTERVENTIONS TO INFLUENCE PHYSICAL INACTIVITY AS A RISK FACTOR: THEORETICAL MODELS AND PRACTICAL EVIDENCE

Wolfgang Schlicht, Martina Kanning, and Klaus Bös

4.1. INTRODUCTION

More than 200 years ago, the medical doctor William Heberden (1710–1801) observed the beneficial effect of physical activity as therapy for coronary heart disease (CHD). In a presentation in 1772, Heberden gave an account of a patient suffering from angina pectoris who forced himself to chop wood for 30 minutes every day (cited in Krasemann, 1990). Heberden deemed this a suitable therapy for the treatment of the symptoms, in addition to bloodletting and purging.

Almost 180 years passed before the effects of physical exercise on cardiac insufficiency and other forms of CHD were explored systematically and physical therapy finally became standard in the therapy and rehabilitation of CHD patients. From a physiological standpoint, the goal of physical therapy interventions is to compensate for the reduction in physical capacity caused by heart disease. Physical exercise triggers adaptive metabolic and hemodynamic processes and central and cardiac adaptation. These physiological adjustments, as well as the associated importance of physical exercise during the rehabilitation and secondary prevention of cardiovascular diseases, have already been sufficiently discussed by various authors (e.g., American College of Sports Medicine, 1995; American Heart Association, 1990; Bouchard, Shephard, Stephens, Sutton, & McPherson, 1994; see also the detailed overview by Weidemann & Meyer, 1991). Thus, physical therapy is commonly regarded as empirically established in the context of rehabilitation and secondary prevention, and physical activity is seen as having a preventative effect and as decreasing the risk of morbidity and mortality.

According to a report from the U.S. Department of Health and Human Services (1998), there is no room for doubt that physical inactivity is a causal factor in cardiovascular illnesses; that correspondingly, increased activity lowers coronary risk; and finally, that physical exercise promotes the rehabilitation of patients with CHD. At the same time, the report noted that only one fifth of all CHD patients for whom physical exercise would be desirable do, in fact, become physically active.

Current epidemiological research shows that unlike smoking, for example, inactivity does not represent a dramatic morbidity and mortality risk when a coronary condition is present. For physically inactive persons, the literature describes a risk that is approximately 1.2 to 1.5 times that for physically active persons (see Blair et al., 1995; K. E. Powell, Thompson, Caspersen, & Kendrick, 1987). Physical inactivity is, however, a type of behavior with a substantial lifetime prevalence. This is valid for primary as well as for secondary prevention.

Preventive intervention is not the topic of this chapter; extensive publications on this subject are readily available (see Bouchard et al., 1994; Fuchs, 1997; Rost, 1998), and meta-analyses (Knoll, 1997; Schlicht, 1994, 1996) have shown that there is no consistent general health-related effect of exercise and that such an effect can be verified only after considering a number of moderating variables (e.g., age, sex, type and intensity of physical activity).

This chapter also does not deal with the physiological effects and adaptations caused by physical exercise; these have been treated sufficiently in sports medicine publications, which have demonstrated not only the clinically negative consequences of physical inactivity but also the implied importance of physical training in appropriate doses.

This chapter explores the reasons for physical inactivity and the potential means to influence these factors in the context of secondary prevention and rehabilitation. Section 4.2 discusses physical activity as it relates to cardiac risk. Section 4.3 reviews the important concepts of motivation to initiate regular physical activity and adherence to this activity once begun, and section 4.4 outlines theoretical models of health-related behavior. Section 4.5 describes strategies for promoting physical activity in persons experiencing CHD risk. Finally, section 4.6 summarizes some conclusions that can be drawn from the current literature.

4.2. PHYSICAL ACTIVITY

This chapter discusses physical activity or exercise, but not sports. This distinction is important because sports are most often associated with competition or high performance. Exercise includes activities such as gardening, cycling, walking, and so on. *Physical activity* is defined as any behavior that elevates energy expenditure in a significant manner. *Exercise therapy* is viewed as a diagnosis-specific intervention implemented in accordance with medical and sports science that is intended to trigger physiological, psychological, and social processes.

Further differentiations concerning the activity discussed in this chapter are necessary. Inpatient cardiological rehabilitation clinics normally have patients participate in supervised exercise therapy that is specifically adapted to their particular disease (for further details, see, e.g., Huonker, 2002). Following subsequent treatment (Phase 2 rehabilitation), which in Germany is also carried out on an inpatient basis, patients can join an outpatient cardiac exercise group (Phase 3 rehabilitation) that offers physical exercise training at various intensities depending on the patient's needs (see Brusis &

Weber-Falkensammer, 1999; C. Halhuber, 1984; Kempf, Reuß, & Brusis, 2000). Phase 4 rehabilitation consists of activity without supervision that patients choose themselves and that, done correctly, becomes part of a healthy way of life (see Grande & Badura, 2001).

4.2.1. Inactivity and Physical Activity

Inactivity and physical activity seem to be opposite sides of a contradictory phenomenon in modern society. Many people say that they exercise, but the number of people who are, in fact, physically active on a regular basis is far too small from a health sciences point of view. In the United States, for example, only about 40% of the adult population is physically active even in a very broad sense of the term (U.S. Department of Health and Human Services, 1999). Few data are available for Germany, and representative studies have been conducted only sporadically. Mensink (2002) found that about a third of the adults they questioned were physically active, a proportion that is comparable to that of the U.S. population.

4.2.2. Physical Activity and Cardiac Risk Reduction

Inactivity is a health risk that has a negative influence on the pathogenesis of CHD. That physical activity leads to a reduction in both general mortality and cardiovascular mortality has been reported time and again in relevant publications (see Huonker, 2002). For example, Blair et al. (1995) reported on a cohort study of 9,777 men whose physical capacity was measured twice at an average interval of 4.9 years. Men who exhibited a level of fitness at both measuring occasions showed the least mortality risk at the second measurement. This study also found a decreased mortality rate among formerly inactive men who had taken up exercising before the second measurement and reached a certain degree of fitness. They reduced their risk by almost half (44%).

A reduction in cardiac risk can be achieved with a relatively small increase in activity. One of the most frequently quoted epidemiological studies highlighted the positive effect of a low dosage of activity: On a sample of about 10,000 Harvard alumni, Paffenbarger, Hyde, Wing, and Hsieh (1986) showed that moderately intensive activity such as walking (6 miles a week) reduced the relative coronary mortality risk by about 0.07 and climbing stairs (36 floors a week) by about 0.34. In the *New England Journal of Medicine,* Manson et al. (1999) reported on a study of 72,488 healthy nurses (no CHD, no cancer), who were first interviewed at between 40 and 65 years of age and followed up at regular intervals over 8 years. In the course of the study, the sample experienced 645 cardiac incidents, 170 of which were fatal. The results demonstrated an inverse connection between moderate physical activity (walking) or intensive exercise and the relative risk of a cardiac incident. As exercise increased in intensity, there was a relative reduction in risk. Intensity was measured in metabolic units (MET) as the rate of energy expenditure. Manson et al. calculated accumulated energy consumption as MET hours per week. In the group with an average intensity of 0.8 MET hours per week, there were 178 cardiac incidents (relative risk 1.00), whereas in the group with 35.4 MET hours per week, there were 89 (relative risk 0.46). Like Blair et al. (1995), Manson et al. proved that even a late entrance into an active lifestyle has a risk-reducing effect. They also showed that the positive effect of an active lifestyle is not reduced by other risk factors (e.g., smoking, obesity, genetic factors).

Ainsworth et al. (2000) listed physical activities and their absolute intensity in MET. Dishwashing, cooking, stretching, and playing miniature golf, for example, use 3 MET. Light to moderate activities, of interest for the purposes of this chapter, include riding a bike (e.g., to work), climbing stairs, and walking rapidly (4–7 km/h) and range from 3 to 6 MET. Measures of intensity do not reflect physical strain, which is to be regarded as a serious barrier to activity both for middle-aged and older people and for people with a cardiac disease. Nevertheless, they are a barrier, as shown by the high prevalence rates for inactivity among CHD patients and CHD risk groups. There is as yet no conclusive evidence for a consistent dose–effect relationship in physical activity. It is possible that independent of a defined duration and intensity of activity, the energy expenditure per week alone is responsible for risk reduction.

Even though available meta-analyses do not describe the physical activity of study interventions in detail and thus fail to provide information on the accumulated energy consumption, they do point to the fact that especially for CHD patients, exercise-based cardiac rehabilitation can lead to a 20% to 24% reduction in both general and cardiovascular mortality (see, e.g., O'Connor et al., 1989; Oldridge, Guyatt, Fischer, & Rimm, 1988; see also the compilation of meta-analyses in Franklin, Bonzheim, Gordon, & Timmis, 1998). A recent meta-analysis by Dusseldorp, van Elderen, Maes, Meulman, and Kraaij (1999) of 37 studies showed a 34% reduction in cardiovascular mortality and a decrease in the reinfarction rate of about 29%. Only 12 of the studies included in the analysis integrated exercise into the intervention measures, however. Interventions typically included stress management or health education, which are also currently considered necessary for comprehensive cardiac rehabilitation. This meta-analysis reveals an interpretation dilemma pointed out by Kollenbaum (1990) 15 years ago: No study proves beyond doubt that exercise therapy significantly improves the rate of survival, because it is impossible to completely rule out the confounding effects of other interventions.

Exercise therapy was not implemented as the sole intervention in any of the studies because it has always been merely one part of a standardized rehabilitation program that also includes educational interventions (see Langosch, Budde, & Linden, 2003). One of the few exceptions is the study by Blumenthal et al. (1997), who investigated the influence of stress management or exercise therapy on recovery from myocardial ischemic injury. They separated 136 patients into two intervention groups (assigned randomly), one that learned stress management techniques and one that participated in an exercise intervention, and they contrasted both groups with a no-treatment control group (not assigned randomly). The group that learned stress management techniques significantly reduced their relative risk of a cardiac incident compared with the control group. Although the exercise group also had a reduced relative risk, neither the difference between the control group and the intervention group nor the differences between the two intervention groups were significant.

Table W4.1 (see the accompanying Web site: http://www.apa.org/books/resources/jordan/) lists studies that examined the effects of cardiac rehabilitation both on morbidity and mortality and on health behavior or psychological variables (see the accompanying Web site). We used no systematic research strategy in selecting studies for inclusion in the table, but we believe it features the most important studies of recent years. The studies, most of all those with higher grades of evidence, demonstrated almost unanimously that cardiac rehabilitation interventions have positive effects on illness-related endpoints (morbidity and mortality), on health behavior, and on psychological variables.

Modifying behavior and health-relevant physical parameters (e.g., blood pressure, cholesterol, triglycerides) is typically thought of as requiring a comprehensive course of rehabilitation that encompasses medical care, exercise therapy, and psychoeducational interventions under professional guidance or supervision. In contrast, Jolliffe et al. (2001) suggested that "exercise-only" rehabilitation is effective in reducing mortality risk, calling into question whether extensive rehabilitation is better for patients than physical activity alone. They found that an exercise-only program reduced cardiovascular mortality 31% (and general mortality 27%), compared with 26% (and 13%) for comprehensive rehabilitation. The study had some methodological problems. For example, the sample was mainly male and middle aged and had low cardiac risk. The authors did not control for possible confounding variables, and it is not clear whether the participants in the exercise-only rehabilitation were randomly assigned or decided themselves to engage in an active lifestyle. This inability to attribute risk reduction to specific variables and the resulting uncertainty about the influence of exercise training on the manifestation and reversibility of CHD has been criticized by other authors (e.g., American Heart Association, 1990; Bjarnason-Wehrens, Kretschmann, Lang, & Rost, 1998; Kollenbaum, 1990).

For most studies, the endpoints of interest were mortality and morbidity; others were more interested in objective physical capacity. Few studies described the benefits of fitness from the subjective viewpoint of the persons affected, so a patient-oriented view of physical activity was insufficiently represented.

Exercise also holds some risk for people with coronary diseases. Studies have shown this risk to be as low as or lower than the risk of sudden death for joggers (see Bartels, 2002). In older studies, 1 death occurred in approximately 120,000 course hours of the outpatient cardiac exercise group (Krasemann & Traenckner, 1989; Laubinger & Krasemann, 1995). Kindermann (2005) defined *sudden cardiac death* as an unexpected death caused by a heart attack. For joggers, the risk is 1 in 15,000 per year. Kallio (1985) reported about 1 death in 250,000 exercise hours. In a more recent study, Unverdorben et al. (1996) found a death rate of 1 in 750,000 exercise hours. In his retrospective analysis, 903 outpatient cardiac rehabilitation patients and 144 doctors responded to a questionnaire about the incidence and type of cardiac complaints. The results indicated that the occurrence of cardiovascular incidents was comparable to that for healthy athletes. Convincing and reliable data on the risk involved in exercise therapy for CHD patients have yet to be produced.

If one relies exclusively on the recommendations of evidence-based medicine, the effect of exercise therapy cannot be proved without doubt. It would be foolish, however, to reject its value on this basis. Inactivity is most probably a risk factor, and physical activity most probably reduces this risk. The same can be said about aggressive invasive treatment of CHD; Grande, Schott, and Badura (1996) observed that it has not been proved that invasive treatments such as percutaneous transluminal coronary angioplasty are superior to conservative treatments (e.g., medication, lifestyle change). Yet refusing to provide invasive treatments would certainly be seen as professional incompetence. In addition, exercise most probably leads to additional benefits not only in health-relevant outcome variables but also in psychological variables (e.g., well-being, quality of life), which in turn may influence other habits or behaviors (e.g., smoking, overconsumption of high-fat foods).

The American College of Cardiology has categorized inactivity as a secondary risk factor that if lowered, like overweight and blood sugar, probably reduces coronary risk (see Fuster & Pearson, 1999). Although a connection between physical inactivity and CHD has been suggested by several studies involving several samples, what is missing in order to define physical inactivity as primary risk factor is consistent evidence of a definite dose–response relationship. Prospective, controlled, and randomized intervention studies with different samples are needed that prove that an increase in physical activity to a defined quantity will most probably lead to a reduction in morbidity and mortality for CHD patients compared with a physically inactive lifestyle.

For the purposes of this chapter, we accept physical inactivity as a secondary risk factor and assume accordingly that almost all CHD patients, provided that there are no contraindications, should undergo exercise therapy. How, then, can patients be motivated to initiate a physically active lifestyle, and how can they be encouraged to adhere to this activity on a long-term basis?

4.3. MOTIVATION AND ADHERENCE

Many people who begin an exercise regimen become inactive again. Compliance with health-promoting and risk-reducing behaviors is low. The pertinent literature uses the term *adherence* instead of *compliance* in regard to exercise to differentiate this activity from a behavior prescribed by a doctor (e.g., taking medications; Dishman, 1993). The term *adherence* has not been used uniformly in the literature; in this chapter we use Dubbert, Rappaport, and Martin's (1987) definition of *adherence* as fulfillment of a predetermined goal. Exercise-related goals are established by doctors or by organizations such as the U.S. Department of Health and Human Services and the American College of Sports Medicine, so the distinction between *adherence* and *compliance*, which means to follow a predetermined course, is easily blurred. In the following section, we will use *adherence* in a wider sense and discuss several studies that examined the adherence of CHD patients to a supervised exercise program or the relapse of such patients from active behavior to inactive behavior.

4.3.1. Method

We undertook a systematic examination of the literature to search for answers to the question of how to promote patient motivation and adherence to exercise therapy. We located studies in the reference lists of pertinent magazines; in reviews, bibliographies, and collections, such as consensus conferences; through abstract services; and through online database searches in Medline, PsycINFO, and PSYNDEXplus. We used search terms individually and in logical connections, including *adherence/compliance*, *lifestyle*, *motivation*, *myocardial and/or coronary heart disease*, and *rehabilitation*. We restricted the search to the years after 1976.

We selected 42 studies for our analysis and evaluated them according to the grading system of the Agency for Health Care Research and Quality (1995; C. M. Clancy, 1997). The methodological quality of many of the studies was rather weak; common faults included missing data on the validity of exercise variables, a one-group-only design with convenience samples, and a lack of statistical validity.

4.3.2. Findings on Motivation and Adherence

The empirical studies we selected to examine participation and dropout rates in exercise therapy are listed in Table W4.2. (See the accompanying Web site. Because these studies also investigated the determinants of dropout or the physical effects of intervention programs, some are also listed in Tables W4.1 and W4.3.)

Although coronary patients are well aware of their health-related risk, their dropout rates are similar to those of primary preventative programs and behaviors. In Germany, 59% to 98% of patients who have had surgery for a coronary condition undergo rehabilitation (see Grande & Badura, 2001), but only 50% of U.S. patients participate in Phase 1 and Phase 2 rehabilitation programs (see Cooper, Lloyd, Weinman, & Jackson, 1999). Dropout from rehabilitation is delayed in Germany; only 20% to 30% of rehabilitated patients join an outpatient cardiac exercise group (Phase 3 rehabilitation), even though, with almost 6,000 such groups, Germany has almost an oversupply (see Deutsche Gesellschaft für Prävention und Rehabilitation, 2002). After 6 to 7 months, about 30% of participants who join a cardiac exercise group leave. Efforts to inspire long-lasting motivation in chronically ill patients to do more exercise do not seem to be working. Rugulies and Siegrist (1999) saw one reason as lack of tutoring support and care, which makes it impossible for patients to transfer the exercise behavior they learned during rehabilitation successfully into their everyday lives.

The problem of motivating patients to engage in physical activity by participating in an outpatient cardiac exercise group has been addressed several times by Budde and Keck (Budde, 1999; Budde, Grün, & Keck, 1988, 1993; Budde & Keck, 1996; Keck & Budde, 1999). These authors' intervention concentrated on motivating patients in Phases 1 and 2 of cardiac rehabilitation to join an outpatient cardiac exercise group. They were able to motivate patients covered by worker's public health insurance—who normally are hard to motivate—to join an outpatient cardiac exercise group. The intervention was an integral part of the health education provided by the entire therapeutic team. It helped patients overcome access barriers to participation in an outpatient cardiac exercise group by involving relatives, providing contact addresses, and giving concrete information about the groups. Participation in an outpatient cardiac exercise group was not the only aim of the program; it also promoted healthy attitudes and lifestyles. Budde and Keck (1999) reported on a prospective study of 1,504 patients (see also Tables W4.2 and W4.3) of outpatient cardiac exercise group participation 4 years after their release from Phase 2 rehabilitation. About half of these patients still attended the heart group.

Hillebrand, Frodermann, Lehr, and Wirth (1995) investigated the effect of an outpatient treatment (Phase 2) following discharge from rehabilitation to promote participation in an outpatient cardiac exercise group by public health insurance patients. The patients were randomized into an intervention group ($n = 46$) and a control group ($n = 41$). The intervention group patients were con-

tacted four times in the following year. The first interview took place before discharge from the clinic; the following interviews were carried out either by telephone or during a home visit after 1, 3, and 6 months. The goals of the intervention were to assess and record patients' current health behaviors, to discuss any difficulties they had in transferring the health-supportive measures they learned in rehabilitation to everyday life, and to work out individual solutions to problems. Patients were also informed about health education, self-help, or psychosocial counseling programs near their homes. The intervention group showed a significantly higher participation rate of 57%, compared with 27% in the control group, and the authors characterized this treatment as a connecting link between Phase 2 and Phase 3 rehabilitation. Castro, King, and Brassington (2001) reported similar success with home-based programs and telephone reminders in the United States.

4.3.3. Reasons for Participation in and Dropout From Exercise Therapy

The relapse rate alone does not explain why patients drop out of exercise therapy. Patients with cardiac disease often reduce their already limited physical activity even more for fear of exacerbating their symptoms (e.g., angina pectoris). Studies have indicated that patients may internalize the recommendations of professional advisers but are unsure how to apply stress reduction and physical activity to the management of their own illness (see U. Frank, 2000).

The Framingham Disability Study (Pinsky, Jette, Branch, Kannel, & Feinleib, 1990) examined the fears of 2,576 men and women between 55 and 88 years of age. CHD patients were more likely than healthy persons to report that they were unable to exercise because of fear of negative consequences. Within the CHD group, such fears were stronger in women and in elderly persons.

Table W4.3 lists subjective and objective factors that discriminate among active and inactive CHD patients and patients who started exercising but became inactive again. The studies listed in the table identify variables that encourage and discourage participation in exercise that can be grouped into more external and more internal reasons; Table 4.1

TABLE 4.1

Matrix of Internal and External Factors That Enhance and Hinder Participation in Physical Activity in the Rehabilitation and Secondary Prevention of Coronary Heart Disease

Locus of control	Factors that enhance participation in exercise	Factors that hinder participation in exercise
Internal	Positive outcome expectations	Lack of interest and motivation to exercise
	Perception of activity as enhancing self-efficacy, providing benefits, and being useful and fun	Perceived barriers (e.g., time, job, transportation difficulties)
	Exercise barrier efficacy (i.e., perceived ability to overcome barriers to engagement in physical activity)	Organizational problems (change of residence, inconvenient training times)
	Employment status: employed	Employment status: unemployed
	Gender: male	Higher age
	Smoking status: nonsmoker	External health-related control beliefs
	Good health (body mass index within norms, cholesterol normal, body fat under control)	Lower education level, lower socioeconomic status
	Engagement in active leisure time activity	
	Desire to reintegrate into job following rehabilitation	
	Low or strong left-ventricular impairment	
External	Social support (e.g., family, professional)	Financial or family-related difficulties
	Treatment results (i.e., after a percutaneous transluminal coronary angioplasty)	Medical contraindications for exercise (e.g., high cholesterol)
		Lack of information and support from the doctor

organizes these variables into a matrix. The variables *perceived self-efficacy* (outcome expectancies), *benefits,* and *barriers,* as well as *social support,* explain 50% of the exercise variance (Bock et al., 1997; Hellmann, 1997). Hellmann (1997) and Bock et al. (1997) found the first three variables, as well as behavioral processes specified in the transtheoretical model of behavior change (see section 4.4.2), to be valid predictors of adherence.

Following Bandura (1977), *self-efficacy* as it relates to exercise is a person's belief that he or she can prepare for and engage in a certain exercise activity. Self-efficacy involves not only personal competence but also a willingness to do the activity despite competing motives (e.g., bad weather, visitors, an interesting television program). K. M. King, Human, Smith, Phan, and Theo (2001) found higher self-efficacy to be a significant predictor of adherence to physical activity, in addition to younger age, lower body mass index values, and shorter distance between home and facility. Carlson et al. (2001) found self-efficacy to be the only significant predictor of long-term participation in physical activity. Vidmar and Rubinson (1994) found a significant correlation between exercise be-

havior and self-efficacy; they also found a correlation with what they called "exercise barrier efficacy," based on Schwarzer and Renner's (2000) concept of "coping efficacy" and defined as a belief in one's ability to overcome barriers.

Burns, Camaione, Froman, and Clark (1998) suggested a close relationship between physical activity in leisure time and exercise-specific self-efficacy. McSweeney (1993) described self-motivation and ongoing participation in exercise as "internal enhancers" that have a beneficial and enhancing effect on exercise; they involve not only a positive attitude toward exercise, but also the capability to judge one's own performance objectively. Self-efficacy also protects patients from straining themselves beyond a medically justifiable level in the different phases of rehabilitation (see Kollenbaum, 1990).

Jeng and Braun (1997) found no covariance between adherence and self-efficacy in their investigation; they ascribed this result to an incorrect method of measuring exercise-specific self-efficacy. They asked patients to judge on a scale from 0 (*not at all able to*) to 5 (*no problem*) whether they trusted themselves to walk or ride a bike a certain distance in 15 minutes. The test did not include questions concerning the exertion and stress the patients had to undergo during the 12-week training. Therefore, the test did not comply with specifically exercise-related self-efficacy.

Social support has proved to be an inconsistent predictor of adherence. Hellmann (1997) found it to be significant, but C. A. Jones, Valle, and Manring (2001) and Carlson et al. (2001) were unable to confirm this finding. Ramm, Robinson, and Sharpe (2001) identified being single (because of the lack of social support) as a significant reason for not participating in exercise.

Oldridge and Spencer (1985) and other authors found active leisure time activity to be an important predictor of adherence, reflecting a widely observed phenomenon in health research: People tend to behave in a way that is consistent to a high degree. As Sutton (1994) observed, "The past predicts the future" (p. 71).

Gainful employment or occupation has been identified as an important predictor of adherence (Ades, Waldmann, McCann, & Weaver, 1992; Budde & Keck, 1996; Evenson, Rosamond, & Luepker, 1998; Oldridge et al., 1983; Oldridge & Spencer, 1985; Tooth, McKenna, & Colquhoun, 1993). Ramm et al. (2001) and Ades et al. (1992) confirmed an observation verified in primary prevention that lower socioeconomic status (operationalized as lower education) is a significant predictor for nonparticipation in an outpatient cardiac exercise group. Oldridge, Rogowski, and Gottlieb (1992) examined the influence of financial reimbursement systems in the United States and found that participation in Medicare was a significant predictor. Exercise training reimbursed by Medicare is increasingly home based, which enhances adherence compared with inpatient or outpatient supervised group care.

According to Dorn, Naughton, Imamura, and Trevisan (2001), adherence was predicted most accurately by considering patients' ability to work or to be employed at the beginning of rehabilitation. Keck, Budde, and Hamerle (1991) also found that a positive prognosis for ability to work was a significant predictor for participation in an outpatient cardiac exercise group.

Budde, Grün, and Keck (1993) described structural barriers to outpatient cardiac exercise group participation and pointed out that adherence can be increased significantly by making organizational improvements (e.g., offering the program on different days at varied times). Emery (1995) observed that adherence in cardiological rehabilitation can be improved only by considering both patient characteristics (e.g., education, depression, fear, dropout from a rehabilitation program) and program and environmental factors (e.g., individual goal setting, use of various media, and flexible scheduling, as well as help integrating techniques into everyday life). Ramm et al. (2001) highlighted difficulties with transportation to the program and inconvenient scheduling as reasons for lack of participation or dropout (see Ades et al., 1992; K. M. King et al., 2001). N. A. Johnson and Heller (1998) identified time barriers as predictors of dropout. DeBusk (1992) estimated that his sample of U.S. patients who attended supervised group training spent more time in the car than on a bicycle ergometer.

Inactivity, unlike many other behavioral risk factors such as smoking or alcohol consumption, does not consist of episodic incidents. Over the life span, most people alternate between phases of physical activity and more or less complete inactivity. Thus, physical inactivity is not a discrete but rather a continuous variable. To counteract the risk factor of physical inactivity effectively and lastingly, it is necessary to overcome considerable motivational and volitional problems.

4.4. MODELS OF HEALTH-RELATED BEHAVIOR

A proximal goal of secondary prevention or rehabilitative intervention is changing behavior. Generally, changing behavior involves changing aspects of one's lifestyle. From a health scientific perspective, secondary prevention involves changing people's way of life; structural forces are not considered. Patients are called on to quit smoking, eat healthier foods, and be more physically active on a regular basis. Behavioral changes, however, are not simply and in every case a matter of exercising one's own will (Schlicht, 2000). People are tied together in social interactions and subjected to structural constraints that may force them into risk behaviors or make risk behaviors appear functional. But these aspects are not the focus of this chapter; rather, the focus is on the constellation of variables that encourage and discourage attitude changes.

The list of variables that influence health behaviors says nothing about the functional connections among them that result in motivation and adherence. Therefore, listing the variables provides only a starting point for the practical work of therapists and health promoters. Most recommendations for behavioral changes follow a heuristic strategy and common sense rather than being structured according to scientifically founded knowledge about change. Research has contributed much to an understanding of the process of promoting behavior change, however. The determinants of motivation and adherence in the context of physical activity and exercise have been the subject of intensive health psychological analysis for more than 15 years (for an overview, see S. E. Taylor, 1990). By using currently available knowledge, health promoters can base practical action on a scientific foundation. The probability that CHD patients can be motivated to initiate exercise and adhere to it over the long term can be increased by building on the theoretical foundations.

Three intentions cause people to change their health risk behaviors: (a) They want to protect themselves from a possible future illness (health management), (b) they want to avoid a worsening of an illness of which they are already experiencing symptoms (crisis management), and (c) they want to restore their health to improve the symptoms of an illness (disease management). Generally, the first intention is considered preventative behavior, whereas the other two intentions are considered disease management (see Mechanic, 1962).

People's cognitive processes differ depending on which of these intentions is given priority. Although people who intend to prevent illness can only imagine the severity of an illness and their vulnerability to it, people who are already ill have experienced its severity and their vulnerability firsthand. Both variables—perceived severity and perceived vulnerability—are significant determinants of behavior change. They are mentioned, among other motivational determinants, in social–psychological continuum theories.

The health belief model was the first of these theories (Rosenstock, 1966). Even though no exact statements about how healthy behavior is initiated and maintained are possible with this model, it did have a considerable influence on newer models, such as protection–motivation theory (Becker, 1974). In both models, the sense of threat that people experience as they become aware of the severity of an illness and their own vulnerability to it is the decisive motivation to change their behavior. The theory of planned behavior stems from another tradition (Ajzen, 1991); it is an extension of the theory of reasoned action, which posits that people's behavior is influenced not only by attitudes and social expectations but also by their perceived ability to control their behavior, which can influence the planned behavior considerably.

In addition to these prominent models, stage models explain the progressive course of behavior change. Stage models emphasize that behavior change is not a static but rather a dynamic process that determines when and how behavior change occurs and which cognitive and behavioral processes accompany the change. According to N. D. Weinstein (1998), complex and novel ways of behavior can be predicted more realistically using stage models. The following sections describe the core assumptions of some of these models.

4.4.1. Continuum Theories

4.4.1.1. Expectancy × Value theory. The health belief model (Rosenstock, 1966) and protection–motivation theory (Becker, 1974) are among the best-known health behavior models. They are based on Expectancy × Value theory, and in the context of health campaigns, are evident in fear appeals. They suggest that a person's behavior depends on (a) the individual's estimate of the likelihood that a given action will achieve his or her goal and (b) the value that the behavioral goal has for the person.

Consequently, people are motivated to be physically active if they expect to prevent a serious illness to which they believe they are vulnerable by being more active (outcome expectancy). In health campaigns, people's sense of vulnerability and severity is provoked mostly by threats and then channeled into action by specific didactic information. Because engagement in many healthy behaviors requires people to acquire abilities and skills and to overcome barriers, overstated threats can lead to rejection processes and reactions if people cannot see a way to avoid the threat (for a summary of this research, see J. Barth & Bengel, 1998). They may be conscious of their vulnerability to a life-threatening illness, and they may know that exercise will lower their risk, but if they perceive that lack of ability or time is an insurmountable barrier, they will not be motivated to become physically active. For this reason, fear appeals should always be connected with a strengthening of self-efficacy expectancies. In empirical testing of these theoretical models, self-efficacy as conceived of by Bandura (1977, 1986) proved to be a significant determinant of behavior (Marcus, King, Bock, Borrelli, & Clark, 1998).

4.4.1.2. Theory of planned behavior.

The theory of planned behavior has proved to be successful in predicting different types of behavior (e.g., condom use, preventative checkups, exercise behavior; Ajzen, 1991). Before people become physically active, they formulate a behavior intention. Ajzen and Madden (1986) defined *intentions* as plans in pursuit of behavioral goals. People plan, for example, to start with walking or to attend the outpatient cardiac exercise group training sessions regularly. The formulation of this intention and the probability that the intended behavior will follow depend on the person's attitudes, subjective norms, and perceived behavior control.

For example, if a person is convinced that a certain behavior will reduce his weight and therefore his health risk (attitude), and if he is convinced that people close to him would be glad to see him behave that way (subjective norm), then he is more likely to formulate an intention. If the person formulates an intention, then he will most probably act on this intention. Strong intentions can compensate for weak subjective norms and vice versa. However, if the person is sure that he does not have the ability to behave in such a way or will not be able to overcome time or other barriers, then he will not formulate an intention.

In empirical examinations, perceived competence or perceived self-efficacy has proved to be a significant variable in predicting intention to exercise (Fuchs & Schwarzer, 1994; Wurtele & Maddux, 1987). Vidmar and Rubinson (1994) found that almost 30% of the variance in exercise behavior of cardiac rehabilitation patients could be explained by differences in barrier-related self-efficacy. This study has weaknesses in terms of evidence criteria, but its results are consistent with those of studies that assessed general self-efficacy (Ewart, Taylor, Reese, & DeBusk, 1983).

Doubts about whether they will be able to exercise regularly especially plague people of middle age (40 to 60 years old), CHD patients, and older adults. They are more likely than younger and healthier groups to believe that they do not have the necessary abilities and skills or to see themselves as hindered by time barriers (e.g., employment and family obligations) as well as situational or social barriers (e.g., lack of opportunities, equipment, sports facilities, social support).

According to Bandura (1986), perceived self-efficacy varies along three dimensions: magnitude, strength, and generalizability. *Magnitude* refers to the difficulty level of the exercise task, *strength* refers to the extent to which the person believes he or she can fulfill the task, and *generalizability* refers to the person's ability to transfer self-efficacy from one task to another. Thus, one cannot simply assume that a patient who experiences self-efficacy in inpatient exercise therapy (i.e., who masters the different intensities of physical training without any problems) will transfer this experience to an outpatient cardiac exercise group or even to supervised home-based training.

Self-efficacy can be learned. The sources of acquired self-efficacy knowledge are one's own experience, models, verbal persuasion, and physiological reactions. Models should be similar to the person (e.g., in age and of the same sex) and should master the behavior in question with effort rather than with ease. Social psychological research has shown that role models are more effective if they are characterized positively (see Caffray & Schneider, 2000). For example, a model who is against the peer norm of smoking who is characterized positively by young persons will be more effective than a model who is characterized negatively. Verbal persuasion is an important strategy; teaching the patient that he or she can be physically active without any cardiac risk is a significant source of self-efficacy and is up to the didactic cleverness of the therapist and training supervisor. Physiological reactions have an influence on the experience of exercise-related self-efficacy, especially when beginning the activity. Patients must learn that shortness of breath, slight indisposition, increased heartbeat, and similar sensations are not cause for alarm.

Attitudes and beliefs are significant determinants of intentions and behaviors. Attitudes can be changed either directly by experiencing positive consequences or indirectly by persuasive communication strategies. Convincing patients that they should change their behavior is one of the primary tasks of any therapeutic intervention. The elaboration likelihood model by Petty and Cacioppo (1986) and the heuristic systematic model by Chaiken (1980) describe strategies for convincing patients to change their attitudes and beliefs. People who possess little knowledge and limited know-how and who are unwilling to follow factual arguments tend to prefer a more peripheral route of persuasion; factual arguments must be presented convincingly and are subject to heuristic processing. The credibility of the carrier of the message and the patient's rapport with him or her are what is important. Changes of attitude prompted in this way are rarely long lasting, however, and do not lead to the desired change in behavior.

Better results are achieved when patients rely more on the strength of the arguments and less on the credibility of the persuader. To be convincing, information must be presented systematically and must be of good quality. A good understanding of the arguments facilitates changes in attitude that are durable and resistant against counterarguments

and that will lead to real behavior change. These theoretical findings support the measures recommended by Budde and Keck (1999) and Hillebrand et al. (1995) to prepare patients for participation in an outpatient cardiac exercise group. Patients should be informed about their vulnerability, they should be informed about the outcome expectancies of their behavior, and their self-efficacy should be strengthened.

4.4.2. Stage Models

A person who has started to exercise is constantly at risk for ceasing to exercise. Only 6 months after they begin to exercise, more than half of patients have stopped. Sallis and Owen (1998) reviewed more than 300 studies dealing with the problem of exercise adherence in primary prevention. They came to the not very encouraging conclusion that about 40 different variables influence adherence to regular exercise. Table W4.3 shows that secondary prevention and rehabilitation efforts encounter the same difficulties. The variables listed in these tables have predictive validity that likely extends to adherence to secondary preventive and rehabilitative exercise.

Stage models divide the process of behavior change into intervention-relevant phases and name the variables that can be influenced to avoid relapse. The transtheoretical model of behavior change (TTM) by the work group of James Prochaska (summarized in Prochaska, Johnson, & Lee, 1998; see also Keller, 1999) is a frequently named and empirically reliable model. Behavior, whether it protects health or places it at risk, is relatively stable, and clear incentives and encouragement are needed to change it permanently (Sutton, 1994). Continuum theories describe health behavior as consisting of action episodes in which patients use motivational and volitional processes to decide whether to engage in the behavior in question. Oldenburg, Glanz, and French (1999) pointed out that behavior-oriented programs are doomed to fail if participants are not aware that their behavior is problematic.

There is an additional difficulty in promoting exercise-related behavior change in CHD patients in particular. Because the emphasis is on invasive treatment, patients who have undergone successful treatment believe that such treatment is enough (Grande, Schott, & Badura, 1996; Jordan, Bardé, & Zeiher, 1998): Why bother with lifestyle changes if, for example, a stenosis can be cured by percutaneous transluminary coronary angioplasty or coronary artery bypass grafting?

Stage models conceive of behavior change as a multiphase process:

- In the beginning phase, the physically inactive person must be made aware of the risks inherent in an inactive lifestyle. Educational and informational interventions that advise patients about the risk involved in inactivity and seek to change their attitudes (e.g., by creating positive consequence expectancies) are more appropriate for this step than interventions that urge patients to act immediately on the recommendation of the American College of Sports Medicine and the Centers for Disease Control and Prevention that they engage in moderate activity for 30 minutes every day (Pate et al., 1995).

- Patients who are aware of their risky behavior and who have recognized and accepted that the new behavior will benefit them still must motivate themselves to actually engage in the new behavior. Encouraging patients' self-efficacy and teaching them the skills necessary to engage in the behavior are appropriate strategies at this stage.

- Once patients have begun participating in the new behavior, they must maintain and adhere to it. They must avoid the old, risky behavior and become accustomed to the new one. Teaching strategies for self-management and for resisting competing motives are helpful in this step.

The different models of behavior change name the stages of behavior differently. The precaution adoption process model of N. D. Weinstein (1988) was conceived for use in encouraging preventative behavior and distinguishes seven stages in moving from a health risk behavior to a permanently health protective behavior:

1. Unaware of the issue
2. Aware of the issue but not personally engaged
3. Engaged and deciding what to do
4. Planning to act but not yet having acted
5. Having decided not to act
6. Acting
7. Maintenance

The best-known theory of change, and one that has received empirical support for a large number of behaviors, is the TTM, which was originally conceived to help people quit smoking. This model differentiates five stages of readiness to change (see Prochaska & DiClemente, 1986):

1. *Precontemplation.* The person is unaware of the need to increase his or her activity level and does not intend, even when asked, to start exercising in the near future (i.e., the next 6 months). Persons at this stage either are not sufficiently informed about the risk or have already made several unsuccessful attempts to change their behavior and simply avoid thinking about the risk.

2. *Contemplation.* The person becomes aware of the problem and formulates the intention to become active within the next 6 months. People at this stage understand the problem and the disadvantages connected with it and see the positive consequences of making the behavior change.

3. *Preparation.* The person informs him- or herself about the options for exercising (e.g., outpatient cardiac exercise group, walking group) and establishes a concrete plan of action for exercising.

4. *Action.* At this stage, the behavior change becomes evident for the first time. The person begins to exercise actively and regularly at an intensity that promotes health and minimizes risk. However, people at this stage must develop metacognitive protection and self-management strategies to guard against competing motives and backsliding (relapse to inactivity).

5. *Maintenance and habituation.* The person has reached the stage of exercising regularly. He or she has engaged in the activity at regular intervals for at least 6 months, but it may take longer for the behavior to become habitual and integrated into daily life. Unexpected disruptions or temptations to neglect the activity may lead to brief lapses but not to a return to inactivity.

Fuchs (2001) observed that when it comes to exercise, many people remain in Stage 4. Their behavior fluctuates; they may attend the outpatient cardiac exercise group, and then they stay away from the group or come only sporadically. The behavior never becomes habitual, and they constantly risk becoming inactive once again.

To help patients establish regular exercise activity, it is not important which terms are used for the stages. More important is an understanding of the attributes (thoughts, feelings, awareness, attitudes, behavior) people exhibit at the different stages and of how to enable people at each stage to go on to the next stage. The TTM describes cognitive–behavioral processes that manifest differently in the separate stages and can be influenced in different ways.

People must first become aware of the problem they create or contribute to by engaging in the health risk behavior (consciousness raising). Medical advice, media campaigns, personal counseling, and other forms of information dissemination can serve to raise consciousness. As soon as the problem becomes apparent, however, people may adopt a fatalistic attitude if they see no possible solution. Providing positive consequence expectancies (persuasive appeals) for health-protective behaviors is an important task of psychosocial intervention. When people can envision a positive outcome, they often experience relief: "Once I become more active, I no longer have to fear my present CHD risk."

The processes of becoming aware of the problem and envisioning a positive outcome are followed by a self-reevaluation and an environmental evaluation. A person who formerly saw him- or herself as needing to feel comfortable now begins to explore a new identity as a person who is active and who takes care of his or her physical well-being. Because this change of self-image has an effect on the social environment, the person will also think about the impression this change will make on others and about the consequences. Referring to U. Lehr and Thomae (1991), Schlicht (2000) posited that behavior is determined socially to a much larger extent than it is determined by one's own deliberate control. The predominant mentalities in the different social groups may present restrictions

that work against behavior change in their constituent members. For example, some groups feel that it is not appropriate for older women to exercise in public, and some groups view the body mechanistically and delegate control over bodily functions to religious powers or to professional personnel.

After reevaluating their self-image and social environment, some people must also undergo self-liberation and social liberation. They must learn to say, "I am the one who is responsible for my physical condition, and I can be physically active if I want," or "Nowadays, people are physically active at an older age, and therefore it is appropriate if I am physically active in public."

Taking action consistent with the new cognitions is made easier when structural supports are in place—for example, campaigns that advertise Nordic walking or other endurance sports, introductory workshops on exercise for beginners, media campaigns using older people as models, and movement and meeting points in city districts. Bös, Woll, and colleagues described several community health projects and showed how public information campaigns and structural measures can increase the prevalence of exercise in the population (Bös, Woll, Bösing, & Huber, 1994; Woll & Bös, 1994.

The cognitive–behavioral processes described so far must be in place before people can take action. Once they reach the action stage, other processes become important. The theoretical models applicable beginning in Stage 4 are based primarily on learning theories. Like other behaviors, physical activity can be created and maintained by controlling or modifying antecedent (stimulus) and consequent (intensifier) conditions (see A. C. King et al., 1992). Stimulus control involves removing stimuli for physically inactive behavior and substituting stimuli for physically active behavior. For example, people can learn to avoid turning on the television (i.e., stimulus removal) in order to give priority to going to their outpatient cardiac exercise group appointment over watching television. Structural supports that provide stimuli to engage in physical activity include stairways of public buildings that are designed more attractively than the elevators and parking lots laid out so that the entrances to public, office, commercial, and residential buildings can be reached only after a walk of 1 to 2 minutes.

Counterconditioning is another process founded on learning theories. It is easier to engage in a health-promoting behavior if it appears to be a functional replacement for the risk behavior. Every problematic behavior is rewarding: Smoking reduces stress, and inactivity is comfortable. People need to learn that moderate physical activity induces positive feelings, reduces stress, stabilizes body weight, or makes everyday movements easier.

Contingency management promotes behavior change by rewarding engagement in the targeted behavior. Reward appears to be more effective than punishment, and classical tactics and strategies of behavior modification, such as self-binding contracts, tokens, and contingency and consequence control, have achieved good results (see the summary by Reinecker & Lakatos, 1999). Finally, helping relationships support behavior change: For example, friends may accompany patients to exercise therapy, family members may state that they find the behavior change to be positive, and training supervisors may follow up if someone misses sessions.

C. S. Rosen (2000) analyzed 46 studies on change in different health behaviors. The most pronounced changes from one stage to another are the commitment to the new behavior (self-liberation), the search for relevant information (consciousness raising), stimulus control, and the use of intensifiers (contingency management). Like nutritional behavior but unlike abstinence behavior (i.e., smoking cessation), in exercise behavior, cognitive and behavioral strategies must be emphasized equally across the stages of change. Thus, interventions cannot emphasize cognitive processes (e.g., consciousness raising, self-reevaluation, emotional relief, social liberation) while neglecting behavioral processes (e.g., contingency management, stimulus control, counterconditioning, self-liberation, helpful relationships).

Exercise behavior has to be reinitiated constantly. According to C. S. Rosen (2000), exercising is not a phenomenon that once acquired is always present (i.e., a discrete variable); it relies heavily on

a readiness to engage repeatedly in a behavior (i.e., continuous variable) and therefore must continually be motivationally inspired. Appropriate theoretical models to explain this phenomenon adequately have yet to be developed.

According to Prochaska et al. (1998), these cognitive–behavioral processes reflect a decisional balance in which the relative weight of positive and negative consequence expectancies (e.g., benefits vs. costs and barriers) are compared at each stage (this cost–benefit balance also forms part of the health belief model of Becker, 1974). On the basis of several studies, Prochaska (1994) postulated two diagnostic criteria for the transition from the precontemplation to action: A quantifiable change in the decisional balance of the consequence expectancies is observed, and the self-efficacy expectancy increases throughout the stages. Positive consequence expectancies (*pros*), Prochaska found, should increase by 1 standard deviation, and negative consequence expectancies (*cons*) should decrease by 0.5 standard deviation. Marcus, Rakowski, and Rossi (1992) similarly showed that for sports-related behavior, in the stages of action and maintenance people express more pros than cons. Prochaska et al. (1998) concluded from their review of studies that the pros are twice as important as the cons and therefore that interventions should place more emphasis on raising positive consequence expectancies than on removing barriers.

Schmid, Keller, Jäkle, Baum, and Basler (1999) supported this model in a prospective longitudinal study. In their samples of consecutively recruited patients of general practitioners, the decisional balance changed in favor of the pros and self-efficacy increased as patients reached a higher stage of readiness to change. Comparable changes can be found, as shown in Table W4.3, in samples motivated by secondary preventative or rehabilitative efforts to increase their physical activity. In summary, interventions to encourage the exercise behavior of CHD patients are well supported by empirical findings; such interventions are most effective when they strengthen patients' motivation by referring to the positive gains of exercise and highlight the emotional benefits of exercise.

4.5. STRATEGIES FOR PROMOTING PHYSICAL ACTIVITY

4.5.1. Social Marketing

The theoretical models discussed in this chapter operate at the level of intervention with individuals. Public health campaigns appeal to larger population groups to promote healthy lifestyles in general or to publicize intervention strategies for risk groups. Such campaigns are educational interventions that more or less explicitly follow the strategies of social marketing.

Social marketing evolved to help health promoters and others "sell" a "product" that is intangible but valuable—for example, a healthier, more risk-free life—through media campaigns in the right place, in the right amount, and at the right time so that the target group will perceive the benefits of purchasing the product to be high and the costs and effort to seem appropriate. Social marketing does not involve content development, which is also important to successful campaigns. Social marketing instead provides a strategy that supports the conception, planning, implementation, and evaluation of health promotion campaigns.

Social marketing favors a client orientation over a product orientation and, similarly, bottom-up processing over top-down processing. In the context of changing health-related behaviors, therapists must avoid the not atypical attitude of knowing what is good for the patient, what the patient needs, and what he or she therefore should take to heart. Such an attitude also involves selling a finished program and expecting unquestioning compliance. Social marketing, in contrast, requires the health promoter to know what customers want, what needs they have, and which information and programs they require to fulfill these needs. Programs to promote lifestyle changes are therefore adapted and geared specifically to target groups.

In accordance with the customer orientation, a voluntary exchange takes place between the health promoter and the CHD patient. Both sides invest, and both want to profit. The promoter invests money, personnel, ideas, and expertise and pursues organizational goals; the customer invests time and effort and gains a personal profit in the form of im-proved health. Monetary profit plays a minor role in social marketing; the organizations are usually public facilities (e.g., Bundeszentrale für gesundheitliche Aufklärung [Federal Center for Health Education], health insurance) for whom maximizing profits is not a primary goal, and in Germany, customers as a rule do not have to pay the full amount to use the offerings (e.g., because of health insurance, cost-free offers). As social–psychological exchange theories and equity theories teach, the exchange of goods must be just. Consumers must be convinced that they do not invest more than seems useful. Campaigns that threaten customers with negative consequences or chide them for not being reasonable and stopping their risky behaviors attempt to force the exchange; they violate the principle of voluntariness and are not very effective in the long run.

The targeted population is segmented into goal groups for whom interventions can be specifically designed. Goal groups can be established on the basis of region, demographics, psychometrics, or risk exposure. Unfortunately, generalized campaigns to promote more activity on a daily basis often appeal only to persons who are already active. According to the U.S. Department of Health and Human Services, "individuals at greatest risk for inactivity include women (especially black women), less educated persons, overweight individuals, blue-collar workers, and elderly persons" (U.S. Department of Health and Human Services, 1998, p. 34). All sectors of society have the same problem—the risks presented by physical inactivity—but they do not all perceive the same necessity to overcome this problem. For members of the middle class, exercise and sports are typical behaviors that are part of their social identity. Members of some other groups do not share this mentality, however. In Germany, for example, for traditionally raised Turkish women it is unthinkable to participate in an outpatient cardiac exercise group, in which they would be physically active in the presence of men, or to walk in public to lower their CHD risk. Much remains unknown about which stimuli increase the probability that less active groups will become physically more active.

Once goal groups have been specified, information media and channels are carefully analyzed and approached for use in disseminating messages to change attitudes and, ultimately, behaviors. Bruhn and Tilmes (1994) reviewed evidence of the effectiveness of different mass media (television, radio, magazines, and newspapers) in public health campaigns. In addition to the costs, health promoters must consider the audience targeted by the media venue, ways to attract attention, and perhaps the use of differentiated messages. In a cultural sociological study, Schulze (2000) showed that different social groups prefer different information channels. The health psychological literature cites the telephone as a preferred medium for disseminating specific information to goal groups; Castro et al. (2001) demonstrated in a study conducted with 140 men and women 50 to 60 years of age that the telephone was an effective medium in improving compliance with a low-dosage home-based exercise program. To help patients maintain a program over the long term, a monthly mailing may be sufficient.

4.5.2. Campaigns and Projects

Community education programs that are often cited and that used components of social marketing include the Stanford Five-City Project (e.g., Farquhar et al., 1990), which influenced the German Heart Prevention Study (von Troschke, Klaes, & Maschewsky-Schneider, 1991); the Minnesota Heart Health Program (Crow et al., 1986); and the Pawtucket Heart Health Program (see Elder et al., 1986). These primary prevention programs sought to increase the amount of activity in the targeted population. In this section we provide a brief overview of the Stanford Five-City Project.

The Stanford Five-City Project, which combined media campaigns and face-to-face-interventions, took place over 9 years (1979–1980 to 1985–1986, with a follow-up in 1989–1990). Two cities formed the intervention group, and three cities formed the reference group. In the intervention cities, community health education was disseminated via local radio and television stations, and exercise programs, such as walking groups, were established. The campaign was aimed at lowering the cardiac risk factors of cholesterol, high blood pressure, over-weight, smoking, and physical inactivity. Reductions in inactivity were reflected both in the level of exercise in participants' everyday lives (e.g., using the stairs instead of the elevator) and in participation in exercise programs. In the intervention cities, the project contributed to a significant decrease in general mortality and CHD risk factors. Knowledge, attitudes, and physical activity, however, changed only slightly (D. R. Young, Haskell, Taylor, & Fortmann, 1996). Only male participants in the treatment cities experienced a significant change in knowledge. Attitudes toward physical activity remained unchanged in both men and women, and there was no improvement in sports- or exercise-oriented behavior. Everyday activity by participants increased, however, and significantly so for women. Compared with the interventions to lower high blood pressure or improve eating habits, the results of interventions to influence physical inactivity were relatively weak. Usually, community education projects are aimed at a wider audience than just the target group, and messages delivered through the media must be brief. This project's messages could provide only limited information on how people could increase their physical activity.

More effective as secondary preventative interventions are projects that cooperate with doctors, who have contact with and some authority over patients, in disseminating behavioral recommendations. However, doctors often lack sufficient knowledge to give the specific information needed to inspire a change in patient behavior.

Provider-Based Assessment and Counseling for Exercise (PACE; see Long et al., 1996) is a project that systematically instructs doctors in giving their patients exercise-related advice that addresses the patient's specific need for behavior change. The doctor uses a diagnostic procedure to identify the patient's current stage of change; help the patient consider exercise-related barriers, self-efficacy, and social support; and provide instruction in self-adhering contracts, reinforcement management, and other techniques. Fifty percent of pre-contemplating patients and 66% of contemplating patients decided to become active following the intervention, and almost 90% of active patients kept up their activity.

Calfas et al. (1996) examined the effects of the PACE program in a nonrandomized but controlled trial. Ninety-eight patients took part in PACE interventions intended to influence the social and psychological factors that hinder or facilitate physical activity. The participants in the precontemplation phase were asked to concentrate on the benefits of mild endurance training, such as walking, and participants in the action phase received advice on how they could counteract lapses in order to avoid a return to inactivity. Significant differences between the intervention group and the control group ($n = 114$) were shown for the walking activity. After 6 weeks, 52% of the experimental group, compared with 12% of the control group, was still active, even though the willingness to become active was identically high in both groups at the beginning. The PACE program proved to be an effective strategy to motivate patients to increase their physical activity.

4.6. CONCLUSION

Research on psychosocial interventions to address physical inactivity as a risk factor in CHD has made a number of advances. Increased physical activity has been proved to reduce cardiac risk under certain conditions; reasons have been identified for the lack of motivation of CHD risk groups to engage in regular exercise and the lack of adherence to an exercise program once initiated; and study findings have supported health behavior models that can inform the development of effective interventions. Medical therapy must be based on the available evidence, and no less is demanded of programs to promote exercise-related behavior change. Research has identified the variables that make motivation and adherence more probable, and it has established the important distinction that exercise is not an episodic event that becomes habitual and automatic, but rather is subject to permanent voluntary control. Implementing secondary prevention programs without a basis in current theory and knowledge regarding the determinants of behavior is, at the very least, unprofessional.

Before implementing an intervention to promote physical activity in patients at risk for CHD, health promoters must examine the attitudes, knowledge, and needs of the people concerned. This information can then be used to focus the intervention as closely as possible on the factors that will increase the patients' willingness and motivation to engage in physical activity. Stage-specific interventions should be promoted as an offer rather than being prescribed from the top down.

The content of interventions should be chosen carefully to have a positive effect on motivation and adherence. An important component is to create positive consequence expectancies and attitudes regarding the new behavior and, most of all, to strengthen patients' experienced self-efficacy. The more people are convinced that they can organize themselves to engage in the exercise activity, the more they will see themselves as capable of succeeding in this effort in spite of the psychosocial and structural difficulties they face. CHD patients are best supported by resource people who can help them find solutions to their problems and, if it seems necessary, who can provide mild warnings about the consequences of physical inactivity. When warnings are necessary, appeals should be positively formulated to anticipate a relatively safe and desirable outcome (A. J. Rothman & Salovey, 1997); people are more likely to want to avoid a risk if they can also expect benefits or gains by changing their behavior. CHD patients generally see an active lifestyle as beneficial, so negative or risk-emphasizing appeals are not often effective as motivators.

Social networks and social support are likely conducive to behavior change, but the results of studies in this field are inconclusive, so we can offer no concrete recommendations. Structural prerequisites also influence behavior change; if exercise programs are available only in one area and always at the same time, patients are more likely to find participation too inconvenient. Interventions must respond to both individual and structural conditions to promote behavior change that results in more active lifestyles for patients with CHD.

CHAPTER 5

ANXIETY AND DEPRESSION IN PATIENTS WITH CORONARY HEART DISEASE

Christoph Herrmann-Lingen and Ullrich Buss

5.1. INTRODUCTION

In addition to pain, shame, and mortality, anxiety and despondence are basic features of human suffering, the "pathic categories or modalities of existence" (Hartmann, 1984, p. 11). Perhaps because these ubiquitous dimensions of emotional experience are not in any way specific to coronary heart disease (CHD), and because CHD patients tend to deny their anxiety and depressive feelings and, in comparison with other patient groups (e.g., patients with noncardiac chest pain), have lower scores on instruments measuring these domains, it is often easy to disregard anxiety and depression in CHD patients.

Anxiety and depression, however, are common among CHD patients, but obtaining consistent data on the prevalence of anxiety and depression is problematic for several methodological reasons. A wide variety of instruments and thresholds are used to determine the presence of depressive or anxiety disorders and to quantify the intensity of anxious or depressive feelings. Anxiety and depression also show heterogeneous distribution at different stages of the disease or in specific patient subgroups. The analyses in this chapter will take these problems into account.

After describing our literature search methodology in section 5.2, we discuss studies that provide criterion-, situation-, and subgroup-related prevalence data for categorically understood abnormal anxiety and depression in section 5.3 (see also section W5.1 on the accompanying Web site for data

on depression in the narrower sense; http://www.apa.org/books/resources/jordan/). We first explain the usefulness of these data for the differential diagnosis of chest complaints and then turn to anxiety and depression as dimensional state variables that are cross-sectionally associated with other environmental and disease factors.

In section 5.4, we examine how anxiety and depressive mood change as heart disease progresses. We also explore the predictive meaning of anxiety and depressive mood in CHD, both subjectively (e.g., mood, quality of life, illness behavior, return to work) and objectively (e.g., cardiac events, mortality). Such considerations are important in cardiac care: In what ways are these factors risk or even protective factors for the progression of the disease? This section also deals with possible psychophysiological relationships that may mediate the effects of anxiety and depressive mood on the course of CHD.

Section 5.5 deals with the effects of specific psychosocial, psychotherapeutic, and psychopharmacological interventions for anxious and depressive CHD patients. We review the few existing studies on the treatment of clinically diagnosed anxiety or depression disorders; psychosocial intervention studies in the field of cardiac rehabilitation are discussed in chapter 10 of this volume.

5.2. METHOD

In autumn 1999, we did a literature search of the Medline and PsycLIT databases for journal articles dating back to 1980. The key words we entered were *anxiety* (*anxi**) and *depression* (*depressi* and psych**); the limitation to *psych* was necessary to reduce the number of false positive hits on topics like *ST-segment depression*). Other terms we searched on were *coronary heart disease* (*coronary*; no additional limitations to find terms such as *coronary events*), *ischemic heart disease* (*ischemic near1 heart*; by leaving out the word *disease,* we covered terms such as *ischemic heart events*, and the code word *near1* helped avoid hits where both search words, *ischemic* and *heart*, showed up but were not connected to each other in any way), and *myocardial infarction* (*myocardial near1 infarct**).

Linking together the search words as follows—*anxi** or (*depressi** and *psych**) and *coronary* or (*ischemic near1 heart*) or (*myocardial near1 infarct**)—resulted in 2,055 hits. We thoroughly reviewed all of these titles and, when available, the abstracts as well. False positive articles, single case studies, and other obviously unsuitable studies were removed from the analysis. We further eliminated studies that examined CHD risk factors exclusively in patients who had not yet shown manifestations of CHD. We used roughly 500 publications in our analysis. We used the reviews relevant to our topic only to complete our bibliography; our analysis is based only on the original publications.

To analyze and weight the selected studies on the prevalence, progression, and predictive value of anxiety and depressive mood, the evidence-based medicine criteria (Hadorn, Baker, Hodges, & Hicks, 1996) did not prove to be helpful, because evaluating therapy was not our purpose. We classified the studies using the best possible objective criteria for the issues in question, an adaptation of the approach described by Wulsin, Vaillant, and Wells (1999). Current methods for measuring anxiety and depression differ in suitability in the cardiological setting, and because data provided in the articles were insufficient for comparison, the necessarily partly subjective judgment of these methods was left out of the qualification index. Table 5.1 shows how we assigned points within each dimension of assessment.

In evaluating the documentation of results, it was frequently necessary to transform the data pro-

vided into suitable effect sizes or to compute significance from frequency distributions (e.g., odds ratios [ORs] and chi-square tests from 2 × 2 cross-tabulations). Group comparisons or courses over time, including mean values and standard deviations, were partly transformed into effect sizes by expressing differences as parts or multiples of the standard deviations of either the reference group or the baseline measurement.

By summing up these aspects of methodological quality, we were able to compute a methodological sum score for each study in a fairly objective way. We divided each sum score (to which extra points could be added, if applicable) by the number of relevant categories (2 or 3; i.e., quality of psychological assessment, quality of outcome assessment if applicable, quality of data reporting); our final result was thus an average methodological mean score. Multiplying this score by the score we computed for the sample size, we arrived at a cumulative qualification index for each study. Studies with indexes >8 were classified as very well-qualified, indexes >6 but ≤8 as well-qualified, indexes of 4 to 6 as partially qualified, and indexes <4 as less qualified. We will discuss in detail only the very well-qualified and well-qualified studies; the remaining studies are summarized on the accompanying Web site as noted in each section.

This ranking was not intended as a judgment of the general quality of the studies; it was made solely for the purposes of applicability to the special objectives of each section of this chapter. It also enabled us to give studies that examined multiple aspects of our investigation separate rankings for each aspect.

5.3. CROSS-SECTIONAL STUDIES ON ANXIETY AND DEPRESSIVE MOOD IN CORONARY HEART PATIENTS

We located about 500 cross-sectional and longitudinal studies on the varying aspects of anxiety and depressive mood in CHD patients; to analyze them completely was beyond the scope of our project. In this section we review longitudinal studies and studies on psychophysiological relationships in patients with documented CHD. Because of space

TABLE 5.1

Computing the Index of Studies' Qualifications

Study characteristic	No. of points				
	1	2	3	4	Other
Sample size: relevant *n*	<30	30–99	100–499	≥500	
Methodological score					
Quality of anxiety/depression measurement	Ad hoc instrument	Unusual or modified questionnaires/interviews	Standard questionnaires or interviews	Standard questionnaires and interviews	In-between categories possible with multiple instruments
Quality of outcome measurement					
Studies on prevalence and correlational studies	*M*s only	(*M* + *SD*), *r*s, or %s	(*M* + *SD*), *r*s, or %s + significance	—	
Longitudinal studies (quality of reporting the course)	*M*s only	(*M* + *SD*) or %s	(*M* + *SD*) or %s + significance	—	In-between categories possible
Predictive studies with subjective endpoints					
Quality of outcome measurement	Ad hoc instrument	Unusual or modified questionnaires/interviews	Standard questionnaires or interviews; objective data	Standard questionnaires and interviews	In-between categories possible with multiple instruments
Quality of reporting the results	Minimal data	Univariate effect size + significance/multivariate without significance	Multivariate effect size + significance	Univariate + multivariate effect size + significance	Because of 3 classes of criteria: division of raw scores by 3
Predictive studies with objective endpoints (quality of prediction)	Univariate effect size + significance	Minimal covariate adjustment (age, gender, etc.)	Adjustment for single (up to 3) cardiac covariates	Adjustment for multiple (>3) cardiac covariates	In-between categories possible (e.g., cardiac covariates without adjustment for age)
Psychophysiological studies	Univariate effect size + significance	Minimal covariate adjustment (age, gender, etc.)	Adjustment for single (up to 3) cardiac covariates	Adjustment for multiple (>3) cardiac covariates	
Additional points	1 point each for separate analysis of subgroups, experimental studies				−1 point each for ▪ Dropouts (>30%) ▪ No precise or consistent diagnosis of CHD ▪ Cross-sectional study design only ▪ Specific or serious methodological deficits

Note. Dashes in cells indicate no applicable data. CHD = coronary heart disease.

constraints, we limit our detailed discussion of the cross-sectional studies to a few essential points.

5.3.1. Anxiety and Depression in the Differential Diagnosis of Chest Complaints

In diagnosing chest complaints, CHD must be differentiated from noncardiac chest pain. Identifying the cause of chest symptoms—cardiac, noncardiac, or psychological—and at the same time addressing the significant comorbidity of psychological symptoms in patients with manifest CHD poses a considerable differential diagnostic challenge. Of 27 studies we identified, 5 (mean N = 480) were very well qualified, 10 (mean N = 111) were well qualified, 10 (mean N = 127) were partially qualified, and 2 (mean N = 70) were less qualified (see Table W5.1 on the Web site).

5.3.1.1. Very well qualified studies. The five very well qualified studies (N = 2,400) demonstrated considerable power because of either large samples or combined psychometric and interview methods (see Table W5.1). They accentuated various aspects of the differential diagnosis of patients with chest symptoms. In a study of a large group of patients that included coronary angiographic examination and multivariate analysis, C. Herrmann, Buss, Breuker, Gonska, and Kreuzer (1994) illustrated the discriminative effects of anxiety and its predictive significance for normal coronary findings. They further found that normal coronary anatomy (NCA) and CHD patients experienced no difference in depressive mood. In his psychometric comparison, Buss (1999) found that higher anxiety scores initially discriminated NCA patients from chronic CHD patients and that later in the course, anxiety and depressive mood showed parallel changes in both groups. Lumley, Torosian, Ketterer, and Pickard (1997) found only a tendency toward a stronger depressive mood in NCA patients; they also found significant discriminative effects for anger control and for physical (hypochondriac) attention. They did not specify their reasons for not testing for anxiety.

Studies by the work groups of Fleet (Fleet et al., 1996, 1998) and Beitman (Beitman, DeRosear,

Basha, & Flaker, 1987; Beitman et al., 1987) examined the comorbidity of psychopathology, especially panic disorder, and CHD. They failed to show a significant difference between CHD and non-CHD patients using the criterion of panic disorder. They found that prevalences were high yet clearly underdiagnosed in both groups; for example, they found that 75% of patients with panic disorder were discharged from the emergency room with a diagnosis of noncardiac chest pain. However, the study group's definition of the criteria for panic disorder in the *Diagnostic and Statistical Manual of Mental Disorders* (3rd ed.; American Psychiatric Association, 1980) was very liberal; their extensive subtotaling of each paroxysmal cardiac complaint under the panic spectrum probably led to an overestimation of panic disorder in a narrower sense.

5.3.1.2. Well-qualified studies. Among the 10 studies we found to be well-qualified (N = 1,107) were several that used angiographic CHD criteria in addition to interview and psychometric methods. These studies consistently showed significantly more anxiety disorders (via a clinical interview or diagnostic checklist), especially panic disorders, in NCA patients compared with patients with established CHD (Bass, Cawley, et al., 1983; Bass & Wade, 1984; Cormier, Katon, Russo, & Hollifield, 1988; Katon et al., 1988; Leibing, Schünemann, Herrmann, & Rüger, 1998). However, depressive mood disorders were not consistently more strongly associated with NCA. Psychometric analysis reveals a similar scenario, in that elevated anxiety scores may differentiate univariately between NCA and CHD (Cormier et al., 1988; C. Herrmann, Scholz, & Kreuzer, 1991; Katon et al., 1988; Leibing et al., 1998; Schocken, Worden, Harrison, & Spielberger, 1984; Serlie et al., 1996) and in that anxiety symptoms and syndromes can still be viewed as predictive of a negative angiography result, even after adjustment for other variables. This scenario does not, however, apply to corresponding depression scales.

The negative and nondiscriminative study results of Zachariae, Melchiorsen, Frøbert, Bjerring, and Bagger (2001) might be attributed to the timing of the psychometric test immediately after angiography. The results might also be due to the short-term relaxation effect of the NCA group.

5.3.1.3. Partially and less qualified studies.
For a discussion of the partially qualified and less qualified studies we located, see section W5.1 on the accompanying Web site.

5.3.1.4. Summary of anxiety and depression in the differential diagnosis of chest complaints.
The analysis of the significance of anxiety and depressive mood in patients who have noncardiac chest pain or angiographically clear coronary arteries leads to fairly consistent results: Anxiety and panic disorders are, in that order, the most commonly seen psychological disorders in NCA patients. Thus, NCA patients differ statistically from CHD patients. Nevertheless, panic attacks are still common and relevant in CHD patients, either as a comorbidity or as a form of secondary neuroticism. The difference in the prevalences of depressive symptoms or disorders between NCA and CHD patients is not substantial and thus cannot be used for differential diagnostic purposes.

Overall, the prevalence of psychologically or psychiatrically abnormal test results—indicating mostly anxiety and depression—proved to be higher in NCA patients compared with CHD patients and with the general population. On the basis of those studies we analyzed that used a "hard" CHD criterion (e.g., angiography; Beitman, Basha, et al., 1987; Cormier et al., 1988; Katon et al., 1988; C. Herrmann et al. 1991; Leibing et al., 1998), the average frequency of high anxiety scores or panic was roughly 43% in NCA versus 13% in CHD, and the average frequency of high depression scores was 30% in NCA versus 9% in CHD

Patients with NCA can be differentiated, at least partially, from those with CHD by their psychological test results. Studies by Fleet et al. (1996, 1998), Ladwig, Hoberg, and Busch (1998), and Buss (1999) show that time is a criterion on its own— that is, the chronicity of recurrent chest pain has a substantial effect: The ability to predict coronary status using psychodiagnostic tests seems to be strongest in patients with a brief history of chest

pain or angina whose symptoms have occurred for the first time and are fairly new, such as in CHD patients during the first wave of diagnostic tests. In patients whose symptoms are of longer duration, certain psychological changes occur in both groups; such patients develop a tendency for a more anxious or depressive way of coping with their CHD- or NCA-associated complaints. According to Ladwig et al. (1998, p. 52), pain symptoms serve to homogenize the patient groups within the disease course much more than the etiology serves to differentiate the groups. Table W5.1 lists the studies on anxiety and depressive mood in the differential diagnosis of chest complaints.

5.3.2. Prevalence of Anxiety and Depressive Mood in Certain CHD-Specific Situations and Their Correlates

5.3.2.1. Relation between anxiety and depressive mood and angina pectoris or silent ischemia.
The phenomenon of silent ischemia (SI) reflects an apparent contradiction between an objective and instrumental (i.e., organically related) test result and a subjective symptomatic complaint. Attempts have been made to explain this contradiction through the physiology of pain, but because of repeated observations that psychological processes were involved in some way in SI pathogenesis, researchers set out to investigate them. A continuum in the manifestation and documentation of angina pectoris (AP) and other symptoms has been developed in which psychological factors such as anxiety and depression are substantially involved. These findings contradict the dichotomy between abnormal psychological morbidity (with AP) on one hand and psychological normality (with SI) on the other.

Studies on psychological morbidity in CHD patients can be separated into two groups: those that exploratively investigate the possible influence of psychological variables of distress (e.g., anxiety and depressive mood) on AP symptoms and those that attempt to psychometrically discriminate between CHD patients with SI and those with already manifest anginal symptoms in a comparative study design (see Table W5.2). In most of the latter studies, the design connects an ergometrically induced proof of ischemia (e.g., significant ST depression in the electrocardiogram [ECG]) and a patient's self-assessment of psychological well-being on a questionnaire. Of a total of 17 studies identified, 6 (mean N = 225) were very well qualified, 8 (mean N = 63) were partially qualified, and 3 (mean N = 1,323, including one very large sample) were less qualified.

5.3.2.1.1. Very well qualified studies. Of the very well qualified studies (n = 1,352), those providing a multivariate analysis (Davies et al., 1993; Herrmann-Lingen, 2001) differ qualitatively from those providing a univariate analysis (Ahto et al., 1997; Buss & Herrmann, 2000; Freedland, Carney, Krone, Case, & Case, 1996; Torosian, Lumley, Pickard, & Ketterer, 1997). With a relatively large number of patients, Herrmann-Lingen (2001) demonstrated that depressive mood and anxiety can predict the manifestation of AP symptoms during ergometrically induced ischemia. This effect was independent of somatic CHD factors (including the severity of ECG ischemia); it proved to be stronger in depressed patients than in anxious ones. As depression scores increased by 1 standard deviation, the incidence of AP symptoms increased by 50%.

Davies et al. (1993) found that univariately minimal depressive mood loses its predictive significance when analyzed multivariately. However, the variable of symptom sensitivity and some ergometric parameters (e.g., duration of physical strain, threshold for ischemia) showed good predictive results multivariately. From univariate analyses of lowered psychological strain in SI cases, Buss and Herrmann (2000) were able to reproduce their results in the form of lower anxiety and depression scores, even over time. The remaining studies (Freedland et al., 1996; Torosian et al., 1997) were able to confirm only nonsignificantly lowered scores. Ahto et al. (1997) found no association between depressive mood and AP symptoms in a Finnish study.

5.3.2.1.2. Partially and less qualified studies. For a discussion of the partially qualified and less quali-

fied studies we located, see section W5.2 on the accompanying Web site.

5.3.2.1.3. Summary of relation between anxiety and depression and angina pectoris or silent ischemia. The study results on depression and anxiety in SI patients are inconsistent. The studies we evaluated failed to either test for or sufficiently consider the existence of anxiety symptoms; for this reason we were able to reach a conclusion only on depressive mood: The various study results show a tendency toward relatively normal psychometric results in SI patients compared with symptomatic AP patients. The same phenomenon occurs in exercise tests—SI patients were able to exercise more and longer. Davies et al. (1993) highlighted the advantage of multivariate analysis, the results of which suggest that anxiety and depression are confounded with exercise test behavior.

The results of lower depression scores in SI patients correspond to the positive association between depressive mood and angina symptoms. It most likely reflects the influence of psychological stress factors on both perception of pain and general sensitivity to physical symptoms. This phenomenon has also been demonstrated in longitudinal studies (see also section 5.4.2.6) for the incidence of AP or the differential diagnosis of chest pain (see also section 5.3.1). The fact that one can predict the incidence of symptomatic ischemic episodes on an ergometric test using depression scores (Herrmann-Lingen, 2001)—independent of sociodemographic and somatic variables—indicates a higher level of vulnerability and symptom-related attention in depressive CHD patients.

AP as a specific manifestation of CHD symptoms seems to be more strongly dependent on subjective than on objective CHD-associated somatic factors. Depressive mood and—although on a weaker scientific base—anxiety contribute as noncardiac psychological variables. Because of methodological difficulties (e.g., operationalization of denial processes), we cannot validly estimate the extent to which the comparably low depression and anxiety scores in SI patients are associated with further reaching mechanisms of denial that affect the perception of symptoms. Table W5.2 lists the studies on the associations of anxiety and depressive mood with AP or SI in CHD patients (see the Web site).

5.3.2.2. Association between anxiety and depressive mood and coronary atherosclerosis.

Costa's work group (Costa et al., 1985) found an association between neurotic symptoms and increased noncardiac chest pain. Some authors referred explicitly to these results, trying to elucidate the association between psychosocial factors and the severity of coronary atherosclerosis. Of the 10 studies we identified, 3 (mean $N = 1,262$) were very well qualified, 5 (mean $N = 64$) were partially qualified, and 2 (mean $N = 469$) were less qualified.

5.3.2.2.1. Very well qualified studies. Of the 10 studies we identified, we rated 3 of them as especially well qualified because of their high test power (Barefoot, Beckham, Peterson, Haney, & Williams, 1992; C. Herrmann et al., 1994; Herrmann-Lingen, 2001; Tennant, Langeluddecke, Fulcher, & Wilby, 1987). All 3 studies found no relevant (positive) association between anxiety or depressive mood and CHD severity. C. Herrmann et al. showed (although without targeted post hoc comparisons for each degree of stenosis) a negative correlation between anxiety on one hand and the number of narrowed blood vessels and extent of left ventricular impairment (as an indirect CHD criterion of severity) on the other. Although Herrmann-Lingen (2001) had a large sample, these results could not be confirmed in the subsample of CHD patients.

5.3.2.2.2. Partially and less qualified studies. For a discussion of the partially qualified and less qualified studies we located, see section W5.3 on the accompanying Web site.

5.3.2.2.3. Summary of the association between anxiety and depression and coronary atherosclerosis. The publications we analyzed could prove no substantial association between the variables of anxiety and depressive mood and the extent of coronary artery blockage; indeed, they failed to show even a hint of a positive association. There were, on the contrary, indications of an inverse association: Anxious patients who also manifested hypochondriac or somatoform symptoms tended to receive more invasive diagnostic tests and to have a comparatively lower

degree of CHD (in the more extreme cases, NCA; see also section 5.3.1). Anxiety and fear thus apparently influence the patient's decision to consult a physician and the physician's decision to do a coronary angiography. Anxiety in CHD patients therefore has a primarily protective function and acts to "select" these patients to survive. Whether the earlier or more frequent use of health care services consequently leads to better treatment and thus a more favorable disease course we cannot comment on; prospective studies are required to validate this. Table W5.3 lists studies investigating associations of anxiety and depressive mood with measures of coronary atherosclerosis (see the Web site).

5.3.2.3. Anxiety and depressive mood and other CHD-related topics.
Many studies have investigated the prevalence or correlations of anxiety and depression in a variety of specific CHD contexts. We have commented briefly on these studies on the Web site but do not analyze them in detail in this chapter (see section W5.4).

5.4. DISEASE PROGRESSION AND PROGNOSIS MODELS

5.4.1. Temporal Course of Anxiety and Depressive Mood in CHD Patients

In this section, we analyze studies on the natural course of anxiety and depressive mood in CHD patients. We have taken this information from explicit progression studies (see Table W5.4) and from descriptions of routinely treated control groups from different intervention studies (Table W5.5). Although the study reports do not describe the control groups in sufficient detail and focus too much on the differences between the control and intervention groups, such studies are so numerous that we would like to analyze them as far as possible within our scope. For this chapter we added brief mentions of 14 recently published studies that we were unable to analyze in detail because they appeared after we had completed our detailed analyses.

Of the 71 studies we identified, 11 naturalistic follow-up studies (described in 12 individual publications and 1 intervention study, mean $N = 327$)

were very well qualified, 7 naturalistic and 5 intervention studies (mean $N = 651$) were well qualified, and 17 observational and 12 intervention studies (mean $N = 81$) were partially qualified. Two observational and 16 intervention studies (mean $N = 45$) were less qualified. The mean N for the more recent studies was 163.

5.4.1.1. Very well qualified studies. These studies can be differentiated by situational aspects of disease manifestations such as the dramatic event of myocardial infarction or interventional procedures, which may differently impact on psychological well-being.

5.4.1.1.1. Disease course after myocardial infarction. Of the 13 very well qualified studies (usable studies $N = 3,925$; the study by Lésperance, Frasure-Smith, & Talajic, 1996, refers to the subgroup of Frasure-Smith et al., 2000b), the basic diagnostic methods used in 5 of them were implemented during treatment of the acute phase of myocardial infarction (MI). They suggest that CHD patients, on average, experience a decrease in anxiety and depression during the first phase after discharge from the hospital, possibly even within the first 3 days (Sykes, Evans, Boyle, McIlmoyle, & Salathia, 1989). This decrease applied only to patients with initially increased scores (Frasure-Smith et al., 2000b; Mayou et al., 2000; Sykes et al., 1989) and to patients with good somatic prognosis. The number of patients with a depressive disorder decreased significantly during the first 3 months after inpatient treatment of the acute phase (Schleifer et al., 1989). However, 50% to 75% of patients with initial major depression or increased depression scores showed the same high depression scores after 3 to 12 months (Frasure-Smith et al., 2000b; Lespérance et al., 1996; Schleifer et al., 1989). In addition, 15% to 20% of patients who showed subthreshold or no depression had at least one depressive episode or abnormal values within a year.

5.4.1.1.2. Perioperative progression in patients with coronary bypass surgery. The peri- and postoperative progression of patients' subjective well-being following coronary bypass surgery was the topic of scrutiny in three studies (Duits et al., 1998; C. D. Jenkins, Stanton, Savageau, Denlinger, & Klein,

1983; Timberlake et al., 1997). In contrast to studies on MI patients, these studies were able to collect preliminary data on their patients *before* the beginning of the coronary event in question. Duits et al. found that during the 2 weeks preceding the operation, a small decrease in state anxiety was already present (SD around −0.27), especially in women, who tended to show initially high scores. All three studies uniformly described the considerable decrease in anxiety or depression, on average, during postoperative progress. For anxiety, the effect measure after 6 months was between −0.66 and −1.14; again, women evinced higher scores than men (Duits et al., 1998; C. D. Jenkins et al., 1983). Duits et al. found an early total improvement of anxiety scores during the first postoperative week with stable scores thereafter.

The progress of depressive mood scores after a bypass operation showed a different trend: The decrease in depression scores after 6 months was smaller, with a standard deviation of −0.35 and −0.55 (Duits et al., 1998; C. D. Jenkins et al., 1983). An interesting point is that the decrease in depression scores, in contrast to the findings on anxiety, was not consistent in the first postoperative week. Instead, abnormal depressive mood scores possibly increased during this period over the limit of the preoperative scores (significantly, according to Timberlake et al., 1997, from 37% to 50%) or remained unchanged (Duits et al., 1998, men only). Only the women in Duits et al.'s study showed a decrease in depressive mood during the early phase after operation compared with 2 weeks before the operation. Timberlake et al. found a sharp decrease in depressive mood after bypass surgery beginning in the 8th postoperative week at the earliest. The prevalence stayed stable, however, until 1-year follow-up.

5.4.1.1.3. Anxiety and depression after coronary angiography. In coronary heart patients treated conservatively, Brummett et al. (1998) found a sharp decrease in depressive mood of roughly 0.4 standard deviations within a single month. This decrease corresponds to the fall of abnormal values from 42% to 27%.

5.4.1.1.4. Determinants of the dynamics of anxiety and depression. The progression of anxiety and depression over time in CHD patients is not yet fully explained and understood. It is likely to depend on the characteristics of the patient base, the situation, and subgroup characteristics. Mayou et al. (2000) described a slight increase later in the disease course after a strong decrease in anxiety and depression "cases" within the first 3 months after infarct. Van Elderen, Maes, and Dusseldorp (1999) found a continual decrease in anxiety and vital exhaustion scores of up to 0.25 standard deviations between admission into a rehabilitation program a month after the coronary event (i.e., infarct or revascularization) and at 1-year follow-up.

Denollet and de Potter (1992) observed subgroup-specific progressions in a comparable rehabilitation setting: Whereas the subgroup with average initial trait anxiety scores showed only a slight, statistically insignificant decrease in state anxiety scores of −0.1 to −0.3 standard deviations until the end of rehabilitation or 1-year follow-up, anxiety in patients initially categorized as "not very anxious" increased fractionally. State anxiety improved in the initially "very anxious" group with a standard deviation of −0.7 at the end of the program. The group improved considerably after a year, with a statistically significant −1.0 standard deviation. The scores were, indeed, significantly higher than those of the other subgroups.

In chronic CHD patients, Buss (1999) and Buss and Herrmann (2000) found differing anxiety and depression progressions between subgroups with initially silent versus symptomatic ischemia. The patients with initially SI and lower anxiety and depression showed significantly increased average anxiety (and a tendency toward increased depression as well) over a 3-year period. In initially symptomatic patients, anxiety scores tended to fall. Kemper (1997) and Herrmann-Lingen (2001) found significant rises in anxiety and depression averages in a study of men with three-vessel coronary blockage during the chronic postinfarct phase

after 2.6 years. In addition, their studies detected a significant increase in the percentage of abnormally depressive patients. Overall, the percentage of patients with abnormal anxiety and depression increased from roughly 20% to about 30%. Over 50% of initially depressed patients showed the same scores at the end of the postobservation phase.

Thus, we can draw the provisional conclusion that during the first treatment phase of an acute MI, after coronary angiography, or after bypass surgery, the psychological strain of the coronary event improves somewhat. For anxiety scores, this is most likely due to a certain leveling off in the regression to the mean. Initially increased anxiety scores fail to normalize completely—instead, they cache the risk of a continually increased level of anxiousness. At least a third to half of initially depressed patients, as well as a certain percentage of initially nondepressive patients, exhibited an abnormally depressive mood when tested again after 6 months or 1 year. During the chronic CHD phase, an increased level of anxiety and depression has been shown, at least in certain subgroups (e.g., SI, collapse of maladaptive denial, three-vessel coronary blockage).

5.4.1.2. Well-qualified studies. We identified 12 well-qualified studies (usable studies; number of subjects, $N = 7{,}809$) that did not show a very promising picture for the early postinfarct phase. Neither D. A. Jones and West (1996, using an assessment instrument with questionable validity)[1] nor Campbell and colleagues (Campbell, Ritchie, et al., 1998; Campbell, Thain, Deans, Ritchie, & Rawles, 1998) found any change in anxiety and depression 6 months or 1 year after the infarct. The Montreal Heart Attack Readjustment Trial (Frasure-Smith et al., 1997) also found that anxiety and depression in postinfarct control patients decreased only marginally after a year. Schott's (1987a, 1987b) results in Germany demonstrated a

---

[1] We classified the seemingly impressive intervention study by D. A. Jones and West (1996) with its negative results as well-qualified. However, a more detailed analysis of the methods and results reported raises severe doubts about the validity of that study. The instrument used for assessing anxiety and depressive symptoms is of unknown validity. Some doubt is also justified regarding the credibility of the results. For example, in an intervention study of that size, it is unbelievable that no refusals occurred; obviously, patients were randomized without their informed consent. In addition, for the 73% of randomized patients actually entering the intervention, no data on participation and dropout rates are reported.

significant increase in anxiety and depression within the first 6 months after the heart attack and only limited improvement thereafter. The deterioration of these patients was the worst in those who were not formally employed after the heart attack.

An interesting issue is whether specific cultural factors are responsible for the discrepant results. The German social welfare system constitutes a strong safety net, which may lead patients to adopt an anxious avoidance strategy with regard to the heart attack; Kemper's (1997) and Herrmann-Lingen's (2001) studies were done on German patients, including the ones done during the chronic CHD phase.

Additional evidence for subgroup-specific anxiety and depression courses can be found in Schleifer et al.'s (1991) study on infarct patients taking digitalis. The initially high prevalence for depression of 61% remained the same after 3 months. The patients not on digitalis experienced a regression in depression prevalence (including minor depression) from 45% to 30%. In terms of regression to the mean, one would expect the digitalis subgroup to improve more strongly than the less depressed subgroup because the digitalis patients' psychological test scores were initially worse. It is possible that some aspect of the physical disease plays a vital role in depression with digitalis therapy or, more likely, in the cardiac problems (e.g., heart failure, tachyarrhythmia) that lie at the heart of its prescription, preventing any natural improvement in patients. By contrast, Oldridge and colleagues found strong average drops in strain–anxiety and dejection–depression in both their sample not receiving any therapy and a sample of postinfarct patients receiving the usual care (Oldridge et al., 1991; Oldridge, Streiner, Hoffmann, & Guyatt, 1995). The postinfarct group was chosen according to the patients' initially above average psychological test scores. Within this study, the strongest improvements were seen in the subgroup with the highest initial scores (Crowe, Runions, Ebbesen, Oldridge, & Streiner, 1996); these results are consistent with the studies discussed previously in this section. Van Elderen, Maes, Seegers, et al. (1994) found minimal improvement in anxiety or vital exhaustion, or both,

during the CHD rehabilitation phase after 11 months (roughly −0.1 standard deviations) and no improvement after 4 months.

Mental strain reflected in a slight increase on the MOS 36-item Short Form Health Survey (SF–36; Ware & Sherbourne, 1992) mental health subscale, which the authors interpreted as depressive mood, was found during a 3-month period in outpatient, nonconfirmed CHD patients (Spertus, McDonell, Woodman, & Fihn, 2000). Initially abnormal scores persisted in 70% of the cases. Hance, Carney, Freedland, and Skala (1996) also observed a 50% persistence of major depression over 1 year following an elective coronary angiography. Two studies done by this group investigated the progression of peri- and postoperative well-being in patients following coronary artery bypass grafting (CABG) surgery (Sjöland et al., 1997; Sokol, Folks, Herrick, & Freeman, 1987). Sjöland et al. confirmed a postoperative decrease in anxiety and depression (which proved relatively steady). Sokol et al.'s (1987) study showed that depression scores in men during the early postoperative phase did not tend to decrease and later were reduced only very slightly. Sokol et al.'s study found significant decreases in anxiety and depression mostly in women, who, however, showed initially higher scores than the men. Women's depression scores partially reached men's scores over time. Yet women's scores generally tended to be higher.

5.4.1.3. Partially and less qualified studies.
For a discussion of the partially qualified and less qualified studies we located, see section W5.14.1 on the accompanying Web site.

5.4.1.4. New studies.
Of the 14 studies we identified that were published in 2000 and 2001, 8 concerned the progression of anxiety or depression, or both, following a coronary bypass operation (Andrew, Baker, Kneebone, & Knight, 2000; Boudrez & De Backer, 2001; Döring et al., 2001; Fraguas, Ramadan, Pereira, & Wajngarten, 2000; Karlsson, Berglin, & Larsson, 2000; McCrone, Lenz, Tarzian, & Perkins, 2001; Parent & Fortin, 2000; Silbert et al., 2001). The 2 largest studies (Boudrez & De Backer, 2001, N = 330; Karlsson et al., 2000, N = 147) described strong improvements in anxiety and

depression from before the operation to 1 year after the operation. Andrew et al. (*N* = 147) described considerably higher anxiety scores and unaltered depression scores before hospital discharge. The rest of the studies showed varying results with small patient numbers (*N*s < 100) and differing objectives. Three small studies (all *N* < 100; H. Lee, Kohlman, Lee, & Schiller, 2000; van Jaarsveld, Sanderman, Miedema, Ranchor, & Kempen, 2001; Yoshida et al., 2001) described disease progressions after an acute heart attack; the information they imparted is not new and hence is not described here. Three studies are on cardiac rehabilitation (Priebe & Sinning, 2001, *N* = 21) or the chronic CHD phase (Plevier et al., 2001, *N* = 99; Stewart et al., 2000, *N* = 1,130); the latter two found stable anxiety and depression scores over time, both during the natural progression of chronic CHD and during long-term medication with pravastatin.

5.4.1.5. Summary of the temporal course of anxiety and depression in CHD patients.
We found extensive results showing that anxiety and depression improve only slightly after an MI. Initially stressed subgroups showed a certain natural improvement, but they exhibited a higher prevalence of abnormal values.

Strong improvements, especially in patients who had elevated anxiety preoperatively, can often be expected shortly after a CABG. Depression scores, on the other hand, improved only following a slight delay, and not as much as did anxiety. An appreciable percentage of perioperative disorders persisted.

Some subgroups, especially during the chronic CHD phase, experienced considerable increases in psychological strain but did not receive any specific treatment. We have described the subgroups with the worst prognoses individually. Most likely, the severity of functional limitations, gender, and initial psychological status played a role in determining prognosis. Table W5.4 lists the specific naturalistic studies we located on the course of anxiety and depression in CHD patients, and Table W5.5 lists studies examining the course of anxiety and depression in the control groups of intervention trials on CHD patients (see the Web site).

5.4.2. Predicting Subsequent Self-Rated Emotions and Quality of Life Using Initial Anxiety and Depression

This section concentrates on the predictability of certain emotions in the broader sense in CHD patients. We look at two important aspects of predictability. First, we examine whether one can truly predict general anxiety and depression scores over time. We mentioned in section 5.4.1 that anxiety and depression demonstrate a relatively high degree of stability over time, which would suggest that anxiety should be a predictive factor for anxiety, and depression for depression. Cross-sectionally, both anxiety and depression are also associated with several different measures of physical and psychological complaints. Second, therefore, we will address whether, longitudinally, anxiety and depression are also able to predict other subjective outcomes at any particular point in time (see Table W5.6 on the Web site). To answer these questions, we studied 46 publications, of which 14 publications describing 11 different studies (mean *N* = 293) were very well qualified, 12 (mean *N* = 264) were well qualified, 15 (mean *N* = 84) were partially qualified, and 5 (mean *N* = 110) were less qualified. We will also cite 14 recently published studies (mean *N* = 215) that we unfortunately could not analyze in detail.

Among the 11 very well qualified studies (*N* = 3,224), Lespérance et al. (1996) reported the results of a subgroup from Frasure-Smith et al.'s (2000b) sample. The two studies by Ladwig and colleagues (Ladwig, Roll, Breithardt, & Borggrefe, 1999; Ladwig, Roll, Breithardt, Budde, & Borggrefe, 1994), as well as those by M. D. Sullivan and colleagues (M. D. Sullivan, LaCroix, Russo, & Katon, 1998; M. D. Sullivan et al., 1999), obviously were done on the same samples. These studies dealt with both predicting anxiety and depression or depressive disorders and predicting physical activity, cardiac symptoms, health-related quality of life, and other endpoints. In the majority of these studies, the patients were included in the trial following an MI, mostly during the acute treatment phase. They were followed up over a 3- to 12-month period. A smaller number of studies examined the predictability of subjective endpoints after coronary angiography (Brummett et al., 1998; M. D. Sullivan et al., 1998, 1999) or after bypass surgery (Duits et al., 1998; Timberlake et al., 1997). Other studies looked at mixed CHD samples (Moser & Dracup, 1995; van Elderen et al., 1999).

The 12 well-qualified studies (*N* = 3,174) reported on predicting anxiety and depression in postinfarct patients during both the acute phase (Barr-Taylor, Houston-Miller, Ahn, Haskell, & DeBusk, 1997; Mayou et al., 2000; Schleifer et al., 1989; Sykes et al., 1989) and at the beginning of rehabilitation (Denollet & de Potter, 1992; Duivenvoorden & van Dixhoorn, 1991). Some investigated the prediction of anxiety and depression in patients before heart surgery (mostly CABG; C. D. Jenkins, Stanton, & Jono, 1994; Perski et al., 1998; Vingerhoets, 1998), exercise testing (Buss, 1999; Buss & Herrmann, 2000), or elective heart catheterization (de Jong et al., 1994; Hance et al., 1996).

Schleifer et al. (1989) studied the prediction of depressive disorders. Sykes et al. (1989), Denollet and de Potter (1992), de Jong et al. (1994), Barr-Taylor et al. (1997), Vingerhoets (1998), and Mayou et al. (2000) attempted to predict cardiac symptoms through initial anxiety or depression. Sykes et al. (1989), Duivenvoorden and van Dixhoorn (1991), Perski et al. (1998), Buss (1999), and Buss and Herrmann (2000) predicted general emotional well-being or quality of life in their studies.

We looked at the very well qualified and well-qualified studies and analyzed them together with respect to the predictability of different endpoints. Each of the following sections discusses the very well qualified and then the well-qualified studies.

5.4.2.1. Predicting a depressive disorder or major depression.

In CHD patients with initially increased depression scores and a positive history of depression, major depression was more likely to be present a year after the infarct (Lespérance et al., 1996). In a multivariate analysis, only the initial number of clusters of depressive symptoms from diagnostic interviews in combination with older age was able to significantly predict independent com-

ponents of the incidence of major depression. Increased depression scores in questionnaires and a history of depression only approached significance in predicting independent components of the incidence of major depression. Pathological cardiac findings and social support showed no significant predictive value (Lespérance et al., 1996).

Schleifer et al. (1989) found that initial depression persisted in 77% of their infarct patients, at least in a broader sense of depression (including minor depression). This result corresponds to a highly significant OR of 5.1. Initial major depression, minor depression during the acute phase, and digitalis medication proved to be predictive of future depression (Schleifer et al., 1991). Hance et al. (1996) found a higher rate of remission for major depression in chronic CHD patients if their depression questionnaire scores were relatively low. Minor depression, however, decreased for elderly patients and those who had more severe CHD, independent of questionnaire scores. In any case, severe organic pathology was not related to a higher persistence of depression.

5.4.2.2. Predicting depressive mood, vital exhaustion, and anxiety.

Initial anxiety and depression scores on questionnaires proved to be the best predictors of corresponding follow-up scores in almost all the studies (Barr-Taylor et al., 1997; Brummett et al., 1998; de Jong et al., 1994; Denollet & de Potter, 1992; Duits et al., 1999; Frasure-Smith et al., 2000b; Mayou et al., 2000; Perski et al., 1998; Timberlake et al., 1997; Vingerhoets, 1998).

5.4.2.3. Depressive mood.

Timberlake et al. (1997) found a predictive effect of preoperative trait anxiety in a post-CABG sample for subsequent occurrence of depression. In some of their analyses, they also found a predictive effect of both older age and lower number of implanted grafts for incident depression. Brummett et al. (1998) found age to be negatively associated with depression occurring within 1 month after coronary angiography. After adjusting for age, initial depression scores, gender, and CHD severity, they found an independent protective effect of social support and an indirect negative effect of hostility; this hostility effect was mediated by low social support.

Frasure-Smith et al. (2000b) were able to shed some light on the residual variance of depressive mood in postinfarct patients through the interaction of initial depressive mood with different measures of social support. Their findings show that a good social support system favorably influences the course of depression only in initially depressive patients. In a subgroup of this study reported by Lespérance et al. (1996), there was no association between cardiac severity markers and the occurrence of major depression. Frasure-Smith et al. (2000b), conversely, found that they might significantly predict depressive mood in their larger patient group using the initial Killip class (a measure of the severity of heart failure) and the existence of diabetes. In diabetes patients, those who were initially depressive were at high risk for reporting depressive mood later on. The predictive interaction between measures of social support and initial depressive mood persisted at least as a tendency, even after adjustment was made for somatic predictors. In contrast to these studies, Barr-Taylor et al. (1997) described being female as an independent predictor for increased depressive mood a year after MI.

5.4.2.4. Anxiety. Ladwig et al. (1994) predicted increased anxiety scores after 6 months using moderately (relative risk [RR] = 1.9) and severely (RR = 4.6) elevated depression scores during the acute post-MI treatment phase. In doing so, however, they did not monitor the predictive effect of initial anxiety scores. Sykes et al. (1989) identified the interaction between severity of infarct and time of hospital discharge as a predictor for state anxiety 3 days after discharge and for a positive answer to an ad hoc anxiety item 3 months after discharge. Early rather than late hospital discharge prompted a stronger short-term decrease in anxiety scores in patients with a good cardiac prognosis. Yet in patients with a poorer prognosis, early hospital discharge led to a higher prevalence of anxiety. Given the unvalidated items and very low cutoff, this finding can also be interpreted otherwise—that the patients discharged earlier perhaps denied less and thus were able to express a moderate but adaptive degree of anxiety.

De Jong et al. (1994) predicted state anxiety measured 1 day before coronary angiography in multivariate analyses. Independent predictors were initial level of anxiety (measured 3 weeks before the procedure), age, and gender. Pathologic cardiac test results and medication showed no effect.

5.4.2.5. Anxiety and depressive mood (vital exhaustion, distress). Depressive mood or vital exhaustion and additional anxiety were investigated by Denollet and de Potter (1992), de Jong et al. (1994), Moser and Dracup (1995), Kemper (1997), Herrmann-Lingen (2001), van Elderen et al. (1999), and M. D. Sullivan et al. (1999) for their predictability in coronary heart patients beyond the acute phase. These studies reported relatively high longitudinal correlations of anxiety and depression scores, which rose to roughly $r = .6$ and even higher over 3 weeks to 2.6 years, even in multivariate analyses. M. D. Sullivan et al. were able to predict extremely high (up to +1.7 SD) anxiety and depression scores in a 6-month follow-up of patients who had depressive disorders early after coronary angiography. Vingerhoets (1998) and Duits et al. (1999) were able to predict postoperative anxiety and depression using baseline anxiety measured before CABG or heart surgery in general. Mayou et al. (2000) identified "psychological distress" (i.e., increased anxiety or depression, or both) 3 months after an infarct as the best predictor of distress after a year. Distress persisted in 53% of the patients with initially abnormal values.

Beyond the expected retest correlations, most of these studies found further independent predictors of anxiety and depressive mood: In heterogeneous samples from Phase 2 (postacute care) to Phase 3 (chronic phase) rehabilitation, Denollet and de Potter (1992), van Elderen et al. (1999), and Moser and Dracup (1995) reported an additional longitudinal effect of initial coping style and locus of control. Denollet and de Potter identified four patient clusters on the basis of trait anxiety (or negative affectivity), self-deception, and social inhibition. They found the cluster with higher trait anxiety and social inhibition and decreased self-deception to be at risk for higher state anxiety later on. Avoidance coping was associated with somewhat lower anxiety in a cross-sectional study by van Elderen et al. However, longitudinally it showed no effect. By contrast, approach coping was initially associated with increased anxiety and vital exhaustion, yet longitudinally it predicted lower scores on both anxiety and vital exhaustion scales ($r = -.20$ to $-.26$), independent of initial scores. The findings in a subgroup of postinfarct patients were basically the same. Moser and Dracup identified a low perceived sense of control over illness as the only independent predictor for anxiety and depression after MI. Sociodemographic variables, severity of disease, and medication did not show any effect.

Kemper (1997) and Herrmann-Lingen (2001) examined extensive initial cardiac data for predictability of anxiety and depression in a chronic post-MI sample over a 2.6-year follow-up. However, they found few significant effects. After examining initial anxiety and depression scores, they concluded that anxiety could additionally be predicted by large ventricular diameter as measured by echocardiography. Depressive mood could be predicted only using cardiac events occurring during the interim ($\beta = 0.19$ for prediction of both anxiety and depression).

Duits et al. (1999) predicted anxiety and depression after open heart surgery (mainly CABG) using internal longitudinal correlations, cross-correlations between anxiety and depressive mood, and initial neuroticism. Vingerhoets (1998) also found preoperative anxiety and depression to predict postoperative results. Early postoperative depressive mood was more difficult (but not significantly so) to predict than follow-up depressive mood (Timberlake et al., 1997, showed the same results).

5.4.2.6. Predicting cardiac symptoms using anxiety and depression. Denollet and de Potter (1992), Ladwig et al. (1994, 1999), and the studies by Kemper (1997) and Herrmann-Lingen (2001) were able to predict cardiac symptoms using anxiety and depression; their studies were, however, limited to men. Schleifer et al. (1989) and Mayou et al. (2000) tested men and women after an acute infarct. C. D. Jenkins et al. (1994) and Perski et al. (1998) worked with both men and women before

heart surgery. M. D. Sullivan et al. (1999) and Buss (1999) assessed patients during a routine cardiologic checkup.

In Ladwig et al.'s (1994) sample of acute infarct patients, initially abnormal depressive mood was predictive of AP symptoms 6 months later (RR = 2.3). Moderately to highly abnormal depression scores were predictive of AP both at rest and during exercise (RR = 2.8). This prediction was valid not only for the persistence of preexisting angina symptoms but also for its occurrence in initially asymptomatic patients. The variables depressive mood, preinfarct angina, and low professional status were able to predict angina symptoms after 6 months in a multivariate prediction model (multivariate OR = 3.0).

By contrast, Schleifer et al.'s (1989) results showed only insignificantly more frequent chest pain 3 months after an infarct in initially depressive versus nondepressive patients. Mayou et al.'s (2000) results also showed mainly insignificantly increased angina and dyspnea in initially anxious or depressive patients after 3 months. They found a significantly increased percentage only of (mostly atypical) chest pain among initially anxious or depressive patients after 1 year. Denollet and de Potter (1992) found angina complaints to be significantly more frequent after a year among CHD rehabilitation patients with high initial trait anxiety compared with other subgroups.

Kemper's (1997) and Herrmann-Lingen's (2001) chronic postinfarct sample showed a predictability of cardiac symptoms after 2.6 years using diverse cardiac predictors as well as initial depressive mood ($\rho = 0.27$) and especially using initial anxiety ($\rho = 0.42$). Initial frequency of cardiac complaints, low left ventricular ejection fraction, and increased anxiety ($\beta = 0.23$) all contributed independently to predicting cardiac symptoms in multivariate analyses. Other initial cardiac findings and cardiac treatments received during the follow-up interval did not show any independent predictive effect.

C. D. Jenkins et al.'s (1994) results showed that trait anxiety and depressive mood were bivariately predictive of cardiac complaints 6 months after a heart operation. Trait anxiety proved to be the best predictor in a multivariate model. Additionally, these cardiological symptoms were independently predictable by initial dyspnea, preoperative hospitalization, sleep disorders, lack of friends, and number of *pack years* (total number of years smoked multiplied by number of packs of cigarettes smoked per day) smoked. Perski et al. (1998) were able to predict, using preoperative emotional distress, a higher rate of spontaneously occurring and exercise test–induced angina symptoms, as well as patients' intake of nitroglycerine medication.

M. D. Sullivan et al. (1999) found stronger heart-related symptoms at 1-year follow-up in patients who received a diagnosis of depression shortly after a coronary angiography showing CHD. This effect was stronger for initial major depression but could also be observed in minor depression.

Buss (1999) and Buss and Herrmann (2000) compared chronic CHD patients with initially symptomatic versus SI during a 3.3-year period. During this period, they found more frequent angina symptoms in initially asymptomatic patients with very low depression scores. Concurrently, these patients' average follow-up anxiety and depression scores surpassed the mean. We thus interpreted the initial findings as a possible effect of denial that, over time, became maladaptive or at least broke down partially. This, in turn, determined the occurrence of AP and the more frequent reporting of physical and psychological symptoms. These findings are similar to those of van Elderen et al. (1999): Avoidance coping accompanied low psychological strain only on a short-term basis. In the medium term, approach coping resulted in better well-being.

5.4.2.7. Predicting physical activity and quality of life using anxiety and depression. Kemper (1997), Herrmann-Lingen (2001), Perski et al. (1998), and M. D. Sullivan et al. (1998, 1999) reported on predictors of quality of life; Sykes et al. (1989), Denollet and de Potter (1992), Duivenvoorden and van Dixhoorn (1991), Buss (1999), and Buss and Herrmann (2000) also briefly touched on this subject. Kemper found that chronic postinfarct patients' initial anxiety and de-

pression scores were able to bivariately predict six targeted quality of life dimensions ($\rho = 0.3–0.5$). The effects of initial depressive mood were, on average, 0.1 standard deviation above those of initial anxiety. Multivariately, the depression scores entered the prediction models for five of the six subscales as well as for global quality of life. Only "negative mood" was mainly predicted using initial anxiety instead of depressive mood. "Psychological capacity" was equally predictable using anxiety and depression, both of which remained in the multivariate model. Aside from depressive mood and anxiety, the other predictor variables were of minor predictive significance. Objective cardiac findings figured into the prediction only of general capacity (predictors: maximum exercise test performance, occurrence of cardiac events during the follow-up period), negative mood (predictor: initially negative exercise ECG), and socioemotional well-being (predictor: revascularization before baseline assessment), with standardized regression coefficients of about 0.2 for each of these predictors. A larger effect was obtained for the initially perceived cardiac symptom load. This effect was independent of the effect found for depressive mood, and especially predicted general quality of life ($\beta = -0.28$) and social capacity. M. D. Sullivan et al. (1998, 1999) found several dimensions of social and functional impairment 1 year after coronary angiography predicted by initial depressive disorders, level of education, low self-efficacy, and—independently of these variables—initial anxiety.

In an acute treatment setting, Huijbrechts et al. (1997), using several questionnaires, examined first-time infarct patients in the acute care hospital without severe psychological disorders, who completed several questionnaires. Five months after the event, they explored patients' physical activity. Patients who limited their physical activity level after the heart attack (15%) had been significantly more anxious, depressed, and vitally exhausted (0.5–0.7 standard deviations) at initial assessment than patients who remained more active. Vitality (as the extreme opposite of depression and vital exhaustion) and state anxiety were able to independently predict the activity level reported at follow-up assessment. In a multivariate discriminant model, additional significant predictors included initial impairment, age, and gender.

Sykes et al.'s (1989) infarct patients, who demonstrated higher anxiety 6 to 11 days after infarct, showed much less "return to normal life" 3 months after infarct. Over time, Denollet and de Potter's (1992) rehabilitation patients perceived themselves to be more handicapped than others if they belonged to the habitually anxious cluster (see section 5.4.1.1.4). They also felt a subjectively more limited sense of well-being. By contrast, Duivenvoorden and van Dixhoorn (1991) were unable to use initial anxiety to predict the composite score of six self-assessment questionnaires at the end of a 5-week rehabilitation period. The questionnaires included items on anxiety, sleep, physical limitations, and functional complaints to operationalize "psychological well-being." In addition to several other predictors, vital exhaustion, self-reported psychological stress, and "functional complaints" were significantly associated with a worse outcome.

Buss (1999) and Buss and Herrmann (2000) demonstrated that increased anxiety in chronic CHD patients with initially silent or symptomatic ischemia was associated with a more negative general appraisal of disease progression over a 3.3-year period. In initially symptomatic patients, increased depressive mood predicted a perceived poorer quality of life as rated by single items on a questionnaire. Initially anxious patients with AP felt cardiologically more vulnerable at follow-up than nonanxious patients did. In the subgroup with AP, anxiety and depression were predictive of less willingness on the part of friends and family to accept and support the patient in his or her sick role.

5.4.2.8. Partially and less qualified studies. For information on the partially and less qualified studies we located, see section W5.14.2 on the accompanying Web site.

5.4.2.9. New studies on predicting subjective endpoints. Fourteen studies published in 2000 and 2001 touched on the prediction of different subjective endpoints. We were unable to analyze them in detail for this chapter. Most of the eight medium-sized studies (Ns = 100–500) on the per-

ceived progression of anxiety and depression after CABG found that early psychological well-being predicted psychological well-being at a later point in time (Andrew et al., 2000; Boudrez & De Backer, 2001; Hamalainen et al., 2000; Saur et al., 2001). Two of these studies described predictive correlations between anxiety and depressive mood and coping (Döring et al., 2001) or sense of coherence (Karlsson et al., 2000). Two further studies examined the influence of age and gender (McCrone et al., 2001) or differing operation techniques (hypothermia vs. normothermia; Khatri et al., 2001) on postoperative anxiety and depressive mood.

Five studies investigated predictions of perceived progression of anxiety and depression after an infarct or coronary event (Cossette, Frasure-Smith, & Lespérance, 2001; Fritz, 2000; Hämäläinen et al., 2000; Lane, Carroll, Ring, Beevers, & Lip, 2000a, 2001a). These studies documented predictions of anxiety or depressive mood using baseline scores and personality variables and using short-term reactions to psychosocial intervention. Anxiety and depressive mood also predicted quality of life 4 to 12 months after infarct. One study (Denollet, Vaes, & Brutsaert, 2000) demonstrated that quality of life over 5 years could be predicted using depressive mood at the beginning of CHD rehabilitation (following different coronary events or procedures). M. D. Sullivan, LaCroix, Russo, and Walker (2001) were able to predict the self-assessment of physical health 5 years after infarct using depression scores obtained 1 year after coronary angiography. They were additionally able to identify mediators of this association.

5.4.2.10. Summary of predicting physical activity and quality of life using anxiety and depression. The available literature makes four major points on prediction. First, a depressive disorder is often seen in heart patients when a depressive episode has already occurred in the patient's medical history or during the early postinfarct phase. In initially nondepressive infarct patients, subthreshold depressive symptoms prove to be a further relevant predictor. The predictive significance of severe pathological organic findings is uncertain, however. A depressive episode occurring soon after an infarct is likely to persist, especially when self-assessed depression scores are also high.

Second, anxiety and depressive mood can best be predicted following a coronary event by their initial scores. For initially depressed patients, a good social support system can be especially advantageous for the remission of depressive mood. Personality traits, coping styles, physical sensations, measures of disease severity, duration of hospital treatment, surgical techniques, age, and gender are possibly relevant for the course of anxiety and depressive mood in coronary heart patients. The findings discussed in this section draw on a few sometimes contradictory studies and cannot therefore be viewed as conclusive. However, the literature suggests that large effects of, for example, physical severity markers cannot be expected for this question.

Third, in patients who are depressive during the acute phase, cardiac complaints, especially (sometimes atypical) AP, occur more frequently during the 6 to 12 months after heart surgery or an acute MI. This observation may be valid for initially anxious patients as well. During the chronic postinfarct phase, the level of cardiac symptoms is predictable through initial depression and especially through anxiety scores. However, extraordinarily low depression scores in patients with silent myocardial ischemia appear to hint at maladaptive denial that, in turn, favors the new occurrence of AP. This isolated result is, however, in need of confirmation by future studies.

Fourth, the different physical, psychological, and social dimensions of health-related quality of life all demonstrate nearly identical, distinct dependencies on initial anxiety and depression. The effect of depression is, on average, larger than that of anxiety. The depression effect usually strongly surpasses the influence of more "solid" physical findings when it comes to predicting quality of life. Depressive mood thus reduces the quality of life of heart patients to a much greater extent than does the cardiac organic defect. Table W5.6 lists studies on anxiety and depression as predictors of subjective endpoints in CHD patients, including predic-

tion of future anxiety and depression (see the Web site).

5.4.3. Predicting Illness Behavior Using Anxiety and Depression

Twenty-six of the studies we analyzed investigated objectively observed aspects of sick role behavior for predictability using anxiety or depression. We do not include studies that attempted to predict solely return to work, which are the topic of section 5.4.4. In the current section, we examine the predictability of various aspects of health care utilization—for example, compliance with medication and participation in rehabilitation programs (see Table W5.7 on the Web site). Of the 26 publications we identified, 12 (reporting on 9 different studies; mean N = 824) were very well qualified, 8 (mean N = 234) were well qualified, 5 (mean N = 166) were partially qualified, and one (N = 42) was less qualified.

5.4.3.1. Very well qualified studies. The very well qualified studies (N = 7,415) mainly investigated aspects of health care utilization. Frasure-Smith et al. (2000a) showed that infarct patients with increased depression scores during the acute treatment phase stayed in the hospital significantly longer than nondepressive patients. The effect size for length of stay was moderate, at 0.19 standard deviations. These depressive patients caused increased costs (an average increase of 718 Canadian dollars). After a year, the difference in total costs for a depressive patient from the time of discharge onward increased to 822 Canadian dollars. These authors also found a similar result for initially anxious versus nonanxious infarct patients (Frasure-Smith & Lespérance, 1998). The increased costs after hospital discharge were caused by more frequent and longer cardiac rehospitalizations and more visits to emergency rooms and primary care physicians. Part of the total costs for depressive patients was accounted for by the initial severity of infarct, gender, level of education, and high blood pressure; however, even after adjusting for these factors, total medical costs after hospital stay were 11% higher for depressive than for nondepressive patients.

Scheier et al. (1999) and J. B. Levine et al. (1996) found results similar to those of Frasure-Smith et al. (2000a): They identified a relationship between initial depressive mood and cardiac rehospitalization in patients who experienced an acute infarct or coronary intervention, and effect sizes were much larger than those of previous studies. Scheier et al. compared the depression scores of cardiac surgery patients in the highest and lowest quartiles. The OR for rehospitalization for treatment of wound infection was 5.4, with higher rates in the most depressed subgroup even after adjusting for other predictor variables. Levine et al. examined the interaction between depressive mood and the *ejection fraction* (i.e., the percentage of ventricular filling volume ejected into the circulation by the heart during each contraction) as independent predictors of rehospitalization. Ejection fraction alone was not a predictor. On average, depressive patients were hospitalized for cardiac reasons more than 3 times (i.e., 6 days) longer than nondepressive patients. Anxiety was not a significant predictor.

Herrmann-Lingen (2001), Buss (1999), and Buss and Herrmann (2000) sought to predict outpatient health care use. Herrmann-Lingen demonstrated that in CHD patients undergoing an exercise test, increased depressive mood or elevated scores on at least one subscale of the hospital anxiety and depression instrument predicted the need for a second exercise test within 2 years. This effect was especially strong in women. Isolated high anxiety scores did not have the same effect. Even after controlling for somatic and sociodemographic factors, this effect was still significant: Initially anxious or depressive (or both) patients showed an adjusted probability for a second exercise test of 27% above patients with normal psychological scores.

Buss (1999) and Buss and Herrmann (2000) found a significant association between number of physician visits over 3.3 years and initial depression and anxiety among patients with silent myocardial ischemia. Patients with initially symptomatic (vs. silent) ischemia and increased anxiety showed a higher risk for a second coronary angiography during the follow-up period. Moreover, Kemper (1997) and Herrmann-Lingen (2001)

showed that initial anxiety and depression could predict the type, but not the absolute number, of coronary interventions needed in men during the postinfarct phase (as did Frasure-Smith et al., 2000a, during the acute infarct phase). Initially depressive patients subsequently underwent fewer bypass operations. However, anxious and depressive patients had coronary dilatations done more frequently.

Five of the very well qualified studies looked into other aspects of sick role behavior. Huijbrechts et al. (1996) and Ladwig et al. (1994) demonstrated that a larger percentage of patients who were depressive after an infarct continued to smoke 5 to 6 months afterwards; these results held true even in multivariate analyses. The predictive role of anxiety turned out to be less significant in Huijbrecht et al.'s analyses. Ladwig et al. did not investigate this particular point. Ziegelstein et al. (2000) confirmed the rough direction of the effect of depression on abstinence from nicotine, but it was not statistically significant. The authors found, however, that abnormal depressive mood was significantly inversely related not only to global measures of adherence 4 months after infarct, but also to poorer indicators in diverse behavioral aspects such as regular exercise, low-fat diet, stress reduction, and social contacts. The initial presence of major depression or dysthymia additionally served to predict worse adherence to prescription medications and, when applicable, to a diabetic diet.

Irvine, Baker, et al. (1999) examined compliance with medication in the randomized Canadian Amiodarone Myocardial Infarction Arrhythmia (CAMIAT) study on amiodarone medication in postinfarct patients. They observed no effect of depression on compliance with medication in either the amiodarone or the placebo group. However, compliance with medication proved to be an independent factor of prognosis in both groups; in the placebo group, patient prognosis additionally depended on the level of social activity before the infarct.

In a univariate analysis of low trait anxiety and depression, Lane, Carroll, Ring, Beevers, and Lip (2001b) were able to predict whether a heart patient would participate in a rehabilitation program or not. This effect lost its statistical significance after adjusting for sociodemographic factors, cardiac factors, and the level of activity before infarct.

5.4.3.2. Well-qualified studies. The well-qualified studies ($N = 1,872$) partly confirmed and partly refuted the results of the very well qualified studies. Mayou et al. (2000) found that anxious and depressive infarct patients used more hospital hours during the acute phase and visited their physicians significantly more often during the 3- to 12-month study period. Yet these patients were not rehospitalized more frequently. Schleifer et al. (1989) observed that initial depression did not influence the rate of rehospitalization 3 months after acute infarct. This negative result should be interpreted with caution because of the relatively small sample, high dropout rate, and short follow-up interval. Contrary to these studies, Westin et al. (1997) found significantly more revascularizations in their subgroup of initially depressive infarct patients within a year compared with nondepressive patients. Their findings also showed that depressive and nondepressive patients visited the emergency room with roughly the same frequency.

Habitually anxious patients in Denollet and de Potter's (1992) rehabilitation sample showed a higher intake of sedatives after 15 months. In CABG patients, Wachter et al. (2000) could not prove any effect of preoperative anxiety or depression on various measures of medical service use (e.g., medication, clinical examination) during the acute inpatient treatment phase.

Several studies in this category examined the predictability of behavior modifications, especially to control risk factors. Mayou et al. (2000) found a larger percentage of smokers among infarct patients who showed acute psychological distress after 3 to 12 months. These patients also did less physical exercise and showed significant constraints in general activities. In an early study, Guiry, Conroy, Hickey, and Mulcahy (1987) reported that anxiety as well as depression after infarct predicted less compliance with exercise and tended to predict less weight reduction. Only depression predicted less abstinence from nicotine with borderline significance. Blumenthal, Williams, Wallace, Williams,

and Needles (1982) found more anxiety and depression among patients who subsequently quit a cardiac rehabilitation program. Habitually anxious and socially inhibited patients tended to prematurely quit rehabilitation treatment more often (Denollet & de Potter, 1992). On the other hand, Petrie, Weinman, Sharpe, and Buckley (1996) found that patients with a low mental health index on the SF–36, which they interpreted as an expression of increased anxiety, tended to participate in rehabilitation programs more often after infarct (they provided no data on successful completion of the program).

5.4.3.3. Partially or less qualified studies. For a discussion of the partially qualified and less qualified studies we located, see section W5.15.1 on the accompanying Web site.

5.4.3.4. Summary of predicting illness behavior using anxiety and depression. These studies show that depressive and anxious infarct patients are hospitalized longer than psychologically normal patients, resulting in higher costs. Initial depression and possibly anxiety are associated with high medical costs after the acute treatment phase; it is not yet clear whether this is an independent effect or where these higher costs come from. Depressive mood (but not anxiety) seems to predict more frequent or longer cardiac rehospitalizations not only after an infarct but also after coronary revascularization, but most results show no effect on total rehospitalizations.

Anxious and depressive heart patients visit outpatient clinics and general practitioners frequently. One study found increased sedative intake by anxious and depressive postinfarct patients. The data from the few large trials on the use of outpatient cardiological treatment or repeat exercise tests are contradictory, as are data on emergency room admissions and coronary interventions. Only a few smaller studies provide data on the use of initial anxiety to predict need for a renewed angiography or participation in a rehabilitation program. Nevertheless, three studies indicate a higher percentage of initially anxious or depressive patients who quit rehabilitation, even though this effect proved to be multivariately significant in only one of the studies.

In the five largest studies, initially more depressive infarct patients abstained from smoking less often during the first year following infarct. The effect of anxiety on smoking behavior was not often examined separately; in the few studies that did so, the effect was not consistently significant.

Other aspects of compliance (e.g., following through with recommendations on physical exercise), including the successful completion of a rehabilitation treatment program, also seem to be predictable using anxiety or depression scores. The data for predicting compliance with medication, despite several positive findings, were on the whole inconsistent. Table W5.7 lists studies examining anxiety and depression as predictors of illness behavior in CHD patients (see the Web site).

5.4.4. Predicting Return to Work Using Anxiety and Depression

A series of trials have been done examining the prediction of return to work for coronary heart patients. We examined return to work in the context of whether anxiety and depression are potential predictors (Table W5.8). Of 17 studies we identified, 4 (mean N = 454) were very well qualified, 7 (mean N = 246) were well qualified, 5 (mean N = 130) were partially qualified, and 1 (mean N = 28) was less qualified.

5.4.4.1. Very well qualified and well-qualified studies.
We discuss the very well qualified (N = 1,814) and well-qualified (N = 1,726) studies together because there are few. Schleifer et al. (1989) and Ladwig et al. (1994) identified major depression or a strongly abnormal depression score (interpreted as severe depression) as a predictor of lower probability of return to work. For depressive patients who were employed before their infarct, Schleifer et al. calculated an OR of 0.36 for return to work within 3 months. Ladwig et al. found a probability of return to work of 0.39 in their depressive sample. This value increased in a multivariate model to 0.54, however, and thus was no longer significant. Guiry et al. (1987) also found a tendency toward decreased return to work in patients assessed as depressive using a semistructured interview. Soejima, Steptoe, Nozoe, and Tei (1999)

studied Japanese men with a high overall return-to-work rate. The relatively few patients who showed any depressive symptoms had significantly reduced rates of return to work in univariate (OR = 0.22) and multivariate (OR = 0.15) analyses. These authors did not monitor for cardiac severity markers.

Dimsdale, Hackett, Hutter, and Block (1982); Schott (1987a, 1987b); and Budde and Keck (2001) examined depressive mood (as a dimensional variable) as a predictor of return to work. Dimsdale et al. did not find any effect of initial depressive mood in their heterogeneous sample of coronary angiography patients. Among Schott et al.'s patients, those who were initially highly depressive either retired early or were still on sick leave. In their Oldenburg Longitudinal Study sample in Germany, initial anxiety scores had an even stronger effect. Anxiety scores were also significantly increased in patients who were on sick leave, who retired early, and (unlike depressive mood) who temporarily retired later. Neither basic cardiac data nor rehabilitation participation proved to play a major role in return to work. However, the findings on anxiety as a return-to-work predictor were not uniform: Budde and Keck found that in a (not purely CHD) sample of cardiac rehabilitation patients, anxiety and depressive mood in both genders predicted a lower 6-month rating of "positive work situation" (meaning that they had returned to work or were participating in employment rehabilitation). Multivariately, women's depression and men's anxiety, depending on the control variables included in the analyses, remained significant predictors but partly lost their independent significance to predict anticipation of occupational problems. Denollet and de Potter (1992) in Belgium and Petrie et al. (1996) in New Zealand also found increased anxiety to be associated with lower return-to-work rates in the first 6 weeks to 3 months after infarct (again, physical fitness or participation in rehabilitation did not play a major role). In contrast, Guiry et al. (1987) in Ireland and Sykes et al. (1989) in Northern Ireland did not find a predictive effect for anxiety.

Maeland and Havik (1987) in Norway did not differentiate between anxiety and depression in their study. They measured anxiety and depression on a 4-point scale. Their results showed a linear association between anxiety and depression (measured on Day 9 after infarct) and 6-month return to work in previously employed infarct patients. Multivariate analysis confirmed this association and additionally identified work expectation, knowledge of cardiac risk factors, area of residence, and occurrence of cardiac complications as further predictors.

5.4.4.2. Partially and less qualified studies.
For a discussion of the partially qualified and less qualified studies we located, see section W5.15 on the accompanying Web site.

5.4.4.3. Summary of predicting return to work using anxiety and depression.
Clinical depression or depressive mood is uniformly associated with lower rates of return to work after an acute heart attack. In other coronary heart patient samples, this result is not as clear-cut. The predictive significance of anxiety is uncertain; it was shown to be significant in only two isolated (i.e., without concurrently measured depression) samples that were both German; features of the German social welfare system may be factors in this finding.

The studies on predicting return to work have a stronger focus on men than any other group of predictive studies. Hence, no conclusion is possible on predicting return to work in women. There is, however, preliminary evidence that depression also holds predictive significance in women. Table W5.8 lists studies of anxiety and depression as predictors of employment or return to work (see the Web site).

5.4.5. Predicting Hard Somatic Endpoints Using Anxiety and Depression
We identified 47 publications that investigated the prediction of "hard" somatic endpoints (i.e., determinable somatic events, such as death or MI; "semihard" endpoints include clearly observable events that are to some degree influenced by physician–patient interaction, such as cardiac surgery) through anxiety or depression in CHD patients, of which more than half were very well or well qualified for our purposes. Of the publications we identified, 22 (reporting on 16 different studies;

mean $N = 725$) were very well qualified, 6 (5 different studies; mean $N = 276$) were well qualified, 10 (9 different studies; mean $N = 489$) were partially qualified, and 9 (mean $N = 568$) were less qualified.

5.4.5.1. Very well qualified studies.
The predictive power of depression and anxiety for somatic endpoints differs among different stages of disease and also depends on interactions with other predictive factors. Thus, it will be analyzed by setting, at least for the very well qualified studies.

5.4.5.1.1. Predictive significance of depression and depressive mood after an acute heart attack. Twenty-two publications reporting on 16 studies were very well qualified (effective $N = 11,600$). Fourteen of these publications examined the predictability of clear-cut, hard endpoints (i.e., sudden or cardiac death, survived cardiac arrest) using depressive disorders or depressive mood in patients shortly following an infarct. Frasure-Smith and colleagues (Frasure-Smith et al., 2000b; Frasure-Smith, Lespérance, Juneau, Talajic, & Bourassa, 1999; Frasure-Smith, Lespérance, & Talajic, 1993, 1995a, 1995b) reported results from the Emotions and Prognosis Post-Infarct (EPPI) study and the Montreal Heart Attack Readjustment Trial (MHART). Three studies on antiarrhythmics, Cardiac Arrhythmic Pilot Study (CAPS; Ahern et al., 1990), Cardiac Arrhythmic Suppression Trial (CAST; S. A. Thomas, Friedmann, Wimbush, & Schron, 1997), and CAMIAT (Irvine, Basinski, et al., 1999), and the Post-Infarction Late Potential study (PILP; Ladwig, Kieser, Konig, Breithardt, & Borggrefe, 1991) also are relevant to this discussion. Recent studies by Kaufmann et al. (1999); Bush et al. (2001); and Lane, Carroll, Ring, Beevers, and Lip (2000a, 2000b, 2001a) mostly confirm, at least univariately, the unfavorable significance of depression in predicting the principal endpoints.

The effects for the prediction of cardiac mortality or cardiac arrest are presented in Table W5.9; for major depression, the reported ORs are between 6.2 and 3.6, with a decreasing tendency over increasing follow-up intervals of up to 18 months. These data are from the EPPI study, which is the only relevant source for this issue. However, only deaths within the first 6 months were factually predicted; the longer term effect arose solely from the delayed decrease in early differences (Frasure-Smith et al., 1995a). In contrast, abnormal questionnaire depression scores (Beck Depression Inventory [BDI] > 10; Beck & Steer, 1987; Beck, Steer, & Brown, 1988) in this study also predicted (with an OR of 13.0) cardiac mortality after more than 6 months. Hence, the predictive effect of these scores actually increased with the duration of follow-up from OR = 5.6 at 6 months to OR = 7.8 at 18 months. The ORs in two publications by the same group reporting on the pooled EPPI and MHART (control group) samples were lower, between 3.0 and 3.3 over 1 year. The authors additionally demonstrated that the effect held for both men and women (Frasure-Smith et al., 1999) and was very strong for patients with low social support (Frasure-Smith et al., 2000b). Ladwig et al. (1991) found significant depressive mood effects with similar figures (ORs = 2.8–4.9) on 6-month cardiac mortality.

Irvine, Basinski, et al. (1999) calculated a relative risk of 2.45 for sudden cardiac death in initially depressive versus nondepressive patients without antiarrhythmic medication with amiodarone. Ahern et al. (1990) and S. A. Thomas et al. (1997) found initial differences in dimensional depression scores of between 0.65 and 0.36 standard deviations in CAPS or CAST patients who had died after 1 to 1.5 years. When separately analyzed, the CAST placebo group reached a univariately significant predictability, but not using initial depression scores; mortality was predicted only by an increase in depression scores toward the 3-month follow-up or by high depression scores obtained after 3 months. Bush et al.'s (2001) results showed that the diagnosis of a depressive disorder was associated with an increased 4-month total mortality but did not reach significance. Abnormal depressive mood (depressive disorder or BDI score > 10 or both), on the contrary, was associated with a significant increase in 4-month total mortality (OR = 4.0). Deaths occurred mostly in patients older than 65 years; in this subgroup, a significant increase in total mortality occurred in patients with BDI scores of higher than 4 points, the score usually viewed as

normal. Lane et al. (2000a, 2001a) found that depressive mood measured with the BDI was not predictive, although patients with abnormal values did show a slight, but not statistically significant, increase in risk for cardiac death (OR = 1.31 after 4 months to OR = 1.15 after 15 months).

Multivariate risk adjustments for important sociodemographic and cardiac predictors did not alter any of the statistical relationships in Frasure-Smith et al.'s (1993, 1995a, 1995b, 1999, 2000a), Irvine, Basinski, et al.'s (1999), and Bush et al.'s (2001) publications. Even Ahern et al. (1990) were able to confirm a significant independent effect of depressive mood in the multivariate analysis. Ladwig et al. (1991) found an only marginally significant effect of depressive mood ($p = .07$). S. A. Thomas et al. (1997) found no multivariate effect for depressive mood in either the total sample or the control group. Table W5.9 lists studies that examined risk estimators for initially depressive or anxious postinfarct patients using the clinical endpoints of cardiac mortality or cardiac arrest over 4 to 24 months (see the Web site).

Frasure-Smith et al. (1995b) attempted to ascertain the effects of depressive mood and anxiety not only on mortality, but also on other cardiac outcomes. Increased depression scores proved to be significantly predictive of total cardiac events and of acute coronary syndromes and arrhythmias. Similarly, in the combined EPPI–MHART sample, initially elevated depression scores predicted the incidence of total cardiac events and arrhythmias and showed a tendency to predict recurrent infarctions. The number of revascularizations could not, however, be predicted. By contrast, Lane et al. (2000b) were not able to prove a clustering of cardiac events in initially depressive patients. Ladwig et al. were able to predict the incidence of arrhythmia through initial depressive mood as early as 1991. Frasure-Smith et al. (1995a) suggested that this finding may have been a mechanism of raised mortality, given the massively increased 18-month mortality seen especially in patients with initially frequent extrasystoles and high depression scores.

5.4.5.1.2. Interaction between depressive mood and other cardiac event predictors. In addition to depressive mood, Frasure-Smith et al. (1995b) examined some other psychological predictors of cardiac events. They showed that major depression shortly after MI was predictive only of the total incidence of cardiac events during the following year. An earlier major depression additionally predicted the occurrence of acute coronary syndromes. Initial state anxiety was able to predict both endpoints even more strongly (OR = 3.1 or 3.6). The coexistence of several psychological risk factors seemed to have a partially additive effect.

Irvine, Basinski, et al. (1999) additionally investigated the predictive role of a perceived decrease in physical capacity ("fatigue" as a combined measure of a functional cardiac impairment and a subjective tendency to complain). They found it to be associated even more strongly than depressive mood with sudden cardiac death; the mathematical model, however, was not adjusted for ejection fraction or the size of infarct. In addition, in the placebo group a statistical trend linked cognitive and affective symptoms of depression with increased cardiac risk; this finding might indicate an arrhythmogenic effect of depression that was somehow suppressed in the amiodarone group. Unexpectedly, depressive mood was not associated with total mortality in the total sample. In the amiodarone group, depressive mood showed a trend toward a negative association with the rate of sudden cardiac deaths; the reason for this association is unclear and might be due to chance. What is conspicuous is that the average initial depression scores (2 weeks after beginning medication) in the amiodarone group were significantly higher than those of the placebo group. Yet later on, the rate of cardiac events was considerably lower. It is conceivable that the side effects of the medication caused increased depression scores (amiodarone is known to cause sleeplessness and nightmares). Thus, the results might have indicated, instead of depression, adherence to the study medication, which by itself favorably improved prognosis; this will remain speculation until further results are available.

5.4.5.1.3. Predictive significance of anxiety after an acute infarct. In contrast to the negative results on depression, the CAST's placebo group showed a significant multivariate predictive effect, especially in men, of initial state anxiety for increased

18-month mortality (S. A. Thomas et al., 1997). However, the available publications demonstrate few and contradictory results on the significance of anxiety in predicting mortality after a myocardial infarct. Even the CAST study showed only small and statistically nonsignificant effects of state and trait anxiety on 18-month mortality in the total sample. Frasure-Smith et al.'s (1999) results showed a significantly adverse univariate effect of state anxiety in men over 1 year. Yet in multivariate analysis they were unable to confirm this finding. Ahern et al. (1990) in the CAPS and Lane et al. (2001a) did not find a 1-year effect of state or trait anxiety. The patients who died later initially showed an even lower (though not significantly so) state anxiety than the surviving patients. Sykes et al. (1989) observed a significantly lower mortality after 3 months in the subgroup of more severely ill cardiac patients who initially showed increased anxiety scores.

5.4.5.1.4. Prediction in other CHD samples. Six very well qualified studies reported on the prediction of cardiac events or mortality in other coronary heart patient samples. Lespérance et al. (2000) confirmed the predictive effect of depressive mood on cardiac and total mortality as well as on nonlethal infarcts in patients with unstable AP. The odds ratio for cardiac events over 1 year in patients with initially increased BDI scores was between 3.8 and 6.7, depending on the covariates.

In rehabilitation patients recovering from a cardiac event, Denollet et al. (2000) identified high scores on a "dejection" scale as a predictor of cardiac events over a 5-year period. The State–Trait Anxiety Inventory scale (Spielberger, Gorsuch, & Lushene, 1970) was not predictive in this study. In the multivariate analysis, depressive mood lost its predictive significance to Type D personality. This so-called "distressed personality" is defined by the combination of *negative affectivity* (i.e., a habitual tendency to experience negative emotions) and *social inhibition* (i.e., the habitual inhibition of self-expression in social interactions).

Welin, Lappas, and Wilhelmsen (2000) found increased cardiac and total mortality over 10 years in patients who were depressive 1 month after infarct. These patients had a multivariate hazard ratio of 3.2 for cardiac mortality and 1.8 for total mortality. Yet anxiety once again was not predictive.

Barefoot et al. (1996) followed patients for up to 15 years after the primary angiographic CHD diagnosis. They found significantly higher total and cardiac mortality in the subgroups with slightly to severely increased depression scores. This association remained significant in a largely well-adjusted multivariate model. On a critical note, the severely depressed group was initially, on average, 1 year older (not statistically significant) than the nondepressive group, which might partially explain the long-term effect; it was unfortunately not recognizably accounted for in the original publication. The authors (Barefoot et al., 2000) adjusted for age only in a more recent publication; they examined the same data for the predictive significance of Self-Rating Depression Scale subscales (Zung, 1965) defined by content. What they found predictive in a multivariate analysis was negative affect; the item on hopelessness tended toward significance. Yet this effect was principally limited to the group of patients less than 50 years old at baseline.

C. Herrmann, Brand-Driehorst, Buss, and Rüger (2000) were unable to prove a univariate effect of depressive mood on 5-year total mortality in patients undergoing routine exercise tests. Among them, 2,455 had a documented diagnosis of CHD. Raised anxiety scores were significantly predictive for a longer survival rate, however, with a moderate effect size. After statistical adjustment for anxiety scores, the multivariate model showed a negative effect of depression scores, indicating an unfavorable prognosis of depressed patients. This effect was small but could also be separately demonstrated in the CHD subgroup. After adjusting for a very efficient cardiac risk index, the negative predictive significance remained. In the CHD subgroup, however, the size of this effect diminished and lost its statistical significance.

Kop et al. (1994) succeeded in predicting new cardiac events over 1.5 years following coronary angioplasty. They used increased scores for vital exhaustion on the Maastricht questionnaire (Appels, Hoppener, & Mulder, 1987) as predictors, which turned out to be independent of cardiac predictors. This group used only semihard outcome criteria

with endpoints such as renewed vascularizations; these endpoints were partly influenced by subjective decisions. Perski et al. (1998) also predicted a mixture of cardiac events. Emotional "distress" proved to be the best and sole multivariate predictor before a coronary bypass operation, with a relative risk of about 1.9.

5.4.5.1.5. Preliminary summary on predicting hard somatic endpoints. The results of the very well qualified studies can be preliminarily summarized as follows: After an acute coronary syndrome (e.g., infarct, unstable AP), depressive mood is a predictor for middle-term mortality and presumably other cardiac endpoints. This prediction is independent of a specific psychiatric diagnosis and, most likely, even of acknowledged somatic markers of prognosis. Findings on the effects of anxiety on mortality and cardiac events rates were, however, inconsistent. During the chronic CHD phase, the effect of depressive mood is most likely lower, and perhaps it is then worsened by accompanying anxiety; the causality of this dynamic has yet to be proved. It is possible that the statistical effect of anxiety is at least in part an artifact of age, higher health care utilization, or referral behavior—all of which bring anxious patients into cardiological institutions more often, even when their prognosis is still good. The prediction of a cardiac event after a coronary artery revascularization using initial distress or vital exhaustion has, until now, rested on a weak database that has also been flawed by partially subjective endpoints.

5.4.5.2. Well-qualified studies. Among the six well-qualified studies (*N* = 1,378 from five different samples), three studies involved acute infarct patients. A succinct article by Silverstone (1987) confirmed the predictive significance of observer-rated depression 1 day after infarct on mortality (OR = 11.8) and cardiac events (OR = 11.9). Although depressive and nondepressive patients seemed comparable on cardiac severity markers, no multivariate analysis was done, and unfortunately the length of the follow-up interval was not indicated. Mayou et al. (2000), on the other hand, could not prove any significant effect of mortality for the Hospital Anxiety and Depression Scale (Zigmond &

Snaith, 1983) total score (anxiety + depressive mood) completed 3 days after infarct; in a univariate analysis they observed a trend in the expected direction with an OR of 1.6. Kaufmann et al. (1999) described a univariate effect that was marginally significant after 6 months and strongly significant after 12 months of "clinical depression" diagnosed through a modified Diagnostic Interview Schedule (Robins, Helzer, Croughan, & Ratcliff, 1981) interview on total mortality. The diagnostic significance of a positive interview result is not clear, because lifetime diagnoses were also included in the interview. In addition, the prevalence rate for depression was found to be relatively high at 27%. Possibly patients who did not suffer from depression at the time were also included and then experienced a recurrence of depression later. This scenario might have been responsible for the significantly increased mortality, which was observed only after more than 6 months. It is also unclear how large the effect of depression was on mortality; this effect was no longer statistically significant in a multivariate model including cardiological predictors.

Gender-specific studies by Denollet and colleagues (Denollet & Brutsaert, 1998; Denollet et al., 1996; men only) and Horsten, Mittleman, Wamala, Schenck-Gustafsson, and Orth-Gomér (2000; women only) examined heterogeneous samples during the interval following a coronary event. Horsten et al. found that in a purely female sample including patients without a confirmed diagnosis of CHD, depression scores taken 3 to 6 months later only approached significance in predicting the 5-year incidence of cardiac events. The scale they used, however, was not comparable to those used in other studies. Only women who were in the lowest quartile for depressive mood showed a significantly lowered risk for a cardiac event compared with all other women. Yet even this significance was partially lost after adjusting for social support and became only marginally significant.

The remarkable studies by Denollet et al. (1996; Denollet & Brutsaert, 1998) do not appear in the very well qualified category because they measured anxiety and depressive mood only as marginal parameters; their primary emphasis was on evaluating the predictive significance of the Type D construct. In a purely male sample from a cardiological rehabilitation program, no significant trait anxiety effect on 8-year mortality was found in univariate analysis. However, they demonstrated a significant prediction of total mortality (OR = 2.7) and cardiac mortality using depressive mood (measured, unfortunately, with unusual methods). This effect was independent of cardiac variables, although it was superseded in the prediction models by the Type D personality (Denollet et al., 1996). Initial state anxiety predicted the occurrence of cancer in a univariate model over a period of almost 8 years in patients who had not died of cardiac disease. Depression scores were not mentioned; in a multivariate model, Type D personality turned out to be, again, the sole significant predictor (Denollet, 1998b).

5.4.5.3. Partially and less qualified studies. For a discussion of the partially qualified and less qualified studies we located, see section W5.17 on the accompanying Web site.

5.4.5.4. Summary. The following summarizes methods of predicting hard somatic endpoints using anxiety and depression.

5.4.5.4.1. Depressive mood as a predictor. The studies we identified clearly prove that depressive mood during the early postinfarct phase (Phase 1) is a significant predictor of prognosis and, especially, of cardiac mortality. Nine of the very well and well-qualified studies, as well as even more high-quality single publications, confirm this association. Only the sample studied by Lane et al. (2000a, 2001a) and the amiodarone-treated subgroup of the CAMIAT study did not exhibit such an effect. The partially qualified studies found an association approaching significance in one case; the result of the other study was negative. Among the less-qualified studies, we found two studies with negative results: In one, a small effect on a small sample pointed toward a trend in the expected direction, although it proved statistically insignificant. The other study could not prove an effect, which may be because of the unvalidated (and presumably not very valid) instrument for measuring depressive mood.

For patients with unstable AP, we found only one study—though very well qualified—that described a predictive significance of depressive mood similar to that described for acute infarct patients. Interestingly, unlike studies investigating anxiety, not a single study shows significantly lower mortality for depressive patients with acute coronary syndrome. We would expect this, however, if the results of the studies were to coincidentally fluctuate around a real 0 correlation. We cannot draw any conclusion about the highly charged issue of independent causal relevance, even with the proof of an assured statistical association, a topic to which we will return later on (see section 5.6).

Six studies investigated depressive mood as a predictor for mortality during Phase 2 after a coronary event. Three very well qualified studies (Denollet et al., 2000; S. A. Thomas et al., 1997, in a subgroup analysis; Welin et al., 2000), one well-qualified study, and one partially qualified study by Denollet and Brutsaert (1998; Denollet et al., 1996; from a shared older patient sample) confirmed such an association. The two less qualified studies were unable to prove any effect with the limitations mentioned above (such as unvalidated assessment of depression). The data thus do not allow us to draw an unequivocal conclusion.

Depressive mood 6 or more months after infarct or in other chronic CHD samples was examined as a mortality or cardiac event predictor. Two of the four very well qualified and well-qualified studies showed clearly positive results, and the other two showed positive results with limitations. The two partially qualified and less qualified studies did not really aid us further because they had relatively small samples and hence cardiac events; they showed one positive and one nonpredictive result.

The remaining six studies on prognosis after a coronary intervention or on prognosis for a population cohort with diverse cardiovascular illnesses demonstrate largely positive results. However, they do so with clear limitations: Three of these studies did not examine depressive mood per se, but rather some related construct (e.g., vital exhaustion, depressive coping, "poor mental health"), and three studied only semihard mixed endpoints.

5.4.5.4.2. Anxiety as a predictor. In one study, anxiety retrospectively appeared to be a trigger for the cardiac event in patients with acute infarct; this association is, however, in no way proved. Anxiety was observed to be a predictor for cardiac events after an acute infarct in two very well qualified and one partially qualified study. Another very well qualified study demonstrated the same results in at least one subgroup. Conversely, a subgroup of another very well qualified study showed its anxious patients to have a significantly better prognosis. Three very well qualified studies and one partially qualified study were unable to prove any effect.

Denollet and colleagues investigated anxiety during Phase 2 following a coronary event in five publications using two samples (one very well qualified, two well-qualified, and two partially qualified studies; Denollet, 1998b; Denollet & Brutsaert, 1998; Denollet et al., 1996, 2000; Denollet, Sys, & Brutsaert, 1995). They found that Phase 2 anxiety in the total sample was either not associated or partially negatively associated with coronary events during the course of illness. However, among those who did not die of cardiological causes, anxiety was able to predict the incidence of cancer. In a subgroup with limited ventricular function, anxiety also predicted the rate of cardiac events or mortality or both. The two less qualified publications on this topic did not yield any indication of a predictive role for anxiety. The sole but especially large and very well qualified study on the prognostic significance of anxiety in chronic CHD patients reported a distinctly more favorable prognosis for the more anxious patients.

One partially qualified and three less qualified studies examined anxiety as a predictor in patients undergoing coronary interventions. None of the studies demonstrated a significant result for the prediction of restenosis after coronary angioplasty using peri-interventional anxiety. A study on the course of illness after coronary bypass surgery, however, was able to predict subjectively influenced, heterogeneous outcome variables using preoperative and early postoperative anxiety.

On the basis of these findings, anxiety cannot be viewed as a general risk marker for hard endpoints in coronary heart disease patients. This finding does not rule out the possible importance of anxiety within the context of more complex constructs, such as the Type D personality, or in certain subgroups. In addition, the few indications of the possible protective significance of anxiety in specific samples or situations need to be examined more closely.

5.4.5.4.3. Psychological distress as a predictor. One very well qualified and one well-qualified study investigated the predictive significance of a general distress score calculated from anxiety and depression scores. One of the studies (Perski et al., 1998) was able to significantly predict the 3-year rate of cardiac events following bypass surgery. The other publication (Mayou et al., 2000) demonstrated only an insignificant trend toward increased 18-month mortality in psychologically distressed patients during the acute infarct phase. These two results do not allow any sort of generalization.

5.4.5.4.4. Association between the effects observed and physical or psychosocial factors. In discussing the well-proven role of depressive mood as a risk indicator shortly after infarct, it would be interesting to address the extent to which it is also risk factor in a stricter sense, independent of the organic lesion. We do not believe that depressive mood would become significant independent of physical processes; both the behavioral effects of depressive mood and possible direct effects are certainly physiologically mediated, and physiological factors also exert an influence on depressive mood. It is important, however, to review the extent to which depressive mood reflects only easily accessible measures of cardiac severity or actually explains independent portions of variance. The extent to which hidden parameters of cardiac illness that are not measured routinely—for example, activation of the neuroendocrine system or of inflammatory pathways—are associated with both myocardial damage and depressive mood has not yet been explained. These processes might be important background variables influencing the observed associations.

Ten publications show that clinically diagnosed depression or depressive mood shortly after infarct at least tends toward predictive significance. One study compared depressive and nondepressive pa-

tients on cardiac variables and found no significant differences; in the nine remaining studies, significant somatic predictors were multivariately controlled. The risk for patients with major depression and, even more strongly, with self-rated depressive mood was confirmed to be partially independent of the cardiac findings measured in the Montreal (EPPI subsample + MHART), CAPS, CAMIAT, and Gruppo Italiano per lo Studio della Sopravvivenza nell' Infarto Miocardico—2 (Carinci et al., 1997) samples and in the study by Bush et al. (2001). It even remained significant in the fully adjusted models. In the PILP study, the multivariate effect of depressive mood at least tended toward significance in multivariate analyses. Only in Kaufmann et al.'s (1999) sample and in the CAST study did the effect of depression or depressive mood lose its significance after adjusting for the cardiac risk markers.

In Denollet and colleagues' studies (Denollet, 1998b; Denollet & Brutsaert, 1998; Denollet et al., 1995, 1996, 2000) from Phase 2 rehabilitation, in Barefoot et al.'s (1996) chronic CHD sample, and in C. Herrmann et al.'s (2000) total patient population, the effect of depressive mood remained significant, even apart from cardiac predictor variables. We can thus assume that depressive mood prognostically influences the disease course, just as the usual CHD or infarct severity markers do. It is plausible that patients in specific cardiac situations would be especially prone to a depressive mood effect, especially those who suffer from an acute coronary syndrome with, for example, increased electric (Frasure-Smith et al., 1995a) or hemodynamic instability. The effect in stable, typically chronic CHD patients would, on average, not be as big.

In addition to its interaction with physical variables, the interaction between the prognostic effect of depressive mood and other psychosocial factors is also of special interest, as well as the issue of which components are actually "toxic." Irvine, Basinski, et al. (1999) and Barefoot et al. (2000) suggested that general fatigue as well as specific cognitive and affective symptoms are prognostically unfavorable components of depression. The best-proved protective factor is actual or perceived social integration and support, which, according to Frasure-Smith et al. (2000b), completely counteracted the effect of depressive mood, especially when such support is particularly strong. Similarly, Denollet and colleagues (Denollet, 1998b; Denollet & Brutsaert, 1998; Denollet et al., 1995, 1996, 2000) found that the significant effect of depressive mood was always less than that of the Type D pattern, with its components of negative affectivity and social inhibition. C. Herrmann et al. (2000) argued similarly that anxious CHD patients seek more help and human contact, a finding also demonstrated in other studies. They completed this line of thought by further arguing that this help seeking might explain why in their study (generalized) anxiety exercised a counteracting effect on depressive mood in chronic CHD patients. This hypothesis easily conforms to the results of Sykes et al. (1989) showing a higher rate of survival in the subgroup of more anxious patients.

Denollet and colleagues' (Denollet, 1998b; Denollet & Brutsaert, 1998; Denollet et al., 1995, 1996, 2000) findings also support this hypothesis: Among his Phase 2 rehabilitation patients who were habitually anxious but not socially inhibited, there was not a single death. Beyond very unstable cardiac situations, isolated negative affect might prove prognostically less important, becoming a problem only when coupled with social inhibition or lack of social support. Because depressive mood is typically (though not always) connected with social withdrawal, its effect is larger than that of isolated anxiety but (as far as it has been studied) smaller than that of Type D personality. This is perhaps also the key to interpreting Mayou et al.'s (2000) negative findings: The total score calculated from the depression and anxiety scores could unintentionally have counteracted part of the depressive mood effect by strengthening its negative affect component at the cost of reducing the social withdrawal dimension. Finally, our hypothesis fits perfectly with the Beta-Blocker Heart Attack Trial (Ruberman, Weinblatt, Goldberg, & Chaudhary, 1984) and Anglo-Scandinavian Study of Early Thrombolysis (Jenkinson, Madeley, Mitchell, & Turner, 1993) study results showing that three "depression" items (hopelessness, morning fatigue,

and sadness) measured reduced negative affect (emotion) but not social withdrawal or inhibition. Table W5.10 lists studies examining anxiety and depression as predictors of hard somatic endpoints in CHD patients (see the Web site).

5.4.6. Association Between Anxiety and Depression and Relevant Physiological Variables of Potential Prognostic Significance

In view of the associations mentioned in this chapter, especially between depressive mood (or Type D personality) and cardiac events in coronary patients, we questioned whether there were possible mediating mechanisms. We have already mentioned (in section 5.4.3) behavioral effects of depressive mood. Some studies address the resulting indirect (behaviorally mediated) and direct (mediated by the autonomic nervous system or neuroendocrine mechanisms) psychological influences on physiological variables. Such psychophysiological investigations have often been undertaken on cardiologically healthy subjects, but the quality of most such studies has not been high, and studies in samples with confirmed CHD diagnoses have been few. Considering the very small number of proper longitudinal studies on this topic, we prefer to include the corresponding cross-sectional studies in our discussion, even though this may be contrary to the general structure of our analysis. Of a total of 21 studies identified, 2 (mean N = 2,912) were very well qualified, 4 (mean N = 739) were well qualified, 9 (mean N = 80) were partially qualified, and 6 (mean N = 53) were less qualified.

5.4.6.1. Very well qualified and well-qualified studies.
There were only two very well qualified and four well-qualified studies (N = 8,780). Buss, Wydra, and Herrmann-Lingen (2001a) demonstrated in a very large sample that heart rate changes during and after an exercise test were inversely correlated with depressive mood. Depressive patients showed a relatively low (sympathetically mediated) increase in heart rate and consequently a somewhat slower heart rate recovery. After adjusting for maximum heart rate, the (vagally mediated) heart rate recovery did not show

an independent association with depressive mood. In a follow-up study, they found that a multivariately significant effect of depressive mood on 5-year mortality was obviously mediated by the reduced (motivation-dependent) increase in heart rate and not by impaired vagal counterregulation.

Additional data are available from the cross-sectional analysis of the Enhancing Recovery in Coronary Heart Disease (ENRICHD) study by Carney et al. (2001). In comparing more than 300 depressive and a similar number of nondepressive infarct patients, the depressed group showed significantly decreased heart rate variability in all four spectral components of the Fast Fourier Transformation. Patients with major depression did not differ on these measures from those with minor depression or dysthymia; nonetheless, after adjustment for somatic group differences, log-transformed spectral power values from the different frequency bands correlated significantly, if weakly, with BDI depression scores. Only the high-frequency power, predominantly vagally mediated, lost its significance in a comparison of depressive and nondepressive groups when adjusting for somatic variables. What is not yet clear is to what extent the differences observed reflect direct effects of depression on the autonomic nervous system or are alternatively related to direct (reduced frequency spectrum due to current inactivity) or indirect (physical deconditioning due to persistent inactivity) behavioral effects. This ambiguity holds true for most of the other studies on depression and heart rate variability as well.

Among the well-qualified studies, Carney et al. (2000) found significantly increased average heart rates and significantly decreased midfrequency heart rate variabilities in a 24-hour Holter ECG in 12 severely depressed chronic CHD patients compared with 22 nondepressed patients. After cognitive–behavioral therapy, the depression had markedly abated in the initially depressed patients. Concurrently, the average heart rate declined significantly; during daytime, midfrequency heart rate variability increased to an extent approaching significance, and the increase in high-frequency heart rate variability was significant—all this without perceived changes in activity levels or medication

(e.g., beta-blockers, antidepressants). Because of the small sample size, however, these results must be interpreted with caution.

Pitzalis et al. (2001) also found significantly decreased heart rate variability in a group of depressive versus nondepressive coronary patients, but only in the subgroup not taking beta-blockers. They could not demonstrate a comparable effect for anxiety. Their very global measure of 24-hour variability (standard deviation of normal-to-normal intervals; see Task Force of the European Society of Cardiology and the North American Society of Pacing and Electrophysiology, 1996) was definitely activity dependent and thus difficult to interpret. However, the authors additionally found reduced baroreceptor reflex activity after phenylephrine administration under resting conditions. This most probably points toward reduced (and thus less protective) vagal activity in the depressive patients of this sample.

Another study allows certain conclusions to be made about the association between anxiety and depressive mood and noninvasive hemodynamic measurements before and during an exercise test in CHD patients (Herrmann-Lingen, 2001). This study found neither anxiety nor depression to be associated with resting heart rate. The systolic resting blood pressure was significantly lower in anxious men and tended to be lower in anxious women, with a similar effect size (around 0.2), compared with nonanxious patients. In women, abnormal depression scores were coupled with significantly lower systolic resting blood pressure. During exercise, both anxious men and depressive men showed a reduced maximum heart rate (about −0.20 standard deviations for both) and lower maximum systolic blood pressure (−0.12 standard deviations for both) compared with nonanxious or nondepressive men. In addition, depressive patients reached a lower maximum exercise performance and a shorter exercise time (−0.19 standard deviations for both). By contrast, in women, anxiety did not have any significant effect; depressive mood was coupled with less endurance (−0.26 SD) and lower maximum blood pressure (−0.30 SD).

Follick et al. (1990) looked for correlations between anxiety and depression and ventricular extrasystoles and their suppression via medication in infarct patients in the Cardiac Arrhythmia Pilot study. They were unable to prove any association.

5.4.6.2. Partially and less qualified studies. For a discussion of the partially qualified and less qualified studies we located, see section W5.18 on the accompanying Web site.

5.4.6.3. Summary of association between anxiety and depression and relevant physiological variables of potential prognostic significance.

The data on physiological variables as a function of anxiety and depressive mood in CHD samples are, for the present, still sketchy and contradictory. Heart rate and heart rate variability seem to be independent of anxiety and depressive mood under resting conditions. By contrast, during the course of the day, depressive CHD patients often show an increased average heart rate and, concurrently, decreased general and low-frequency heart rate variability markers. The reasons for this are still unclear (e.g., effect of nicotine consumption or limited physical activity vs. direct autonomic effects). Likewise, only isolated data are available on the relationship between depressive mood and high-frequency heart rate variability markers. Information on the limited baroreceptor reflex activity of depressive coronary patients indicated an actual vagal deficit. The largest study on this subject matter was unable to verify the presence of any independent association with depressive mood of a prognostically relevant vagal marker (early heart rate recovery after exercise testing). The finding that psychotherapy (and, apparently, sertraline; see McFarlane et al., 2001, and section 5.5) can possibly normalize increased 24-hour heart rate and decreased heart rate variability is worthy of research attention.

Results from the early postinfarct phase suggest an association between anxiety and depressive mood and clinically diagnosed arrhythmia (see section 5.4.5). C. Herrmann et al. (1999) were successful in predicting arrhythmia episodes documented by the implanted cardiac defibrillator arrhythmia memory function in a mixed sample with implanted cardioverter defibrillators. Such an association was confirmed with 24-hour long-term ECG recordings in a small group of CHD patients,

but in a larger study no such association could be found.

Only one study currently exists on the associations between depressive mood and Holter ECG–registered ischemic episodes, increased plasma levels of inflammatory markers, and thrombocyte activation; it obtained positive results for each of these factors. These results should be viewed as preliminary, however, and the same applies to isolated results that relate increased anxiety scores with more favorable and greater depression with less favorable lipid profiles. Table W5.11 lists studies examining associations of anxiety and depression with relevant physiological variables of potential prognostic significance (see the Web site).

5.5. INTERVENTIONS FOR ANXIETY AND DEPRESSIVE DISORDERS IN CHD PATIENTS

A huge body of psychiatric and psychotherapeutic literature on the general treatment of anxiety and depressive disorders demonstrates proved effects of psychotherapeutic and psychopharmacological therapies. A full discussion of this literature is beyond the scope of this chapter; we refer readers to the guidelines of the American Psychiatric Association (2000) on depression and a survey on the psychotherapy of depression by Schauenburg et al. (1999). Guidelines for the treatment of panic disorders are available from the American Psychiatric Association (1998). Although there is no basis for arguments against the transferability of these guidelines to CHD patients with a few modifications (e.g., cardiological side effects of antidepressant medications), few studies have specifically targeted the treatment of diagnosed depression or anxiety disorders in coronary patients. (The numerous "nonspecific" psychosocial intervention studies in coronary patients with or without abnormal psychological questionnaire scores but without diagnosed anxiety or depressive disorders are discussed in chap. 9 of this volume by Langosch, Budde, & Linden.)

A few studies have evaluated the administration of antidepressants in depressed CHD patients. Veith et al. (1982) found in an older double-blind study that imipramine and doxepin significantly improved 24 patients' self- and observer-rated depression by >1 standard deviation in the short term; the control group showed only small, insignificant improvements. Relevant cardiological side effects did not occur. They did not report on long-term effects. Roose et al. (1998) compared a selective serotonin reuptake inhibitor (SSRI), paroxetine, with a tricyclic antidepressant, nortriptyline, in a randomized controlled double-blind study on 81 CHD patients with a *Diagnostic and Statistical Manual of Mental Disorders* (4th ed.; American Psychiatric Association, 1994) diagnosis of major depression. They found that for both drugs, more than 50% of the patients experienced a normalization of observer-rated depressive mood. Paroxetine showed fewer side effects. They did not include a placebo group, nor were any follow-up data reported.

Shapiro et al. (1999) treated 26 depressive infarct patients with sertraline in the open-label Sertraline Antidepressant Heart Attack Trial (SADHAT). They found a good antidepressant effect with an acceptable rate of side effects and no relevant cardiological effects. Strik et al. (2000) randomized postinfarct patients with major depression into a treatment group with the SSRI fluoxetine and a placebo control group. They demonstrated that during both the acute treatment phase and the 25-week study period, fluoxetine possessed an advantage over placebo that only approached significance in influencing the average severity of depressive symptoms. However, in categorical analyses, patients were significantly more responsive to fluoxetine treatment ($p = .05$; 48% vs. 26%). Especially in a subgroup with less severe depression, depressive symptoms improved. Cardiological side effects of the medication were not demonstrated.

As a general rule, coronary patients receive SSRI treatment rather than tricyclics (Coupland, Wilson, & Nutt, 1997; A. H. Glassman, 1998a, 1998b; A. H. Glassman, Rodriguez, & Shapiro, 1998; Roose, Devenand, & Suthers, 1999), although the basis of this recommendation lies in theoretical considerations and not in studies comparing the use of different antidepressants in CHD patients. Compared

with SSRIs, tricyclics may lead to a higher incidence of CHD in cardiologically healthy individuals. They were not able to lower the increased risk for a primary occurrence of CHD, especially MI, in patients with a history of depression (H. W. Cohen, Gibson, & Alderman, 2000; H. W. Cohen, Madhavan, & Alderman, 2001; Hippisley-Cox et al., 2001; Sauer, Berlin, & Kimmel, 2001). Recent data on coronary patients lead us to believe that SSRIs are able to inhibit thrombocyte aggregation (Serebruany, O'Connor, & Gurbel, 2001) and normalize heart rate variability, which is usually reduced after infarct (McFarlane et al., 2001). Both might lead to a more favorable course of cardiac disease.

We will better be able to assess differential drug treatment strategies once the results of the Dutch Myocardial Infarction and Depression—Intervention Trial (mirtazapine or citalopram vs. placebo in depressive postinfarct patients; van Melle et al., 2000) and the successor to SADHAT, the recently completed Sertraline Antidepressant Heart Attack Randomized Trial (SADHART) study (sertraline vs. placebo in depressive patients following an acute coronary syndrome) have been published (A. H. Glassman et al., 2002). The first, positive conference presentation of the SADHART results (O'Connor, Glassman, & Harrison, 2001) raised high expectations. The first published SADHART findings (A. H. Glassman et al., 2002), which appeared after this review was completed, confirmed the beneficial effect of sertraline over placebo at least for the subgroups with severe or recurrent depression. Cardiac side effects were infrequent. However, no effect on heart rate variability was observed.

Surprisingly, specific psychotherapy for depression in CHD patients has until recently been examined only in small uncontrolled studies (M. A. Brown & Munford, 1984, $N = 9$; Mandke, Mishra, Kumaraiah, & Yavagal, 1996, $N = 5$; Sunil Dath, Mishra, Kumaraiah, & Yavagal, 1997, $N = 5$). Carney et al. (2000) treated the largest sample so far, with 8 to 16 single sessions of cognitive–behavioral therapy. Of their 18 chronic CHD patients with mild depression, 28% reached full remission and 56% reached partial remission after 17 weeks of therapy. Of 12 severely depressed patients, three reached full remission and eight reached partial remission. The average BDI depression scores fell from 15.2 to 5.5 (SD = 2.7) in the mildly depressive group. In the severely depressive group, scores fell from 27.9 to 10.2 (SD = 2.5). However, no control group was included in the study.

Recently, the large multicenter randomized ENRICHD trial (Berkman et al., 2003; ENRICHD Investigators, 2000, 2001) attempted to improve prognosis by using cognitive behavioral psychotherapy for treating depression or low perceived social support in post-MI patients. However, treatment effect sizes on psychological endpoints were only moderate and did not translate into reduced cardiac event rates.

5.6. CONCLUSION AND FUTURE PERSPECTIVES

Although a final evaluation remains to be made, in this section we will draw some conclusions, even given the enormous, indeed almost unmanageable, number of publications; the heterogeneous operationalizations of anxiety, depressive mood, and depression (in a nosological sense); and the widely varying methodological standards of the publications studied.

Anxiety and depressive mood are among the most common psychological symptoms not only among the general public, but also in coronary patients. Anxiety is less pronounced in recently diagnosed CHD patients without a previous history of infarct than in patients with ongoing cardiac complaints; the latter demonstrate a high level of anxiety that statistically differentiates them from recently diagnosed CHD patients.

Temporary episodes of sustained anxiety occur during the long course of coronary heart disease, often in connection to MIs or invasive procedures. One in every five or six postinfarct patients experiences a major depressive episode. Depressive symptoms or episodes of clinical depression following infarct tend to persist longer than episodes of anxiety. Anxiety and depressive mood are thus useful in predicting far-reaching impairments in well-being, sick role behavior, and quality of life. This

prognostic effect is mainly independent of cardiac pathology. Depressive mood or the typical depression-related combination of negative affect and social inhibition presents a marker of poor prognosis that is at least partly independent of cardiac pathology. This effect is mainly found in unstable cardiac conditions (e.g., during the first few months following MI) and can probably be counteracted by good social support.

The literature provides evidence that depression is a causal risk factor, that the mediators are both the behavioral consequences (e.g., poorer adherence) and the psychophysiological effects of depressive mood, and that affected patients engage in more health care utilization. Comparable effects could not be unequivocally demonstrated for anxiety, despite partially similar physiological consequences. The prognostic significance of depression in stable chronic CHD patients also is not clear, again hinting at the paramount importance of the balance and interactions among cardiac vulnerability, psychophysiological processes, and behavioral factors in individual prognoses. The need for a multidimensional, biopsychosocial risk conceptualization is clear.

Considering the colossal amount of data on the rate and subjective and objective consequences of anxiety and depression in CHD patients, the lack of sufficient data on the treatment of comorbid anxiety or depressive disorders in these patients is astonishing. So far, mainly small, less qualified studies on the psychopharmacological and psychotherapeutic treatment of anxiety and depressive disorders are available; their results indicate that these therapies, the effectiveness of which has been shown in many noncardiac patient samples, probably work in CHD patients as well. A well-known limitation is, of course, the cardiac side effects of antidepressants, principally the older tricyclic antidepressants. However, we have yet to see convincing results for the effectiveness of specific psychotherapeutic methods in specific CHD patient groups or for the differential indication of various treatment options.

In the coming years, this clinical field of CHD research could be the largest in psychosomatic medicine. Such research might address the effectiveness of therapeutic interventions for improving morbid anxiety and depressive symptoms in CHD patients and examine to what extent the unfavorable behavioral, economic, and physiological consequences of anxiety and depression can be positively influenced. Without doubt, the improvement of subjective well-being, sick role behavior, and quality of life are all worthy goals for therapy in themselves. But it would also be of great interest to explore whether and which psychotherapeutic and pharmacological interventions could improve the somatic prognosis, including the survival rate, of anxious and especially depressive CHD patients. This would be an important link in the chain of results, helping to clarify the possible causal role of depression in unfavorable somatic CHD endpoints.

Obviously, the complexity of the issue demands carefully planned, large, multicenter studies, the costs of which will be great. However, given the enormous epidemiological relevance of the co-morbidity of CHD and depression, it is definitely justified. The results of such studies would potentially allow health care systems to realize huge savings. We hope that such studies will not be limited to the North American continent—where the ENRICHD and SADHART studies are currently expending tens of millions of dollars—but that research foundations, health insurance providers, and pension funds all over the world will also free up sufficient funding for independent contributions to this vital issue.

CHAPTER 6

TYPE A BEHAVIOR AND HOSTILITY AS INDEPENDENT RISK FACTORS FOR CORONARY HEART DISEASE

Michael Myrtek

6.1. INTRODUCTION

6.1.1. History of Type A Behavior

Beginning during World War I, coronary heart disease (CHD) became the leading cause of mortality in the United States. An urgent search began for the origins of this disease, and extensive prospective studies were undertaken. Studies such as the well-known Framingham Heart Study, initiated in 1948 in the U.S. city of Framingham, Massachusetts (Kannel, Castelli, Gordon, & McNamara, 1971), developed the concept of risk factors, such as sex, age, smoking, cholesterol, hypertension, family history, and diabetes. In Germany, a strong increase in CHD was observed only after the 1950s, with the onset of the economic boom.

Only 50% of the CHD variance can be explained with the so-called "classic" risk factors (Epstein, 1979). Therefore, the search for other risk factors, especially for psychosocial risk factors, has continued. The search for psychosocial risk factors was fostered through the popularization of the stress concept by Selye (1956) and with the emergence of stress and life event research (e.g., Rahe, 1972, 1974; Theorell, Lind, & Floderus, 1975). The term *manager's disease* gained popularity in referring to CHD because of its initially higher incidence in higher socioeconomic groups, who were believed to have higher psychosocial stress than lower socioeconomic groups. In subsequent years, however, the highest incidence of CHD shifted to the middle class and subsequently to the lower socioeconomic groups. During this period, the

incidence of CHD decreased in the higher socioeconomic groups, who developed heightened health consciousness and made improvements in their diet, nicotine consumption, and exercise habits. On the whole, stress research was not very successful and was heavily criticized (e.g., C. D. Jenkins, 1976, 1978a). A more recent large-scale prospective study with 12,866 men, the Multiple Risk Factor Intervention Trial, also found no correlation between life events and CHD mortality or myocardial infarction rates (Hollis, Connett, Stevens, & Greenlick, 1990). However, this study investigated a high-risk sample drawn from a larger sample of 360,000 persons on the basis of cholesterol level. It is at least conceivable that the influence of life events on CHD in this sample was so small that it was no longer observable but that this influence would have been shown in a nonselected group.

The relative failure to identify psychosocial factors as risk factors for CHD seemed to vanish with the emergence of the Type A concept. The prospective Western Collaborative Group Study (WCGS; Rosenman et al., 1975) pioneered research on this concept. In this study, 3,200 healthy men from different companies in California were first examined in 1960 and were reexamined at intervals thereafter. After 8.5 years, 257 men had been diagnosed with CHD. Even after taking the classic risk factors into account, the incidence rate of CHD was 1.9 times higher for Type A than for Type B men. Type A men are characterized by competitive drive, enhanced aggressiveness, preoccupation with deadlines, impatience, and a sense of time urgency. Type B men are more relaxed and less hurried.

The results of the WCGS initiated a dramatic increase in Type A research. A book by M. Friedman and Rosenman (American edition; 1974) entitled *Type A Behavior and Your Heart* further increased the popularization of the Type A concept. In the German edition of this book, we can read the following in the Preface:

> People without Type A behavior will almost never get CHD before the age of 70, irrespective of how much fat is in their diet, how many cigarettes they smoke, and how little physical activity they have. However, if they demonstrate Type A behavior, CHD will occur in their thirties or forties. (Friedman & Rosenman, 1975, p. 9; German edition; my translation)

In 1981, the Review Panel on Coronary-Prone Behavior and Coronary Heart Disease (1981), initiated by the National Heart, Lung, and Blood Institute of the National Institutes of Health in the United States, acknowledged Type A behavior as a risk factor for CHD. Subsequent prospective studies with other samples, however, failed to confirm or only partially confirmed the WCGS results. At first the conceptual weakness of Type A behavior and its diagnosis was blamed for these negative results. However, as early as 1983 there were already signs that the Type A concept was no longer tenable (Myrtek, 1983). A second review panel in 1987 was forced to relativize the correlation between Type A behavior and CHD (Costa et al., 1987).

The concept was once and for all thrown into doubt in a study of the survival of the 257 patients with CHD from the initial 8.5-year phase of the WCGS (Ragland & Brand, 1988a). Type A behavior was not related to mortality in 26 patients who died within 24 hours of the coronary event. Of the 231 patients who survived for at least 24 hours, the relative risk for CHD mortality was 0.58 for Type A men compared with 1.00 for Type B men. This meant that Type B men were at nearly double the risk of dying from CHD during the prospective interval of more than 20 years. This study used CHD patients and unhealthy men; as shown by the meta-analyses described in this chapter, the association between Type A and CHD differs for healthy men and CHD patients.

Hostility, the most important concept to succeed the Type A concept, concentrated on subcomponents of Type A behavior (R. B. Williams, 1987). Other studies tried to find an association between negative emotions, such as anger, and CHD. Research on both concepts, Type A behavior and hostility, has found a higher psychophysiological reactivity for Type A or hostile subjects as compared with Type B or nonhostile subjects (Myrtek, 1995). This chapter presents meta-analyses that summarize and evaluate the extensive research on Type A and hostility.

6.1.2. Definitions and Operationalization

6.1.2.1. Type A behavior. According to Rosenman et al. (1966), Type A behavior is

> characterized particularly by excessive drive, aggressiveness, and ambition, frequently in association with a relatively greater preoccupation with competitive activity, vocational deadlines, and similar pressures. An enhanced sense of time urgency is usually also exhibited by subjects possessing this interplay of endogenous behavioral factors and exogenous pressures, with various resulting characteristic motor mannerisms and stylistics. The relative absence of this emotional interplay has been designated as characterizing the subjects with behavior pattern B. (p. 130)

Persons with Type A personalities are more prone to stressful situations. In stressful situations, they experience a psychophysiological activation that is quantitatively and qualitatively different than that of Type B persons. Through this activation, hormonal processes, such as an increase of catecholamines and of hormones from the adrenal cortex, and neural processes, such as activation of the sympathetic autonomic nervous system, are initiated.

In turn, these processes lead to a negative influence on blood pressure, cholesterol, blood sugar, and blood clotting, which in the long run results in atherosclerosis of the coronary vessels. Type A behavior has been described in detail by Dembroski, Schmidt, and Blümchen (1983); Dembroski, Weiss, Shields, Haynes, and Feinleib (1978); Langosch (1989); Myrtek (1997); V. A. Price (1982); and Schmidt, Dembroski, and Blümchen (1986).

The structured interview (SI) is the classic method for assessing Type A behavior (Rosenman, 1978). Trained interviewers ask subjects standardized questions to elicit subjects' aggression and impatience. The interview is recorded on tape and subsequently evaluated. For this evaluation, the content of the answers is of minor importance; more important is the expression of the subject's answers (i.e., tone of speech). In addition to fully developed Type A behavior (A1) and Type B behavior (B), two other types have been designated. Type A2 denotes a weaker display of the Type A behavior, and Type X designates the absence of both Type A2 and B behavior (i.e., not classifiable). For group comparisons, the four categories are usually dichotomized, with Types A1 and A2 forming Group A and Types X and B forming Group B. Sometimes, Type X subjects are omitted from the analysis.

Little is known about the test–retest reliability of the SI. According to Rosenman (1978), 80% of the subjects participating in the WCGS were classified in the same category after 12 to 20 months. Using the results of seven studies (N = 2,311), the interrater reliability of the SI was 70% for all four behavior categories and 78% using only two categories (i.e., Group A and Group B; Myrtek, 1983). In most studies, however, more than 60% of subjects were rated as Type A (A1 and A2), so this interrater reliability does not exceed chance by very much.

As early as 1964, C. D. Jenkins (1978b) began to develop a questionnaire for the assessment of Type A behavior. For the Jenkins Activity Survey (JAS–A/B), item selection and item weights were established using the results of the WCGS, which based its assessment of Type A on the SI. Furthermore, three other scales for the determination of special aspects of

Type A behavior were constructed using factor analyses (Zyzanski & Jenkins, 1970). These scales were called Hard Driving and Competitive (H), Job Involvement (J), and Speed and Impatience (S). These scales are not relevant for the present analyses, because most studies on Type A behavior and hostility used only the JAS–A/B scale. C. D. Jenkins, Zyzanski, and Rosenman (1971) investigated the test–retest reliability of the JAS–A/B scale with 2,800 participants of the WCGS for an interval of 1 year. The coefficient of .66 is satisfactory. A later study by Sprafka, Folsom, Burke, Hahn, and Pirie (1990) with 140 subjects showed a comparable test–retest reliability of .69 (interval of 1 year).

Nine studies (N = 1,856) used the SI as well as the JAS–A/B scale to assess Type A behavior. The weighted mean correlation between the methods was .34 (Myrtek, 1983). A test of homogeneity for this coefficient revealed significant heterogeneity. The correspondence of the methods for assessing Type A behavior, therefore, is small, because the common variance is only 11%. The reason for this might lie in the poor psychometric properties of the JAS–A/B scale. The developers of the scale attempted to imitate the SI categorization of the subjects optimally (i.e., discriminant functions with the SI categories as criteria). This procedure resulted in unusual weights for the answers given to the items of the JAS–A/B scale. For example, the four possible answers to one of the items of the JAS–A/B scale are allocated the weights 81, 67, 9, and 4. The power of the items (i.e., correlation of an item with the total score of the respective scale) is thus decreased, and correspondingly, the internal consistency is low. In our own studies, mean power coefficients between r_{it} = .07 and r_{it} = .12 were observed for four different samples (N = 209, N = 55, N = 53, N = 78). Internal consistency (Cronbach's alpha) of the JAS–A/B scale was between α = 0.59 and α = 0.75 (Myrtek, Schmidt, & Schwab, 1984). Some other prospective studies used questionnaires other than the JAS–A/B for the assessment of Type A behavior, such as the Framingham Type A Scale (Haynes, Levine, Scotch, Feinleib, & Kannel, 1978) or the Bortner Short Rating Scale (Bortner, 1969). The first scale was exclusively used in the Framingham Heart Study;

therefore, no correlations with the JAS–A/B have been done. Kittel, Kornitzer, De Backer, and Dramaix (1982) used both the Bortner scale and the JAS–A/B (N = 4,297 men), and the two scales correlated at .62.

6.1.2.2. Hostility. At the beginning of the 1980s, some authors claimed that hostility and anger were important risk factors for CHD (see Dembroski & Costa, 1987; Vögele & Steptoe, 1993; R. B. Williams, 1987). Like the Type A concept, hostility is not unidimensional. Prospective studies used several components of hostility: cynical hostility, with mistrust and ill feeling; overt hostility, or "anger-out"; and suppressed hostility, or "anger-in." In this chapter, we deal with cynical hostility, because most prospective studies used this concept. Cynical hostility is usually operationalized using the Hostility Scale (Ho Scale) developed by W. Cook and Medley (1954). Another way to operationalize hostility is the so-called "component analysis" (Dembroski, 1978), which was used to reanalyze the WCGS (Dembroski & Costa, 1987).

The Cook–Medley Ho Scale consists of 50 items taken from the Minnesota Multiphasic Personality Inventory (MMPI; Hathaway & McKinley, 1943). Originally, the Ho Scale was used to identify teachers who had problems with their students (W. Cook & Medley, 1954). According to Cook and Medley, the internal consistency, estimated by a variance analytic method, is 0.86. R. B. Williams et al. (1980) performed a study with 424 patients who underwent a diagnostic coronary angiography and used the SI and the Ho Scale simultaneously. Both the SI and the Ho Scale correlated with the angiographic findings; Type A patients and hostile patients showed a greater degree of coronary stenosis. These findings prompted a search for former university students who had taken the MMPI during their studies. With the help of university alumni files, these former students were questioned about CHD by mail. The prospective studies by Barefoot, Dahlstrom, and Williams (1983); Hearn, Murray, and Luepker (1989); and McCranie, Watkins, Brandsma, and Sisson (1986) examined the results.

Hostility measured using the Cook–Medley Ho Scale is not a unidimensional construct. Costa, Zonderman, McCrae, and Williams (1986) investigated 1,002 patients with the MMPI and conducted a factor analysis with the 50 items of the Ho Scale. Two factors emerged that they named Cynicism and Paranoid Alienation. Cynicism was assessed using 24 items (Cronbach's α = 0.83) and Paranoid Alienation was assessed using 15 items (Cronbach's α = 0.70). The Cynicism scale contains items that indicate a low opinion of human nature, such as "I think most people would lie to get ahead." The Paranoid Alienation scale includes feelings of persecution, such as "Someone has it in for me," and emotional distance from others, such as "No one cares much what happens to you." The scales were correlated at .54. The authors stressed that the Ho Scale has nothing to do with anger and its expression. Therefore, the term *hostility* is somewhat misleading; a better term might be *cynical mistrust.*

Barefoot, Dodge, Peterson, Dahlstrom, and Williams (1989) suggested six subscales for the Cook–Medley Ho Scale: Cynicism, Hostile Attributions, Aggressive Responding, Hostile Affect, Social Avoidance, and Other. However, all of these scales were positively correlated with each other. In a prospective study, 128 law students were followed up after 29 years (Barefoot, Dodge, et al., 1989). Total mortality was differently predicted by the subscales Hostile Affect (p = .007), Aggressive Responding (p = .016), and Cynicism (p = .031); the other subscales were not significant. In this study, the total Ho Scale (p = .012) and the Cynicism (p = .026) and Paranoid Alienation (p = .021) scales proposed by Costa et al. (1986) also showed significant results. In the large-scale prospective Coronary Artery Risk Development in Young Adults (CARDIA) study, 5,115 young adults were administered the Ho Scale and the SI (Scherwitz, Perkins, Chesney, & Hughes, 1991). Results showed that Type A behavior was almost completely uncorrelated with hostility (r = −.02).

The component analysis of the SI was used to try to identify the "toxic" components of global Type A behavior. Using the WCGS, it was established that CHD patients mainly differed from persons who remained healthy in the prospective interval in the components Potential for Hostility, Anger-Out, and Competitiveness (Dembroski & Costa, 1987). Dembroski (1978) systematically analyzed the components of the SI and found that Potential for Hostility was the most important. Potential for Hostility denotes the tendency to feel anger, irritation, and other negative affects in frustrating situations in normal everyday life, such as waiting in lines and waiting to be seated at a restaurant, or to react to such situations with expressions of antagonism, disagreeableness, rudeness, and uncooperativeness. The operationalization of Potential for Hostility from the SI is based on the content of the response to the questions asked by the interviewer (e.g., frequent reports of annoyance, anger, and irritation), on the intensity of response (e.g., use of emotionally laden words), and on the style of interaction with the interviewer (e.g., arrogance, argumentativeness). Each of the categories is scored on a 5-point scale. Interrater reliability of SI ratings of total Potential for Hostility ranges between 70% and 85%, and test–retest reliability after 6 to 18 months was $r = .55$. The correlation between Potential for Hostility and the Cook–Medley Ho Scale, however, was only .37 ($p < .01$; Dembroski & Costa, 1987).

6.1.3. Correlation of Type A Behavior and Hostility With Other Personality Dimensions and Bodily Complaints

The correlations between Type A behavior or hostility and bodily complaints and other personality dimensions are important because certain correlations may be critical for the evaluation of results derived from prospective studies. The disease endpoint of angina pectoris, often used in prospective studies, ultimately represents a bodily complaint that does not lend itself to being unequivocally objectified. Kannel and Sorlie (1978; Kannel was one of the founders of the Framingham Heart Study), described the diagnosis of angina pectoris as follows:

> Angina is a subjective phenomenon, and its diagnosis is uniquely dependent on a history of chest discomfort and based on an evaluation of symptoms little different from the original description by Heberden in 1772. Although physical findings during the attack, the exercise electrocardiogram [ECG] and the associated coronary risk profile may all help to clarify the problem, the diagnosis of angina ultimately depends on a careful evaluation of symptoms. (p. 120)

In the WCGS, too, angina pectoris was conceptualized as a mere complaint. Rosenman et al. (1964) reported,

> The diagnosis of manifest CHD was made solely by the senior medical referee and designated as group I (myocardial infarction confirmed by history and ECG), group II (myocardial infarction confirmed by diagnostic QRS changes in the ECG, but without history, i.e., "silent"), group III (angina pectoris without manifest myocardial infarction), and group IV (suspect CHD, based upon ECG thus classified). (p. 105)

Rightly, therefore, angina pectoris is considered a "soft" criterion. In contrast, myocardial infarction as confirmed by ECG or enzymatic diagnosis and coronary death is a "hard" criterion. An analysis of Type A behavior or hostility and bodily complaints might result in spurious correlations if angina pectoris is used as disease endpoint in a prospective study. Billing, Hjemdahl, and Rehnqvist (1997) compared 767 patients suffering from angina pectoris with 50 healthy persons, with groups matched for sex and age. Compared with the healthy group, patients with angina pectoris reported having bodily complaints ($p < .001$) and sleep disturbances ($p < .001$) more frequently. Moreover, patients were less satisfied with their lives ($p < .001$) and more hostile ($p < .05$) and more often reported adverse life events ($p < .001$). It is important in this context to mention that aside from acute bodily complaints, the reporting of bodily complaints represents a facet of personality that is extremely constant over time. In the Baltimore Longitudinal Study of Aging with 386 healthy men, the Cornell Medical Index (Brodman, Erdmann, & Wolff, 1949), a well-known list of bodily complaints, was completed a second time after 5 to 8 years. The correlation of both scores was .74 (Costa & McCrae, 1985). Prospective studies with healthy persons in which angina pectoris is used as a disease endpoint should assess the propensity for reporting bodily complaints at the beginning of the study to better evaluate subsequent angina pectoris. However, none of the studies took this step.

Myrtek (1998a) conducted meta-analyses of psychophysiological personality research. These analyses assessed the correlations between Type A behavior (SI and questionnaires were analyzed separately) or hostility and different personality dimensions. The studies forming the basis for the meta-analyses used healthy adults of both sexes (Table 6.1). Type A behavior is correlated with extraversion and neuroticism for both SI and questionnaires. Accordingly, Type A persons describe themselves as more extroverted and more emotionally labile than Type B persons. At least a small positive correlation with bodily complaints is observed when using Type A questionnaires. Hostility and Type A behavior assessed with questionnaires are correlated at .257 (population effect size [weighted average of all correlation coefficients]). Therefore, the correspondence between both concepts is not high. Furthermore, hostility is correlated negatively with extraversion and positively with neuroticism. Hostile persons are more emotionally labile and introverted than persons with low scores on hostility. A small positive correlation exists, moreover, between hostility and psychoticism.

Costa et al. (1986) had 1,002 patients complete the full MMPI and then examined the correlations between the Cook–Medley Ho Scale and other personality dimensions. The Ho Scale correlated with cynicism ($r = .91$), neuroticism ($r = .69$), psychoticism ($r = .49$), bodily complaints ($r = .33$), and extraversion ($r = -.06$). This study confirms the results of the meta-analyses. Therefore, a positive correlation exists between hostility on one hand and neuroticism and psychoticism on the other.

The correlation between hostility and extraversion is more likely to be negative.

Potential for Hostility derived from the component analysis of the SI also correlates positively with neuroticism (Dembroski & Costa, 1987). T. Q. Miller, Markides, Chiriboga, and Ray (1995) examined 373 Americans of Mexican heritage. In this study, hostility and bodily complaints correlated at .29. Eleven years after the first examination, 251 persons were reexamined. Hostility assessed 11 years previously correlated with present bodily complaints at .09.

There is also direct evidence of a correlation between Type A behavior and angina pectoris, in that Type A persons complain more frequently of angina pectoris. L. D. Young, Barboriak, Hoffman, and Anderson (1984) investigated 2,433 men who underwent coronary angiography for diagnostic reasons. A significant positive association between Type A, assessed with a newly developed questionnaire, and angina pectoris was observed ($p = .01$). However, no correlation between Type A and the extent of coronary stenosis was detected. A highly significant association between Type A, assessed with the Bortner scale, and a questionnaire about angina pectoris ($p = .00001$) was observed in 5,936 men by D. W. Johnston, Cook, and Shaper (1987). In a prospective study by Appels et al. (1987) with 2,414 men, a tendency for an association between Type A (measured using a Dutch adaptation of the JAS–A/B) and future angina pectoris in the 9.5-year follow-up interval was observed ($p = .080$). Within the scope of the Framingham Heart Study, Eaker, Abbott, and Kannel (1989) investigated 570 healthy men and 719 healthy women over a period of 20 years. A significant association between Type A behavior, assessed with a questionnaire, and future angina pectoris was found; Type A persons showed angina more frequently. No association, however, was observed between Type A and future myocardial infarction or coronary death. Shekelle, Vernon, and Ostfeld (1991) conducted the Western Electric Study on 2,003 healthy men with a follow-up interval of 10 years. The authors were interested in the correlation between bodily complaints or neuroticism and the incidence of angina pectoris, myocardial infarction, and coronary death. Regres-

TABLE 6.1							

Meta-Analyses of the Correlations Between Type A Behavior or Hostility and Personality Dimensions

Correlation	N	K	R	z	p	SD	Hp
Extraversion							
With Type A (structured interview)	334	5	0.214	3.95	.00004	0.082	*ns*
With Type A (questionnaire)	5,494	20	0.207	15.52	.00000	0.172	*
With hostility	2,015	2	−0.180	8.17	.00000	0.000	*ns*
Neuroticism							
With Type A (structured interview)	462	6	0.160	3.45	.00028	0.088	*ns*
With Type A (questionnaire)	5,812	23	0.248	19.21	.00000	0.155	*
With hostility	2,015	2	0.275	12.59	.00000	0.004	*ns*
Bodily complaints							
With Type A (structured interview)	365	3	0.007	0.14	.44132	0.044	*ns*
With Type A (questionnaire)	1,370	11	0.121	4.52	.00000	0.094	*
Psychoticism with Type A (questionnaire)	1,383	7	0.089	3.34	.00041	0.042	*ns*
Type A (questionnaire) with hostility	2,015	2	0.257	11.72	.00000	0.026	*ns*

Note. N = total population of all samples; K = number of combined effect sizes; R = population effect size (weighted average of all correlation coefficients); z = overall z score of the standard normal distribution; p = significance of this z score (one-tailed); SD = residual standard deviation (95% confidence interval = R ± 1.96 * SD); Hp = significance of the chi-square test for heterogeneity of the effect sizes. From *Enzyklopädie der Psychologie: Themenbereich C, Theorie und Forschung, Serie I, Biologische Psychologie, Band 5: Ergebnisse und Anwendungen der Psychophysiologie* (pp. 297–298) by F. Rösler (Ed.), 1998, Göttingen, Germany: Hogrefe. Copyright 1998 by Hogrefe-Verlag. Adapted with permission.
*p < .05.

sion analyses with several risk factors as covariates revealed significant associations between bodily complaints and angina pectoris (p < .001) and neuroticism and angina (p = .011). However, no significant associations between the incidence of myocardial infarction or coronary death and bodily complaints (p = .978) or neuroticism (p = .340) were observed.

Altogether, a host of results demonstrates the correlation between Type A behavior or hostility on one hand and angina pectoris, bodily complaints, and neuroticism on the other. All prospective studies that included angina pectoris as a disease endpoint may be erroneous to an unknown degree and must be viewed with great caution. The rather small correlations between Type A or hostility and future CHD (when angina pectoris is included as disease endpoint) could be caused by the associa-

tions described above and may, therefore, be spurious.

6.1.4. Correlation of Type A Behavior and Hostility With Risk Factors for Coronary Heart Disease

Aside from the correlations between Type A or hostility on the one hand and personality dimensions or angina pectoris on the other, there is information indicating a correlation of Type A or hostility with different risk factors for CHD. In the Aspirin Myocardial Infarction Study conducted by Shekelle, Gale, and Norusis (1985) with 244 women and 2,070 men using the JAS–A/B, women had significantly lower Type A scores than men (p = .012). Higher education was significantly correlated in both women (r = .14) and men (r = .16) with higher Type A scores. Moreover, younger men scored higher on Type A than older men ($r = -0.12$). For men, small but significant correlations were seen between Type A and body mass index ($r = .05$), working full time ($r = .09$), current cigarette smoking ($r = .06$), and current consumption of alcohol ($r = .07$). Sprafka et al. (1990) examined 1,074 Black and White women and 1,083 Black and White men with the JAS–A/B. As observed in the foregoing study, women had significantly lower Type A scores than men. Again, significant correlations between Type A and education emerged, at .12 for 849 Black subjects and .19 for 1,308 White subjects, with persons with higher education revealing higher Type A scores. The correlation between age and Type A was replicated, too, yielding coefficients of $-.09$ and $-.05$ for Black and White subjects, respectively. In this study, younger persons had higher Type A scores. In the sample of White persons, a significant association between Type A and smoking ($r = .11$) was observed. There were no significant Type A correlations for the risk factors of blood pressure and cholesterol.

Studies with 816 adolescents of both sexes using the JAS–A/B showed that men were classified more frequently than women as displaying Type A behavior ($p < .01$; D. J. Lee, Gomez-Marin, & Prineas, 1996). In the study by Eaker et al. (1989) with 570 men and 719 women, Type A behavior in men increased with increasing education ($p < .001$). For both sexes, white-collar workers were classified more often as showing Type A behavior than blue-collar workers ($p < .001$). An association between higher education and higher Type A scores was also found in a study with 551 women using the Framingham Type A Scale (Matthews, Kelsey, Meilahn, Kuller, & Wing, 1989). An indirect association between Type A and education was also observed in a German sample. A large-scale prevention study with 16,430 women and men revealed an association between Type A behavior (measured using the Bortner scale) and socioeconomic status (SES; $p < .001$) and that the higher SES subjects were more often classified as displaying Type A behavior (Helmert, Herman, Joeckel, Greiser, & Madans, 1989). In this study, significant associations were observed between SES and physical activity (higher

activity levels for higher SES groups; $p < .001$), smoking (lower rates for higher SES groups; $p < .001$), and obesity (lower rates for higher SES groups; $p < .001$). In a cross-sectional study with 2,187 men by J. B. Cohen and Reed (1985), significant associations between Type A behavior (measured using the JAS–A/B) and several CHD risk factors were established. Type A men had higher cholesterol levels ($p < .05$), higher body weight ($p < .01$), and lower physical activity levels ($p < .01$) than Type B men. In 1,305 healthy men, Kawachi et al. (1998) investigated the association between Type A (using a Type A scale derived from the MMPI) and risk factors for CHD. Persons who were classified as displaying Type A behavior showed a higher body mass index ($p = .0001$) and were more likely to have a family history of CHD ($p = .010$).

C. C. Johnson, Hunter, Amos, Elder, and Berenson (1989) reported in their study of adolescents a significant association between the hostility component of Type A behavior and smoking; subjects who smoked showed higher scores on the Ho Scale. The correlation for adolescents under age 14 was .11 ($N = 462$, $p = .003$) and for those over age 14, it was .13 ($N = 237$, $p = .008$). Räikkönen and Keltikangas-Järvinen (1991) conducted a representative study with 1,609 adolescents and young adults in Finland. Higher hostility scores (assessed with a three-item scale) were observed for women ($p < .001$) and younger persons ($p < .01$). An association between hostility and smoking ($p < .001$) and lack of physical activity ($p < .05$) was also evident in women. No associations of this kind were observed for men. Men revealed a correlation only between hostility and alcohol consumption, hostile men showing higher consumption. In a study with 4,646 women and men who as students had taken the Cook–Medley Ho Scale 20 years earlier (Lipkus, Barefoot, Williams, & Siegler, 1994), smokers also demonstrated higher hostility scores than nonsmokers ($p < .0001$). This study also asked whether former nonsmokers had subsequently begun smoking. Results showed that persons who had begun smoking displayed higher scores on the Ho Scale ($p < .01$).

In the CARDIA study (Scherwitz et al., 1991), 5,115 persons were stratified into 16 groups according to age (18–24 and 25–30 years), sex, race (White and Black), and education (higher education or less than high school). Several associations between the Cook–Medley Ho Scale and the stratifications emerged. Hostility scores were higher in Black subjects compared with White subjects ($p < .001$), higher in less educated compared with well-educated persons ($p < .001$), higher in men compared with women ($p < .001$), and higher in younger compared with older persons ($p < .001$). According to these findings, young Black men with low education have the highest hostility scores, whereas older White women with a good education display the lowest scores. In another publication from this study (Scherwitz et al., 1992), the authors reported that persons scoring high on the Ho Scale smoked significantly more cigarettes, had higher alcohol consumption, and had a higher calorie intake (all $ps < .001$). Maruta et al. (1993) examined 366 women and 254 men with the Ho Scale and observed several correlations with risk factors for CHD. Hostile persons were characterized by higher age ($p < .001$), were more often men ($p = .002$), had a higher relative body weight ($p = .001$), and were more likely to suffer from diabetes ($p = .018$). In a study by Barefoot, Larsen, von der Lieth, and Schroll (1995) with 740 healthy women and men, a positive association between hostility and body mass index was observed ($p = .030$).

In summary, several studies showed associations between Type A behavior or hostility and risk factors for CHD. Both for Type A and for hostility, significant positive correlations were observed with smoking in several studies. Moreover, for both factors, positive associations between overweight (measured using body mass index, adiposity, calorie intake, or body weight) and low levels of physical activity were found repeatedly. The correlation between alcohol consumption and Type A behavior or hostility cannot be evaluated unequivocally, because moderate alcohol consumption may be protective for CHD (Hulley, Cohen, & Widdowson, 1977; Ricci & Angelico, 1979). Substantial correlations for both factors were also observed for sex and age. Higher scores for Type A and hostility are seen in younger persons and men. Persons with

better education or higher SES score higher for Type A but reveal lower hostility scores. Prospective studies examining Type A or hostility have to take these results into account to avoid misinterpretations.

6.1.5. Previous Meta-Analyses

6.1.5.1. Meta-analysis by Booth-Kewley and Friedman (1987).

Booth-Kewley and Friedman (1987) conducted the first meta-analysis of the association between Type A behavior or other personality dimensions and different manifestations of CHD. Unfortunately, in most of their analyses the authors combined the results from prospective and retrospective studies. They therefore provided no evidence for the most important questions, such as the prospective association between personality and myocardial infarction. Moreover, the effect sizes used in the meta-analysis were not weighted by the number of subjects; S. V. Stone and Costa (1990) also criticized this flaw. Finally, the meta-analysis mixed all of the disease endpoints in the prospective studies, including myocardial infarction, angina pectoris, positive ECG findings, cardiac death, and atherosclerosis. A mean effect size of $r = .045$ emerged (10 effect sizes with a total $N = 6,907$, $p = .00009$, one-tailed) between CHD defined in this way and Type A behavior.

6.1.5.2. Meta-analysis by Matthews (1988).

Matthews (1988) conducted a second meta-analysis dealing with this issue. The results diverged greatly from those of Booth-Kewley and Friedman (1987). Matthews considered only prospective studies and weighted the results according to the number of subjects. However, instead of using effect sizes, this author aggregated the significance values from the studies. The association between Type A behavior and CHD was no longer significant in the studies considered (16 independent tests from the prospective studies; $p = .261$). However, the analyses of studies using the SI for assessment (5 tests; $p = .008$) and the studies with healthy persons (6 tests; $p = .001$) showed significant results. No significance was found for studies using the JAS–A/B (11 tests; $p = .464$) or for studies with CHD patients (9 tests; $p = .552$).

6.1.5.3. Meta-analyses by T. Q. Miller, Turner, Tindale, Posavac, and Dugoni (1991) and by T. Q. Miller, Smith, Turner, Guijarro, and Hallet (1996).

Large-scale meta-analyses by T. Q. Miller et al. (1991, 1996) examined Type A behavior and hostility, respectively. Unfortunately, the authors used not only the normal Pearson correlation coefficient, but also the so-called "tetrachoric" correlation coefficient to describe effect size. With the latter coefficient, the correlation increases with increasing skewness of the distribution. Because skewness of the distribution is very frequent in prospective studies, the results of these meta-analyses are inflated to an unknown degree. The tetrachoric correlation coefficient is defined as follows: $r_{tet} = \cos (180°/1 + \sqrt{a*d/b*c})$, where a, b, c, and d are the frequencies in a four-field table.

To illustrate the effects of this coefficient, we analyzed the prospective study by Barefoot et al. (1983). In this study, 255 medical students completed the Cook–Medley Ho Scale in the period from 1954 to 1959. After 25 years, 15 of the respondents, then physicians, suffered from CHD. The following frequencies for hostility (median split of the Ho score) and CHD were observed: (a) healthy and low hostility, $n = 133$; (b) CHD and low hostility, $n = 3$; (c) healthy and high hostility, $n = 107$; and (d) CHD and high hostility, $n = 12$. For the association between hostility and CHD, Barefoot et al. computed $z = 2.7$ ($p = .007$), resulting in $\chi^2(1, N = 255) = 7.11$, $p = .007$, or Pearson's $r = .169$ ($p = .007$). Using the formula for the tetrachoric correlation coefficient, however, yields $r_{tet} = .560$. The standard error of $r_{tet} = .1572$, resulting in $z = 3.56$ ($p < .0004$). Considering the common variance between hostility and CHD, the Pearson's r yields 2.9%, but the $r_{tet} = 31.4$ %, thus grossly inflating the association.

Considering the binomial effect size display more closely, the association between hostility and CHD can be further elucidated. If one assumes a disease rate of 50%, then of 100 persons with low hostility scores and $r_{tet} = .560$, 78 persons would remain healthy, and 22 persons would suffer from CHD. In the reverse case of 100 persons with high hostility scores, 22 would remain healthy, and 78

would develop CHD. This result would portray hostility as an extremely important risk factor. Using the Pearson $r = .169$, the result of the binomial effect size display is modest. Of 100 persons with low hostility, 58 would remain healthy, and 42 would develop CHD. In the high hostility group, 42 would remain healthy, and 58 would suffer from CHD. The relative risk (RR) of persons with high hostility scores as opposed to persons with low scores would be 3.55 (tetrachoric) or 1.41 (Pearson). In addition to the tetrachoric correlation coefficient, T. Q. Miller et al. (1991, 1996) also mixed biserial and normal Pearson coefficients in the meta-analyses.

It is not possible to directly compare the tetrachoric correlation with the Pearson correlation. As stated earlier in this section, $r_{tet} = .56$ yields $z = 3.56$ ($p < .0004$), whereas a Pearson coefficient of .56 would yield $z > 6.0$ ($p < .000000005$). The editor of *Psychological Bulletin*, in which the meta-analyses by Miller et al. were published, replied to a letter I wrote commenting on the meta-analyses that "although it would be useful to alert people to the problem of using tetrachoric *r*s, the contribution of doing so is not sufficient to merit publication in *Psychological Bulletin*" (Nancy Eisenberg, personal communication, April 22, 1998).

6.1.5.4. Meta-analysis by Hemingway and Marmot (1999).

During the work on the meta-analyses in this chapter, Hemingway and Marmot (1999) also published a meta-analysis on this topic. These authors analyzed 14 prospective studies with healthy persons and 5 studies with CHD patients. This meta-analysis did not differentiate between Type A and hostility. The studies were evaluated as follows: 0 = no association between Type A or hostility and CHD, + = small association (RR > 1 ≤ 2), and ++ = strong association (RR > 2). The 10 studies yielded 20 evaluations: 14 of 0, 3 of +, and 3 of ++. All studies with CHD patients yielded null as a result. According to this evaluation, the authors stated, "In healthy populations, prospective cohort studies suggest a possible etiological role for: Type-A/hostility (6/14 studies)" (p. 1462).

This analysis is open to criticism on several fronts. As the meta-analyses in this chapter will show, at least 35 prospective studies exist for Type A behavior and hostility with 53 independent effect sizes. Therefore, the analysis by Hemingway and Marmot (1999) takes only 38% of the available effect sizes into account. Moreover, the results of the WCGS are entered into the analysis three times; the same sample is used in the publications by C. D. Jenkins, Rosenman, and Zyzanski (1974); Rosenman, Brand, Sholtz, and Friedman (1976); and Ragland and Brand (1988b). Subsequently, the authors assigned one + evaluation too many, reducing the evaluation to 5 positive and 14 negative studies. Finally, the method used is open to criticism. The authors did not indicate why the relation of 6 positive to 14 negative studies is significant. They apparently conducted no statistical analysis, and a critical evaluation of the primary studies is missing; there is no comment on the different disease endpoints, the confounding variables, or the different methods of assessing Type A behavior.

Petticrew, Gilbody, and Sheldon (1999) criticized Hemingway and Marmot's (1999) analysis in a letter to the editor of the *British Medical Journal*. Petticrew et al. especially pointed to the confounding variables such as the classic risk factors that modify the association between Type A or hostility and CHD. In a direct reply to this letter, Hemingway and Marmot argued,

> As discussed in our review, psychosocial factors may have effects on disease which are mediated by health related behaviours. Thus if the causal chain involved hostile people being more likely to smoke, then adjusting for smoking as a confounder would be misguided. (Petticrew et al., 1999, p. 917)

Hemingway and Marmot had already recognized this point in their original article. It follows that in the end, all acute or chronic diseases and accidents can be traced back to psychosocial factors and personality dimensions.

To illustrate this point, we provide a fictional example. On a vacation, J and his partner traveled to West Africa. J bought ice cream from a vendor in the street, and after eating the ice cream, he became ill from an unknown virus and soon died. What was the cause of J's death? According to Hemingway and Marmot, psychosocial factors and personality dimensions were the cause of death. Some friends of J confirmed that he was always seeking out adventure. A psychologist who once tested J confirmed this inclination; "venturesomeness" is a personality trait and denotes a facet of extraversion (Eysenck & Eysenck, 1978). Furthermore, J's friends reported that when J was under stress, he suffered from ravenous hunger that he could not resist. J's partner, once again at home, said that she had ended the relationship a few hours before J ate the deadly ice cream.

The explanation of J's death is unequivocal. If J had not been so daring, he presumably would have traveled not to Africa but perhaps, instead, to a destination closer to home. The critical point was the social isolation caused by the separation from his partner: J could cope with this situation only by eating something. Therefore, J's death can be attributed to his personality and to special psychosocial factors. Before these events took place, preventative psychotherapy for J's extreme daring would have been indicated. Training to improve J's ability to cope with stress would have been beneficial, too. More examples of this sort are unnecessary to demonstrate the fruitlessness of giving primacy to soft psychosocial and personality risk factors over hard physiological risk factors.

6.2. METHOD

6.2.1. Literature Search

The gold standard in research on risk factors for CHD are prospective studies with healthy persons. These studies represent Level I of the quality evaluation created for studies on therapeutic interventions. The value of prospective studies with CHD patients is somewhat lower (Level II-1). Correlation studies that describe the association between the degree of coronary atherosclerosis and Type A behavior are of still lesser quality (Level II-2). It is therefore clear that meta-analyses should concentrate on prospective studies. Case control studies must be evaluated differently for Type A behavior and hostility. The stress concept is more critical for results concerning Type A behavior than for results on hostility, because the items of the JAS–A/B are more closely related to the stress concept than the items of the Cook–Medley Ho Scale. The need for causal attributions in CHD patients is surely much stronger than in controls. The stress concept allows patients to externalize the cause of disease, thus mitigating their own responsibility. CHD patients are therefore more likely to reveal Type A behavior than controls. This chapter does not consider case control studies of Type A behavior, but case control studies of hostility will enter the analysis.

The literature search was done using the Medline (Index Medicus) database of the U.S. National Library of Medicine for 1966 to 1998. The combination of the terms *Type A personality* (exploded) and *coronary disease* (exploded) yielded 559 citations. A further combination of the terms *Type A personality* (exploded) and *prospective studies* (exploded) yielded 59 citations. The literature search with the American Psychological Association's PsycLIT database for the interval 1967 to September 1998 was less successful. Instead of *Type A personality*, this database uses the term *coronary prone behavior*. The combination of this term with *coronary disease* yielded 52 citations, and *coronary prone behavior* with *prospective studies* yielded 9 citations. The literature search was carried out in the same manner for the term *hostility*. Medline yielded 241 citations for the combination of *hostility* (exploded) and *coronary disease* (exploded) for 1966 to 1998 and 85 citations for the combination of *hostility* (exploded) and *prospective studies* (exploded) for 1967 to September 1998. PsycLIT, again, was not as productive, yielding only 24 and 8 citations, respectively.

Using the abstracts of all citations, I screened studies for their suitability and obtained the original articles. I believe that this literature search detected practically all prospective studies dealing with Type A behavior or hostility, because the enormous costs of such studies surely guarantees that an article in English is published in an interna-

tional journal. In addition, I screened the reference lists of articles describing meta-analyses on the issue in question (see section 6.1.5). Of the correlation studies dealing with the association between Type A behavior and coronary atherosclerosis, only the largest studies (*N* > 100) were included; this criterion also applied to the case control studies dealing with hostility.

6.2.2. Determination of Effect Sizes
The present meta-analyses essentially follow the rules proposed by Matthews (1988): Only prospective studies, but no case control studies, are to be used for the meta-analysis of Type A behavior. For case control studies, the risk factor in question might be a consequence of CHD, and not a cause of CHD. Additionally, in studies of this kind patients who have died obviously are lost to follow-up, possibly distorting the results.

In the framework of a prospective study, often several intermediate results are published. It is therefore important to include only the publication with the longest prospective interval or the final publication in the analysis. Type A behavior is often operationalized differently (depending on whether it was measured using the SI or questionnaire), implying different results. Moreover, results might vary according to the study population (healthy persons or CHD patients). Finally, the criteria defining the disease endpoint for CHD are important (hard criterion vs. soft criterion). For these reasons, it is necessary to compute different meta-analyses with all combinations of the different factors (data-gathering method, study population, and endpoint criterion).

Moreover, certain rules are important for the analyses themselves. Effect sizes must be weighted according to the number of subjects in the study. In addition, insignificant results, which are typically downplayed, must be considered. In the present meta-analyses, unspecified insignificant results are assumed to have the values of $p = .500$ or $r = .0000$, respectively.

6.2.3. Meta-Analytic Method
All meta-analyses were conducted with the program Meta-Analysis (Schwarzer, 1987). The

Pearson correlation coefficient was used for the effect size; because it was rarely included in correlation studies, I mostly computed it from p values by transforming the p value to the z value of the standard normal distribution and using the formula $r = z/\sqrt{N}$ (N = number of subjects in the study). I calculated the variance of the population effect size R according to the Schmidt–Hunter method using Fisher's z-transformed r values. More information about the method was provided by Schwarzer (1987). The tables for this chapter include the following parameters:

- N = total population of all samples.
- K = number of combined effect sizes or studies; some studies have more than one effect size.
- R = population effect size as the weighted average of all correlation coefficients: $R = \Sigma N_i r_i / \Sigma N$ (r_i = correlation coefficient of sample i). The evaluation of this population effect size is important. According to J. Cohen (1977), a population effect size of $R = .100$ is considered small, $R = .300$ moderate, and $R = .500$ high.
- z = overall z score of the standard normal distribution (z): $z = R * \sqrt{N}$.
- p = significance of this z score (one-tailed). If many studies are combined, yielding a very high sample size, a highly significant overall z score does not necessarily provide useful information.
- SD = residual standard deviation: The square of the standard deviation represents the population variance, or residual variance ($S^2\text{res}$), of the effect sizes. The residual variance is computed by the formula $S^2\text{res} = S^2_r - S^2_e$, where $S^2_r = \Sigma N_i (r_i - R)^2 / \Sigma N_i$ is the observed variance of the effect sizes and $S^2_e = (1 - R^2)^2 * K/N$ the sampling error, according to the Schmidt–Hunter method. The 95% confidence interval of the population effect size is defined as $R \pm 1.96 * SD$. If $SD = 0$, the observed variance is explained solely by the sampling error, meaning that the confidence interval will be 0 as well. Alternatively, a large standard deviation indicates heterogeneity of the underlying data set. In this case, moderator variables must be assumed—for example, different effect sizes for women and men.

- Hp = significance of the chi-square test for heterogeneity; should be significant at $p < .05$.

6.3. RESULTS

6.3.1. Type A Behavior and Coronary Heart Disease

6.3.1.1. Prospective studies on Type A behavior and coronary heart disease. I analyzed each prospective study systematically and ordered all studies according to the publication date (see Table W6.1 on the accompanying Web site: http://www.apa.org/books/resources/jordan/). The sections that follow first describe the samples, including sample size, sex, and age of the subjects. Especially relevant is the designation of healthy persons or CHD patients. Next, information is provided on the method used for assessing the Type A behavior. As already mentioned, assessment using the SI is more important than assessment with questionnaires. In the studies using questionnaires, the JAS–A/B was usually used. The disease endpoints of each study, the hard or soft criterion, are also noted. The term *interval* denotes the prospective time interval from the beginning of the study to the last examination. The kind and number of control variables vary greatly from study to study; it can be assumed that studies with few or sometimes even no control variables must be judged more negatively. Important control variables include confirmed risk factors such as age, sex, smoking, cholesterol, family history of blood pressure, diabetes, lack of physical activity, and overweight. In studies using the soft criterion, bodily complaints and neuroticism should also be controlled (see section 6.1.3). Discussion of the results indicates the number of persons diagnosed with CHD in the prospective interval and the significance level as published by the authors of the study; the latter information enables the computation of the effect size r. Positive effect sizes signify that Type A behavior is a risk factor for CHD; negative effect sizes indicate that Type A might be a protective factor. Table W6.2 describes all 25 prospective studies on Type A behavior and CHD (see the accompanying Web site; for references, see Appendix W6A).

TABLE 6.2

Meta-Analyses of Prospective Studies Using the Structured Interview

Study characteristic	N	K	R	z	p	SD	Hp
Soft criterion, healthy persons	3,264	3	.08625	4.93	.00000	0.01399	*ns*
Hard criterion, healthy persons	1,110	2	.03361	1.12	.13163	0.00000	*ns*
Hard criterion, coronary heart disease patients	7,954	10	−.01370	1.22	.11098	0.02960	*
All studies with hard criterion	9,064	12	−.00790	0.75	.22596	0.03150	*
All studies with the structured interview	12,328	15	.01708	1.90	.02896	0.04996	*

Note. N = total population of all samples; K = number of combined effect sizes; R = population effect size (weighted average of all correlation coefficients); z = overall z score of the standard normal distribution; p = significance of this z score (one-tailed); SD = residual standard deviation (95% confidence interval = $R \pm 1.96 * SD$); Hp = significance of the chi-square test for heterogeneity of the effect sizes.
*$p < .05$.

6.3.1.2. Meta-analyses of prospective studies on Type A behavior and coronary heart disease.

First, prospective studies with the SI are analyzed followed by prospective studies using questionnaires. Within each method, analyses are ordered according to the disease endpoint. Finally, analyses are ordered by the study population.

6.3.1.2.1. Prospective studies using the structured interview. Studies using the soft criterion with healthy persons. Apart from a small study with 100 subjects (Schaubroeck, Ganster, & Kemmerer, 1994), the meta-analysis is based on 3,154 healthy persons in the WCGS (Rosenman et al., 1976), which represents the starting point for all studies dealing with Type A behavior (Table 6.2). The population effect size of R = .086 is the highest of all analyses conducted for Type A behavior and statistically highly significant. The binomial effect size display gives an impression of this effect size. If the probability for CHD is 50% in a population, 54% of the Type A persons, but only 46% of the Type B persons, would be diagnosed with CHD. Presumably, the computed effect size still represents an underestimation, because the meta-analysis can use only the levels of significance published by the authors. When only p values up to .001 are published, then the meta-analysis must use this value, regardless of the fact that the significance level might be even better than .001. On the other hand, in the WCGS, a soft criterion (i.e., inclusion of angina pectoris)

was used that might inflate the effect size spuriously, as pointed out in section 6.1.3.

Studies using the soft criterion with CHD patients. No prospective studies were identified for CHD patients with the soft criterion.

Studies using the hard criterion with healthy persons. Prospective studies with healthy persons using the hard criterion have the best possible design. However, the meta-analysis of the two studies with this design (Appels & Mulder, 1985; Kittel, 1986) showed no significant results.

Studies using the hard criterion with CHD patients. Compared with studies with healthy persons, the bulk of studies using the SI were conducted with CHD patients. In this analysis, seven studies with a total of 10 effect sizes were considered. In two studies with four samples, positive correlations or no correlations between Type A and CHD were observed (Brackett & Powell, 1988; Orth-Gomer & Unden, 1990). However, five studies with six samples showed negative correlations between Type A and CHD (Barefoot, Peterson, et al., 1989; De Leo, Caracciolo, Berto, & Mauro, 1986; Palmer, Langeluddecke, Jones, & Tennant, 1992; Ragland & Brand, 1988a; Shekelle et al., 1986). Taken together, therefore, Type A is negatively related to the criterion, although not significantly. This finding means that Type A behavior is not a risk factor in patients already suffering from CHD. The test for heterogeneity is significant, revealing that the results of

TABLE 6.3

Meta-Analyses of Prospective Studies Using Questionnaires

Study characteristic	N	K	R	z	p	SD	Hp
Soft criterion, healthy persons	7,851	6	.02908	2.58	.00499	0.03357	*
Soft criterion, CHD patients	886	3	.00000	0.00	1.00000	0.00000	ns
All studies with soft criterion	8,737	9	.02613	2.44	.00729	0.02731	*
Hard criterion, healthy persons	28,013	8	−.00433	0.72	.23453	0.01290	ns
Hard criterion, CHD patients	25,248	7	−.00399	0.63	.26313	0.00000	ns
All studies with hard criterion	53,261	15	−.00417	0.96	.16817	0.00866	ns
All studies with questionnaires	61,998	24	.00010	0.03	.48962	0.01673	*

Note. N = total population of all samples; K = number of combined effect sizes; R = population effect size (weighted average of all correlation coefficients); z = overall z score of the standard normal distribution; p = significance of this z score (one-tailed); SD = residual standard deviation (95% confidence interval = R ± 1.96 * SD); Hp = significance of the chi-square test for heterogeneity of the effect sizes; CHD = coronary heart disease.
*p < .05.

the different studies are heterogeneous; the correlation coefficients range from $r = -.3070$ to $r = .0687$.

All studies using the hard criterion. The meta-analysis with all studies using a hard criterion for both healthy persons and CHD patients does not yield a significant correlation between Type A and CHD.

All studies with the structured interview. With a total N of 12,328 in the prospective studies, the correlation between Type A and CHD yields only $R = .017$. In the one-tailed test, this coefficient is still significant but practically meaningless. Moreover, it must be considered that the WCGS, which contributed most to this result, used a soft criterion. According to the effect size display, 50.85% of Type A persons and 49.15% of Type B persons would develop CHD in the prospective interval.

6.3.1.2.2. *Prospective studies using questionnaires.* *Studies using the soft criterion with healthy persons.* This meta-analysis is based on five studies with six effect sizes (Table 6.3). Two studies showed a positive relation between Type A and CHD (Haynes, Feinleib, & Kannel, 1980; Kawachi et al., 1998), whereas in the other studies, no relation was found (J. B. Cohen & Reed, 1985; Koskenvuo et al., 1988; Leon, Finn, Murray, & Bailey, 1988). The effect size in this analysis is small but significant. In particular, the study by Haynes et al. reveals two

rather high correlation coefficients ($r > .10$) causing significant heterogeneity.

Studies using the soft criterion with CHD patients. Two studies (Julkunen, Idänpään-Heikkilä, & Saarinen, 1993; Koskenvuo et al., 1988) with three effect sizes were analyzed. Because all effect sizes are zero, the population effect size is zero as well.

All studies using the soft criterion. As we might expect from the foregoing analyses, the population effect size is small ($R = .026$) but significant. However, the criterion is a soft one, and the small effect size might also reflect the tendency of Type A subjects to report bodily complaints more frequently than Type B subjects (see Table 6.1).

Studies using the hard criterion with healthy persons. The result of this meta-analysis is especially important because of the very high N—more than 28,000 subjects—and the hard criterion. Three studies revealed a positive correlation between Type A and CHD (Haynes et al., 1980; Kawachi et al., 1998; Kittel, 1986), two studies no correlation (Appels et al., 1987; Tunstall-Pedoe, Woodward, Tavendale, A'Brook, & McCluskey, 1997), and three studies a negative correlation (Brackett & Powell, 1988; Haynes et al., 1980; Tunstall-Pedoe et al., 1997). The population effect size of $R = -.004$ is negligible and not significant.

Studies using the hard criterion with CHD patients. In this analysis, the *N* of more than 25,000 patients is also very high. None of the six studies showed a positive correlation between Type A and subsequent CHD. Three studies revealed no correlation (Mann & Brennan, 1987; Ruberman, Weinblatt, Goldberg, & Chaudhary, 1984; Shekelle et al., 1986), and three others showed small negative correlations (Ahern et al., 1990; Case, Heller, Case, & Moss, 1985; Shekelle, Gale, & Norusis, 1985). In this analysis, the population effect size is also negligible and far from being significant. It is interesting that in these patients, the correlation between Type A and CHD is also numerically negative.

All studies using the hard criterion. The summary of all studies using the hard criterion with healthy persons or CHD patients yields a 0 correlation.

All studies with questionnaires. The meta-analysis of all prospective studies that used questionnaires yields an extremely small and insignificant population effect size of $R = .0001$. The heterogeneity of this analysis is caused by the criteria used. The population effect size yields $R = .026$ with the soft criterion but $R = -.004$ with the hard criterion. This discrepancy can most certainly be ascribed to the correlation between Type A (using the questionnaire) and bodily complaints (using angina pectoris), as already described in section 6.1.3. Therefore, the correlation between Type A and CHD assessed with the soft criterion can be considered a methodological artifact.

6.3.1.2.3. Prospective studies with healthy persons. The meta-analyses described in the preceding section have shown that the prospective studies conducted either with healthy persons or CHD patients might be evaluated differently. I conducted a separate analysis for healthy persons and patients (Table 6.4).

The summary of all prospective studies conducted with healthy persons, regardless of the method of assessment or the criterion, yields a significant population effect size of $R = .011$. Omitting the WCGS in this analysis yields an effect size of $R = .005$, which is no longer significant ($p = .1873$). Because studies with the soft criterion reveal higher effect sizes than studies using the hard criterion, I conducted separate analyses. The meta-analysis

with studies using the soft criterion yields a highly significant population effect size of $R = .046$, whereas the analysis with studies using the hard criterion is not significant. Therefore, prospective studies with healthy persons show significant results only if angina pectoris is included as a disease endpoint.

6.3.1.2.4. Prospective studies with coronary heart disease patients. The analysis of all studies with CHD patients without considering the criterion or the method of assessment yields a very small population effect size that is not significant. Compared with studies with healthy persons, the effect size is numerically negative (Table 6.4).

6.3.1.2.5. All prospective studies on Type A behavior and coronary heart disease. Figure W6.1 (see the accompanying Web site) graphically displays the effect sizes of all prospective Type A studies according to their publication date. There is no significant correlation between the date of publication and the magnitude of the effect size ($N = 39$, $r = .209$, $p = .202$). Similarly, no significant correlation between the effect sizes and the magnitude of the samples can be observed ($N = 39$, $r = .018$, $p = .913$). Finally, the sample magnitudes are not significantly correlated with the year of publication (Figure W6.2 on the Web site; $N = 39$, $r = -.107$, $p = .518$).

Of the 25 prospective studies, the samples of 11 studies included both men and women. A separate analysis for men and women, however, was done only in the studies by Shekelle et al. (1985), Haynes et al. (1980), and Tunstall-Pedoe et al. (1997). In Shekelle et al. and Haynes et al., the effect sizes for men and women were comparable—that is, there were no significant correlations using the hard criterion. Tunstall-Pedoe et al. revealed no significant correlation between Type A and CHD for men but a significant negative correlation for women. Of the 74,326 persons examined in the prospective studies, only 10,847 (14.6%) were women.

In summarizing all prospective studies for Type A and CHD, there is a population effect size of $R = .00292$, which is not significant in the one-tailed test ($N = 74,326$, $K = 39$, $z = 0.80$, $p = .21297$, $SD = 0.02621$, *Hp* significant at $p < .05$). The omission of the WCGS from the meta-analysis yields a

TABLE 6.4

Meta-Analyses of Prospective Studies on Healthy Persons and CHD Patients

Study characteristic	N	K	R	z	p	SD	Hp
All studies with healthy persons	40,238	19	.01060	2.13	0.01670	0.03233	s
Soft criterion, healthy persons	11,115	9	.04590	4.84	0.00000	0.03909	*
Hard criterion, healthy persons	29,123	10	−.00288	0.49	0.31157	0.01442	ns
All studies with CHD patients	34,088	20	−.00615	1.14	0.12810	0.01068	ns

Note. CHD = coronary heart disease; N = total population of all samples; K = number of combined effect sizes; R = population effect size (weighted average of all correlation coefficients); z = overall z score of the standard normal distribution; p = significance of this z score (one-tailed); SD = residual standard deviation (95% confidence interval = $R \pm 1.96 * SD$); Hp = significance of the chi-square test for heterogeneity of the effect sizes.
*$p < .05$.

correlation close to 0 with a negative sign ($R = -.00054$, $N = 71,172$, $K = 37$, $z = 0.14$, $p = .44237$, $SD = 0.02121$, Hp significant at $p < .05$). Both analyses reveal that the combined 39 or 37 effect sizes are heterogeneous, again caused by the discrepancy between the soft criterion and the hard criterion, but also by the discrepancy between healthy and CHD subjects. Studies with healthy persons tend to show a positive correlation and studies with CHD patients a negative correlation between Type A and CHD.

6.3.1.3. Correlation studies on Type A behavior and coronary atherosclerosis.
The design of this analysis is similar to that used with the prospective studies. Instead of endpoints, however, dependent variables are used, in this case usually the degree of coronary atherosclerosis. In such studies, there is no prospective interval. Positive effect sizes denote a correlation between Type A and coronary atherosclerosis. Table W6.2 describes the four studies on Type A behavior and coronary atherosclerosis (see the Web site; for references, see Appendix W6A, also on the Web site).

6.3.1.4. Meta-analyses of correlative studies on Type A behavior and coronary atherosclerosis.
Studies using the structured interview. Two studies used the SI to assess Type A behavior (Dimsdale, Hackett, Hutter, & Block, 1980; R. B. Williams, Barefoot, Haney, & Harrell, 1988). The correlation between Type A and the degree of coronary stenosis is very small and not significant ($R = .00689$,

$N = 2,392$, $K = 2$, $z = 0.34$, $p = .36813$, $SD = 0.00000$, $Hp = ns$).

Studies using a questionnaire. Three studies with four effect sizes used questionnaires to assess Type A behavior (Dimsdale et al., 1980; Hayano et al., 1997; Young et al., 1984). No study revealed a significant correlation ($R = .00000$, $N = 3,055$, $K = 4$, $z = 0.00$, $p = 1.00000$, $SD = 0.00000$, $Hp = ns$).

All studies. As one might expect from the foregoing analyses, a significant correlation between Type A and the degree of coronary stenosis cannot be confirmed ($R = .00303$, $N = 5,447$, $K = 6$, $z = 0.22$, $p = .41167$, $SD = 0.00000$, $Hp = ns$).

6.3.1.5. Intervention studies for Type A behavior.
After the identification of Type A behavior as a risk factor for CHD, it seemed worthwhile to modify Type A behavior in CHD patients through planned interventions. In this context, the intervention study by M. Friedman et al. (1984) is important. This study is often cited as proving the relevance of Type A behavior as a risk factor for CHD. It is, therefore, important to look at this study more closely.

Nunes, Frank, and Kornfeld (1987) conducted a meta-analysis with 10 controlled studies. The authors computed an average effect size of $d = 0.61$ ($N = 1,484$, $p < .001$) for the successful alteration of Type A behavior. The transformation of d to r yields $r = .085$. Still more important is the reduction of myocardial infarction and cardiac death by about 50% in the 3-year interval after the psychological intervention. However, this result is based on only two studies. One of these studies stems from M. Friedman et al. (1984) with $N = 1,012$ (according to Nunes et al., 1987). The second study had an N of only 44. In considering the total N of 1,484 of this meta-analysis, the study by M. Friedman et al. accounts for 68% of the whole data base. This study, however, is problematic.

Within the framework of the Recurrent Coronary Prevention Project, M. Friedman et al. (1984) conducted an intervention study with 862 CHD patients. The control group comprised 270 patients (Group 1, cardiac treatment only), and the intervention group comprised 592 patients (Group 2, special training to reduce Type A behavior). At follow-up after 3 years, five patients in Group 1 and eight patients in Group 2 could no longer be contacted. Of the remaining 265 Group 1 patients, 164 adhered to the treatment, and 101 voluntarily dropped out during the prospective interval. In Group 2, 203 patients dropped out, and 381 adhered to the treatment. As might be expected and as Nunes et al. (1987) showed, active patients of Group 2 showed a significant reduction in Type A behavior compared with active patients of Group 1. The cumulative rate of myocardial infarction and cardiac death was 13.2% for the 265 Group 1 patients and 7.2% for the 584 Group 2 patients. This difference, of course, is highly significant.

At first glance, these figures support the special training and were interpreted by M. Friedman et al. (1984) correspondingly. However, on closer inspection of the tables, when differentiating between active patients and dropouts, a remarkable finding emerges: Of the 545 active patients ($N = 164$ from Group 1 and $N = 381$ from Group 2), 65 (11.9%) experienced a myocardial infarction; of the 304 dropouts, however, only 12 (3.9%) experienced an MI. This difference is highly significant, $\chi^2(1, N = 849) = 15.1$, $p < .0003$. Thus, in this study patients who voluntarily quit the treatment were less likely to experience an MI.

Because the authors did not mention this highly important finding, I asked them in a letter to the editor of the *American Heart Journal* to comment on this result (Myrtek, 1986). Unfortunately, M. Friedman, who together with Rosenman is regarded as one of the founders of the Type A concept, could

not explain this finding. In summing up, he made the following statement: "I believe that this article of his (Myrtek) and that of Case et al. (N Engl J Med 312:737, 1985) and Shekelle et al. (Am J Cardiol 56:221, 1985), serve as prime examples of how clinical studies can be irretrievably flawed when investigators attempt to substitute statistical quasi-expertise for clinical acumen and common sense" (M. Friedman, 1986, p. 1216). This statement implies that the concept of Type A behavior is grounded on "clinical acumen" and on "common sense" but not on statistically analyzed studies.

The question remains of how to explain the finding that treatment dropouts experienced fewer myocardial infarctions. Presumably, more Type A patients quit the treatment because of their impatience and aggressiveness. This interpretation is reminiscent of the study by Thoresen, Friedman, Gill, and Ulmer (1982, p. 183) and would also support the study by Ragland and Brand (1988a), in which the recurrent infarction rate was lower in Type A than in Type B patients. It is also conceivable that the healthier patients dropped out.

An intervention study was conducted in Sweden with 261 patients after coronary bypass surgery (Burell, 1996). The intervention group consisted of 128 patients, and 133 patients were assigned to the control group. The intervention group participated in group psychotherapy every third week for 1 year to reduce Type A behavior. Moreover, patients practiced a relaxation procedure and were given homework assignments related to healthy behaviors (e.g., eating healthy foods, drinking less, and smoking less). Follow-up was made after 6 to 6.5 years; 7 patients in the intervention group and 16 patients in the control group had died ($p = .020$, according to the author); $\chi^2(1, N = 261) = 3.49$, $p = .058$. For total mortality, therefore, a marginally significant difference between the groups existed, but not for cardiovascular mortality (5 patients in the intervention and 8 patients in the control group); $\chi^2(1, N = 261) = 0.61$, $p = .440$. The author did not address this difference in mortality rates. Because the intervention comprised different treatment elements, it is not clear whether the difference in total mortality can be ascribed to a reduction in Type A behavior.

TABLE 6.5

Meta-Analyses of Prospective Studies on Hostility and Coronary Heart Disease (CHD)

Study characteristic	N	K	R	z	p	SD	Hp
Soft criterion, healthy persons	4,496	5	.00502	0.34	0.36837	0.02823	ns
Soft criterion, CHD patients	794	2	.02549	0.72	0.23664	0.04110	ns
All studies with soft criterion	5,290	7	.00809	0.59	0.27821	0.03135	ns
Hard criterion, healthy persons	8,281	6	.03490	3.18	0.00074	0.00000	ns
All studies with hard criterion	9,748	7	.02965	2.93	0.00170	0.00000	ns
All studies on hostility and CHD	15,038	14	.02207	2.71	0.00340	0.01860	ns

Note. N = total population of all samples; K = number of combined effect sizes; R = population effect size (weighted average of all correlation coefficients); z = overall z score of the standard normal distribution; p = significance of this z score (one-tailed); SD = residual standard deviation (95% confidence interval = $R \pm 1.96 * SD$); Hp = significance of the chi-square test for heterogeneity of the effect sizes.

6.3.2. Hostility and Coronary Heart Disease

6.3.2.1. Prospective studies on hostility and coronary heart disease. The sections that follow describe the studies on hostility using the same scheme as that used for the prospective studies on Type A behavior (see section 6.3.1). The studies were ordered according to the publication date, and a distinction is drawn between healthy persons and CHD patients on one hand and hard or soft criterion on the other. In all studies, questionnaires, usually the Cook–Medley Ho Scale, were used to operationalize hostility. Therefore, differentiation according to the data-gathering method is not possible. Positive effect sizes denote hostility as a risk factor for CHD. Table W6.3 summarizes the 10 prospective studies on hostility and CHD (see the accompanying Web site; for references, see Appendix W6B, also on the Web site).

6.3.2.2. Meta-analyses of prospective studies on hostility and coronary heart disease. *Studies using the soft criterion with healthy persons.* Five studies were used for the meta-analysis (Barefoot et al., 1983; Koskenvuo et al., 1988; Leon et al., 1988; Maruta et al., 1993; McCranie et al., 1986; Table 6.5). The population effect size is extremely small and not significant.

Studies using the soft criterion with CHD patients. The study by Koskenvuo et al. (1988) with CHD patients and the soft criterion yielded two effect

sizes. No significant correlation between hostility and CHD in the prospective interval emerged.

All studies using the soft criterion. As one might expect from the foregoing analyses, no significant correlation can be shown when combining all studies with the soft criterion.

Studies using the hard criterion with healthy persons. Prospective studies with healthy persons using the hard criterion are the most useful. Four studies with six effect sizes used this design (Barefoot, et al., 1995; Everson et al., 1997; Hearn et al., 1989; Shekelle, Gale, Ostfeld, & Paul, 1983). The effect size of $R = .035$ is small but significant.

Studies using the hard criterion with CHD patients. A hard criterion was used only in the study by Barefoot et al. (1989) with CHD patients. Therefore, it is not possible to conduct a meta-analysis. The correlation between hostility and later CHD yields $r = .000$ ($N = 1,467$).

All studies using the hard criterion. As expected, the combination of all studies using the hard criterion yields a small but significant effect size.

All prospective studies on hostility and CHD. The combination of all prospective studies examining the correlation between hostility and later CHD reveals a significant result, too. The effect size of $R = .022$, however, is of no practical importance.

6.3.2.3. Case control studies on hostility and coronary heart disease. Two studies used the component analysis of the SI for the assessment of

177

hostility (see section 6.1.2.2), and all other studies used questionnaires. The studies can be differentiated by hard or soft criterion, too. Positive effect sizes denote hostility as a risk factor for CHD. Table W6.4 describes the eight case control studies on hostility and CHD (see the accompanying Web site; for references, see Appendix W6B).

6.3.2.4. Meta-analyses of case control studies on hostility and coronary heart disease.
First, case control studies with the component analysis of the SI are presented, followed by case control studies using questionnaires. Within each method analyses are ordered according to the disease endpoint.

6.3.2.4.1. Studies using the component analysis of the SI. Studies with the soft criterion. Only the study by Hecker, Chesney, Black, and Frautschi (1988) used the component analysis of the SI with the soft criterion. The study yields a significant $r = .120$ ($N = 750$). According to this result, CHD patients are higher in hostility than healthy controls. This positive result is not surprising, because the study is a later analysis of the WCGS.

Studies with the hard criterion. Only one study with the hard criterion exists (Dembroski, MacDougall, Costa, & Grandits, 1989). The effect size is $r = .077$ ($N = 576$) and is significant at $p < .01$.

All studies using the component analysis of the SI. The two case control studies using the component analysis of the SI to assess hostility yield a highly significant population effect size of $R = .10157$ ($N = 1,326$, $K = 2$, $z = 3.70$, $p = .00011$, $SD = 0.00000$, $Hp = ns$).

6.3.2.4.2. Studies using questionnaires. Studies with the soft criterion. This meta-analysis is based on three studies with eight effect sizes (Atchison & Condon, 1993; Lichtenstein, Pedersen, Plomin, De Faire, & McClearn, 1989; Van Dijl, 1982; Table 6.6). The result of the meta-analysis with a population effect size of $R = .111$ is highly significant.

Studies with the hard criterion. Another three studies with four effect sizes used the hard criterion (Lahad, Heckbert, Koepsell, Psaty, & Patrick, 1997; Meesters & Smulders, 1994; Ranchor, Sanderman, Bouma, Buunk, & van den Heuvel, 1997). Compared with the population effect size of the meta-analysis with studies using the soft criterion, the

effect size of $R = .018$ for studies that used the hard criterion is very small and not significant.

All studies using questionnaires. The combination of all case control studies that used questionnaires for hostility assessment results in a small but significant effect size of $R = .048$. The chi-square test for heterogeneity is significant for the analysis because of the rather different effect sizes of studies with the soft criterion ($R = .111$) compared with studies with the hard criterion ($R = .018$). The difference might be well explained by the correlation between angina pectoris (soft criterion) and hostility (questionnaire). To this extent, the correlation between hostility and CHD would be spurious.

6.3.2.4.3. All case control studies on hostility and coronary heart disease. Combining all case control studies that have addressed the correlation between hostility and CHD yields a population effect size of $R = .056$ (Table 6.6). According to the binomial effect size with an assumed disease rate of 50%, of 100 persons with high hostility scores, 52.8% would suffer CHD and 47.2% would remain healthy. In the reverse case of 100 persons with low hostility scores, 47.2% would get the disease and 52.8% would remain healthy. The significant test for heterogeneity denotes that the effect sizes of the different studies are rather heterogeneous.

6.3.2.5. Correlation studies on hostility and coronary atherosclerosis.
Three more recent studies dealing with hostility and coronary atherosclerosis, among others, are worthy of mention. Helmer, Ragland, and Syme (1991) investigated 118 men and 40 women undergoing coronary angiography. Hostility was assessed both with the component analysis of the SI and with the Cook–Medley Ho Scale. No significant correlations were shown between the degree of coronary atherosclerosis and hostility. In a small study with 49 men (Air Force personnel) by Barefoot et al. (1994), no relation between the Ho Scale and the result of the coronary angiography was detected. Haney et al. (1996), however, reported a very high correlation of .57 between coronary atherosclerosis and a self-developed Hostile Behavior Index in 136 men. This index is similar to the component analysis of the SI as suggested by Dembroski (1978).

TABLE 6.6							
Meta-Analyses of Case Control Studies on Hostility and Coronary Heart Disease							
Study characteristic	**N**	**K**	**R**	**z**	**p**	**SD**	**Hp**
Soft criterion	2,529	8	.11114	5.60	.00000	0.04107	*ns*
Hard criterion	5,322	4	.01795	1.31	.09518	0.00919	*ns*
All studies with questionnaires	7,851	12	.04809	4.26	.00001	0.04947	*
All case control studies	9,177	14	.05584	5.35	.00000	0.04799	*

Note. N = total population of all samples; K = number of combined effect sizes; R = population effect size (weighted average of all correlation coefficients); z = overall z score of the standard normal distribution; p = significance of this z score (one-tailed); SD = residual standard deviation (95% confidence interval = $R \pm 1.96 * SD$); Hp = significance of the chi-square test for heterogeneity of the effect sizes.
*$p < .05$.

6.3.3. Hostility and Total Mortality

6.3.3.1. Prospective studies on hostility and total mortality.
The studies dealing with hostility and CHD often analyzed the correlation between hostility and total mortality. Therefore, I conducted a meta-analysis for this issue. The description of the analysis is the same as in section 6.3.2.1. Positive effect sizes denote hostility as a risk factor for total mortality. Table W6.5 describes the 10 prospective studies on hostility and total mortality (see the accompanying Web site; for references, see Appendix W6B).

6.3.3.2. Meta-analysis of prospective studies on hostility and total mortality.
With the exception of the study by Houston, Babyak, Chesney, Black, & Ragland (1997), all studies used questionnaires to assess hostility, mostly the Cook–Medley Ho Scale. Therefore, only the result of the meta-analysis based on all studies will be described. Of the 10 studies, 6 revealed a significant relation between hostility and total mortality. The results of 3 other studies are not significant, but the numerical tendency does not contradict the hypothesis. Only the study by McCranie et al. (1986) shows a tendency incongruent with the hypothesis. The population effect size of $R = .05998$ is relatively high, and the different effect sizes are homogeneous ($N = 8,693$, $K = 10$, $z = 5.60$, $p = .00000$, $SD = 0.02316$, $Hp = ns$). Therefore, a correlation exists between hostility and total mortality.

6.4. DISCUSSION

Section 6.3 documented in detail the basic data of all studies forming the starting point of the meta-analysis and described all important formulas for the meta-analyses. If, against expectation, a prospective study has been overlooked, this would have little influence on the results, because the large number of studies in the analyses is such that an additional study would change the population effect sizes very little. It is noteworthy that no study—on either Type A behavior or hostility—was conducted in a German-speaking country. Moreover, about 85% of all persons studied were men.

6.4.1. Evaluation of the Results on Type A Behavior
The database for Type A behavior is excellent. The relationship between Type A behavior and CHD was investigated in 25 prospective studies with 74,326 persons. In 12,328 persons, Type A behavior was assessed with the SI; in the rest, it was assessed using questionnaires. Separate analyses were conducted for the different methods. Important sources of variance are the endpoints of the prospective studies (soft or hard criterion) and the samples investigated (healthy persons or CHD patients). The best possible study design involves healthy persons assessed with the SI and the hard criterion. However, only two studies met these requirements. The population effect size of $R = .034$

(N = 1,110) is not significant. Two other studies with healthy persons and the SI also used angina pectoris (soft criterion) as an endpoint. The population effect size of R = .086 (N = 3,264) is highly significant, establishing Type A behavior as a risk factor for CHD. However, this meta-analysis, with 3,154 persons, is heavily based on the WCGS, which represents the starting point of the Type A hypothesis.

The inclusion of angina pectoris as a CHD endpoint in a prospective study is problematic. As shown in section 6.1.3, Type A behavior assessed with the SI is significantly correlated with neuroticism. This personality dimension correlates substantially with bodily complaints (r = .39, N = 4,104), as has often been shown (Myrtek, 1998b). Therefore, it cannot be ruled out that persons with high scores in neuroticism complain of angina pectoris more often. This would establish a spurious correlation between Type A behavior and CHD.

A considerable number of studies using the SI were conducted with CHD patients. The meta-analysis with 7,954 patients yields an insignificant population effect size of R = −.014. It is interesting that the correlation between Type A and CHD is negative, meaning that Type A behavior in persons with concurrent CHD seems more likely to be a protective factor. In the study by Barefoot, Peterson, et al. (1989) with 1,467 CHD patients, a significant interaction between Type A and cardiac risk was observed. In the prospective interval, Type A patients with high cardiac risk (i.e., congestive heart failure) had a better chance of survival than Type B patients with high cardiac risk. This difference was not found in patients with low cardiac risk.

The meta-analytic summary of all studies conducted with the SI yields a population effect size of R = .017 (N = 12,328). In the one-tailed test, this result is statistically significant but numerically negligible. With the exception of the WCGS, all other prospective studies conducted with the SI yield no significant relation between Type A and CHD.

With a total of 61,998 persons, studies using questionnaires (mostly the JAS–A/B) to assess Type A behavior are much more extensive. Studies with healthy persons and the hard criterion are the most important. The population effect size of R = −.004 (N = 28,013) is not significant and numerically negligible. Using the soft criterion in healthy persons yields a significant population effect size of R = .029 (N = 7,851). However, the argument against the soft criterion still carries more weight in studies with questionnaires than in studies with the SI. Type A questionnaires substantially correlate with neuroticism and bodily complaints (see section 6.1.3). The small population effect size may well be traced to this correlation.

The analysis of all questionnaire studies conducted with CHD patients and using the hard criterion yields a population effect size of R = −.004 (N = 25,248), which is not significant. Two smaller studies with CHD patients used the soft criterion. The population effect size is R = .000 (N = 886). The analysis of all studies conducted with questionnaires in healthy persons and CHD patients yields an insignificant population effect size of R = .0001 (N = 61,998). Adding the studies conducted with the SI to the questionnaire studies yields R = .003 (N = 74,326). This population effect size is not significant (p = .213) in the one-tailed test. The exclusion of the WCGS from the analysis results in a 0 correlation (R = −.0005; N = 71,172; p = .442). The correlation studies of Type A behavior and coronary atherosclerosis are no more favorable. Studies with the SI yielded an insignificant population effect size of R = .007 (N = 2,392). Questionnaire studies resulted in a population effect size of R = .000 (N = 3,055).

To summarize, Type A behavior is not an independent risk factor for CHD. The relation between Type A and CHD detected by the WCGS could not be replicated in a large number of prospective studies. This is true independent of the method used for Type A assessment (i.e., SI or questionnaire).

Ragland and Brand (1988b) conducted a subsequent analysis of the WCGS data based on all coronary deaths of the 3,154 participants until the end of 1983; thus, the prospective interval amounts to 22 years. Significant risk factors for coronary death were systolic blood pressure, cholesterol, smoking, and age. Taking these risk factors into account, Type A behavior was not significant (RR = .98; 95% confidence interval 0.85–1.12). It follows, therefore, that when using the hard criterion in the WCGS, Type A is not a risk factor. The assumption that the positive result in the WCGS is caused by the use of the soft criterion is affirmed.

6.4.2. Evaluation of the Results on Hostility

The database for hostility and CHD is much smaller than that for Type A behavior and CHD. Only 10 prospective studies could be found with 15,038 persons. Four studies used the hard criterion in healthy persons. The population effect size yields $R = .035$ ($N = 8,281$), which is significant. When evaluating this result, it must be taken into account that hostility correlates with several CHD risk factors (see section 6.1.4), including smoking, low physical activity, adiposity, and low SES. However, in the studies not all of these risk factors were taken into account. The studies by Shekelle et al. (1983) and Hearn et al. (1989) did not consider the risk factors of physical activity, adiposity, and SES. In the study by Barefoot et al. (1995), adiposity and SES were neglected, and in the study by Everson et al. (1997), SES was omitted. Everson et al. made the following assumption on the relation between hostility and CHD: "These findings suggest that hostility itself may not be pathogenic; rather, hostility may be a marker for behaviors that increase risk for mortality and morbidity. Alternatively, hostility may be associated with the development and maintenance of such behaviors" (p. 149).

The relation between hostility and CHD is not significant in healthy persons when using the soft criterion ($R = .005$, $N = 4,496$). The studies with CHD patients show a similar result. Using the hard criterion, an effect size of $r = .000$ ($N = 1,467$; only one study) is observed, and with the soft criterion an insignificant population effect size of $R = .025$ ($N = 794$) is obtained. All prospective studies analyzed together yield a significant population effect size of $R = .022$ ($N = 15,038$). According to the binomial effect size display, if one assumes a CHD base rate of 50% in the population, 51% of hostile persons and 49% of nonhostile persons would get the disease. The relative risk amounts to 1.04.

Somewhat more favorable is the result in the case control studies. However, the quality of case control studies is only Level II-2, according to the quality evaluation created for studies on therapeutic interventions. Eight case control studies were found with a total N of 9,177. These studies, too, can be differentiated according to the method used to assess hostility (SI or questionnaire). However, only two studies used the component analysis of the SI; one study used the hard criterion and the other study the soft criterion. The meta-analysis of these two studies yields a significant population effect size of $R = .102$ ($N = 1,326$). However, the study with the soft criterion is the WCGS ($r = .120$, $N = 750$, $p = .001$), and the study with the hard criterion is not significant ($r = .077$, $N = 576$, $p = .064$).

In studies with questionnaires, those with the hard criterion are more important than those with the soft criterion. For studies with the hard criterion, an insignificant population effect size of $R = .018$ ($N = 5,322$) is observed. Studies with the soft criterion show a highly significant population effect size of $R = .111$ ($N = 2,529$). However, tone must consider the correlation between hostility on one hand and neuroticism and bodily complaints on the other. Moreover, the three studies with the soft criterion did not take the risk factors into account. The studies by Van Dijl (1982) and Lichtenstein et al. (1989) did not control for the risk factors smoking, physical activity, adiposity, and SES. Only smoking and SES were controlled in the study by Atchison and Condon (1993). For the reasons mentioned, the studies with the soft criterion are not very telling. The correlative studies on hostility and coronary atherosclerosis are heterogeneous. Two studies established no relation, whereas in the third study the relation was very high.

The correlation between hostility and total mortality investigated in 10 prospective studies seems to be more substantial. The meta-analysis found a highly significant population effect size of $R = .060$ ($N = 8,693$). The relative risk amounts to 1.13. One might assume that hostile persons exhibit hazardous behaviors in everyday life more often than nonhostile persons and that they therefore have a higher mortality risk. In a study with 202 young adults, Leiker and Hailey (1988) observed that those high in hostility (Cook–Medley Ho Scale) exhibited more risky health-related behaviors (e.g., drug use, unsafe driving). The longitudinal study by Pakiz, Reinherz, and Giaconia (1997) with 375 adults showed a relation between high hostility scores and subsequent deviant behavior.

To sum up the findings for hostility and CHD, the prospective studies reveal a significant but questionable result. Moreover, the population effect size is so small as to be practically meaningless. The significant result of the case control study using WCGS data is not surprising. This study included a subsequent analysis of the toxic component of Type A behavior. More convincing would have been the second study using the component analysis of the SI, but the result is not significant. The case control studies with the soft criterion are not relevant, because neither the correlation between hostility and bodily complaints nor the correlations between hostility and the CHD risk factors were taken into account. The result of the questionnaire studies with the hard criterion is not significant. Therefore, for the time being, hostility cannot be considered an independent risk factor for CHD.

6.4.3. Evaluation of Intervention Programs

Type A behavior is not a risk factor for CHD and must not be regarded as an issue in CHD prevention. Similarly, for patients with existing CHD, an intervention to alter Type A behavior is not indicated. Indeed, as shown by the population effect sizes of the prospective studies, a tendency toward a negative correlation between Type A and subsequent CHD exists.

The intervention study by M. Friedman et al. (1984), described in detail in section 6.3.1.5, is remarkable for its paradoxical result that patients who dropped out of the intervention had a significantly lower reinfarction rate than those who adhered to the intervention program. The assumption that Type A patients left the program because of impatience would provide indirect proof that Type A behavior is more likely to be a protective factor. The mechanism underlying this fact is open to speculation. Perhaps the more hardworking Type A patients alter the classic risk factors more energeti-

cally than Type B patients, leading to a lower rate of cardiac events.

No intervention in hostile patients with CHD can be considered necessary at present, because hostility is not a risk factor for CHD. Moreover, one might pose the question whether preventive reduction of hostility would be meaningful at all. Colligan and Offord (1988) investigated more than 14,000 persons stratified by age and sex with the MMPI. Most of these persons were above the cutoff value proposed by hostility researchers and, therefore, ought to be treated. However, it might not be possible to carry out interventions in more than 70% of the population. To date there have been virtually no intervention trials to reduce hostility. Gidron and Davidson (1996) proposed an intervention program to reduce the pathogenic components of hostility and conducted a small study with 22 healthy men to test their program. There have been no large-scale intervention studies that could prove the benefit of interventions to alter hostility.

6.4.4. Discrepancy With the Evaluation in a U.S. Report

The National Heart, Lung, and Blood Institute (1998) published a report that dealt with the relationship between Type A or hostility and CHD. The report stated the following:

> Reports from several epidemiological studies show that individuals with a Type A behavior pattern . . . have about twice the risk of CHD as individuals with non–Type A behavior patterns. . . . In a number of recent studies, however, researchers report no effect of Type A behavior on risk of CHD. . . . Recent meta-analytic evaluations of the epidemiological literature indicate definite associations between hostility and risk for CHD. After controlling for other risk factors, the researchers have found that cognitive measures of hostility were most predictive of all-cause mortality and, to a lesser degree, morbidity from CHD. (p. 44)

This report is essentially a narrative review; references are largely missing. Studies that do not support the hypotheses are not mentioned. Questionable studies, such as M. Friedman et al. (1984), are not analyzed critically. When the report cites meta-analytic results, it cites the wrong results from the meta-analyses by T. Q. Miller et al. (1991, 1996; see section 6.1.5.3).

6.4.5. Benefits of Type A Behavior and Hostility

The report by the National Heart, Lung, and Blood Institute (1998) sought to support the Type A concept, or at least the hostility concept. This same endeavor is also obvious in many articles by other authors. It may therefore be assumed that concepts of this sort are of great benefit for all parties concerned, including patients, clinical psychologists, and physicians. Many years ago, a physician involved in cardiac rehabilitation summed up this fact as follows: "If we did not already have Type A, we would have had to invent it" (M. J. Halhuber, personal communication, 1977).

For patients, concepts such as stress, Type A, and hostility have the benefit of enabling them to form an external causal attribution. Patients are thereby relieved from responsibility for their CHD risk factors including smoking, poor diet, or lack of physical activity. Such concepts enable patients to see the causes of their disease as external factors that can be influenced only to a minor extent. Many articles dealing with the issue of causal attribution in patients support this opinion (Myrtek, 1998b). These concepts benefit physicians when none of the classic risk factors in CHD patients can be established. The concepts offer simple causal attributions that all patients can accept.

Finally, the concepts render a special legitimization to the clinical psychologist, who is the specialist of choice to treat related problems. A controversy triggered by these conjectures some years ago showed that important and sensitive interests were at stake (M. J. Halhuber, 1985; Mittag, 1987; Myrtek, 1985a, 1985b). The work of clinical psychologists is obviously necessary. Many of my own studies and those of other authors have shown that somatic findings—for example, the severity of a myocardial infarction—and subjective well-being—for example, bodily complaints and subjective physical fitness—are not correlated (Myrtek, 1998b). Many somatically severely diseased patients do not perceive bodily complaints and are able to resume work, whereas other patients with a relatively low severity of disease have bodily complaints that lead them to retire. It is the work of the clinical psychologist to analyze the risks and lifestyles of individual patients and to guide them in making the right decisions.

CHAPTER 7

CHEST PAIN, ANGINA PECTORIS, PANIC DISORDER, AND SYNDROME X

Kurt Laederach-Hofmann and Nadine Messerli-Buergy

7.1. INTRODUCTION

Chest pain is one of the prevalent physical symptoms in medicine. The Epidemiologic Catchment Area Program Study (Kroenke & Price, 1993) inquired about physical symptoms in general populations in Baltimore, Maryland; St. Louis, Missouri; Durham, North Carolina; and Los Angeles, California (United States). On the basis of the information supplied by 13,538 individuals, a catalogue of the 26 major symptoms was elaborated. The most common ones were menstrual symptoms and joint pain followed by back pain, headache, and chest pain (24.6%); arm or leg pain; abdominal pain; fatigue; and dizziness. At some point in their lives, the respondents had considered 84% of their symptoms to be so distressing that they sought medical assistance. One third of their symptoms were either psychiatric or medically unexplained, and most symptoms were associated with an increased lifetime risk of a common psychiatric disorder.

Studies conducted in Europe have revealed figures regarding the lifetime likelihood of chest pain similar to those found in surveys conducted in the United States (Schuler, Epstein, & Stransky, 1978). On the other hand, a U.S. health survey that focused on specific symptoms (the Health and Nutrition Examination Survey) revealed that 17.4% of the respondents suffered from chest pain symptoms, 13.8% complained of chest pressure, and 7.6% reported strong pain that lasted 30 minutes or longer (Costa, Fleg, McCrae, & Lakatta, 1982).

In a representative survey about the state of health among the population of Germany conducted in 1990 to 1991, 7,443 people aged 25 to 69 years were interviewed. A total of 11.1% of the men and 9.1% of the women reported angina pectoris (Ladwig, Lehmacher, Roth, & Breithardt, 1992; see Figure 7.1).

However, studies on the prevalence of chest pain in clinical patient samples have yielded other results. For instance, Rose et al. (1968) interviewed a cohort of 818 middle-aged men once a year over a period of 4 consecutive years using a standardized questionnaire to measure stress-related angina pectoris. They found that the overall prevalence remained stable over the course of time, even though there was substantial interpersonal variability among the cohorts regarding the stress caused by pain. The result was that the number of patients who reported pain rose from 3.8% to 10.4% by the fourth interview. According to health surveys, patients with chest pain do not evidence a clinical picture of chronic pain. Instead, they suffer from acute and remitting pain, which would be typical of ambulatory angina pectoris—a finding that casts doubt on its cardiac etiology. Gerstenkorn (1990) screened 4,734 men and women over the age of 18 and found stress-dependent chest pain complaints diagnosed according to criteria used in Rose et al.'s questionnaire in 5.5% of the male and 8.7% of the female respondents, respectively. Of the patients who complained of pain, 38.4% had not sought any medical help in the 12 months prior to the interview. Retrospective analysis of the receipts of

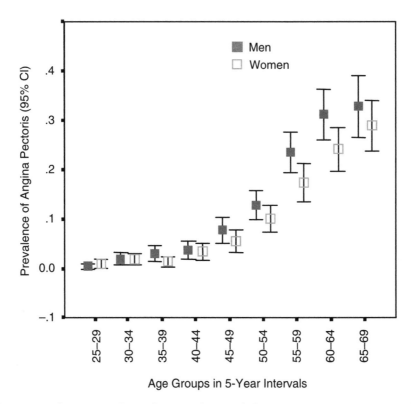

FIGURE 7.1. Subjective information about the prevalence of chest pain in a German population (ages 25–69 years) by age and gender. CI = confidence interval.

payments conducted by the Bundesinstitut für Bevölkerungsforschung (Federal Institute for Populations Surveys) in Germany revealed that barely 36% of patients who had had a stroke had received antianginal therapy 180 days prior to acute infarction (Ladwig, Hoberg, & Busch, 1998). A retrospective study of 652 male postinfarction patients showed that the most common prodromal symptom was angina pectoris (77%). Even so, only 32% of the patients who had had a history of angina pectoris had obtained effective medical therapy for cardiovascular problems (Ladwig et al., 1992).

Despite the restrictive utilization of medical services on the part of patients suffering from chest pain, the high incidence of chest pain symptoms among the general population does have an influence on the health system. In the above-mentioned survey conducted in Germany, a relatively high percentage of persons with positive angina pectoris were on ongoing oral heart medication: 54.2% of the men and 56.2% of the women with a history of chest pain explained that they were on regular heart medication (Bormann, 1994). In a study on

the prevalence and classification of symptoms in medical outpatients, 45% of the respondents complained of chest pain that led 14% of them to seek medical attention (Gutzwiller, 1980; Gutzwiller, Junod, Epstein, Jeanneret, & Schweizer, 1980). Noren, Frazier, Altman, and DeLozier (1980) revealed that internists in North America devote an average of 5.4% of their time to making differential diagnoses of chest pain.

There are also quite a number of patients who evidence abnormal findings in noninvasive investigations (e.g., suspicious ST-segment depression in electrocardiograms [ECGs] testing for ischemia, abnormalities in nuclear imaging studies) and at the same time complain of both typical and atypical stress-dependent chest pains. As a result, most of these patients undergo coronary angiography, which is at present the only accurate method of diagnosing pathoanatomy of the coronary arteries. Apparently normal coronary arteries are found in 30% of the patients who undergo invasive tests because of typical angina pectoris and an ergometer that documents a suspicion of ischemia (Cannon,

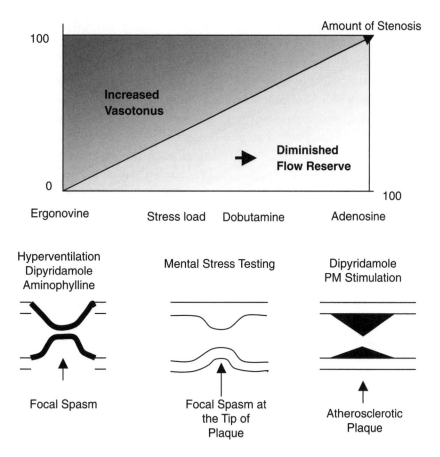

FIGURE 7.2. Comparison between different pathophysiological concepts in cardiac ischemia. PM = pacemaker.

1991; Carvalho & Carrageta, 1990; Laederach-Hofmann, 1994). If, however, macroscopic changes are revealed in coronary angiography, stress-dependent pain is usually associated with coronary-related ischemia that is caused by possible stenoses, even though a link between symptoms and test results is not as stringent as initially postulated (see Figure 7.2).

7.2. PATHOPHYSIOLOGY OF ANGINA PECTORIS

Even though many cardiologists regard ST-segment depression recorded in ECG exercise stress testing as evidence of cardiac ischemia, a specificity of approximately only 70% and a sensitivity of about 80% was found in a review conducted by Gibbons et al. (1997). All the same, there seem to be patients whose ECGs show typical ST-segment depression in stress tests but that do not reveal any

cardiovascular dysfunction when measured with invasive examination procedures (i.e., coronary sinus; Flugelman et al., 1991).

The important question of whether there is a direct relationship between the prevalence of ischemia and angina pectoris has remained unanswered to date (Crea, Gaspardone, Kaski, Davies, & Maseri, 1992; Davies et al., 1993; Mody et al., 1988). Angina pectoris presumably corresponds to a change in the heart, in neural transmission or in central nervous integration. Stress dependence and reproductivity are probably likely organic etiologies. On the other hand, typical or atypical localization of angina pectoris is of lesser—if any—importance in differential diagnosis. Psychological factors such as anxiety, depression, and hostility influence the strength, severity, and recurrence of the pain caused by angina pectoris. Furthermore, other mechanisms, in particular psychological factors, must also be assumed to lead to complaints that are indistinguishable from angina pectoris (Light et al., 1991; Rutledge, Linden, & Davies, 1999). Research on this subject has provided evidence that there is a linear relationship between the height of surrogate markers (e.g., ST-segment depression) or products of ischemia (e.g., lactate overabundance in coronary sinus) and the chronicity or severity of angina pectoris.

Despite the fact that these methods have been used by a wide range of authors (Bory et al., 1996; Pratt, Francis, Divine, & Young, 1989; Roeters van Lennep, Zwinderman, & van der Wall, 2000; A. K. Sullivan et al., 1994; Walling & Crawford, 1993), a viable clinical algorithm has not been constructed to date. Particular problems have arisen in attempts to distinguish typical (i.e., related to coronary sclerosis) or atypical (in relation to localization, contributing factors, or pathology) pain from vasospastic (in normal coronary arteries) angina or even from angina pectoris in *syndrome X* (a common designation for chest pain with normal coronary arteries, but see discussion later in this chapter; Song et al., 1996). Patients who underwent echocardiography were initially administered ergonovine. The relatively ischemic-specific myocardial-related changes that were detected in sonography (in particular diastolic dysfunction) were found to have a specificity and a sensitivity of 88% and 91%, respectively, so that patients with coronary sclerotic abnormalities could be distinguished from those with vasospastic etiology. This in itself does not predict anything about the symptom angina pectoris, which in this chapter is not classified as typical or atypical before a diagnosis has been established. Even though 24-hour ECG screening (Holter ECG) is a good method of distinguishing organic heart disorders from normal heart arteries, the specificity and the sensitivity of this method amounted to only 80% and 40%, respectively (Marinoni, Perotti, & Specchia, 1987).

There is conclusive evidence that psychological tests fail to predict which patients will be stricken by unstable angina—an enormous danger—or to distinguish between patients who will suffer from myocardial infarction and those who will not. Ladwig's research group in Munich, Germany (Ladwig et al., 1998) investigated patients who had to undergo coronary angiography on an emergency basis because of suspicion of a preinfarction syndrome (that had been provoked by symptoms of unstable angina pectoris) despite the patients having no history of heart disease. Although approximately 37% of the respondents had a normal coronary artery condition, the remaining respondents actually had very severe heart dysfunction. The measures used to appraise psychological morbidity failed to differentiate between the two groups of patients with chest pain. One of the main reasons why psychological factors failed to distinguish between coronary artery disease and normal coronary artery condition was that both groups suffered to the same extent from anxiety, feelings of helplessness, depressive symptoms, and somatic preoccupation.

In addition, noncoronary chest pain has been referred to in the literature by terms such as *noncoronary, atypical, (post hoc) angiographically negative,* and *heart neurosis,* or by psychiatric classifications such as *somatization disorder* and *somatic depression* (cf. Castell, 1992). One cannot do justice to the complex nature of reality by merely distinguishing between underlying somatic and psychological causes. There are also other illnesses that cannot be detected so easily. For instance, the syndrome of angina pectoris without evidence of coronary stenosis, which is more likely to have an organic origin as in the case of chest pain due to aortic stenosis (onset due to increased intracardiac pressure) or in severe hypertension (with a similar pathological mechanism) needs to be compared with an absence of macroscopic changes in the heart arteries. The latter possibility is also referred to as *functional* heart symptoms, whereby a wide range of disorders may be diagnosed (depending on the physician's area of specialization), such as Barlow syndrome, irritable heart syndrome, sensitive heart, neurasthenia, heart neurosis, vegetative heart syndrome or—so as to include extracardiac explanations—esophageal dysfunction or esophagus spasms (cf. Hegglin, 1975).

Because the scope of this chapter is limited to patients with angina pectoris who do not evidence any macroscopically stenosed coronary arteries, we are faced with the problem of the validity of the concept of syndrome X—one that is unfortunately used to describe manifold clinical manifestations in the literature. To date, there is a lack of conclusive evidence about the origins of the pathophysiology of angina in patients without macroscopic coronary stenosed changes or in those with syndrome X (Cannon, 1998; Dotson, 1997; Lorenz & Bromm, 1997), and it has remained the subject of widespread speculation. In addition, there has been a lack of consensus as to whether patients with syndrome X manifest ischemia at all. Although many authors (Cannon, Camici, & Epstein, 1992; Chierchia & Fragasso, 1996; S. D. Rosen & Camici, 1994) have found that patients with syndrome X do not actually display any signs of myocardial ischemia, other abnormalities have also been detected in blood flow similar to those in cardiomyopathy (Chen et al., 1999), ischemia-specific increase of lactic acid in coronary sinus (Virtanen, 1985), decreased O2 in the analysis of arterial veins (Botker et al., 1993), abnormalities of the clotting system with increased platelet aggregability (Lanza et al., 2001), or other abnormalities of coronary hemodynamics and myocardial metabolism (Camici et al., 1991).

Another matter of controversy is *noncardiac chest pain*—a newer term used to refer to pain that is not attributable to coronary sclerotic etiology—and the related question of how chest pain can occur in the first place. My own research (Laederach-Hofmann, 1994) has revealed that about 20% of chest pain symptoms are caused by esophageal abnormalities, most of which are of functional origin (Maunder, 1998); about 60% of noncardiac chest pain can be associated exclusively with esophageal dysfunction (J. E. Richter & the Working Team for Functional Esophageal Disorders, 1994). A review of the literature (Maunder, 1998) reported comorbidity of noncardiac chest pain and panic disorder ranging from 16% to 76%.

7.2.1. Pain Sensation

There is conclusive evidence that the perception of pain is influenced by study design and by psychological factors, in particular by psychiatric diseases such as depressive and anxiety disorders as well as by altered perception of pain—for example, preoc-

cupation with pain. In light of the fact that the lifetime risk of anxiety or panic disorders is 3.6% (Escobar, Swartz, Rubio-Stipec, & Manu, 1991), these disorders must be assumed to have an effect on symptom presentation in general and on pain presentation in particular. At the same time, the fact must be taken into account that patients who feel ill are more anxious than the general population (Katon, 1990) and that the perception of pain can be attenuated by stigmatized pain localization such as chest pain (Arntz & de Jong, 1993). On the other hand, the effect of depressive reactions or depression on bodily sensations has been a proven fact for a long time (Corruble & Guelfi, 2000). Psychopathological processes have repeatedly been assumed to contribute to symptom manifestation and to reactions to pain (Cormier, Katon, Russo, & Hollifield, 1988). There is evidence that such patients tend to suffer from anxiety disorders (Bass, 1989; Beitman, Mukerji, Russell, & Grafting, 1993; Cannon, 1998; Cannon et al., 1992; Cormier et al., 1988) or other psychiatric disorders (Costa et al., 1985), such as neuroticism according to the Cornell Medical Index (Weaver, Ko, Alexander, Pao, & Ting, 1980), anxiety (Schocken, Greene, Worden, & Harrison, 1987), or tension (Beck, Taegtmeyer, Berisford, & Bennett, 1989; Elias, Robbins, Blow, Rice, & Edgecomb, 1982). At the same time, a history of sexual abuse in women has also been shown to predispose them to perceiving chest pain more often later in life (Scarinci, McDonald-Haile, Bradley, & Richter, 1994).

Although Roy-Byrne, Uhde, Post, King, and Buchsbaum (1984) found evidence of normal pain reactions in patients with panic disorder, other authors have postulated abnormally strong reactions to pain in comorbid anxiety or panic disorders (L. A. Bradley, Richter, Scarinci, Haile, & Schan, 1992; Numata, Ogata, Oike, Matsumura, & Shimada, 1998; Ruggeri et al., 1996). The prospects seem small for reaching consensus in the future about the significance of pain reactions, the mechanism of the development of pain, and the method of coping with pain (Ladwig et al., 1998), in particular in connection with patients with syndrome X—the subject of this chapter. Mention should also be made of the observation that a substantial proportion of patients with panic disorder (between 24% and 89%) eventually develop major depression (Breier, Charney, & Heninger, 1984; Uhde et al., 1985), which, in turn, often has undeterminable effects on clinical presentation and poses a large methodological problem in long-term follow-up studies of this group of patients.

7.2.2. Trimodal Conceptualization of Pain

In angina pectoris, physiological indicators should be experienced as correlates of pain, not as its underlying cause (Chapman et al., 1985). Although a dichotomous distinction between *sensory* (sensation of pain) and *affective* (evaluation of pain) components of the sensation of pain (Thiery, 1988) is firmly established in daily clinical practice, heuristic approaches to pain (e.g., Beitman et al., 1993; Birdwell, Herbers, & Kroenke, 1993) are to be found as well, despite the fact that the meaning of communication has been poorly understood to date. Sensory components have been shown to play as important a role (F. Nelson, Zimmerman, Barnason, Nieveen, & Schmaderer, 1998) as emotional ones (D. Price, 1984; Wade, Dougherty, Hart, Rafii, & Price, 1992). Pain self-schemas are dependent on the context in which patients experience pain. F. Nelson et al. (1998) interviewed patients who had undergone a bypass operation and found that sensory discriminative components were considerably less context-related than affective ones. The components themselves—despite the fact that they are basically not interrelated—are not independent factors in the theoretical framework presented. Instead, they are to be considered as integral and closely interconnected parts of a whole. As a result, the more intense pain becomes (an expression of sensory components of pain), the stronger the emotion (aversion, etc.) that is associated with pain.

For every clinical form of pain, including angina pectoris, the impression of pain and the sensation of pain can be said to be made up of both sensory and affective characteristics (that often happen to be exclusive of one another when clinically presented). Affective processes of coping might be expected to have a greater long-term effect on patients with syndrome X—the exact pathophysiology of which has been examined with conventional methods and is still poorly understood—than on patients with coronary artery disease. To our knowledge, to date no research except that of Laederach-Hofmann, Truniger, Mussgay, and Jürgensen (2001) has reported differences in the intensity or quality of pain in patients with angina pectoris caused by coronary artery disease or syndrome X.

7.2.3. The Problem of the Symptom Angina Pectoris

English-speaking authors define *angina pectoris* as heart pain that is specifically related to ischemia (Matthews & Julian, 1985) and systematically distinguish between chest pain, nonanginal pain, and angina pectoris (Braunwald, 1988). On the other hand, German-speaking authors have defined *angina pectoris* as pain that feels like pressure, which—if of cardiac etiology—is referred to either as *typical* (stress dependent) or *atypical* (i.e., not stress dependent) angina pectoris and otherwise as *pseudo-angina pectoris* (subsumption of all functional artery complaints that do not have an organic cause; Hegglin, 1975). Both English- and German-speaking authors use this term to describe extracardial chest (thoracic) pain or noncardiac chest pain. Other authors included both types of chest pain under cardiac etiologies, making it unnecessary to distinguish between functional and organic etiology. In addition, the term *chest pain* is used to describe functional, gastrointestinal pain (e.g., esophagus spasms) as well as organic-associated pain such as a lung embolism.

7.2.4. Definition of *Angina Pectoris*

The following definition is used in this chapter according to the newest international releases on syndrome X. In this review, the term *angina pectoris* is used as in English-speaking countries as in the following definition:

> Angina pectoris in its most common form is defined as pain in the chest (usually localized to the retrosternal area), neck, shoulder, or left arm in patients with organic artery disease which

is usually produced by effort and relieved by rest or nitrates. (New York Heart Association, 1979, p. 289)

It is clear that this definition of chest pain is based on an assumption that has not always been confirmed in clinical practice: that pain symptoms can be accounted for by organic factors (J. E. Richter, 1991; A. K. Sullivan et al., 1994). In this chapter, the definition cited above will be supplemented to include all symptoms that are closely (i.e., organic ones) and loosely (i.e., psychological ones) associated with heart physiology insofar as they present as angina pectoris. However, the definition of angina pectoris presented here will not cover any thoracic origins of pain, such as costal, costo-diaphragmal, pulmonal, pleural, perivascular-related, or extrathoracic, which are projected onto the thorax (e.g., subdiaphragmatic, abdominal, neck, or muscular pain). Despite the fact that pain symptomatology (often concurrently or alternately present in panic disorder, depression, or posttraumatic stress disorder) and esophageal pain (here, exclusively functional, nonorganic) are not triggered by the same pathophysiological mechanism, they have similar presenting problems.

7.2.5. The Problem of Chest Pain Without Coronary Macropathology: Angina Pectoris Without Coronary Artery Disease

Although coronary stenotic changes usually lead to reactions to pain that are uniquely experienced by each individual, as outlined above in the definition of angina pectoris, this only applies to some "nonorganic" cardiac complaints. These include "heart neuroses"; panic, depressive, and anxiety disorders as well as posttraumatic stress disorder that lack comorbidity with organic heart disease of any etiology; and others such as microvascular angina pectoris, vasospastic angina pectoris, variant angina (so-called "Prinzmetal" angina), and, in a broader sense, syndrome X as well. Diagnosing microvascular angina pectoris poses a problem, because there might be abnormal changes such as arterial wall thickening (primarily of the pars media), which, however, cannot be detected angiographically without the use of special diagnostic procedures. On the other hand, the time of onset or the connection between symptoms and certain activities are often so typical of vasospastic angina or variant angina that these diagnoses have been excluded from our overview.

7.2.6. Anginal Syndrome X

The definition of *anginal syndrome X*—which is still used today—dates back to a research article written in 1967, in which Kemp, Elliott, and Gorlin (1967) interviewed a large sample of patients ($N = 253$) who presented with angina-like symptoms despite normal coronary angiograms. In the same year, a research group (Likoff, Segal, & Kasparian, 1967) published an article in which syndrome X was described in an all-female sample for the first time, even though the concept of syndrome X had not been associated with these authors at the time. Six years later, Kemp (1973) published an editorial on the problem of angina pectoris in normal coronary arteries. He referred to syndrome X for the first time in order to focus attention on the conundrum of the pathophysiological mechanisms, the ischemia-like changes in ECG, and the symptom angina pectoris in these patients.

Our definition of *syndrome X* (also referred to as *cardiac syndrome X*) includes the following trias:

- angina pectoris (often typical);
- altered ECG (in particular ST-segment depression and in coronary-ischemia-related abnormality) related to ergometric stress; and
- macroscopically normal coronary arteries in coronary angiography.

Not included in this definition are dysfunctions that might occur in heart muscle hypertrophy (often with histological evidence of the thickening of the basal membrane, media hypertrophy of coronary arteries, and a subsequent decline in compliance), which can also lead to angina pectoris; silent ischemia, or diseases that can damage the afferents of the cardiac autonomic nervous system (in particular the parasympathetic and vagal system), are also not covered by this term (e.g., diabetes mellitus).

7.2.6.1. Pathogenetic mechanisms in cardiac syndrome X.

An updated and simplified overview of the pathogenetic mechanisms in cardiac syndrome X can be found in a recent article by Kaski and Russo (2000a). Despite the fact that the definition of microvascular angina pectoris is narrower than the definition of syndrome X, considerable overlap occurs between the two pathologies (Vantrappen, 1992). The following symptoms may be present in microvascular angina pectoris: endothelial dysfunction (Abbott, 1993; Agmon, 1993; Gorlin, 1993; Suzuki, Takeyama, Koba, Suwa, & Katagiri, 1994), absence of a specific essential amino acid (L-arginine; Egashira, Hirooka, Kuga, Mohri, & Takeshita, 1996), reduced functional coronary flow reserve (Motz et al., 1991), absence of vasodilatation in response to acetylcholine (Egashira et al., 1993), elevated plasma-endothelial-1 level; decreased endothelial-dependent vasodilatation (Piatti et al., 1999), decreased nitric oxide release in response to insulin infusion (Piatti et al., 1999) characteristic of insulin resistance as common in metabolic syndrome X and other metabolic abnormalities (Botker, Sonne, Frøbert, & Andreasen, 1999; Chierchia & Fragasso, 1996), dysfunction of the autonomic nervous system with hypersympathetic tone (Frøbert, Molgaard, Botker, & Bagger, 1995), and—as in syndrome X—increased pain perception (Cannon, 1991). The question of whether it is simply a case of dynamic ischemia—a mismatch between demand and need (functional ischemia)—has likewise been a bone of contention (W. L. Lee et al., 1998). It is unclear whether there are differences between hibernating and stunning functional ischemia, regardless of their respective etiology.

7.2.6.2. Functional ischemia in syndrome X?

To verify the hypothesis that changes in ST-segment shift (that are identical to those caused by coronary stenosis) are markers of ischemia, research has been conducted to identify substances in the sinus coronary that are also found in patients with significant stenoses. Lactate might be an initial marker that is released by muscle cells when—as in "real" ischemia—there is a lack of O2 to ensure oxydative phosphorylation of the substratum. Varying re-

search results have been reported to date: Virtanen (1985), for instance, was the first to provide evidence for increased lactic acid when patients with chest pain syndromes and normal coronary angiograms were paced. Their normal values were at least 12% higher than those of asymptomatic patients under stress. Ishihara et al. (1990) and Nagayama et al. (1996) substantiated these findings, as opposed to Camici et al. (1991), who identified a change in pyruvate mechanism in syndrome X patients, even though there were no differences in lactate excess between the patient groups. Even though adaptive metabolic changes have been observed in patients with syndrome X on high doses of glutamate that substantially elevated the pain level for angina pectoris during pacing (Thomassen, Nielsen, Bagger, Pedersen, & Henningsen, 1991), because of very limited sample size the results cannot be regarded as conclusive. There is also histological evidence that patients with microvascular angina pectoris display microscopic changes indicative of ischemia, which may occur in stress tests (Suzuki et al., 1994). Egashira et al. (1993) observed reduced coronary blood flow reserve in patients after an intracoronary infusion with acetylcholine, which, in turn, indicates impaired vasodilation in patients with syndrome X. In addition, Zeiher, Krause, Schachinger, Minners, and Moser (1995) found that there was a significant difference between the level of vasodilation in syndrome X patients who exhibited reversible thallium perfusion stress defects and in patients who did not. On the other hand, Cannon (1997) found that differences in vasodilation reactivity do not invariably lead to ischemia during stress in patients with syndrome X, because a wide range of mechanisms (to some extent reflectory, local–hormonal, or intracellular ones) would hinder its onset. Other studies have confirmed this line of thought. Nihoyannopoulos, Kaski, Crake, and Maseri (1991) did not obtain any evidence of ischemia in echocardiography during stress in patients with syndrome X. Nor did Panza et al. (1997) succeed in providing any evidence of significant differences between behavior of the myocardium in patients with syndrome X and healthy control subjects using dobutamine stress echocardiography. Moreover, recent research conducted on a sample of control subjects without angina pectoris (i.e., physicians who were on call) showed ST-segment shifts similar to those in ischemia despite lacking evidence of coronary pathology (Toivonen, Helenius, & Viitasalo, 1997). A recent study using cardiovascular magnetic resonance imaging to detect abnormal subendocardial perfusion provided conclusive evidence that syndrome X patients exhibit inner layer ischemia, in particular of the left ventricle, compared with control subjects (Panting et al., 2002), which has sparked a heated debate (see Bassan, 2002; Collins, 2002). If these findings can be replicated, it may very well resolve the question of ischemia (Huang & Ewy, 2002). All the same, the question of whether there are any other mechanisms that play a part has remained unanswered to date—for example, the fact that there is evidence of a relationship between altered pain perception as frequently noted in clinical vignettes and the frequent occurrence of syndrome X in women (Kaski, 2002).

7.2.6.3. Altered pain perception in syndrome X?

Patients with syndrome X seem to experience pain differently from those without it. For instance, they tend to react with angina pectoris when electric stimulation is applied to the right ventricle and contrast medium (Cannon, 1998) is injected into the coronary artery concurrently during coronary angiography—which basically amounts to temporary O2 withdrawal and thus is equivalent to strain. On the other hand, Bass, Cawley, et al. (1983) found psychiatric comorbidity in a large number of patients. In a study of the psychiatric comorbidity of symptoms in patients with chest pain and normal coronary arteries, Beitman et al. (1989) found panic disorder in 34% of a total of 94 participants. In an effort to ascertain central (i.e., alternating pain processing) pathologies, S. D. Rosen and Camici (2000) recently found out that patients with syndrome X suffer from a central thalamic disorder of pain. Peripheral pain afferents seem to be transmitted from the heart to the brain to a considerable degree. Rosen et al.'s view is that increased pain perception is due to altered activation of the cerebral processing centers (in particular the front

insular cortical area and connections to the frontal operculum). They concluded that the origin of cardiac syndrome X cannot be ischemic. Frøbert, Arendt-Nielsen, Bak, Funch-Jensen, and Bagger's (1996) findings coincided with Rosen et al.'s that central pain processing in patients with syndrome X must be altered.

7.2.6.4. Affected coronary blood flow in syndrome X?

Chen, Hsu, Ting, Lin, and Chang (2000) investigated hemodynamic changes and normal or elevated ventricular contractility in patients with syndrome X. They found reduced coronary flow reserve—which can probably be attributed to diminished microvascular dilatation function in both groups of patients with syndrome X (i.e., those with elevated and with normal contractility) compared with the control subjects. These functional changes and the transitions to coronary stenotic etiologies are illustrated clearly in Figure 7.2. They are depicted as an ongoing process that involves functional determinants on the one hand and macropathological changes in coronary artery stenosis on the other. What this figure does not depict, however, are microvascular factors which are incriminated as central in syndrome X.

In addition, there might be a change in myocardial metabolism, but this has not been described in detail. Goel, Gupta, Agarwal, and Kapoor (2001) confirmed abnormalities of coronary flow. Furthermore, P. M. Elliott, Krzyzowska-Dickinson, Calvino, Hann, and Kaski (1997) found that oral aminophylline (an adenosine receptor blocker) had a beneficial effect on ergometric stress performance in patients with syndrome X. They also noted that patients with syndrome X who had taken aminophylline for longer than 3 weeks reported fewer angina pectoris attacks. Particularly striking was the fact that oral aminophylline had no effect on ST-segment depression in this sample of patients. The contradiction between possible ischemia and a debatable change in perception has, nevertheless, remained a major challenge.

7.2.6.5. Endothelial dysfunction in syndrome X?

In their overview, Kaski and Russo (2000b) defined syndrome X as a disorder of coronary microvascular regulation (the mechanism of endothelial dysfunction being of prime importance) that is triggered by multiple causal mechanisms, including hypertension, hypercholesterolemia, estrogen deficiency, smoking, and other factors that have remained unknown to date.

7.2.6.6. Autonomic dysfunction in syndrome X?
Recent research has also examined changes in autonomic functions in the pathogenesis of syndrome X. For instance, Gulli et al. (2001) identified the activities of the sympathetic and parasympathetic nervous systems by means of noninvasive tests. Although impaired parasympathetic activity was found in a subset of two thirds of syndrome X patients, sympathetic activity had not increased as had always been assumed. Eriksson, Jansson, Kaijser, and Sylvén (1999) went even further by comparing skeletal and cardiac muscle function in 7 women between the ages of 50 and 65 with 5 matched control subjects. They found that ergometric performance in syndrome X patients was impaired even though there was neither evidence of differences in plasma lactate levels nor in fiber typology or the phosphagen content of muscle biopsies of the lateral femoral muscle. The only difference was a higher plasma concentration of norepinephrine in the blood level of patients with syndrome X. Eriksson et al. assumed that individuals with syndrome X might be hypersensitive to catecholamines.

7.2.6.7. Prospects of pathogenetic hypotheses concerning syndrome X.
Syndrome X is a good illustration of the fact that increasingly sophisticated options are being elaborated to gain greater understanding into this disorder. Nevertheless, this progressive fragmentation should not let us forget that syndrome X is a disorder that is difficult to bear and is currently not understood by the medical field. Many (if not all) symptoms are a result of a learning and adjustment process and therefore can only be understood within the patient's unique frame of reference. On the other hand, we are impatiently awaiting new ideas and research findings that will equip us to gain greater understanding of the mechanisms of the pathogenesis of pain and respective methods of coping with it in the future.

7.3. HYPOTHESES

A comparison of patients with syndrome X, panic disorder, coronary artery disease, and noncardiac chest pain and normal subjects will be conducted to test the validity of the following hypotheses:

- *Pain localization.* Patients with coronary artery syndrome locate their pain more accurately than those with syndrome X or panic disorder.
- *Frequency of pain.* Syndrome X patients have pain more frequently than panic disorder patients, coronary artery disease patients, or the normal population.
- *Well-being.* The well-being of syndrome X patients is worse than those with panic disorder, coronary artery disease, or the normal population.
- *Focus of attention.* Syndrome X patients focus more attention on physical symptoms than do patients with coronary artery disease, panic disorder patients, or healthy subjects.
- *Hostility.* Patients with coronary artery disease are more hostile than syndrome X patients, panic patients, those with noncardiac chest pain, or normal controls.
- *Neuroticism and obsessive–compulsive disorder.* Syndrome X patients are more neurotic and more obsessive–compulsive than panic patients; patients with noncardiac chest pain are more neurotic and more obsessive–compulsive than syndrome X patients, patients with a coronary artery disease, or the normal population.
- *Anxiety.* Panic disorder patients are more anxious than syndrome X patients, patients with coronary artery disease, patients with noncardiac chest pain, or the normal population.
- *Depression.* Patients with noncardiac chest pain or panic disorder are more depressed than syndrome X patients, patients with coronary disease, or the normal population.

7.4. METHOD

7.4.1. Literature Search
All of the works considered in this article were collected by means of public databases. To be able to

TABLE 7.1

Results of Literature Search

Search term	Database		
	Medline	PsycINFO	PSYNDEX
heart	420,610	11,790	1,381
psych*	87,447	544'078	125,188
syndrome X	354,320	403	17
cardiac	201,437	3,101	254
cardiac syndrome X	12,567	0	0
angina pectoris	18,763	158	40
chest pain	13,067	292	8
anxiety	46,289	43,810	6,260
panic	6,292	6,795	508
heart + psych*	1,143	7,527	1,259
heart + psych* + chest pain	59	80	1
heart + anxiety	2,336	1,529	240
heart + panic	431	382	60
psych* + chest pain	172	219	8
psych* + angina pectoris	59	100	35
angina pectoris + anxiety	124	23	4
angina pectoris + panic	33	8	0
heart + panic + chest pain	51	27	0
heart + anxiety + chest pain	84	30	1
chest pain + anxiety	264	91	3
chest pain + panic	168	92	1

Note. Medical databases last updated on November 30, 2002. Data represent number of results for each term.

gain a wide-ranging understanding of cardiac syndrome X, we decided to investigate both the medical and the psychological aspects of the syndrome. Medical articles were collected with the help of Medline database published by the U.S. National Library of Medicine. The search for relevant psychological literature was undertaken via PSYNDEX and PsycINFO of the American Psychological Association. The search restricted itself to works published after 1980 and before the end of November 2002. An overview of search terms and the number of articles elicited from the databases are listed in Table 7.1. No mention is made of double or repeated entries.

In addition, the usefulness and relevance of all the documents elicited via the search terms *syndrome X* and *cardiac syndrome X* were examined on the basis of their titles, and whenever available, the respective abstracts were studied as well. Articles dealing with the following topics were not included: the therapeutic setting, effectiveness of medication, theoretical models of bodily perception, isolated panic disorders or isolated coronary artery disease, classification of diseases, and psychosomatic complaints in disorders that were not related to our topic. Studies on children, adolescents, and fringe groups were also excluded. Articles on older theoretical models (e.g., Type A and B behavior) were included provided they were based on relatively up-to-date methods of data evaluation. We also excluded chapters of books that referred to studies that were available in their original form or book articles that were of a narrative and superficial nature that failed to do justice to the topic of interest.

A total of 1,326 publications were elicited by means of combined search procedures, and an additional 42 were found on the basis of the abstract search outlined above. The literature management program Endnote (Version 6) was used to organize the articles cited. The qualitative data from each article were stored and organized in an Excel table using Microsoft Excel 2000. Meta-analysis was undertaken with the help of the Comprehensive Meta-Analysis Program (Biostat, 2002).

7.4.2. Evaluation Procedure

An evaluation sheet was designed to qualitatively rate the various studies included. The studies elicited were sorted on the basis of relevance and evaluated using a questionnaire that was based on the critical appraisal standard for evidence-based medicine of the Cochrane Society (2002). The quality of a study is expressed in the score attained in our appraisal system (see Tables W7.1 and W7.2 on the accompanying Web site: http://www.apa.org/books/resources/jordan/).

7.4.3. Empirical Meta-Analysis

Quantitative synthesis of results was performed using the procedure described by Whitehead and Whitehead (1991). Statistical analysis is driven by the fixed effect model (FEM) as well as by the random effect model (REM). REM analysis is used as sensitivity analysis for the results of FEM analysis. If there is considerable divergence between the two results, the FEM results cannot be trusted. Even though REM is the appropriate model for certain forms of heterogeneity, the REM result does not represent all situations correctly. Of the 1,326 titles referring to cardiac syndrome X that had been ordered in the literature search, 243 publications were sorted according to cardiac and psychological indexing terms (*depression, anxiety, compulsiveness, anger, hostility, neuroticism, general complaints*, and *somatization*). The fact that only 25 references were actually incorporated in the meta-analysis is related to the following problems:

1. In many of the studies, the distinction between coronary artery disease and syndrome X as well as the definitions of both disorders that were exclusively based on noninvasive investigations were unclear or incomplete. The participating patients often suffered from noncardiac chest pain with or without a history of coronary artery disease. These articles were excluded from the meta-analysis because they were not relevant to our research question.

2. The two disorders were not clearly distinguished from each other, nor were the diagnostic groups homogeneous. In some publications, there was overlap between panic disorder and chest pain of noncardiac origin and between patients with coronary artery disease and the normal population.

3. In some publications, the statistical data were incomplete or contradictory, so they could not be used for determining either effect sizes or odds values. It was particularly regrettable that statistical problems could not be resolved even by consulting with the respective authors.

These difficulties seem to suggest that only a limited number of references actually addressed the problem of syndrome X or related aspects (depression, anxiety, hostility, tendency to somatization, and personality factors). This fact cannot be explained either by the current accessibility of relevant data or methodological possibilities. Nevertheless, syndrome X can be said to be a disorder that is distinguishable from others, yet it is not as common in its pure form as narrative reviews have suggested. The incredibly large number of narrative reviews—some of which are highly selective—are characterized by the distinctive features of un-

clearly defined patient groups and basic data that had been published elsewhere (so that new reviews were novelties). The inclusion criteria of our meta-analysis cover reviews of the pure form of angina pectoris (or chest pain),whether typical or atypical, were characterized by a thorough description and physical examination of the patients and fulfillment of the above-mentioned diagnostic criteria— namely, evidence of an abnormal stress test with electrical signs of ischemia and a completely normal coronary angiography, if possible with no coronary reaction to ergonovine (exclusion of vasospastic angina pectoris). In addition, patients were not allowed to display any changes in heart function, in particular no arterial hypertension with left-ventricular hypertrophy, diabetes mellitus, or obesity. Furthermore, participants could not be under 16 or over 70 years old. There is still a great need for studies that fulfill these criteria; all other topics that have been published in this area have had biased patient selection and do not call for replication.

7.5. RESULTS

The results of our research will be presented in the following sections. We describe the overall results by means of odds values and the separate components of effect sizes for the respective variables of the different diagnoses in spider graphs for the psychometric variables depression, hostility, anxiety, neuroticism, anger, compulsiveness, somatization, and frequency of general complaints. Different instruments—although we list them by name, we do not address the question of validity and reliability or their appropriateness—were used by different authors to assess the separate areas. (For detailed results of the meta-analysis, see Table W7.3 on the accompanying Web site.)

7.5.1. Odds Values

Table 7.2 illustrates that the disorders that are associated with syndrome X, in particular with respect to anxiety, differ significantly from each other. On the other hand, no significant differences were found in the area of depression (even though Yingling, Wulsin, Arnold, & Rouan [1993] investigated patients who had been admitted to the emer-

TABLE 7.2

Odds Values of Patients With Cardiac Syndrome X Compared With Others With Panic Disorder or Major Depression

Effect name	Citation	Year	Effect	Lower	Upper	N	p	Treated[a]	Control[a]
Anxiety	Ruggeri et al.	1996	0.029	0.003	0.250	52	.000	10/22	29/30
Fixed anxiety (1)			0.029	0.003	0.250	52	.000	10/22	29/30
Depression	Klimes et al.	1990	1.222	0.0236	5.762	29	.921	0/13	0/16
Depression	Yingling et al.	1993	0.486	0.228	1.035	229	.058	10/53	57/176
Fixed depression			0.501	0.238	1.055	258	.069	10/66	57/192
Panic disorder	Beitman et al.	1987	1.950	0.431	8.828	33	.383	13/17	10/16
Panic disorder	Fleet et al.	1998	1.093	0.614	1.946	250	.762	25/81	49/169
Panic disorder	Kushner et al.	1989	1.055	0.0215	3.707	187	.979	0/91	0/96
Panic disorder	Yingling et al.	1993	1.204	0.578	2.505	229	.620	13/40	54/189
Fixed panic disorder (4)			1.185	0.769	1.824	699	.442	51/229	113/470
Fixed combined (7)			0.862	0.597	1.245	1009	.429	71/317	199/692

Note. Numbers in parentheses represent the number of studies entered into the statistical analysis. Fixed = fixed effects.
[a]Numbers represent the number of patients with the disorder/total number of patients.

gency room with acute, nonspecific chest pain), and the patient group of Klimes, Mayou, Pearce, Coles, and Fagg (1990) was unfortunately extremely heterogeneous. In addition, there is evidence that patients with syndrome X are less depressive than patients with panic disorder. The studies by Kushner, Thomas, Bartels, and Beitman (1992) included in our review, for example, examined patient groups with panic disorder and observed its developmental course, whereas Fleet, Dupuis, Kaczorowski, Marchand, and Beitman (1997) reported on patients with coronary artery disease and patients with chest pain of noncardiac origin—in other words, two groups that are distinguishable from each other on the basis of the spider graphs below. Table 7.2 depicts the selection of detectable odds values for anxiety, depression, and panic disorder.

7.5.2. Summary of Group Comparisons Using Effect Sizes

The different psychological profiles of the participating patient groups are depicted in the network diagrams below. The effect sizes used were obtained by means of the above-mentioned meta-analysis and thus ensure a relatively substantial

sample size, which, in turn, ensures as good a match as possible between the hypotheses we formulated and the diagnostic instruments used. The effect size and rank of an indicator are displayed in bold and fine lines, respectively.

7.5.2.1. Noncardiac chest pain versus coronary artery disease. Figure 7.3 shows that patients with chest pain of noncardiac origin are more neurotic, depressed, and anxious; somewhat more compulsive; and somatize more than patients with coronary artery disease. On the other hand, patients with coronary artery disease are more hostile. To date, no empirical research has been conducted that examined and compared general complaints and anger in these patient groups. All the hypotheses we formulated have been conclusively confirmed. All the differences between patients with and without coronary artery disease were significant.

7.5.2.2. Noncardiac chest pain versus normal population. Patients with chest pain that is not caused by coronary artery disease suffer from significantly more severe forms of somatization disorder, anxiety disorder, and depression than healthy controls, with the exception of general complaints.

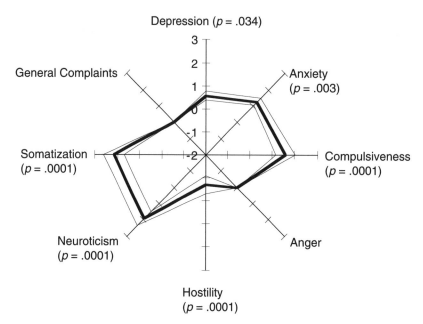

FIGURE 7.3. Noncardiac chest pain versus coronary artery disease.

On the other hand, the only personality trait that significantly distinguished the groups was compulsiveness, whereas anger and hostility did not, and neuroticism just attained the significance level. As we initially postulated, patients with chest pain of noncardiac origin can be characterized as follows in comparison with healthy controls: they are more anxious, more depressed, and more hostile, and they have a greater tendency to develop somatization disorders and to become angry. (See Figure 7.4.) Consequently, the differences we found—aside from the nonsignificant ones mentioned above—correspond to the hypotheses formulated.

7.5.2.3. Panic disorder versus normal population. In Figure 7.5, there is evidence of significant differences between panic disorder patients and healthy controls with regard to depression, anxiety, and the personality traits compulsiveness and anger as well as somatization. The hypotheses concerning general complaints, neuroticism, and hostility could not be tested between these two groups. None of the literature that was reviewed in the meta-analysis was related to that topic.

We have produced a conclusive body of empirical data confirming our hypotheses that panic disorder patients are more depressed, more anxious,

and develop physical complaints to a greater extent than does the normal population. They are also more compulsive and tend to become angrier than controls.

7.5.2.4. Panic disorder versus noncardiac chest pain. In the meta-analysis, patients with panic disorder were compared with patients with chest pain of noncardiac origin (see Figure 7.6). On the one hand, significant differences were found regarding depression, anxiety, and general complaints. Although the groups did not significantly differ in personality factors such as compulsiveness, anger, and hostility, there is evidence—which, however, must be regarded with skepticism, because it is based on a single study on neuroticism—that panic disorder patients are significantly more neurotic.

The assumption elaborated in the hypotheses that panic disorder patients display a higher level of anxiety and more general complaints was confirmed by the data obtained in the meta-analysis. On the other hand, the expectation that panic disorder patients would be less depressed and would score lower on neuroticism indicators than patients with noncardiac chest pain was not fulfilled. Our data show that panic disorder patients were more depressed and more neurotic.

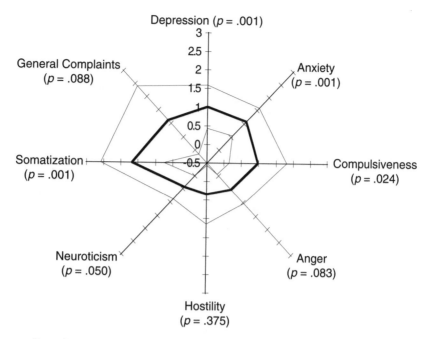

FIGURE 7.4. Noncardiac chest pain versus normal controls.

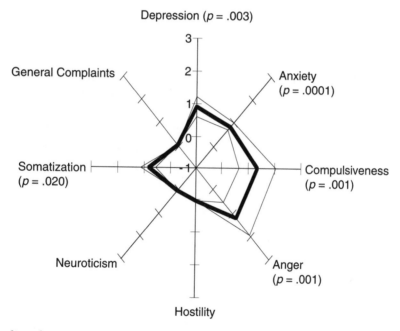

FIGURE 7.5. Panic disorder versus normal controls.

7.5.2.5. Panic disorder versus cardiac syndrome X. There are significant differences between patients with panic disorder and those with syndrome X regarding depression, anxiety, and tendencies to become angry and to develop somatization disorders (see Figure 7.7). On the other

hand, no differences were detectable for personality dimensions such as compulsiveness or hostility. No data were found in the studies reviewed concerning neuroticism and general complaints.

We had initially hypothesized that depression, anger, and somatization would significantly differ

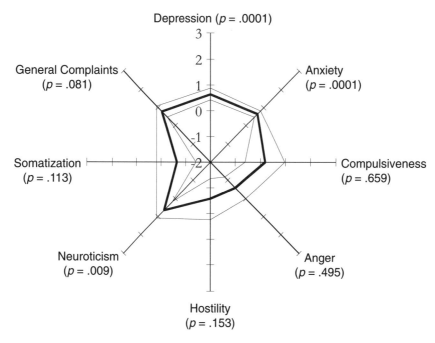

FIGURE 7.6. Panic disorder versus noncardiac chest pain.

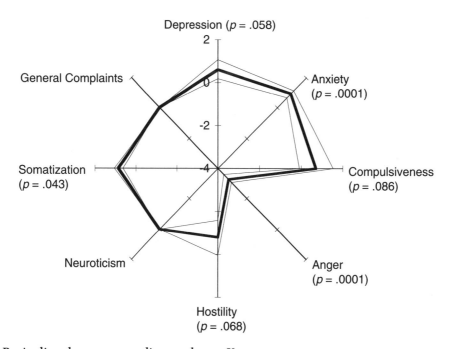

FIGURE 7.7. Panic disorder versus cardiac syndrome X.

in that patients with panic disorder would score higher in all of these areas than patients with syndrome X. The meta-analysis yielded conclusive evidence for this. On the other hand, we were unable to locate any research on the other dimensions.

7.5.2.6. Cardiac syndrome X versus coronary artery disease. There are significant differences between patients with cardiac syndrome X and patients with coronary artery disease regarding depression, anxiety, anger, and general complaints (see Figure 7.8). None of the titles incorporated in

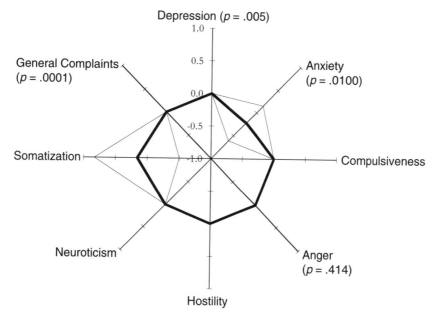

FIGURE 7.8. Cardiac syndrome X versus coronary artery disease.

the meta-analysis yielded data about the dimensions of compulsiveness, hostility, neuroticism, and somatization.

The initial assumption that patients with cardiac syndrome X were more depressed and more anxious than patients with a coronary artery disease was confirmed. In contrast, the hypotheses regarding anger were shown to be untenable. The data indicate that syndrome X patients have a greater tendency to become angry than patients with a coronary artery disease. On the other hand, with regard to general complaints, the result points in the right direction: that patients with syndrome X report more complaints.

7.6. DISCUSSION

An overview of the results of our meta-analysis shows that cardiac syndrome X is an independent disorder that differs significantly in its clinical presentation and psychosomatic and psychological features from coronary artery disease as well as from panic disease and noncardiac chest pain. Pathophysiology and psychological parameters are more useful diagnostically by far than physical complaints such as angina pectoris—which presents exactly the same symptoms in patients with clini-

cally established coronary artery disease. The problematic nature of diagnosis as well as uncertainties in evaluating the incidence of angina pectoris in syndrome X play a role in the area of psychophysiological adaptation. In addition, comorbidity of syndrome X in a substantial proportion of patients might tempt physicians to declare a psychiatric disorder—even if it might not necessarily have been diagnosed beforehand—in patients who do not show any detectable evidence of coronary pathology.

Another well-known phenomenon is that if patients are misdiagnosed the first time they visit a physician, there is an increased risk of morbidity either because patients rightfully feel misunderstood (which is especially likely to occur if an illness is classified exclusively as a psychiatric one) or they feel they have to consult other physicians until the true (i.e., psychosomatic) nature of their illness is ultimately recognized (see Bass & Wade, 1984; Bass, Wade, Hand, & Jackson, 1983; Clancy & Noyes, 1996; Costa et al., 1985; Katon, 1984, 1990; Katon et al., 1986; I. S. Ockene, Shay, Alpert, Weiner, & Dalen, 1980; Sheehan, Ballenger, & Jacobsen, 1980). Many patients who show negative results in coronary angiography complain of persistent chest pain in the course of illness and suffer under decreased social and vocational function in the long term (Bass, Chambers, Kiff, Cooper, & Gardner, 1988; I. S. Ockene et al., 1980).

To date, few studies have been conducted on the relationship between chest pain and personality involving validated, objective evaluation of psychological factors and operationalized procedures to examine chest pain. Although Type A behavior is of particular importance in most of this research, in light of Myrtek's (2001) meta-analysis, we felt that the exclusion of studies referring to the Type A construct was justifiable. Denollet and colleagues recently elaborated a new personality subtype (Denollet & Brutsaert, 1998; Denollet & de Potter, 1992), designated as the *distressed type* or *Type D*, which is characterized by negative affectivity and social inhibition. Although conclusive evidence has shown that the combination of these two factors is a good predictor of cardiac events (Denollet & Brutsaert, 1998), the impact of the distressed personality type on the incidence of chest pain of noncardiac etiology is not reported on. On the one hand, Moustier, Benichou, Giudicelli, and Bory (1984) found significant personality differences between patients who had normal coronary arteries, but who had revealed arterial spasms in angiography and suffered from retrosternal pain of noncardiac origin, and coronary artery disease patients. On the other hand, no differences were found between patients with normal coronary arteries with spasms and their counterparts without spasms. In addition, significant differences were found in personality dimensions such as psychoneuroticism and compulsiveness in a comparison between patients with heart disease and those with chest pain of noncardiac origin (Serlie et al., 1996). J. G. Beck, Berisford, Taegtmeyer, and Bennett (1990) did not find any differences when comparing chest pain patients, panic disorder patients, and a normal population with regard to obsessive–compulsive behavior. Also, Costa (1987) found higher scores in neuroticism in patients with noncardiac chest pain than in coronary artery patients. Roll and Theorell (1987) corroborated these results in a comparison of chest pain patients and healthy controls. There is

substantial evidence from the National Health and Nutrition Examination Survey, a large-scale study of 9,727 people, that neuroticism is related to an increased incidence of somatic symptoms, including chest pain or angina-like complaints (Costa, 1987).

Results of a 10-year cohort study conducted by Shekelle, Vernon, and Ostfeld (1991) show that besides neuroticism, hypochondria and hysteria are also associated with the incidence of uncomplicated angina pectoris, whereas they are not associated with myocardial infarction. In addition, the tendency to report somatic complaints or to experience negative, distressing emotions chronically is related to an increased incidence of a benign, non-atherosclerotic condition that is similar clinically to angina pectoris. Additionally, T. W. Smith, Follick, and Korr (1984) documented the relationship between neuroticism and avoidance behavior. Patients with angina and high neuroticism scores tend to avoid activities because of the possibility of angina more than those with low neuroticism scores. That diffuse somatic complaints and emotional instability are predictors of angina without an atherosclerotic etiology has been reported by Costa et al. (1987) in a long-term retrospective predictive study and henceforth replicated in other prospective studies (Macleod et al., 2002; Marusic & Gudjonsson, 1999).

Tendency to anger and hostility are two of the few personality traits that have been found to be stable constructs in the meta-analysis of the association between Type A personality and coronary artery disease (Myrtek, 2001). With regard to the association between chest pain and these personality factors, Schocken et al. (1987) reported on a study with angina patients in which patients with silent ischemia showed less of a tendency to become angry than patients with ischemia. In addition, patients with angina were rated as more hostile and more neurotic than those without chest pain. J. G. Beck et al. (1989) compared patients with persistent chest pain, panic disorder patients, and control subjects. Neither Beck et al. nor Serlie et al. (1996) found any significant differences with regard to either anger or hostility, nor could

Ruggeri et al. (1996) demonstrate any differences between syndrome X patients' anger and heart patients' anger and related coping and management strategies. On the other hand, Eifert, Hodson, Tracey, and Seville (1996) found significantly higher anger potential in panic disorder patients than in healthy controls. Tennant et al.'s (1994) goal was to distinguish between the two groups on the basis of indices of myocardial thallium scintigraphy. They detected a significant difference in anger between ischemia patients and those with normal thallium scans. T. W. Smith et al. (1984) reported a significant correlation between anxiety and the incidence of anginal complaints.

Various authors have examined the question of anxiety. J. G. Beck et al. (1989) compared chest pain patients, panic disorder patients, and control subjects. Although trait anxiety and phobic fears were strongest among patients with panic disorder, chest pain patients displayed the highest degree of situation-related anxiety. Serlie et al. (1996), on the other hand, could not find any significant differences in state or trait anxiety between patients with chest pain of noncardiac etiology and heart patients. Roy-Byrne et al. (1984) compared panic disorder patients and patients with microvascular angina. The differences in anxiety were thought to suggest either panic disorder comorbidity or two possible categories of microvascular angina.

There is overall consensus that chronic pain leads to depressive mood and depression, which, in turn, contribute to a lower perceived threshold of pain. In patients with chronic depression, estimates of prevalence of comorbidity range from about 30% to nearly 100% (Kramlinger, Swanson, & Maruta, 1983; Romano & Turner, 1985; Skevington, 1983). In addition, anxiety is a frequent concomitant of angina pectoris of cardiac origin and in part even replaces actual pain. Anxiety occurs as an alarm sign in an acute episode of chest pain (Eifert, 1992; Procacci, Zoppi & Maresca, 1986) and is detectable as an independent symptom in exercise-provoked myocardial ischemia by intravenous infusion of adenosine (Sylvén, 1986; Sylvén, Eriksson, Jensen, Geigant, & Hallin, 1996). In a randomized consecutive patient population of 3,705 that had undergone ergometric

investigation, C. Herrmann, Buss, Breuker, Gonska, and Kreuzer (1994) found high anxiety and depression scores in 19.7% and 9.1% of the sample, respectively.

Distinctive personality factors and other psychological factors such as anxiety and panic disorder (Beitman, Mukerji, Flaker, & Basha, 1988; Carter, Servan-Schreiber, & Perlstein, 1997) and depression (Elias et al., 1982) are extremely common in patients with chest pain of noncardiac etiology. The prevalence of anxiety and panic disorders is between 30% and 50% (Beitman, DeRosear, Basha, & Flaker, 1987; Katon, 1990). These disorders—like other psychiatric disorders—often fail to be recognized (Weissman, 1990), which might, in turn, lead to a chronic course or to further psychiatric comorbidities, such as agoraphobia and depression, a development that puts this group of patients at risk for suicidal behavior (Beitman et al., 1991; Fleet et al., 1997).

Serlie et al. (1996), for example, found a significantly higher level of basic anxiety in chest pain patients who had no organic disease—a finding that had already been reported by Elias et al. (1982) more than a decade before. J. G. Beck et al. (1989), on the other hand, found a lower level of anxiety and avoidance in chest pain patients who did not have an organic heart disease than in panic disorder patients. In addition, the former group of patients did not need as much anxiolytic medication to alleviate symptoms. However, both patient groups had higher state and trait anger as well as higher depression and somatization scores than the normal population (J. G. Beck et al., 1989). In a later study, chest pain, dyspnea, and paresthesias as well as substantially greater anxiety prior to myocardial infarction was found significantly more often in both patient groups than in the control group, whereby panic disorder patients' symptoms were the most intense and frequent (J. G. Beck et al., 1990). J. G. Beck, Berisford, and Taegtmeyer (1991) succeeded in lending even greater support to these results by conducting a provocation test with hyperventilation. As opposed to J. G. Beck et al., Beitman et al. (1992, 1993) described a subgroup of panic disorders that met all the diagnostic criteria for panic disorder with the exception of subjective fear. As a result, these patients had been designated as suffering from "nonfear panic disorder." In studies on the family-related prevalence of panic disorders, both groups of patients were found to be at greater risk than the normal population if they had a close relative with panic disorder history (Beitman et al., 1992; Kushner et al., 1992).

Another subject besides the relationship between panic disorder and noncardiac chest pain symptoms that has also attracted research attention is the increased incidence of generalized anxiety disturbances (Carter & Maddock, 1992), which Bass and Wade (1984) had referred to as *anxiety neurosis*. *Heart-focused anxiety* is another term used to describe noncardiac chest pain (Eifert, Zvolensky, & Lejuez, 2000). Eifert et al. (2000) hypothesized that this form of disorder would cause anxiety, because for someone suffering from it, all cardiac-related experiences are perceived and attributed as adverse and dangerous. This can result in a shift of attention away from and avoidance of heart-related stimuli and sensations (McNally, 1990; McNally & Eke, 1996; Reiss, 1997). According to Cox (1996), the relative degree of congruence with the anxiety experienced by the afflicted and the feared object is a decisive individual factor in triggering heart-related fears. Eifert et al. (2000) regarded heart-related fear as a special type of anxiety that occurs predominantly in a clinical medical setting in which chest pain occurs in combination with psychological distress and that supposedly is relevant to cardiac and noncardiac chest pain as well as to panic disturbances. Heart-related fear increases the likelihood—independently of specific preconditions—of responding to chest pain with anxiety or to heart-related perceptions with such reactions as palpitations (Eifert, 1992).

Various attempts have been made to develop a better and simpler method of assessing the symptoms and the psychiatric–psychological problems of persons who experience chest pain. Another approach was developed by Fraenkel, Kindler, and Melmed (1996) to identify the differences in cognitions during chest pain between patients with angina pectoris and those with panic disorder. All patients with normal coronary angiograms

experienced frightening cognitions during chest pain. In 83% of this group, the cognitions were the predominant experience, whereas only 18% of the patients with proven symptomatic coronary artery disease complained of their symptoms, and only 4% of them attributed their frightening cognitions to chest pain. On the other hand, Ladwig et al. (1998) suggested grouping chest pain symptoms of noncardiac origin as a somatoform pain disorder rather than as an anxiety and panic disorder.

There are differences with regard to the localization pattern of angina between patients with chest pain who have angiographically normal coronary arteries and others with coronary artery disease. A significant number in the former group have left-sided, sharp chest pain and palpitations more frequently than in the latter group (Mukerji, Beitman, Alpert, & Hewett, 1987). The question of whether there ought to be differences in pain perception between patients with chest pain and coronary artery disease and syndrome X patients has remained controversial. Cannon (1995) found exaggerated or abnormal cardiac pain perception in patients with chest pain, normal coronary angiograms, and ischemic signs under stress (syndrome X; Cannon, 1995). In a study comparing pain perception in patients with syndrome X, patients with mitral valve disease and coronary artery disease, and heart transplant recipients, Chauhan et al. (1994) found typical anginal chest pain more often in syndrome X patients (94%) than in the other groups (0%–19%) when stimulated intracardially. The authors concluded that the results of their study suggested that abnormal cardiac pain perception is a fundamental abnormality in syndrome X.

A number of constructs deserve mention in the area of somatization and desomatization that play a part in altered sensations of pain. These might include attention-focusing or even personality-related components. There are basically two ways that symptoms of various etiologies can develop or be perceived. First, organs (in this case the heart) can cause specific or unspecific organ-related symptoms because of an emerging pathology attributable to changes in the afferents to perception. The complex processes involved in the transmission of an afferent modality to intrapsychic sensation or emotion (here pain) will add to the complexity of pain perception. Second, intrapsychic processes can provoke emotions of various origins, which might lead to sensations in organs that do not evidence any somatic pathology. An illustration is bereavement, which leads to the sensation of thoracic pressure similar to angina pectoris (tightness in chest) triggered by coronary artery disease. Perception—as an act of consciousness—is probably ultimately identical for the somatic and the intrapsychic causes of a sensation or an emotion and therefore can be regarded as a sort of common final pathway in the developmental process from the onset of any complaint to perception. On the other hand, the act of appraising sensations is a cognitive process and therefore associated with coping. It therefore is a third factor that is merely independent of the others. However, this third factor may have physical and emotional effects on the abstraction of the physiological reaction–that is, on the attempt to understand this reaction or the detectable physical sensations—regardless of the respective developmental mechanism.

Early theories about the development of heart-associated complaints are psychoanalytical. The concept of conversion neurosis was first used by Freud (1915) in "Bemerkungen über die Übertragungsliebe" ("Remarks on Transference") to refer to intrapsychic conflicts that arise because of incongruence between wishes and constraints accompanied by the impossibility of consciously perceiving these conflicts, which causes the physical expression of this conflict to be perceived within the symbolic context of related organs (so-called "conversion mechanism"; see Scheidt, Koester, & Deuschel, 1996). Symptom formation involves a wide range of defense mechanisms as well as symbolic processes. It also involves what is referred to as "somatic adjustment" comparable to an organ-specific vulnerability and the use of earlier processes of identifying with significant others, whereas the conversion mechanism converts conflicts symbolically or deterministically (so-called "somatization"), corresponding to a process of "freeing" oneself in intrapsychic terms from the actual conflict and to the primary gain of illness. The secondary gain provided by illness occurs

in the individual's interaction with his psychosocial environment, including the medical system (Lazare, 1981). In contrast to Scheidt et al. (1996), McDougall (1974) conceptualized fantasy activity as a completely intrapsychic feature. Fantasies are eventually linked to psychosomatic symptoms as time evolves, not as they originally were, but rather in a coincidental manner. Krystal (1978) supplemented McDougall's theories by borrowing insights from developmental psychology, adding the problem of regression, and also conceptualizing a part of the superego, which is externalized from the body and which underlies symptom formation. Marty and de M'Uzan (1962) designed their own theoretical model called *pensée opératoire* (operationalized thinking) to explain conversion disorders. It accounts for the fact that although affects and related somatic expressions are usually linked, they might in certain cases exist separately from each other, side by side. If this were to happen, people would not be able to infer physiological correlates from certain affect patterns (e.g., anxiety and heart palpitations) so that they would have to devote their full attention to physiological processes. These would be operationalized in a certain sense without developing the ability to establish a bridge between complaints and affects. Although the emotional expression can be described in great detail, the contents and the actual reason for the emotional expression, namely, the feeling involved, cannot be linked up with each other. Sifneos (1973) developed a similar concept, called the "alexithymia model" (cf. Defontaine-Catteau, Pedinielle, & Bertagne, 1992).

Another theoretical model that added to our understanding of somatization was designed by Krohne and Hock (1993). They distinguished between "cognitive avoidance" and "vigilance." According to this model, all individuals have both aspects in themselves but to a different extent. Thus, the coping strategies manifested are attributable to person-specific, systematic differences in ways of tolerating uncertainty or emotional arousal. As a consequence, very anxious patients are high in vigilance and in cognitive avoidance, which is characterized by an intolerance of arousal and uncertainty.

7.7. CONCLUSION

All in all, the results of our meta-analysis show that syndrome X is an entity characterized by distinct clinical and psychosomatic–psychological features that can be clearly distinguished from coronary artery disease, panic disease, and noncardiac chest pain. Differences in complaints, such as angina pectoris—which is indistinguishable from coronary artery disease and syndrome X—appear to be less pronounced than in pathophysiology and psychological parameters.

CHAPTER 8

PSYCHOSOCIAL ASPECTS OF CORONARY CATHETERIZATION, ANGIOGRAPHY, AND ANGIOPLASTY

Jochen Jordan and Claudia Lazanowski

8.1. INTRODUCTION

This chapter reviews scientific publications on the psychosocial aspects of cardiac catheterization, coronary angiography, and percutaneous transluminal coronary angioplasty (PTCA). These intervention techniques have greatly and lastingly influenced cardiac diagnostics and therapy in the past several decades.

Because the interventions discussed in this chapter have changed so rapidly, we provide a short historical overview in section 8.2. The chapter is subsequently organized by methodological design; after describing our search methodology in section 8.3, we describe and evaluate in section 8.4 our findings from the cross-sectional, longitudinal, prospective, and intervention studies we located. Because this structure does not allow a presentation based on clinical criteria, in section 8.5 we provide general conclusions from all types of studies. Technological progress has brought many changes to this field, so we did not include studies published before 1990 in our methodological evaluation, except in the case of intervention studies.

8.2. HISTORICAL OVERVIEW

Twenty-five years have passed since Andreas Grüntzig founded interventional cardiology by pioneering the clinical application of PTCA (S. King, 1998). Of course, this technique was based on decades of experience and started with the first cardiac catheterization by Werner Forßmann. In 1959, Mason Sones presented the first coronary angiography at the Cardiology Congress in Philadelphia. X-ray examination of blood vessels after injection of a radiopaque contrast medium produces an angiogram. In 1964, Edward Garrett, and shortly afterward René Favaloro, developed the standard procedure for the direct revascularization of the myocardium: coronary artery bypass grafting (CABG).

Parallel to this development, Charles Dotter tested a dilatation technique for the peripheral arteries, which Eberhardt Zeitler, among others, implemented in Germany. Zeitler worked with Grüntzig, who developed a double-lumen catheter that carried an inflatable balloon on its tip to expand vessel stenoses. After initial difficulties, the first successful coronary angioplasty took place in September 1977. The second successful intervention was accomplished in the same year at the University Clinic of Frankfurt am Main (Germany) by Grüntzig and Martin Kaltenbach. Half a year later, John Myler and Richard Stertzer introduced coronary angioplasty in the United States. The new procedure spread rapidly, from a few thousand applications worldwide before 1980 to more than 30,000 by 1983. The clinical application of cardiac stents since 1986 was a further crucial development in interventional cardiology.

Improvements in the technique resulted not only in an expanded therapy spectrum but also in the reduction of hospital stays; this procedure can now be performed on an outpatient basis. As the rate and rapidity of success procedures have risen, the rates of acute complications and of restenosis have fallen.

8.3. METHOD

There has not yet been a systematic review of the psychosocial implications of cardiac catheterization, coronary angiography, or PTCA. The goal of this chapter is to provide such a review.

Cardiac interventions are stressful for patients for various reasons:

- For coronary angiography and angioplasty, patients are fully conscious throughout the procedure and are not sedated.
- The results of the intervention will determine many important health-related issues, and the occurrence of acute complications may necessitate further treatment (e.g., bypass surgery, intensive care; Jordan, 1991). Because most PTCA patients receive a stent to keep the vessel open and because medications are more effective, however, the risk of complications and of restenosis have dropped significantly.
- The postoperative rest period requires patients to be immobile, which many find unpleasant.
- In many countries, patients must endure a long waiting period before undergoing the intervention. Fortunately, waiting periods have decreased over the years. The ability to perform coronary angiography and PTCA simultaneously, if necessary, has also shortened waiting periods; patients can be instantly dilated after results are obtained and need not wait for a second intervention, thus avoiding further delay.

This chapter focuses on empirical studies investigating psychosocial issues surrounding coronary interventions. The following issues will be explored: emotional and cognitive experiences surrounding a procedure, common psychological symptoms, psychological and social coping with the procedure, quality of life (QoL) before and after the procedure, the predictive ability of psychosocial factors for the disease course after the procedure, and the effects of educational and psychological interventions on patient well-being.

8.3.1. Literature Search

We used the Medline, PSYNDEXplus, and PsycINFO databases for the literature search. To classify and evaluate the publications, we used a set of evidence criteria based on the principles of evidence-based medicine (EBM; see Centre for Evidence-Based Medicine Web site: http://www.cebmnet; see also Canadian Task Force on the Periodic Health Examination, 1979; Cook, Guyatt, Laupacis, Sackett, & Goldberg, 1995; Sackett, 1986, 1996; Yusuf, Cairns, Camm, Fallen, & Gersh, 1998). The search, which covered the period from 1975 to April 2002, used the following key words: *coronar* and PTCA, coronar* and angio* and psych*, coping*, anxiety, depression, quality of life, risk*,* and *patient education.* A total of 1,938 hits resulted from the three databases. After eliminating duplication and performing an initial review, we selected 133 relevant publications. In addition to the database searches, we did an extended search of the reference lists of available publications, relevant journals, overviews, and textbooks, increasing the total publications reviewed for this chapter to 145 (92 were empirical studies).

8.3.2. Exclusion Criteria

We excluded publications from consideration that were not written in English or German; that did not focus on psychosocial variables; that focused on cardiac interventions in children; that compared PTCA, stent, and chest pain; and that examined return to work in the context of PTCA treatment research. Many psychosocial studies of cardiac interventions examined variables that have no direct relation to the intervention itself (e.g., psychological variables of return to work, vital exhaustion as a predictor of the disease process, Type A behavior). Although these studies do not address the main topic of this chapter, we decided to include them in the discussion because they demonstrate the clinical relevance of psychosocial variables in cardiac interventions.

8.3.3. Evidence Criteria

As far as possible, our evaluation of the methodological quality of the selected publications followed the criteria for EBM. We used the classification system developed by Herrmann-Lingen and Buss (see chap. 5, this volume) to assess the qualifications of a publication on the basis of its sample size and methodological quality. Methodological quality encompasses the quality of the instruments used, of the analysis of data, and of the reporting of the results. A qualification index was assigned by calculating the product of the sample size and the mean score for methodological quality. Studies with indexes >8 were classified as very well qualified, those with indexes >6 but ≤8 as well qualified, those with indexes of 4 to 6 as partially qualified, and those with indexes <4 as less qualified.

Herrmann-Lingen and Buss (chap. 5, this volume) developed their evaluation system for their examination of the role of anxiety and depression in coronary heart disease (CHD). Their question requires large samples to answer, which many investigations in this chapter did not have. After calculating the mean sample size of studies selected for this chapter ($N = 132$), we decided for reasons of uniformity to follow the system of Hermann-Lingen and Buss. Table 8.1 describes the system for evaluating the qualifications of the studies we selected, and Table 8.2 reports the number of studies in each qualification and methodological category and mean sample sizes.

8.4. RESULTS

8.4.1. Preliminary Remarks

In this section, we report methodological evaluations and study results for the cross-sectional, longitudinal, prospective, and intervention studies we located. Tables W8.1–W8.4 on the accompanying Web site (http://www.apa.org/books/resources/jordan/) list and summarize all the studies we selected for review. Results of the cross-sectional and longitudinal studies are summarized for three categories: coping studies, QoL studies, and other studies. Prospective studies are reported in two sections: those with hard endpoints (e.g., mortality, later cardiac events) and those with soft endpoints (e.g., psychological variables, angina pectoris). Two categories of intervention study are described: educational and psychological. A brief description of reviews and expert reports follows (an evaluation of

their methodological suitability was not appropriate).

The lack of comparability of the studies we selected made consistent evaluation difficult for at least three reasons. First, many different questions were researched, and some questions were addressed in only a single study, making comparison to other studies impossible. Second, most studies reported insufficient details on the environmental conditions of the cardiac interventions (e.g., waiting time, technical equipment), even though these conditions can significantly influence patients' experiences. A third factor influencing comparability is the rapid development of interventional cardiology technology; studies published before 1980 differ in many ways from those published in the past 15 years. For this reason, we divided the studies into those published before 1990 and those published from 1990 on to reflect major medical and technological developments in coronary procedures. Eighty percent of the studies belong to the latter category; we decided to describe the older studies only briefly and did not include them in the methodological evaluation. However, this could not prevent a small flaw in the results presentation, because many public health systems today still have long waiting periods. In modern medical systems, waiting times are short. In an acute state of the illness, an angiography and, if necessary, a PTCA, are made immediately if possible. Waiting times of days and weeks increase anxiety and are sometimes dangerous.

Of the 92 studies for which origin was apparent, 49% were conducted in the United States, 17% in Germany, 9% in the Netherlands, and 5% in other countries. Twenty-one empirical studies, 2 reviews, and 11 expert reports were published before 1990; from 1990 on, 83 empirical studies, 2 reviews, and 12 expert assessments were published. Eighty-six percent of the cross-sectional studies, 85% of the longitudinal studies, 95% of the prospective studies, and 50% of the intervention studies were published after 1990.

8.4.2. Cross-Sectional Studies

We categorized all empirical studies with only one measurement point as cross-sectional studies. Of

TABLE 8.1

Classification of the Qualification of Selected Studies

Study characteristic	Points assigned			
	1	2	3	4
Relevant *n*	<30	30–99	100–499	≥500
All studies				
Quality of instruments	Ad hoc instrument or single item	Unusual questionnaire or interview	Standard questionnaire or interview	Standard questionnaire and interview
Quality of reporting of the results	Only mean values or percentages	Mean + *SD*, correlations, or percentages	Mean + *SD*, correlations, or percentages + significance	—
Prospective studies				
Quality of reporting of the results (soft endpoints)	Minimal data	Univariate effect sizes + significance or multivariate effect sizes without significance	Multivariate effect sizes + significance	Univariate + multivariate effect sizes + significance
Quality of reporting of the results (hard endpoints)	Univariate effect sizes + significance	Minimal covariate adjustment	Adjustment for single (up to 3) cardiac covariates	Adjustment for multiple (> 3) cardiac covariates
Intervention studies				
Quality of intervention (1 point is assigned for each of the six criteria fulfilled from the list in section 8.4.5)	1 criterion fulfilled	2 or 3 criteria fulfilled	4 or more criteria fulfilled	—
Quality of reporting of the results	Only mean values	*M* + *SD* or percentages	*M* + *SD* or percentages + significance	—
Qualitative studies				
Quality of data gathering	Unstructured interview or descriptive report	Semistructured interview or unusual method	Semistructured interview with established rating system	Semistructured interview with established rating system and independent raters

Note. This table applies only to studies published after 1990. A methodological score was computed by adding the points and dividing by the number of scores. Dash in cell indicates no applicable data.

course, many longitudinal and prospective studies also reported data from specific measurement points. However, we decided for methodological reasons to assign each study to only one category and to evaluate each category separately.

All cross-sectional studies are listed and summarized in Table W8.1 on the accompanying Web site. Three of the 22 cross-sectional studies were published before 1990 (Davies Osterkamp & Salm, 1980; de Bruijn, 1989; Fraser, 1984). These studies

examined the statistical relationship between different coping mechanisms, information distribution during the intervention, and psychological coping with very long waiting periods. The sections that follow describe the studies published after 1990.

8.4.2.1. Coping studies. Three studies were published by a Swedish team (Bengtson, Herlitz, Karlsson, & Hjalmarson, 1994, 1996; Bengtson, Karlsson, & Herlitz, 2000) and were conducted

Number of Studies and Mean Sample Sizes of Selected Studies

	Very well qualified (>8 points)	Well qualified (>6 to ≤8 points)	Partially qualified (≤4 to ≤6 points)	Less qualified (<4 points)	Total number of studies
Cross-sectional studies					
Number of studies	9 (7)[a]	3 (2)[a]	4	3	19
Mean sample size	16,479 (184)[b]	54	137	47	—
Longitudinal studies					
Number of studies	17 (15)[a]	8	6	2	33
Mean sample size	246 (297)[c]	149.5	73.3	26.5	—
Prospective studies					
Number of studies	14	3	1	—	18
Mean sample size	280 (165)[d]	218	41	—	—
Intervention studies					
Number of studies	1 (2)	9	7	7	22
Mean sample size	145	93	50	31	67.7

Note. This table includes data only for studies published after 1990. Dash in cell indicates there are no applicable data. [a]Studies that assessed identical samples were counted only once; numbers in parentheses are the number of studies that used different samples. [b]The number in parentheses refers to the mean sample size excluding the large study by Druss et al. (2000). [c]The number in parentheses refers to the mean sample size excluding the large study by Pocock et al. (1996). [d]The number in parentheses indicates the mean sample size excluding the two large studies by Hlatky et al. (1997) and Pocock et al. (2000).

with a previously examined patient population. These studies, which we evaluated as very well qualified, examined the effects of long waiting periods of an average of 8 months for angiography and 5 months for PTCA (for countries with shorter waiting periods, this study may not reflect current realities): "56% of all patients reported that uncertainty, fear, or other unspecified problems were the most disturbing symptoms, while pain was the worst for 44%" (Bengtson et al., 1996, p. 258). The prevalence of pain was not affected by age, but the intensity of pain correlated significantly with the frequency of other cardiac and psychosomatic symptoms ($p < .001$); the stronger the pain these patients experienced, the more symptoms they reported. The patient group experienced significantly more anxiety than the control group. Patients with waiting periods of more than 6 months were significantly more anxious, experienced more sleep disorders, and consumed more cigarettes and sedatives. Women had significantly higher levels of

stress from cardiac and psychological problems ($p < .007$) compared with men; in particular, women suffered more from sleeping disorders and consumed more sleeping pills ($p < .005$), whereas men suffered more from general unrest, irritability, and inability to act ($p < .03$).

Another very well qualified study by Brezynskie, Pendon, Lindsay, and Adam (1998) found that patients' most important need was for information on PTCA results and on what to do if chest pains recurred after discharge. Information on psychological issues was reported as least important; the authors interpreted this finding as being a result of the need for brevity and simplicity during the intervention and hospitalization. The authors also concluded from their observations that both patients and surgeons downplayed the seriousness of the disease and the intervention.

An additional very well qualified study by Kraft and Werner (1994) examined the subjective illness theories of patients with no previous diagnosis of

CHD for whom a cardiac catheterization found no evidence of pathology. The authors used a semi-structured interview and questionnaires to assess patients' impressions of the procedure. Most patients (84%) were able to clearly describe the results of the intervention. Nevertheless, only 39% felt "heart healthy," whereas the remaining 61% of patients could not understand the results or felt that the results were not accurate. The latter group also reported significantly more cardiac symptoms, but the onset of symptoms proceeded slowly; that is, these patients realized that they had symptoms over periods of weeks or months. In contrast, patients who reported no symptoms perceived specific situations—trigger situations when they felt the symptoms for the first time—as psychologically induced.

Two qualitative studies using the same sample (Gulanick, Bliley, Perino, & Keough, 1997, 1998) were well designed, but we rated them as only well qualified because of their small sample size (*N* = 45). In a single interview 3 to 18 months after the intervention, these authors investigated the impressions of three groups of patients in relation to their coronary angioplasties (i.e., PTCA, simultaneous PTCA and atherectomy, and simultaneous PTCA and stent implantation). Patients were also asked about the problems they encountered in changing their lifestyles. They cited the information and support provided by the treating medical team as important aids for coping with the intervention; possibly for this reason, they reported experiencing low levels of anxiety during the procedure. Many patients also tried to implement lifestyle changes (e.g., improved diet, increased exercise, stress management); they found good social support to be especially helpful but were confused by conflicting information from physicians and the media. Uncertainty about the disease progression and the prognosis were perceived as very stressful. Patients reported interesting and plausible intervention ideas such as telephone hotlines, video rentals, and patient education courses to help them obtain sufficient information and cope with their disease.

We rated a qualitative study by Beattie and Geden (1990), which examined patients' pain symptoms following PTCA from the perspective of nursing staff, and a study by Gaw-Ens and Laing (1994), which investigated patients' efforts to reduce their risk factors after PTCA or myocardial infarction through behavior modification, as partially qualified because of methodological deficits. We also classified three other cross-sectional studies as less qualified because of their small samples and methodological deficiencies (Beckermann, Grossmann, & Marquez, 1995; Hupcey & Gilchrist, 1993; Miracle & Hovekamp, 1994). These studies are summarized in Table W8.1 on the accompanying Web site.

8.4.2.2. Quality of life studies. A very well qualified study by Echtheld, van der Kamp, and van Elderen (2001) using extensive assessment instruments and statistical analyses examined psychological correlates of QoL in patients on a waiting list for PTCA and a healthy control group. The goal of the study was to assess relationships between coping styles (approach vs. avoidant), sociodemographic variables, social support, and other coping variables (e.g., expectations regarding disease progression, unfinished goals, optimism), on the one hand, and dimensions of QoL (e.g., negative or positive affect/mood and health-related QoL) on the other. Some hypotheses of the authors were refuted by the data:

> The relationships between approach coping and QoL are (1) not very strong, and (2) are negative. . . . There are no significant relationships between optimism and approach coping. . . . The data show that optimism is not significantly related to any QoL variable. (Echtheld et al., 2001, p. 496)

Other hypotheses were partly confirmed:

> Chest pain only related to negative QoL variables and goal disturbance had no relationships with positive QoL variables at the .05 level of significance. Chest pain and goal disturbance had fairly strong relationships with the negative QoL variables. (Echtheld et al., 2001, p. 496)

A very well qualified study by Krumholz et al. (1997) compared the health-related QoL of a group of patients after stent implantation with that of a group who underwent PTCA without stenting. The authors found no significant differences in QoL between the groups 6 to 18 months after the intervention. Specifically, the scores for mental health, vitality, and social functioning (using scales from the SF–36 Health Survey, International Quality of Life Assessment Project; Aaronson et al., 1992) did not differ significantly ($p > .6$). Sixty percent of patients from both groups reported having no symptoms; 47% reported their health to be excellent or very good. Stent patients reported significantly fewer pain experiences ($p = .02$) but no fewer chest pain symptoms than PTCA patients, a finding that remains unexplained.

A very well qualified study by Kimble and King (1998) assessed the advantages and side effects of PTCA as perceived by 62 patients 2 weeks after discharge. Eighty percent felt that the intervention had improved their physical and mental status; 39% experienced fewer chest pains, 19% experienced a reduction in dyspnea, 12% were less tired, and 8% felt more optimistic. The remaining 20% of patients were undecided or felt worse than before the PTCA and were more fearful of restenosis. Correlation analysis yielded a significant relationship ($p < .05$) between long-lasting angina symptoms or angina pectoris symptoms after hospital discharge and the feeling of worsened health after PTCA. Fifty-two percent of patients described side effects, particularly pain in the loins, unspecified chest pains, and side effects from medications. Few psychological reactions were reported; only 3% of patients reported experiencing anxiety or depression.

8.4.2.3. Other studies. Druss, Bradford, Rosenheck, Radford, and Krumholz (2000) conducted a very well qualified study with a large sample of 113,653 participants. Unfortunately, they did not address psychological issues in a methodologically sound manner. The study investigated whether psychiatric disorders in an older patient population (>65 years) influenced their access to cardiac treatment. Psychiatric disorders were not diagnosed by psychiatrists, possibly biasing the results.

A sophisticated qualitative study by Philpott, Boynton, Feder, and Hemingway (2001) investigated whether gender-specific differences existed in the reporting of cardiac symptoms that then influenced the rate of revascularization. Women reported significantly fewer chest pains and had a lower rate of CHD diagnosis (via angiography) than men ($p < .01$), but they reported significantly low physical functioning and frequent neck and jaw pain and other symptoms ($p < .01$). The subgroup of women with low physical functioning and angiographically secured cardiac catheters reported these symptoms significantly more often than men. After 18 months, there were no significant gender-specific differences in revasculated patients' descriptions of their symptoms. Nonrevasculated women who had undergone cardiac catheterization described significantly more neck or jaw pain and felt those pains to be more impairing than did men. Thus, no gender differences were found in the description of symptoms (e.g., narrative vs. factual), but they were found in the localization of pain and the reporting of different symptoms. In its conclusion the authors hypothesized that women's descriptions of atypical symptoms contribute to their decision not to undergo a revascularization.

Saha, Stettin, and Redberg (1999) reported an interesting result based on a study from 1994. They found, surprisingly, that women were much more open-minded toward technological cardiac interventions (angiography, PTCA, and bypass surgery) than were men. This result must be interpreted with caution because of the nonstandardized instruments they used and a high dropout rate of 34%. Finally, a partially qualified study by Garachemani et al. (1997) was designed as a longitudinal study but reported psychosocial variables from only one measurement point.

8.4.2.4. Summary of cross-sectional studies. Cross-sectional studies have only a limited explanatory power, because they represent a small time frame. The methodological quality of 50% of the studies is satisfactory.

8.4.2.4.1. Preparation for intervention. Cross-sectional studies have documented that waiting times lead to increased anxiety, stress, and psychosomatic symptoms in patients. Medical staff can use waiting times to provide sensitive and comprehensive information about the process and risks of the intervention to patients and their family members. This information should describe possible pain reactions and their significance for the intervention. Supportive verbalizations by staff are very helpful in reducing anxiety.

8.4.2.4.2. During the intervention. Our review shows clearly that the literature contains no evidence of clinically significant psychological complications or symptoms of psychopathology in patients undergoing these coronary interventions (catheterization, angiography, and PTCA). During the procedure, and particularly during the first few minutes, however, patients experience the highest levels of stress and anxiety, and staff should encourage them to ask questions and to report their sensory experiences. Patient coping is maximized when information seeking is met with responses that promote confidence in the medical procedure and staff.

8.4.2.4.3. After the intervention. Many patients have reported that the intervention was much easier and less stressful than they had anticipated. This relief may lead them to underestimate the continuing danger inherent in the underlying atherosclerotic process (Gaw-Ens & Laing, 1994). Because their symptoms of angina pectoris and breathlessness decreased, nearly 80% of patients experienced an improvement in their somatic and psychological status and report less exhaustion and better spirits (Kimble & King, 1998). Many patients do not sufficiently anticipate the limitations that often exist after PTCA in various spheres (e.g., sexuality, work, recreation). Patients who suffer from angina pectoris symptoms or other complaints after discharge following PTCA report that the procedure had marginal effects (Kimble & King, 1998). A detailed communication of the results and possible consequences following the procedure (e.g., restenosis, complications) can minimize uncertainty for patients and their family members when symptoms appear unexpectedly. Patients need to know exactly which symptoms or circumstances should prompt a medical consultation and which call for immediate hospitalization or emergency care.

Patients who receive inadequate information or who have an avoidant coping style can seriously misinterpret the underlying atherosclerotic illness. Patients who appraise the intervention as easy and undramatic may minimize the symptoms and dangerous consequences of the basic illness and may make less effort to change risky lifestyles or behaviors.

To support lifestyle changes, patients require clear and understandable guidance. Many cardiac patients (30%–60%) are motivated and try hard to establish risk reduction behaviors in their lives (Gaw-Ens & Laing, 1994). If guidance is not communicated repeatedly, patients' efforts lose intensity. Thus, patients should receive repeated contacts by their cardiac unit, cardiologist, or general practitioner. Hotlines, booklets, videotapes, and Web sites are other means of communicating with patients. Those who have uncomfortable symptoms but whose angiography results are negative tend to continue to feel ill and to mistrust the diagnosis, and these patients in particular need intensive and uncomplaining care.

Concerning gender-specific differences, some interesting results should be replicated and revised in future studies. These studies found that women have different symptom presentations and coping mechanisms than men but also, contrary to existing preconceptions, that women do not tend to have negative attitudes toward technical interventions.

8.4.3. Longitudinal Studies

Longitudinal studies are empirical studies for which data are gathered at two or more measurement points. Many available studies have a pretest–posttest design (i.e., variables are measured before and after the cardiac intervention). Longitudinal studies that assess predictive variables are discussed in section 8.4.4 on prospective studies. The terms *comparison group* and *control group* are used synonymously in the literature; in this chapter we will use the term *control group* or *controls.*

All longitudinal studies are briefly summarized in Table W8.2 on the accompanying Web site. Six of the 39 longitudinal studies, dealing with such themes as the influence on patients of anxiety, depression, and stress surrounding the interventions, were published before 1990 and therefore are not described in detail (Blumlein, Anderson, Barboriak, & Rimm, 1977; Davies Osterkamp & Salm, 1980; W. Freeman, Pichard, & Smith, 1981; Raft, McKee, Popio, & Haggerty, 1985; Richter, Richter, Leistner, & Toellner, 1989; Salm, 1982).

8.4.3.1. Coping studies. Coping mechanisms were assessed in 11 longitudinal studies. These studies focused on patient expectations and stress in the context of invasive cardiological diagnosis and therapy. One very well qualified study (Jordan, 1991) and three well-qualified studies involving the same Finnish sample (Heikkila, Paunonen, Laippala, & Virtanen, 1998, 1999; Heikkila, Paunonen, Virtanen, & Laippala, 1998) reported generally low levels of anxiety among patients. Younger and female patients showed higher levels of anxiety during the intervention period than older and male patients. Anxiety decreased steadily in both sexes as soon as the procedure was over. It is interesting that patients who had had previous angiographies showed higher levels of anxiety than patients experiencing the intervention for the first time.

Patient anxiety most frequently involved uncertainty about the course of the illness, the possible necessity of a bypass operation, and even death (Heikkila, Paunonen, Virtanen, & Laippala, 1998; Hütter, 1994). Female patients felt more anxiety about pain and the lack of time spent with the medical staff, and male patients more often reported problems and fears concerning sexuality (Heikkila, Paunonen, Virtanen, & Laippala, 1999).

Jordan (1991) concluded that an anxious or depressive attitude led to increased stress during the intervention; as a consequence, some of Jordan's data suggest worse results and more frequent complications during or following the intervention. These findings must be replicated in future studies. In contrast, another very well qualified study (Röckle, 1999) found no significant differences between patients with depression or anxiety and less anxious patients in regard to PTCA results. They found only a tendency toward increased complications or restenosis in patients with depression or anxiety. This study supports previous results (Hütter, 1994; Jordan, 1991) indicating that stress

and the course of the illness after angiography and PTCA are determined less by objective factors than by psychological parameters. These results also require confirmation in further studies.

Two publications (Gulanick & Naito, 1994; Jordan, 1991) found that most patients have great confidence in their attending physicians and in medical technology. The patients assessed the benefits of PTCA positively (after 1 week, 72% of patients; after 3 months, 86%). These high expectations can lead to problematic illness-related behaviors and could influence the disease course unfavorably. Many patients assess their self-efficacy in regard to cardiac risk factors and restenosis as high, consistent with their reports of significantly improved mood following PTCA (Gulanick & Naito, 1994; S. Perkins & Jenkins, 1998). We will not describe two studies in detail because of their methodological deficiencies (Albrecht, Ostermann, Franzen, & Höpp, 1995; Cason, Russell, & Fincher, 1992; see Table W8.2 for summaries).

8.4.3.2. Quality of life studies. In the 13 publications exploring patients' QoL in the context of an invasive cardiac procedure, various instruments (e.g., questionnaires such as the Functional Status Questionnaire [Jette et al., 1986], General Health Questionnaire [Goldberg, 1978], or Quality of Life Index [Ferrans & Powers, 1985]) were used to investigate both general and health-related QoL and psychological and physical well-being. Four very well qualified and two well-qualified studies reported significantly improved feelings of both physical and psychological health following PTCA (Bliley & Ferrans, 1993; Cleary et al., 1991; Englehart, 1993; Fitzgerald, 1996; McKenna et al., 1992, 1994). Factors in this improvement were a reduction in angina pectoris symptoms and dyspnea, increased physical activity and emotional well-being, and improved social and sexual performance. This improvement in QoL, especially the reduction in angina pectoris, was observed in the early phase ($p < .001$), but 1 year following the PTCA, feelings of health no longer continued to improve (with the exception of a marked reduction in cardiac risk factors; Bliley & Ferrans, 1993; Englehart, 1993; McKenna, 1995; McKenna et al., 1992, 1994). A less qualified study (small sample, high dropout rate) reached the opposite results (Faris & Stotts, 1990); no significant improvement was observed in QoL within the first 6 weeks after the intervention. These authors did, however, find a significant reduction in state anxiety and an increase in performance.

A very well qualified publication focused on the relationship between vital exhaustion and CHD (Kop, Appels, Mendes de Leon, de Swart, & Bar, 1993). Average exhaustion scores (the cutoff score indicating exhaustion is >11) decreased from 20 before the PTCA to 16.5 at 2 weeks following the intervention and 11.7 at 6 months follow-up. Furthermore, a positive correlation existed between vital exhaustion and extent of CHD. The number of exhausted patients did not decrease significantly, however (of 90 patients, only 5 improved substantially), and the presence of angina pectoris symptoms did not influence these results significantly.

Two partially qualified studies (Kähler et al., 1999; Little et al., 1993) showed only minimal differences in risks and costs of PTCA for geriatric (> 80 years) patients compared with younger ones. See Table W8.2 for summaries.

A very well qualified study administered a QoL examination to patients experiencing different cardiac events or procedures. In one of two articles on this study, Westin, Carlsson, Erhardt, Cantor, and McNeil (1999) compared the QoL (after 1 month and 1 year) of female and male patients using nine QoL dimensions. Women displayed significantly worse results in the areas of general health, anxiety, and depression. In comparison with the control groups (acute myocardial infarction, $n = 296$; bypass, $n = 99$; PTCA, $n = 18$; healthy controls, $n = 88$) the patients scored lower in the dimensions of chest pain and arrhythmia. In addition, female patients showed worse results in general health and male patients in sexual matters.

In the other article on this study, Westin et al. (1997) found that the PTCA, CABG, and acute myocardial infarction groups displayed worse results in the dimensions of arrhythmia, chest pain, and self-confidence (after 1 year, in the case of arrhythmia) in comparison with the control group. In the remaining QoL dimensions, the results of the

PTCA patients were similar to those of the control group after 1 month, and there were no significant differences after 1 year. Within the patient groups, the PTCA patients displayed better results in the areas of anxiety, sexual matters, and general health after 1 month, but this difference was no longer significant at 1-year follow-up.

8.4.3.3. Comparison of percutaneous transluminal coronary angioplasty with coronary artery bypass grafting or pharmacological treatment.

Nine studies assessed differences in QoL and functional status between PTCA and bypass surgery patients with partly contradictory results. Three very well qualified and well-qualified studies, among them a multicenter study from Sweden (Allen, Fitzgerald, Swank, & Becker, 1990; Papadantonaki, Stotts, & Paul, 1994; Währborg, 1999), found better physical and social performance and mood in PTCA patients 3 weeks and 6 months after the procedure. However, after 1 year, the bypass patients were not significantly different from the PTCA patients in these aspects or in general well-being; in some aspects they showed a tendency to perform better.

Three studies, two very well qualified (McGee, Graham, Crowe, & Horgan, 1993; Pocock, Henderson, Seed, Treasure, & Hampton, 1996) and one partially qualified (Skaggs & Yates, 1999), concluded that PTCA patients showed a significantly higher prevalence of angina pectoris symptoms than bypass patients (20.0% and 1.4%, respectively) after 1 month and at 1- to 3-year follow-up; PTCA patients also experienced more limitations in everyday activities ($p = .05$). However, bypass patients displayed significantly more general complications. Three months after the intervention, QoL was assessed similarly highly by both groups; of possible scores of 0 to 30, PTCA patients scored an average of 22.3 and bypass patients 25.7. The rates of return to work were about the same in both groups of patients (PTCA 68%, bypass 59%), but PTCA patients resumed work significantly earlier.

A very well qualified study by W. Strauss, Fortin, Hartigan, Folland, and Parisi (1995) investigated QoL, physical capacity, and restenosis in PTCA patients in comparison with those receiving pharmacological treatment. The groups had similar QoL scores, physical activity scores, and rates of restenosis before the start of treatment. At 6-month follow-up, the PTCA patients had significantly higher QoL scores ($p = .02$) and activity scores ($p = .01$) and significantly lower rates of restenosis (55% of PTCA patients vs. 7% of patients treated pharmacologically). Scores on the Physical/Psychological subscale of the Quality of Life Index correlated strongly with physical activity scores ($p < .001$).

A well-qualified study by R. E. White and Frasure-Smith (1995) measured differences in uncertainty and psychological stress between PTCA and bypass patients and the influence of social support on these parameters. PTCA patients were more insecure ($p < .05$) but not significantly more stressed than bypass patients 1 to 3 months after the procedure. A high level of social support led to a significant reduction in psychological stress in PTCA patients ($p < .01$), whereas stress levels in bypass patients remained basically constant. The authors explained the differential effects of social support by citing differences in the types of treatment: PTCA is a relatively uncomplicated procedure requiring little or no social support, whereas patients who undergo bypass surgery require more assistance following the procedure. These results indicate the importance of support from family members and medical staff. The authors concluded that better social support for patients after PTCA could improve their psychological well-being.

A partially qualified study (Blumenthal et al., 1991) tested the cognitive performance of PTCA, bypass, and heart valve surgery patients using five neuropsychological tests; see Table W8.2 on the accompanying Web site for a brief description.

8.4.3.4. Summary of longitudinal studies. The results of the longitudinal studies indicate that the majority of patients showed low levels of anxiety in the context of a coronary angiography and PTCA. Those who reported medium to high levels of anxiety tended to be younger or female. Patients receiving a repeat angiography displayed higher levels of anxiety than patients undergoing the procedure for the first time. Herrmann-Lingen (1998) reported

that clinically relevant anxiety (i.e., general anxiety disorders) appeared in about 10% of internal medicine department patients. This author found that 25% to 30% of cardiac and general medicine patients had elevated results for anxiety and depression on the Hospital Anxiety and Depression Scale (Zigmond & Snaith, 1983). Significantly more female patients displayed anxiety than male patients (27% vs. 16%).

Among the most common feelings concerning the interventions are uncertainty about the future course of the illness and anxiety about the necessity of bypass surgery. Additionally, female patients worry about possible pain and lack of care, whereas male patients worry about sexual matters and lack of mobility after the procedure. Anxious or depressive patients display a higher degree of psychological distress and increased discomfort during PTCA compared with less anxious patients. Anxiety has been shown to negatively influence the results of therapy and the course of illness, but the extent of the influence has been assessed in different ways, so further research is needed to confirm these results.

To reduce patients' anxiety and increase their self-efficacy during a coronary procedure, medical staff should ask targeted questions about their sensory and pain experiences and engage them in dialogue. Additionally, social support by family members can reduce patients' psychological stress considerably. Most patients trust their attending physicians and medical technology to a great degree, and most report a positive assessment of PTCA after the procedure, which may lead to unrealistically high expectations regarding their prognosis and may discourage them from changing risk behaviors. Patients also gauge highly their own efficacy at addressing cardiac risk factors and making the necessary changes in behavior. To maintain a high level of motivation over the long run, regular contact with rehabilitation and other medical personnel is helpful.

The influence of PTCA on QoL has been assessed inconsistently both within and among the different samples. Most publications report a significant improvement in patients' physical and psychological feelings of health, reduced angina pectoris symptoms and dyspnea, better emotional well-being, and improved social and sexual functioning. One publication, however, showed no improvement in QoL in most of its sample.

Comparisons of QoL and functional status in PTCA and bypass patients have showed contradictory results. Some found better physical, social, and emotional functioning in PTCA patients 6 months after the procedure but no significant differences between groups after 1 year. Others found no differences in QoL for the two patient groups even in the early phase but higher rates of complications in bypass patients and of chest pain in PTCA patients.

8.4.4. Prospective Studies

Table 8.1 describes the method we used to evaluate the quality of the prospective studies for soft and hard endpoints. If a study used both soft and hard endpoints, we used the hard endpoints in rating its quality. We eliminated five studies with the endpoint of work status and two with the endpoint of transfer for cardiac catheterization from the review because these fields of research are not applicable to the topic of this chapter. The instruments used, target variables, and endpoints of the selected studies are listed in Table W8.3 on the accompanying Web site.

Only one of the 19 prospective studies was published before 1990. Shaw et al. (1986) focused on whether a disjunction between coping style and appropriateness of information provided was predictive of coronary complications and restenosis within 6 months following PTCA.

8.4.4.1. Studies with hard endpoints. Nine studies published since 1990 used a hard endpoint. Three very well qualified studies from a Dutch work group (Appels, Kop, Bär, de Swart, & Mendes de Leon, 1995; Kop, Appels, Mendes de Leon, de Swart, & Bar, 1994; Mendes de Leon, Kop, de Swart, Bar, & Appels, 1996) focused on vital exhaustion as a risk factor for new cardiac events after PTCA. Twice as many patients with vital exhaustion as without it (35% vs. 17%) experienced a serious cardiac event (e.g., myocardial infarction, bypass surgery), and their illnesses had a significantly more unfavorable course ($p < .02$) than nonexhausted patients. Vital exhaustion and

anger were independent risk factors for recurrent cardiac events following PTCA. Forty-five percent of the patients with both risk factors (i.e., anger and vital exhaustion), 26% of the patients with one of the risk factors, and 7% of the patients with neither factor had recurrent cardiac events.

These articles were based on one empirical study with the same sample. The instrument used to measure vital exhaustion was the Maastricht Questionnaire (Appels, Höppener, & Mulder, 1987), but the authors used different cutoff points for vital exhaustion. Kop et al. (1994) classified patients as exhausted if they exceeded a score of 18; Mendes de Leon et al. (1996) used 19 as the cutoff; and Appels et al. (1995) did not mention a cutoff score.

Three studies examined the predictive influence of psychosocial variables on the occurrence or extent of restenosis after PTCA. A very well qualified study by Joksimovic et al. (1999) investigated whether overcommitment was an independent predictor for restenosis 6 or 12 months after PTCA. Overcommitted men who were older than 55 years and who had a low high-density lipoprotein (HDL) level had the highest risk of restenosis (>70%).

Another very well qualified study by Titscher, Huber, Ambros, Gruska, and Gaul (1996) focused on the relationship between the extent of restenosis and psychosocial factors. Resigned coping, depressive coping, and self-pity correlated significantly with the risk of restenosis. Whether a patient would develop a restenosis within 3 months after PTCA could be predicted significantly ($p = .0024$) using a discrimination analysis of the scales from a coping questionnaire.

A partially qualified study by Goodman, Quigley, Moran, Meilman, and Sherman (1996) investigated the predictive value of hostility for restenosis. In this study, hostility was the only significant predictor for restenosis; other variables, such as sex and ethnicity, were not predictive but correlated highly with hostility. The highest scores were found in male and White patients and the lowest scores in female and African American patients. Notably, African American patients showed a higher rate of restenosis than patients with high hostility scores.

A very well qualified study by van Domburg, Schmidt-Pedersen, and van den Brand (2001) investigated the predictive significance of feelings of powerlessness and despair for 10-year mortality following PTCA. Women scored significantly higher for feelings of powerlessness and despair ($p < .001$) and lower for well-being ($p < .0001$) than men; these differences were minimized after adjusting for other factors. Feelings of powerlessness, age, diabetes, and ejection fraction were predictive of mortality in male patients; in female patients, hypertension and previous myocardial infarction were predictive. Thus, feelings of powerlessness appear to be predictive only for men, and not for women, over a period of 10 years following PTCA.

A very well qualified study by C. Herrmann, Buss, Lingen, and Kreuzer (1998) investigated how well personality and bodily complaints measured before undergoing angiography could predict the course of bodily complaints over 2 years. It is interesting that patients without CHD showed (before the angiography) significantly higher scores on a complaints questionnaire than patients with a CHD diagnosis ($p < .00005$). Somatic parameters, especially heart complaints, could be predicted accurately only in patients without CHD ($p < .00005$; predictors used were variables from a personality questionnaire). For patients with diagnosed CHD, only predictors for anxiety and depression could be determined. In summary, 2 years after angiography, patients with negative results experienced more bodily complaints than did patients diagnosed with CHD.

8.4.4.2. Studies with soft endpoints.

Nine of the prospective studies investigated soft endpoints. In addition to the study by C. Herrmann, et al. (1998), described in section 8.4.4.1, another very well qualified study (Brummett et al., 1998) focused on the predictive significance of depression and social support for depressive symptoms 1 month after PTCA. Both variables predicted depressive symptoms after the procedure; hostility was only an indirect predictor in combination with social support. Factors such as age, sex, and severity of the illness did not influence the development of depressive symptoms significantly.

Various studies assessed factors that determine QoL or state of health and long-term course of CHD following PTCA. In the British multicenter study called Randomized Intervention Treatment of Angina—II (Pocock, Henderson, Clayton, Lyman, & Chamberlain, 2000), QoL of PTCA patients was compared with that of pharmacologically treated patients. Both patient groups showed an improvement in QoL within the 1st year after the procedure or initiation of medication; however, PTCA patients displayed significantly higher QoL scores and less frequent and also less pronounced angina pectoris symptoms, a disparity that after 3 years no longer existed. The differences in QoL scores in the 1st year may have been determined by the occurrence of angina pectoris. The best predictors for the dependent QoL variables bodily function, vitality, and general health were angina pectoris and shortness of breath.

A 5-year multicenter study from the United States (Hlatky et al., 1997) found that the physical stamina of patients who had had bypass surgery improved significantly in the first 3 years after the procedure compared with PTCA patients ($p = .02$). Emotional health improved significantly in both groups without relevant differences ($p < .001$). Predictors for the combination of physical functional status and mental health were sex, education, and age. Predictors for physical status only were cardiac insufficiency and diabetes mellitus.

A study by Schröder et al. (2000) investigated the long-term course of PTCA patients. Four measurement points were reported: before PTCA (medical data from the center), immediately after PTCA (medical data from the center), 3 months after PTCA (medical data from the center), and 38 to 52 months after PTCA (questionnaire). This study had a large sample ($N = 549$), but because of methodological problems, we rated it as only well qualified. Retrospective data were obtained 3 to 4 years after the procedure by questionnaire. Sixty percent of patients complained less of acute angina pectoris symptoms than before the PTCA. The authors concluded that a successful primary intervention is a significant predictor for positive long-term recovery. Furthermore, there was a close positive correlation between angina pectoris symptoms and the subjective assessment of QoL.

Two very well qualified studies investigated the physical health of patients 1 and 3 years following PTCA (Permanyer et al., 1999; Tooth, McKenna, & Maas, 1999). Both studies found significantly improved physical condition (physical and psychological functional status) following PTCA (*p* < .001); physical condition did not change significantly between the early phase (to 4 months post-PTCA) and the late phase of recovery.

Another very well qualified study reached a different conclusion (Franzen, Nicolai, Schannwell, Albrecht, & Höpp, 1993). In this study, 66% of patients without restenosis (4 months after a successful PTCA) felt worse than before the procedure, and only 3% felt better. None of the predictors—angina pectoris symptoms, restenosis, earlier myocardial infarction, risk factors, and comorbidity—were perceived as significant predictors of the subjective well-being of the patients. The authors concluded that objective cardiac parameters are less decisive for feelings of physical well-being and patient rehabilitation than psychosocial factors, which were not a focus of this study.

Permanyer et al. (1999), in a subgroup analysis, ascertained a significantly improved state of health (*p* < .05) only for patients without angina pectoris, myocardial infarction, or recurrent revascularization; patients with rest-related angina, dyspnea, or a second revascularization showed no significant improvement in their state of health. Significant predictors for a change in state of health were the base score of the overall score on the Nottingham Health Profile (Hunt, McKenna, McEwen, Williams, & Papp, 1981), comorbidity, and stable or unstable angina (*p* < .01). Tooth et al. (1999) found four predictors of physical and psychological functional status: chest pain, shortness of breath during stressful situations, vocational status, and duration of CHD (*p* < .01).

In a well-qualified study, Kimble (1998) investigated PTCA patients' cognitive assessment of the procedure in relation to psychological parameters. Patient expectations were generally optimistic

(mean score of 3.46 on a scale of 1 to 5). Patients' assessments of the procedure as positive and physical feelings of well-being increased in the period shortly before the PTCA and remained constant until 2 to 3 weeks afterwards (*p* < .001), whereas the perceived threat from CHD remained unchanged. Perceived threat was also the only significant predictor for physical feelings of well-being (*p* < .01), whereas optimism, assessment of the procedure, and previous PTCA had no significant influence.

In a very well qualified study by Leibing, Schünemann, Herrmann, and Rüger (1998), the authors investigated the incidence of psychological symptoms and disorders in a sample of patients undergoing a coronary angiography and examined which factors predicted a diagnostic finding. Half of the 40 patients examined showed no angiographic finding; of these, 12 had a psychological disorder, usually an anxiety disorder. Of the 20 patients with angiographically confirmed CHD, only 5 had a psychological disorder. Sociodemographic factors (e.g., age), duration of illness, and significant results on psychological questionnaires were significant predictors for a CHD diagnosis and explained 42% of the variance.

Using highly sophisticated methods, de Jong et al. (1994) investigated the extent to which state and trait anxiety, heart rate, and skin resistance could be predicted shortly before cardiac catheterization by measuring anxiety in patients at home 3 weeks before the procedure. Trait anxiety was relatively unchanged at the two measurement points. State anxiety, in contrast, rose significantly shortly before the procedure; this rise was more clearly perceptible in female patients (*p* < .001) than in male patients (*p* < .01). The intercorrelation among psychological and physiological variables was minimal, as was the correlation among the physiological parameters. Heart rate and skin resistance significantly increased during the interview, regardless of sex. Patients' at-home state anxiety, sex, and age were significant predictors of state anxiety shortly before the procedure, accounting for 62% of the variance. Trait anxiety, defense mechanisms, and coping behavior had no noteworthy predictive significance.

8.4.4.3. Summary of prospective studies.

The prospective studies selected for this review provide evidence for the following preliminary conclusions:

- The soft endpoints of depression and social support were found to be independent predictors of depressive symptoms following PTCA. Age and sex played no significant role in depression. Age, sex, and state anxiety 3 weeks before PTCA were predictive of state anxiety just before the procedure.

- The soft endpoints of QoL and state of health, measured using validated QoL questionnaires, were related mainly to cardiac predictors: severity and duration of CHD or angina pectoris symptoms, dyspnea, comorbidity, and the success of the primary intervention. One study found a significant improvement in state of health only for patients without angina, myocardial infarction, or renewed revascularization.

- The hard endpoint of restenosis was predicted using the psychosocial variables of overcommitment in correlation with age and HDL values, coping style (e.g., resigned approach to stress), and hostility in correlation with sex and ethnicity.

- The hard endpoints of cardiac events and mortality were predicted using psychosocial, medical, and sociodemographic factors. About half of patients displaying both vital exhaustion and anger had a renewed cardiac event. In male patients, feelings of powerlessness, age, and diabetes predicted mortality; in female patients, hypertension and previous myocardial infarctions were predictors.

8.4.5. Intervention Studies

We located 22 intervention studies in our literature search. As shown in Table W8.4, these studies show significant deficiencies in methodological quality: We classified half of them as partially or less qualified. Only two publications (from the same study) are very well qualified. No replication studies have been published; future intervention studies will require improvements in methodology to enable replication.

We did not exclude intervention studies published before 1990, as in previous sections of this chapter; 11 of the studies (50%) appeared before 1990. All of the publications that appeared later than 1990 were conducted on patients waiting for an angiography or PTCA. In situations necessitating acute cardiac intervention, it is presumably not possible to conduct a psychological intervention study, at least not with a randomized controlled design. For this reason, we decided to report all available results. Not included in this section are studies initiated shortly after the cardiac interventions (catheter, angiography, PTCA) focusing on secondary prevention (e.g., to reduce cardiovascular risk factors or to increase health-promoting behaviors).

In this section we will examine two types of intervention: educational interventions and psychological interventions. Twelve studies described educational interventions and examined the effects of information provision on patients (Davis, Maguire, Haraphongse, & Schaumberger, 1994a, 1994b; Finesilver, 1978; K. S. Herrmann & Kreuzer, 1989; Hill, Baker, Warner, & Taub, 1988; Lamb, 1984; Lloyd, Cooper, & Jackson, 1997; M. C. Murphy, Fishman, & Shaw, 1989; Peterson, 1991; Rice, Siegreen, Mullin, & Williams, 1988; Tooth, McKenna, & Maas, 1998; Tooth, McKenna, Maas, & McEniery, 1997). Ten studies described interventions that had psychological content and were based on an explicit psychological theory (Appels, Bar, Lasker, Flamm, & Kop, 1997; Black, Allison, Williams, Rummans, & Gau, 1998; Davis et al., 1994b; Frenn, Fehring, & Kartes, 1986; Kendall et al., 1979; Lisspers et al., 1999; Mott, 1999; Rice, Caldwell, Butler, & Robinson, 1986; Schultheis, 1987; E. J. Weinstein & Au, 1991). In both groups of studies, we evaluated half of the selected articles as very well qualified or well qualified and half as partially or less qualified. Table W8.4 provides brief descriptions and lists the qualifications of these studies.

To rate the quality of interventions in a uniform way, we established the following six criteria and assigned points based on the number of criteria met (see Table 8.1):

1. Qualified staff administered the intervention, or qualified materials (e.g., videos, brochures) were used.
2. The intervention is clearly and thoroughly described.
3. The groups were randomly selected.
4. There was a control group or an attention placebo group or both.
5. There were 15 or more persons in each treatment group.
6. Results demonstrated differential outcomes.

The classification of quality was complicated by wide variations in the characteristics of the interventions and the dosages participants received. Interventions ranged in complication from a 10-minute videotape of information about the cardiac procedure to complex psychological interventions with assessment of numerous variables. Most publications provide only short descriptions of the intervention, the qualifications of staff administering the intervention, and the materials or videos presented to participants. They do not provide sufficient detail to allow an evaluation of the clinical quality of the interventions, and replication studies usually are not possible without contacting the authors.

Nearly all studies lacked a so-called "attention placebo group." A simple control group of persons who receive "standard care" is not sufficient for this kind of study, because of the justified assumption that only the attention of an examiner or clinical staff member during the waiting period (or control condition) can comfort and calm the patient. Therefore, well-designed intervention studies have both a classic control group and an attention placebo group to control for this generalized social effect. An attention placebo group is helpful because unspecific social attention influences a patient waiting for a medical intervention, and the effects of a professional psychological intervention can only be measured if results are compared with a control group and an attention placebo group. The attention placebo group is informed, for example, that a person will talk with them to help them relax. The technique of the therapist is nondirective and active listening, focusing on the patients' jobs, families, or interests. The patient is allowed to steer the conversation (Kendall et al., 1979). Because this research design was used in only four of the 22 studies (K. Anderson & Masur, 1989; Hill et al., 1988; Kendall et al., 1979; Peterson, 1991; Hill et al. and Peterson included an attention placebo group but did not name it as such), we have not assessed it as a central criterion, in spite of its importance.

The mean sample size of the 22 studies was 67.7 (SD = 42.8). On the basis of this mean, we would have assigned 1 point for samples of fewer than 25 subjects, 2 points for samples of 26 to 110 subjects, and 3 points for samples of more than 110 subjects. However, because these values are very close to those used in the previous sections and in chapters 2 and 5 of this volume, we decided to follow the established categories for sample size.

Sixteen of the studies examined intervention techniques intended to influence psychological variables. The intervention techniques included audio- and videotaped presentations of medical, procedural, and sensory information and information about risk factors; modeling of positive behaviors, either in person or via audio- or videotape; provision of information brochures; personal counseling at the bedside; personal counseling at home with family members; relaxation techniques; multimodal cognitive–behavioral interventions for relaxation, breathing, or cognitive structuring; discussions; interviews; and individually designed multimodal interventions. Individually designed interventions are clinically quite reasonable but inappropriate for a research study. In some cases, the interventions could be classified as routine or standard care.

The psychological variables assessed included anxiety (before and following the intervention), patients' knowledge about the intervention, QoL of partners, psychological stress, vital exhaustion, questionnaire scores, other psychological variables (e.g., Type A behavior, external locus of control), medical parameters (e.g., body mass index, cholesterol, blood pressure), and external ratings of patient anxiety or stress (by nurses or other medical personnel). Together with the other methodological problems we have described, this variety in intervention strategies and variables makes comparison of the studies very difficult.

Before describing the studies in detail, we provide a short overview of the effects they achieved. Sixteen of the 22 studies at least partially achieved the targeted effects with their interventions, and 6 could show no effects. The studies with no appreciable effects (Frenn et al., 1986; Hill et al., 1988; Peterson, 1991; Rice et al., 1986, 1988; Schultheis, 1987) were predominantly qualified as methodologically insufficient. Two of these studies (Peterson, 1991; Rice et al., 1988) did not target any effects, because they compared two different interventions and had no control group. In both studies one of the intervention groups could be considered an attention placebo group, and their findings indicate that social interaction may produce effects similar to those of a complex psychological intervention. The other four studies with negative findings had very small sample sizes and provided a low intervention dosage (e.g., a 10-minute audiotape or a single relaxation exercise), so only small effects could be expected.

The various interventions described in these studies provided different dosages to bring about the targeted effects. They appear to have provided systematic, planned, and professionally delivered preintervention information about CHD, the necessity of lifestyle modifications, procedural aspects and intervention techniques, and expected sensory experiences. Their results indicate that videotaped presentations, information brochures of high quality, and personally communicated information are very helpful and welcome to patients.

Long-term effects (measured at 6 or more months) on lifestyle cannot be expected from such limited and low-dosage interventions. Several psychological interventions had favorable influences on anxiety, stress, and other variables. However, research results concerning differential therapy indications are contradictory. Questionnaire and interview results can be used to identify subgroups for whom targeted interventions could be developed (see Black et al., 1998). Some studies found measurable effects in the attention placebo group, indicating that social attention by medical staff may produce significant effects. These studies also found that early in the cardiac intervention, patients experience the highest levels of anxiety and

would benefit most from encouragement and support from medical staff.

8.4.5.1. Psychological interventions.

Ten of the 22 intervention studies can be classified as psychological intervention studies. These interventions included cognitive–behavioral interventions to help patients reduce anxiety or learn more effective coping strategies, special relaxation methods or stress management techniques, and even hypnosis. The planning and delivery of these interventions systematically incorporated psychological and scientific knowledge and generally required certain qualifications of the staff.

We categorized five of the psychological intervention studies as methodologically very well qualified or well qualified. The oldest study was published in 1979, the most recent in 1999. Two studies analyzed cardiac catheterization interventions (K. O. Anderson & Masur, 1989; Kendall et al., 1979), two analyzed PTCA patients (Appels, Bär, et al., 1997; Lisspers et al., 1999), and one analyzed a mixed sample of patients after acute myocardial infarction, bypass surgery, or PTCA (Black et al., 1998).

K. O. Anderson and Masur's (1989) study design included four intervention groups and one attention placebo group. The four interventions consisted of 20-minute videotapes providing (a) procedural and sensory information, (b) modeling of positive behaviors, (c) cognitive–behavioral techniques (e.g., coping styles), and (d) a combination of (c) and (d). The combined sample of 60 was relatively small.

In the oldest and methodologically best study, Kendall et al. (1979) compared a group receiving cognitive–behavioral intervention, a group receiving an educational intervention, an attention placebo group, and an additional control group. Unfortunately, the sample was very small ($N = 44$) for such a complex and well-executed examination.

Appels, Bär, et al. (1997) provided a 16-hour multimodal intervention that targeted increased relaxation, lowered hostility, and improvements in psychological state variables to a sample of PTCA patients. In another study on PTCA, Lisspers et al. (1999) offered their intervention group a high-dosage program with different modules; unfortunately, the program description is unclear. The program began with an inpatient intervention over 4 weeks and continued on an outpatient basis for approximately 1 year. This program targeted different variables such as physical activity, nutrition, weight, psychological factors, and QoL in addition to cardiac events.

Black et al. (1998) selected 60 of 380 coronary patients after a clinical screening (using the SCL-90; Derogatis, 2000) and randomized them into an intervention group and a control group. The authors classified the intervention as cognitive–behavioral, but their description is unclear. It seems that a psychiatrist talked with the patients at the bedside, offered relaxation training or stress management if necessary, provided support, and recommended a reduction in risk factors.

Except for the study by Black et al. (1998), these interventions mostly accomplished their intended effects: They reduced anxiety, improved coping during and after the intervention, promoted lifestyle changes, and achieved significant effects in reducing cardiac events after the intervention. The multimodal interventions had better results than the simpler interventions. It is not possible to draw a conclusion about the required dosage because of the differences among the interventions. More studies are needed that not only examine different types of interventions, but also provide dosage–effect guidelines. The studies we classified as partially or less qualified (Frenn et al., 1986; Mott, 1999; Rice et al., 1986; Schultheis, 1987; E. J. Weinstein & Au, 1991) are summarized in Table W8.4.

8.4.5.2. Educational interventions. Educational interventions informed patients about the intervention and described its potential complications using audio- or videotapes, information brochures, and dialogue. Ten of the studies we selected were designed to provide information about the cardiac intervention or illness. Two studies (Frenn et al., 1986; E. J. Weinstein & Au, 1991) measured the effects of the interventions mainly on medical parameters.

We categorized half of the 12 educational intervention studies as very well qualified (Davis et al.,

1994a, 1994b) or well qualified (K. S. Herrmann & Kreuzer, 1989; Rice et al., 1988; Tooth et al., 1997, 1998). The oldest study was published in 1978, the most recent in 1998. Seven studies examined cardiac catheterizations (Davis et al., 1994a, 1994b; Finesilver, 1978; K. S. Herrmann & Kreuzer, 1989; Hill et al., 1988; Lamb, 1984; Peterson, 1991), 2 assessed angiography patients (Lloyd et al., 1997; Rice et al., 1988), and 3 examined PTCA patients (M. C. Murphy et al., 1989; Tooth et al., 1997, 1998).

The very well qualified publications by Davis et al. (1994a, 1994b) used the largest sample of the intervention studies ($N = 145$). They used a questionnaire about self-reported anxiety, nurses' ratings of patient behaviors, and cardiovascular parameters to assess the influence of educational interventions on coping styles and anxiety levels in the course of cardiac catheterization. The patients were randomized into three intervention groups and were assessed with questionnaires to examine their coping styles.

In a randomized controlled study, K. S. Herrmann and Kreuzer (1989) analyzed the extent to which videotaped information contributed to anxiety reduction in cardiac catheterization patients. The treatment and control groups were both informed about the intervention by a cardiologist for about 7 minutes, and the intervention group received an additional 14-minute videotaped introduction before the discussion with the cardiologist.

Rice et al. (1988) randomized a relatively low number of patients about to undergo coronary angiography ($N = 40$) to control and intervention groups. The intervention group listened to a 10-minute audiotape that explained the coronary angiography procedure.

Tooth et al. (1997, 1998) described the effects of an educational and advisory program for two groups of PTCA patients and their spouses ($N = 125$ and $N = 160$). The intervention group participated in a 2-hour multimedia program consisting of an interview, a book, a videotape, and a demonstration of a balloon catheterization. In addition to differences in sociodemographic data between the control and intervention groups, this intervention was provided at each patient's home and thus may not have been uniform. Therefore, it would be difficult to replicate this study to confirm its results.

Davis et al.'s (1994a, 1994b) very well qualified study showed no significant differences in anxiety related to type of intervention or patient coping style. Significant differences were found only with respect to the measurement point: Patients experienced the highest anxiety level at the beginning of the catheterization procedure. K. S. Herrmann and Kreuzer (1989) showed significantly lower anxiety levels in the intervention group (which received an additional video presentation) in comparison to the control group. In addition, the intervention group described the intervention as very helpful. Tooth et al. (1997, 1998) published similar results; their intervention group showed lower anxiety levels than the control group and significantly greater knowledge about the intervention, and their family members also benefited greatly from the educational program. Rice et al. (1988) also found positive effects from an audiotape intervention. The patients experienced less negative mood before and after the intervention compared with the control group.

In conclusion, audio- or videotapes have been found to be a simple and effective way of reducing patient anxiety before a coronary intervention and should be used to complement interviews. Furthermore, the results show that better-informed patients (and family members) can develop more realistic expectations and experience the intervention more positively.

The six partially qualified or less qualified studies (Finesilver, 1978; Hill et al., 1988; Lamb, 1984; Lloyd et al., 1997; M. C. Murphy et al., 1989; Peterson, 1991) are summarized in Table W8.4. Only the study by Peterson used a sufficient design, but because of the small sample size, we classified it as partially qualified. These studies found significantly lower anxiety levels in the intervention and attention placebo groups, providing further evidence that support by medical staff is an important factor in reducing patients' anxiety.

8.4.5.3. Summary of intervention studies. The methodological quality of educational and psycho-logical intervention studies of patients undergoing a cardiac procedure has significant limitations. Many articles are older and may be obsolete, and half of them are insufficiently methodologically qualified; only two articles from the same study were very well qualified. No replication studies have been published. In most cases, the description of the content of the interventions is not sufficiently detailed, and the professional qualifications of the staff are often unclear.

Several tentative conclusions can be drawn, however. The few studies that included an attention placebo group suggest that interpersonal attention by medical personnel beyond the standard care can yield positive effects. Some studies indicate that intended effects can be achieved and that patients profit. Because anxiety levels are highest during the first phase of the cardiac procedure, dialogue, encouragement, and support by medical personnel are indicated.

Various interventions achieved satisfactory levels of targeted change: anxiety reduction, improved coping during and after the procedure, decreases in health risk behaviors, and even considerable and significant effects on physical well-being after the intervention. Multimodal interventions achieved better results. Components of successful interventions include modeling of positive behaviors, provision of information about the procedure and sensory experiences to expect, and above all psychologically oriented videotape presentations. Further studies with improved designs are required to draw more definitive conclusions.

The methodologically soundest studies allow some clinical conclusions. It is helpful to thoroughly inform the patients before the intervention about the following:

- the etiology of coronary heart disease,
- the targets of the intervention and the resulting consequences,
- the techniques involved,
- the procedure used during the intervention, and
- sensory experiences that can be expected during the intervention.

This information can be conveyed in written form or using an audio- or videotape; a combination may be most effective. Written material allows patients to read and reread about the intervention, and videotapes can model positive behaviors. Cognitive–behavioral methods have also proved valuable but are difficult when there are time constraints.

During the intervention, and especially during the first phase, active communication and encouragement by medical personnel are critical. Patients and their family members should be encouraged to ask questions, talk about their fears, and explore the patient's sensory experiences. This support has a calming effect and improves trust. Support for these recommendations comes not from controlled intervention studies, but rather from the results of interviews with the involved patients.

8.4.6. Reviews and Expert Reports

Only four reviews are available regarding psychological aspects of undergoing a coronary procedure. Two reviews addressed the methodologically interesting question of generalizability of results, medically as well as psychologically. Pickering (1985) and Ragland, Helmer, and Seeman (1991) concluded that definite and partially uncontrolled selection effects can be expected.

Two other reviews focused on clinical considerations. K. O. Anderson and Masur (1983) reviewed the state of the research concerning the psychological preparation of patients for medical diagnostic techniques in general; PTCA in particular was mentioned only briefly. The analysis was not based on a systematic search of scientific databases, but it appears to be complete. These authors divided the existing interventions to prepare people for cardiac procedures into information, psychotherapy, modeling, behavioral, cognitive–behavioral, and hypnosis interventions. The authors concluded that the empirical evidence suggests a continuous relationship between anxiety and outcome: The higher the level of anxiety, the worse the coping result. Concerning cardiac catheterization and PTCA, the authors reviewed three articles (Cassell, 1965; Finesilver, 1978; Kendall et al., 1979) and concluded that it is necessary to use an attention placebo group in this field of research, but these

recommendations have had no real influence on study design in subsequent years.

The most recent review, by Gentz (2000), partly meets current methodological criteria. She reported the search terms and databases searched. Unfortunately, she did not analyze the methodological qualifications of the 19 publications she reviewed, but rather treated them as methodologically equivalent. Nevertheless, her conclusions are quite reasonable. She used the Cumulative Index of Nursing and Allied Health Literature database, so many articles were authored by nurses. Her specific interest in this review was the learning needs and impressions of patients undergoing angiography. One important conclusion in her review is that patients and their spouses reported "informational needs on risk factors and feeling prepared for a future cardiac emergency as their most important needs" (p. 169). Another implication from the review is that "PTCA experience was viewed as mostly positive, with low levels of mood disturbance and mild to low levels of heart disease threat. Trust in competent staff members and care exceeding expectations were probably contributing factors to this view" (p. 170).

We classified articles as expert reports if they reported no systematic empirical data and provided no systematic review of the literature. We found 23 expert reports and divided them into three groups: (a) subjective reports of their experience by physicians who underwent PTCA, (b) general information and instructions for the care and nursing of coronary patients, and (c) reports of clinical experiences in caring for coronary patients. The following paragraphs discuss each of the categories in turn.

The four experience reports by physicians undergoing PTCA described how unprepared they were and how stressful they found their angina pectoris attacks or myocardial infarctions (Cahill, 1993; Dean, 1993; Kostka, 1992; Rogers, 1986). Like most patients, they were inclined to minimize their worry, which nevertheless shows through the clinical and professional reporting style; the focus of their reports is on the course of the PTCA and the professionalism of the medical team.

About half of the expert reports (12 of 23) provided recommendations or instructions to nursing personnel in coronary care units to promote excellence in the care of coronary patients (Bouman, 1984; J. Cohen & Hasler, 1987; Dault, Groene, & Herick, 1992; Dolman, 1994; M. Edwards & Payton, 1976; Fields, 1991; Finesilver, 1980; N. Jenkins & Kotrba-Ottoboni, 1991; Jensen, Banwart, Venhaus, Popkess, & Perkins, 1993; Markakis, 1990; Ott, 1982; Teasley, 1982). These reports were published exclusively in North American nursing journals. Some describe the use of specially qualified and educated "angioplasty program nurses," who help patients prepare for their procedure by answering questions, providing additional information, and giving emotional support.

Seven articles described in detail the authors' clinical experiences in caring for coronary patients (H. K. Fischer, 1977; Hussey, 1997; Kendall, 1983; Kendall & Watson, 1982; Mudd, 1986; Pearson, 1994; Tooth & McKenna, 1995). All articles referred to the necessity of preparing the patient not only physically, but also psychologically, for the procedure. Two of the articles supported a cognitive–behavioral intervention to help patients manage stress. Another described the effectiveness of self-efficacy theory in helping patients better cope with the intervention; these authors observed that the more patients believe in their own ability to manage the situation, the more they can cope with their feelings. Another relevant topic was the involvement of the patient's close relatives or partners.

These expert reports provide detailed explanations of the circumstances involved in cardiac procedures and the physical and psychological stressors patients experience. Such detail is largely missing from empirical studies.

8.5. CONCLUSION

This chapter discusses the literature on the psychological aspects of specific cardiac interventions. Much of this literature has examined the emotional and cognitive experiences of patients and has sought to identify the prevalence of certain psychological symptoms within the scope of cardiac procedures. Other publications examined the psychological management of cardiac interventions,

the predictive contributions of psychosocial factors to the course of CHD, and the efficacy of available psychological interventions.

This review includes 92 empirical studies, 50.6% of which we rated as very well qualified and 22.9% of which we rated as well-qualified. Thus, nearly three quarters of these studies were of sufficient methodological quality, which provides a positive evaluation of this research field. Nevertheless, this conclusion is too positive; our evaluation does not reflect whether all important psychological constructs have been analyzed. Many studies have been accomplished with simple psychological instruments such as the Quality of Life Index. Some studies were secondary efforts tacked on to studies that analyzed primarily biomedical parameters. Many possible predictor variables for psychological, as well as cardiac, outcomes of PTCA have not been researched so far. Research from other fields has examined promising variables such as self-efficacy, physician–patient relationships, and social support. Predictors such as anxiety, depression, and vital exhaustion have received attention in psychology research, but protective, compensatory, and stabilizing variables have been disregarded.

Furthermore, research is needed that addresses whether the technological effectiveness and rapidity of PTCA (e.g., same-day or next-day discharge) encourage patients to minimize the severity of the disease and the need for lifestyle changes. Such research could help professionals increase patients' motivation to make lifestyle changes during the weeks after the intervention.

Several studies within the scope of multicenter studies assessed psychological variables using psychosocial questionnaires. Four such studies, rated as very well qualified, were discussed in this chapter (Bypass Angioplasty Revascularization Investigation [Hlatky, 1997]; Randomized Intervention Treatment of Angina—I [Pocock et al., 1996]; Coronary Angioplasty Versus Bypass Revascularization Investigation [W. Strauss et al., 1995; Währborg, 1990]; Randomized Intervention Treatment of Angina—II [Pocock et al., 2000]).

The available data make it possible to draw conclusions about emotional condition, mood, and anxiety and depression in patients before, during, and after the cardiac procedure. Most patients experience the cardiac interventions positively and cope well with the related anxiety. As a result, for instance, sedatives are now administered only in exceptional cases. However, knowledge about the psychosocial predictors of long-term outcomes of PTCA is still unsatisfactory. The development and evaluation of specific psychological interventions also remains unsatisfactory.

An important difficulty in this field of research is the rapid change in the cardiac procedures themselves. Within 20 years, PTCA changed from a major, high-risk intervention with an average hospital stay of 14 days to a routine intervention with a maximum of one overnight stay.

Studies assessing the prevalence of psychological symptoms, subjective experiences, and patient coping have a number of methodological problems. There is considerable variation in the instruments and cutoff points used to assess stress, burden, anxiety, or depression. In many studies, for example, mean values or correlations are reported, but the point prevalence is not. The evidence does not indicate the need for additional or specific psychological interventions; only a small group of patients show clinically significant anxiety and stress scores. There is evidence, however, that standard care can be optimized, and the following sections summarize recommendations based on the findings in this review.

8.5.1. Before the Intervention

Most patients experience a waiting period as stressful. The longer they wait, the more they show symptoms of anxiety, distress, nervousness, and sleep disorders, and the higher their consumption of sedatives is. Most patients (about 70% to 80%) show low anxiety levels, but 4% to 8% have clinically relevant depression before the intervention. Principal causes of anxiety include loss of control, fears of serious complications that could lead to bypass surgery, and uncertainty about prognosis and the success of the therapy. More women than men and more younger patients than older patients show heightened anxiety. Patients having a repeat

angiography have higher anxiety levels than patients having the procedure for the first time.

It is important that medical staff obtain a comprehensive history and provide patients with encouragement and support. Both written information and videotapes that portray the procedure and prepare patients for the sensory experiences they will encounter have been found to be beneficial. In addition to enabling patients to handle their impressions and sensory experiences better, which heightens feelings of control and lowers fears, these measures also increase patients' confidence in their physicians and procedures.

8.5.2. During the Intervention

Patients' highest anxiety levels are measured during the intervention. Anxiety levels decrease quite quickly following the intervention in most patients. Therefore, it is important, especially during the first phase of treatment, to engage the patient verbally by asking for complaints or sensory impressions and to give explanations about the procedure. Supportive contact minimizes patients' strain and anxiety.

Clinically relevant psychological complications have not been reported in the literature. Only anxious and depressive patients (perhaps 8% to 12%) experience more serious disorders and more intervention-related stress. The support of the medical team can help them manage their reactions.

8.5.3. After the Intervention

The anxiety level of most patients decreases significantly following the intervention. Patients continue to need information about the results, possible complications (e.g., a recurrence of cardiac symptoms), and the necessity of secondary prevention.

More than 80% of the PTCA patients experience the intervention as improving their QoL, reducing their cardiac symptoms, and promoting their emotional well-being. Patients over 80 years of age also experience improvements in QoL. But nearly one in four patients still feels restricted in some areas (e.g., sexuality, work, social life) and is disappointed with the results of the procedure. A possible explanation is that some patients misjudge the intervention and believe that it will "cure" them; such patients may disregard new symptoms and may place a low priority on making necessary lifestyle changes.

Most patients report high levels of self-efficacy and high motivation to change cardiac risk factors. Regular contact with rehabilitation or cardiological clinics over the long term can help patients maintain their motivation, which usually decreases over time. Patients can be invited to information sessions and provided with take-home material (e.g., brochures, videotapes, Internet links, telephone hotlines).

Motivation to make lifestyle changes may begin to wane when QoL no longer improves after the first month following PTCA. This phenomenon was highlighted in some studies comparing PTCA and bypass surgery that found that QoL increased more after PTCA than after bypass surgery in the early phase, but that after 1 year the differences in perceived QoL were no longer significant; in some studies bypass patients had better QoL than PTCA patients. In studies comparing PTCA and pharmacological treatment, however, PTCA patients had better QoL after 6 months.

Prospective studies assessing psychosocial variables (anxiety, depression, and QoL) and cardiac variables (restenosis, cardiac events, and mortality) provide data relevant for secondary prevention. Whereas the level of anxiety and depression before PTCA was predictive of level of anxiety and depression following the intervention, results for QoL showed that only cardiac variables (e.g., degree of CHD, angina pectoris symptoms, dyspnea) were predictive. Restenosis was satisfactorily predicted using psychosocial variables such as overcommitment, resignation, and stress. Cardiac events were predicted using both cardiac and psychosocial factors.

8.5.4. Future Research

Psychological interventions that take place while cardiological interventions are under way are a valuable and financially justifiable area for future research. Future research in this area is essential and also financially justifiable. It is necessary to understand, for example, which patients need a targeted psychological intervention in addition to the suggested standard care. The literature as a whole indicates that 10% to 15% of patients experience stress, fearfulness, or depression that would require additional psychological intervention. Adequate screening instruments are needed to identify patients' needs. Once the need for extra help is identified, a short, targeted clinic-based intervention by qualified personnel may be implemented. Because the numbers of patients undergoing coronary angiography and PTCA are increasing, interventions targeting lifestyle changes will also be increasingly necessary. Integrating spouses and other significant others is essential.

In the future, research is needed to identify the best interventions to use in assisting the small subgroup of patients who experience undue fear, depression, and stress before a cardiac intervention. Future research is also needed to clarify gender-specific differences in intervention experiences and demands for information procurement and patient guidance. In addition, prospective studies are needed to investigate a wide spectrum of psychological constructs and their effects on patient prognosis.

Finally, a considerable research goal is the systematic integration of secondary preventive measures following PTCA. Changes of lifestyle that are effective and that improve prognosis and QoL are seldom systematically targeted, and the available research results provide little concrete information to support such programs.

CHAPTER 9

PSYCHOLOGICAL INTERVENTIONS FOR CORONARY HEART DISEASE: STRESS MANAGEMENT, RELAXATION, AND ORNISH GROUPS

Wolfgang Langosch, Hans-Günter Budde, and Wolfgang Linden

9.1. INTRODUCTION

The common view of coronary heart disease (CHD) is that it has multiple causes. The most important ones are the "classic" risk factors: diet, smoking, lack of exercise, and high blood pressure. In consequence, the practical rehabilitation of patients with CHD includes cardiological diagnosis, exercise therapy, and pharmacological treatment as primary approaches (Ades, 2001; W. Linden, 2000; Völler, 1999). The effectiveness of this approach regarding cardiac mortality and morbidity is considered solid. Nevertheless, the positive predictive power of the classic risk factors is limited, and this provides opportunities to consider other risk factors.

If patients themselves are asked about the presumed reasons for their disease, classic risk factors are not the ones first mentioned. More than anything, patients themselves will indicate "stress" as a likely cause or contributor for their disease (Myrtek, 2000). In the past few years, there has been accumulating evidence that psychological and social factors are indeed critical for the etiology of CHD (Rozanski, Blumenthal, & Kaplan, 1999). In particular, research has focused on the importance of psychological disturbances, psychological symptoms, personality features, coping strategies, risky behaviors, and physical stress reactivity (Budde, 2000). Rozanski et al. (1999) provided a diligent overview in which they discussed the relationships among CHD and depression, anxiety, and social isolation as well as acute and chronic stress. These

writers concurred that psychosocial risk factors tend to coexist and that their aggregated existence also increases the probability of disease. They subdivided the pathophysiological mechanisms for these relationships into intermediate mechanisms (e.g., neuroendocrine changes or modified platelet activation) and behaviorally related mechanisms (e.g., health risk behaviors like cigarette smoking, poor nutrition, etc.). Rozanski et al. concluded from these results that research should focus on the modification of chronic stress as a potential cardiac risk factor. Denollet (2000) concurred and also emphasized that it is highly relevant to identify those patients for whom the greatest risk exists and test predictions about high risk for cardiac events that are due to psychological stress.

The development of psychological interventions and their evaluation for patients with CHD are not new and have long been considered promising. Following the observations of Blumenthal and Emery (1988), such interventions can be divided into behavioral approaches for risk reduction, such as reduction of cigarette smoking, improved nutrition, and exercise training on the one hand, and approaches that are more generally directed at the reduction of psychosocial distress on the other hand. In the following text, we investigate whether these interventions do indeed lead to the expected secondary prevention and rehabilitation results that are hoped for. In particular, we want to investigate what evidence exists that psychological treatment is able to reduce cardiac mortality and morbidity in CHD patients.

9.2. METHOD

A hierarchy of scientific evidence for the classification of publications by scientific value was established by the Agency for Health Care Policy and Research; it consists of a scheme of evidence classes that was published in 1992 (Flagle & Cahn, 1992). In this scheme, studies can be classified regarding their trustworthiness and relevance for clinical practice by the type of evidence they provide. The lowest numbers present the highest quality evidence.

1a. Evidence based on meta-analyses of randomized controlled studies.

1b. Evidence based on at least one randomized controlled study.

2a. Evidence based on at least one high quality controlled study without randomization.

2b. Evidence based on at least one high quality quasi-experimental study.

3. Evidence based on high quality, non-experimental, descriptive studies that may be case controlled comparative or correlational in nature.

4. Evidence based on comments of experts or consensus groups.

Consistent with this category system, we are placing the greatest emphasis here on randomized controlled studies and aggregations of such studies via meta-analysis. Meta-analysis has the advantage of going beyond the evidentiary possibilities inherent in narrative reviews and of allowing aggregation of nonsignificant singular results, which when pooled may show clinically meaningful and statistically significant effects after all, but it also has a variety of limitations that need to be carefully considered in order to arrive at meaningful conclusions. We will not provide a detailed criticism of all potential flaws of meta-analysis, but we refer the reader to Rosenthal (1984). Note that the most critical features to be considered are issues around publication and retrieval bias; meaningful extraction of truly comparable studies; clear definitions of target populations; and basic methodological features like randomization, drop-out analysis, issues of selectivity, follow-up, description of potential confounds, blinding, and treatment integrity.

9.3. LITERATURE SEARCH

The review and systematic analyses of literature for this chapter were greatly facilitated by two published articles that have appeared in highly respected journals. W. Linden, Stossel, and Maurice (1996) published a meta-analysis in the *Archives of Internal Medicine* that evaluated all studies up to the middle of the year 1995; it assessed the effectiveness of psychosocial interventions in patients with CHD over and above the effects of other rehabilitation efforts. The W. Linden et al. review covered sufficient numbers of randomized studies to be classified 1a in the hierarchy scheme outlined above. A few years later, a second meta-analysis appeared in *Health Psychology* that also investigated the effects of psychoeducational programs for patients with CHD (Dusseldorp, van Elderen, Maes, Meulmann, & Kraaij, 1999). This meta-analysis is similarly based on a very diligent and thorough search and analysis of the literature and qualifies as 1a. Both articles are particularly relevant for the questions posed here and will be described in detail below. The results of these two analyses are to a fair degree consistent, but there also are differences. Some of the differences can be attributed to the fact that because of their publication dates, two large studies (Frasure-Smith et al., 1997; D. A. Jones & West, 1996) that showed that psychological treatments were not effective were available to Dusseldorp et al. (1999) but not to W. Linden et al. The results from these large controlled trials were in contrast to earlier findings, thus requiring a balanced discussion of findings, and these are discussed in considerable detail because they allow highlighting of critical methodological issues that affect the question of effectiveness posed here. In addition Blumenthal et al. described a psychological intervention that led to more positive results. Note, however, that this study did not include full randomization, which may limit its generalizability.

For the time period of 1998 to 2001, when we originally surveyed the literature (main report published in German; Langosch, Budde, & Linden, 2003), no new experimental studies for the topic covered here could be identified. That notwithstanding, since 2001, the results from the largest trial to date have been published (the Writing Committee for the ENRICHD Investigators, 2003) and will be discussed here as well. In addition, we cover the work by the Ornish group (Ornish et al., 1990), which is a multicomponent program for lifestyle changes. Although this study does not allow separate evaluation of the effectiveness of the psychosocial treatment when provided alone, the research is important in that it has shaped the interventions offered in many locations and has promised considerable improvement of quality of life and possibly improved prognosis for many patients with CHD.

9.4. DESCRIPTION OF PSYCHOLOGICAL INTERVENTION IN VARIOUS STUDIES

Most authors do not describe the exact type of psychological intervention in great detail. They do indicate the length of the intervention and the number of sessions but do not necessarily justify why these time periods were chosen. This continues to be true for the Enhancing Recovery in Coronary Heart Disease (ENRICHD) study (Writing Committee for the ENRICHD Investigators, 2003), which was a multicenter trial that focused on CHD patients who had an elevated risk for a cardiac event because of elevated depressive symptomatology or who were socially isolated. The study evaluated the effects of a reduction of these risk factors regarding mortality and morbidity. One criterion for the successful conclusion of treatment was a minimum participation in six sessions of therapy in either group or individual format, but treatment confounds via parallel drug treatment were permitted, and the treatment of social isolation was minimally described.

Widespread among psychological treatment studies of cardiac patients is a lack of detail regarding qualification of therapists. Most of these interventions used a cognitive–behavioral approach, and this was at times based on the use of manuals. The most typically used methods can be considered derivates of clinical practice approaches developed in the 1970s that are of a behavioral and cognitive nature.

9.5. META-ANALYSES

9.5.1. W. Linden et al. (1996)

W. Linden et al. (1996) accepted the premise that the effectiveness of cardiac rehabilitation with core components of cardiac medication, exercise training, and nutrition counseling has been documented as effective for the reduction of mortality and morbidity (Lau et al., 1992). The explicit intention of their meta-analysis was to quantify whether the effectiveness of this type of cardiac rehabilitation could be augmented through additional psychological treatment.

Their literature search was based on a Medline database search and the exploration of all secondary references. The study selection was based on the following criteria: (a) inclusion of patients with documented CHD, (b) inclusion of one or more controlled conditions, (c) at least one treatment condition in which patients were offered psychological treatment over and above standard care for another controlled condition, and (d) randomized assignment to experimental and control conditions.

The psychological treatment of the experimental conditions varied considerably regarding the techniques used; the length of treatment sessions and overall study length also varied, and included psychotherapeutic group sessions, teaching of cognitive and behavioral coping strategies, and relaxation techniques and health education. W. Linden et al. (1996) reported that the great majority of all studies were cognitive–behavioral in their orientation, and they considered the interventions to be subsumable under the umbrella of "stress management." These labels will be maintained in the following description of the meta-analysis.

The interventions of the control conditions comprised cardiology drugs as well as exercise and nutrition recommendations or skill training. The original intent to separate studies into drug therapy alone and drug therapy plus exercise therapy was abandoned in favor of having a category labeled "usual care." This was justified by W. Linden et al. (1996) by the fact that in the majority of analyzed studies, patients were typically instructed in or given recommendations for controlled exercise training and that there was little evidence of patients only using drug treatments. Furthermore, there is generally insufficient information about the degree of the adherence to these recommendations. There are only a few studies available in which the exercise intervention component could be analyzed as a distinct additional condition.

Endpoints (or treatment targets) were only considered for the analysis if they had been investigated in at least four studies. Endpoints were distinguished as being either "hard" endpoints like mortality or morbidity; "subjective measures" like anxiety and depression; or "biological intermediary goals" like blood pressure, heart rate, and lipid levels. The terms *biological intermediary endpoint* and *hard endpoint* were considered separately, because treatment effects on mortality were thought to have low probability and, therefore, that they would be difficult to study unless very large samples were available. On the other hand, it was possible to compare psychological and behavioral interventions in smaller sample studies, because intermediary biological endpoints were often tested, and other interesting outcomes (like cost savings due to quicker return to work) could also be effectively studied even in studies with small sample sizes.

Effect sizes were determined using Cohen's *d* (J. Cohen, 1977) within each category for each individual study. W. Linden et al. (1996) only displayed effect sizes that referred to change occurring from pre- to posttest. This selection was justified because effect size calculations for long-term changes would be greatly affected and diffused by the fact that follow-up length and patient adherence were highly variable and thus difficult to contrast with each other. When no indices of variability had been provided in the original studies, these were estimated on the basis of available indices in similar studies using the same measurement instruments. Given the pronounced variability of sample sizes, each study was weighted according to its degree of freedom using the formula Weight = $N - 3$. Statistical comparisons were based on two-sided *t* tests for unequal variances. The testing of hypotheses was thus made rather conservative and protected for violations of the homogeneity of variance requirement. The potential problem of a different

number of available variables per study was resolved by computing only an average effect size for each category of endpoints for each study. This was particularly relevant for the measurement of anxiety and depression, because it is well known that these two variables intercorrelate highly (often in the range of $r = .06$ to $.80$). This was seen as justifiable, because both factors clearly are indicative of psychological distress. If there were distortions because of this aggregation principle, then these distortions would ultimately underestimate resulting effect sizes. Mortality and morbidity data were presented. The follow-up data were clustered into follow-up that was less than 2 years versus follow-up longer than 2 years. Using the contingency tables, odds ratios (ORs) were computed using the Mantel-Haenszel procedure. The mortality and morbidity data of the experimental conditions were expressed such that a risk ratio of 1.0 was considered the base. If a risk ratio was greater than 1.0, this meant that the risk was greater because a treatment did not include stress management.

A total of 23 studies were included in the meta-analysis, and these studies involved a total of 2,024 patients who received psychology therapy and 1,156 control patients. The data from the Recurrent Coronary Prevention Project (RCPP; M. Friedman et al., 1984) were included in some of the analyses, although they were not completely based on randomization principles. The two active treatment groups had been randomized to their respective conditions, but the standard control groups were not fully randomized for ethical reasons. Given the considerable importance and prominence of this study, and to prevent loss of this critical information, W. Linden et al. (1996) decided to conduct all statistical analyses first with and then without the RCPP data. In about 80% of all included studies, only those patients that had been diagnosed with CHD had been accepted for a study. The average length for a follow-up less than 2 years was 12 months, and the average length for the longer term follow-up was 63 months.

The addition of stress management to usual care had a beneficial effect for nonfatal cardiac events. The reduction for the shorter follow-up translated into a 46% benefit (OR = 1.84). The long-term follow-up period led to a benefit of a 39% risk reduction (OR = 1.64). Therefore, the short and medium length long-term effects can be considered well established whether the RCPP data were used or not.

Regarding mortality, the results were affected by inclusion or exclusion of the RCPP data. For the short-term interval, the OR of 1.7 reflected a 41% reduced mortality of psychologically treated patients relative to those of the control group. However, the mortality reduction of 26% observed in the psychological treatment condition translated into an OR of 1.39 and was not statistically significant. When, however, the RCPP data were included, the mortality reduction for the shorter term follow-up remained pretty much the same (OR = 1.76), but for the long-term follow-up, it increased to 28%, and this exceeded the statistical significance cutoff. Hence, it was concluded that on the whole, longer follow-up was associated with a decreasing effect size.

Although there were no changes in the control conditions regarding psychological distress, the experimental conditions showed significant reductions. These reductions reflected an effect size of $d = 0.3$, and given that in control patients a reduction of 0.04 was observed, a statistically significant difference at the level of $p < .001$ was determined.

The differences between control and experimental groups regarding systolic and diastolic blood pressure as well as heart rate were very small; however, they consistently pointed in the same direction, namely, that stress management participants showed improvements. Other than for diastolic blood pressure reduction, the observed effect sizes were statistically significant. In the usual care conditions, no change in blood pressure or heart rate was observed. The rather large decrease in lipid levels was striking; however, it was based on a very low number of studies and might be difficult to replicate.

9.5.2. Dusseldorp et al. (1999)

The second major meta-analysis of relevance was the one by Dusseldorp and her colleagues (Dusseldorp et al., 1999), who tried to differentially assess the effect of psychoeducational relative to psychosocial interventions. *Psychoeducational intervention* is understood as systematic teaching by health professionals to patients and their families regarding cardiac disease risk factors and their modification. *Psychosocial intervention* comprises various forms of psychotherapy and relaxation and can also be conceptualized as *stress management intervention*. Both types of interventions share the underlying rationale that the disease itself is a stressor that may elicit affective distress, that affective distress interferes with rehabilitation (partly by interfering with adherence to healthy lifestyle prescriptions), and that distress may increase risk for new events and mortality. Stress reduction is held to facilitate or accelerate the rehabilitation process. Important features of the Dusseldorp et al. analysis were the systematic test of a moderator model (i.e., will there be health benefits only if existing distress is effectively reduced?) as well as the determination of the influence of various study characteristics on differential outcomes.

The literature search embraced the years 1974 to 1998, and the PsycLIT and Medline search engines were supplied with these key words: *myocardial infarction, coronary bypass, percutaneous transluminal coronary angioplasty, heart disease,* and *cardiovascular disease.* Other search terms regarding outcomes were *mortality, morbidity, blood pressure, cholesterol, overweight, weight, obesity, distress, well-being, physical exercise, nutrition, food, anxiety, depression, anger, emotional distress,* and *quality of life.* Regarding program type, these terms were used: *cardiac rehabilitation, psychological intervention, psycho-educational intervention, education, stress management, training, therapy, counseling,* and *relaxation.* Additional studies were identified via use of secondary sources. Included were only those studies where patients had documented heart disease, with an event occurring within 6 months prior to the psychological intervention. Psychological interventions were only considered for inclusion if they had been tested for effect on morbidity, mortality, or biological risk factors. Screening was conducted for design quality, randomization (or matching strategies), presence of control groups, and availability of pre- and posttest data. In nine studies, more than one comparison of treatment outcomes was possible because there had been multiple active treatments, but only one comparison was extracted, namely, the one with the most intensive intervention relative to standard care control. Face-to-face contact of therapist and patient was also a requirement for inclusion. Endpoints were differentiated as either being distal (cardiac mortality, reinfarction, bypass surgery, angina) or proximal (affective distress, biological risk factors [like blood pressure and cholesterol], smoking, exercise, nutritional habits). Length of follow-up was classified as short term (<1 year), medium term (1–2 years), or long term (>2 years). When multiple follow-up tests had been conducted, only the longest interval was used. Treatment types were classified as fitting into five clusters: stress management only, stress management plus health education, stress management plus health education plus exercise conditioning, health education only, and health education plus exercise conditioning. Also coded were numerous study and patient characteristics, including publication year, male–female ratio within samples, program setting, participation of partners, and so forth.

Studies were labeled "successful" when at the end of treatment a significant improvement in the desired proximal goal was reached, that is, reduction of anxiety, subjective stress, or depression. Results were displayed as Cohen's *d*. In the case of missing detailed data but reported statistical significance, an estimated *d* = 0.5 was substituted. The resulting findings were evaluated for homogeneity of variance, and if heterogeneity was detected, then the researchers attempted to identify the moderators that might account for heterogeneity. No such tests were conducted for subsamples of five or fewer studies.

9.5.2.1. Results. The researchers identified 37 relevant studies with a total of 8,988 patients. The study sample comprised 8 studies classified as stress management only, 14 stress management plus health education packages, 9 studies with stress management plus health education plus exercise, 3 health education only, and 3 health education plus exercise interventions. Pretest measures had on average been obtained within 4 weeks of a

cardiac event. Program length varied from 1 week to 234 weeks and averaged 28 weeks, although the modal number was about 12 weeks. The mean number of actual sessions was 18; about half of all programs included 12 sessions or fewer. Interventions were usually multidisciplinary and offered by a team, and about half of all studies had employed specifically trained mental health professionals (i.e., psychologists or psychiatrists).

Studies with a sample size of less than 100 were not considered for inclusion because of the heterogeneity of effect sizes. The follow-up length for determination of nondeadly reinfarction lasted from 6 months to 10 years. For the follow-up period of less than 1 year, the effect sizes were not significant. However, significant effect sizes were determined for follow-up periods of 1 year and longer, and the variable "success with proximal endpoints" served as a moderator. With regard to effect size estimations, the larger studies and those with partially successful outcomes represented a homogeneous group. The effect sizes were only statistically significant for the "success group" such that a reduction of reinfarction was observed that translated into a 42% reduction (OR = 1.71), and for the long-term follow-up, a reduction in mortality of 41% (OR = 1.69) was observed. For the total follow-up period, the group that had successfully reduced distress as an intermediary endpoint also showed a significant reduction in reinfarction of 36% (OR = 1.56), whereas a 2% reduction in risk was observed in patient groups in which psychological distress reduction had been only partially successful or failed altogether (OR = 1.02). The short-term success of studies regarding emotional distress, systolic pressure, smoking, and physical exercise were considered. Of the total of 16 studies that had been included in this analysis, 13 contained at least some stress management program elements or were primarily conceived of as stress management.

9.5.2.2. Mortality. All studies that explicitly studied the effect on mortality contained stress management elements. The follow-up periods covered a time period of 6 months to 10 years. For the short and medium follow-up length, the effect sizes were not statistically relevant. For the longer follow-up periods of more than 2 years, a substantial reduction in mortality of 34% (OR = 1.52) was demonstrated. The effect sizes were not homogeneous regarding this length of follow-up. The variable "success in reaching intermediary goals" was identified as a moderator such that immortality reduction of 31% was observed when the intermediary endpoints had also been reached, and this translated into an OR of 1.44. The follow-up period for the analyses of patients with bypass surgery covered a time period of 1 to 10 years and revealed no statistically significant benefit. The follow-up for patients with angina pectoris covered a time period from 6 weeks to 3 years. Six of the eight studies included stress management. The total effect size was significantly reduced only for the short follow-up period, with a 19% reduction (OR = 1.22).

9.5.2.3. Anxiety and depression.

All the effect sizes were based on or met the criteria of homogeneity, and there were no statistically significant effects. Regarding biological intermediary endpoints, there was a significant reduction of systolic blood pressure for the total follow-up period and for the period from 1 to 2 years posttreatment. A large reduction in cholesterol levels was determined for experimental treatments. The reduction of weight was relevant at all follow-up measurement time points. The total effect size regarding reduction of smoking was larger for the total measurement period and for the intermediate follow-up length. Overall, a 63% reduction in smoking had been reported (OR = 2.71).

9.5.3. Comments on the Meta-Analyses

The meta-analysis of W. Linden et al. (1996) was designed so that potential distortions would act against the possibility of finding positive effects for stress management interventions. This is at least in part due to the possibility that patients in controlled conditions may have received confounding treatments and help with lifestyle modification using their own initiative. Furthermore, it was presumed that even minimal exposure, training, and educational components could lead to improved perceptions of social support that translated into potentially valuable nonspecific treatment benefits. All such distortions would render results conservative. Differences between control and experimental conditions would, therefore, be difficult to show, and that would lead to an underestimation of the effects of stress management interventions. Additional psychological treatment relative to control conditions showed significant reductions in morbidity of 46% and a mortality of 41% for the shorter term follow-up period, whereas for the long-term follow-up period, the morbidity reduction was 41% and the mortality reduction 26%, which, in the latter case, no longer met the statistical significance criterion. Substantial benefits were also apparent for biological risk factor reduction regarding cholesterol level, heart rate, and systolic blood pressure changes. Similarly, the reduction of psychological distress at the end of the intervention was statistically greater in the experimental relative to the control condition. The results of the meta-analyses of W. Linden et al. and Dusseldorp et al. (1999) are largely similar, in particular as regards morbidity outcomes. W. Linden et al. documented a significant reduction in nondeadly reinfarction for the shorter and longer term follow-up period, and Dusseldorp et al. reported similar results, but only for those patients who achieved the proximal target, namely, reduction of distress. This led to the conclusion that moderator effects—in this case, the success or failure of achieving psychological stress reduction—accounted for the observed benefits on morbidity. Although psychological distress on the whole was not reduced because of treatment, there was a higher mortality in the experimental group than the control group (OR = 0.88), and morbidity was essentially the same for both groups (OR= 1.03). However, in studies in which psychological distress was reduced, mortality (OR = 1.52) and morbidity (OR = 1.96) were also reduced (for further discussion of this moderator effect, see W. Linden, 2000). The explicit proximal goal of the programs were reduction of classic risk factors like smoking, sedentary activity, or hypertension, as well as psychological distress, as is apparent on anxiety and depression measures. About 80% of all programs contained at least some stress management components. All studies that were used to estimate effects regarding mortality reductions contained stress management interventions or were at least predominantly directed at stress management.

Although the meta-analysis of W. Linden et al. (1996) showed clear benefits for reduction of psychological distress, this was not apparent in the Dusseldorp et al. (1999) review. These latter authors explained the negative effects for psychological distress as being due to the inclusion of two large and more recent trials in which no reduction of anxiety and depression had been demonstrated. Both these studies will be discussed in more detail because their large size gives them a particularly critical role in the literature and because the nature of the protocol and the results are very useful for exploring moderator effects and showing how critical protocol features affect outcomes.

One of these studies was a multicenter study in which treatment was only activated in a crisis; nurses without special training in clinical psychology or diagnosis executed the intervention as required (Frasure-Smith et al., 1997). The second study was also a multicenter study in which the effects of a psychological treatment program combining counseling and psychotherapy in a group form were evaluated in the context of standard cardiological care (D. A. Jones & West, 1996). The randomization to treatment conditions was executed in a nonspecified population of heart patients. In the present chapter, the results of these studies will be compared with each other and also one additional study, which included stress management, physical exercise, and standard care for the purpose of reducing mental stress in myocardial ischemia patients (Blumenthal et al., 1997).

9.6. STUDY BY FRASURE-SMITH ET AL. (1997)

Earlier studies by Frasure-Smith's research team have shown that a nursing intervention for emotional adaptation for male cardiac patients could reduce cardiac morbidity and mortality (Frasure-Smith & Prince, 1985, 1986, 1989). Encouraged by these results, Frasure-Smith et al. (1997) compared the effects of a similar intervention with a

standard cardiac rehabilitation package and made a particular effort to also include a large number of female cardiac patients. This was a multicenter study with participation of 10 clinics. The primary question was whether or not the intervention was effective and could be integrated into clinical routines in an economical fashion.

9.6.1. Method

The exclusion criteria were other life-threatening conditions, more than 32 kilometers distance between home and the clinic, lack of telephone access, deafness, lack of English or French language skills necessary for participation, refusal of participation by the treating physician, and participation in other studies. During the recruitment period (from January 1991 to September 1994), a total of 4,047 patients with documented myocardial infarction were contacted, and 2,483 met the inclusion criteria. Of these, 2,180 were invited to participate, and 61.3% consented (54.4% of the female and 68.9% of the male patients). Significantly more women than men refused participation. The refusers were typically older (mean age 65.1 years, $SD = 12.0$) than the participants (mean age 59.3 years, $SD = 11.4$). After release from the hospital, 234 female and 458 male patients were randomized to the intervention condition, and 239 female and 445 male patients were randomized to the control condition.

Patients first provided consent to allow access to their medical chart information; next, interviews were conducted during which demographics, medical process, and psychological variables were assessed. This was done via use of standardized tools measuring depression, trait anxiety, anger expression, and social support.

The treatment consisted of one telephone call per week following release from the hospital and after the initial treatment phase. The intervention continued for a 1-year period with additional calls at 1-month intervals. These calls were conducted by a research assistant, and it was not clear whether patients always interacted with the same caller. The patients, when called, responded to the same 20 items of the General Health Questionnaire (Goldberg & Williams, 1988) that were read to them. If a value of greater than 5 was obtained or a new hospitalization had occurred, the research assistant contacted the nurse assigned to the program. As quickly as possible, this nurse arranged a direct contact with the patient either in their residence or at another location, and such visits typically lasted 1 hour. The nurse reviewed current psychological problems and needs as well as the cardiac status quo of the patient and then proceeded to deal with the problems at hand. If patients agreed, a second appointment within the next month was set up. After a second contact, visits were only arranged until the nurse and the project team were of the opinion that the patient no longer needed any treatment. Each of the participating nurses cared for patients in one or two of the centers. The content of each intervention was individually tailored and consisted of a combination of emotional support, reassurance, education, and advice as well as referrals to the family physician, cardiologist, or other health resources. In weekly team meetings with three or four nurses and one of three participating psychiatrists, the problems of patients and treatment plans were discussed. If treatment was perceived as necessary beyond the 1-year project length, referrals to other resources were made. The participating nurses had been in the profession for at least 10 years and possessed considerable experience in cardiology. Ten of these nurses had university degrees. They had been trained in the study protocol and had acquired special knowledge and experience through weekly team meetings. None of these nurses had received any special training in psychological intervention prior to initiation of the study. This was justified with the explanation that the rationale for the project was to test the implementability of this approach in standard care in which nurses are not routinely trained as psychotherapists.

Patients in the control condition received the usual standard care and were not contacted throughout the study except for follow-up interviews at 3 and 12 months postevent. The General Health Questionnaire was not given to patients in the control group.

Mortality within 1 year after release from the hospital as well as later revascularization were assessed by contacting patients or family members at 3 and 12 months or were extracted from medical charts. To evaluate the cause of death, hospital or ambulatory care records as well as death certificates were used. The differentiation between cardiac and noncardiac death was made in a blinded fashion and corroborated by two independent working cardiologists. Nonfatal myocardial infarction was defined by the same criteria as had been used for study inclusion. Three and 12 months postrelease from the hospital, all patients were contacted and completed the depression and trait anxiety measures.

9.6.2. Results

In 584 (82.9%) members of the intervention group, there was at least one postrelease visit of a nurse. This applied to 86.3% of the female and 81.2% of the male patients ($p = .09$). This contact came about because of elevated general health questionnaire scores in about 90% of all incidences ($n = 502$). The median interval between first telephone call and nurse visit was 12 days, with a range of 2 to 350 days. For most patients receiving the intervention, the total contact period extended over 7 to 8 months. Within this interval, there typically were five to six visits and 12 to 13 telephone calls by the nurse. Women had more contacts than men, with a mean of six visits, relative to four visits for men. Experts outside of the core team were consulted in less than half of all cases. In the 1st year, there were 65 deaths (4.7%), of which 56 (86.0%) were cardiac in nature. The intervention overall had no effect on total mortality or cardiac mortality. Inferential statistical testing showed that female patients had a significantly greater risk for overall mortality (OR = 1.99) and for cardiac mortality (OR = 1.96). There were no equivalent effects for male patients. The results appeared consistent across the different participation centers. Especially impressive was the finding of greater frequency of arrhythmia for the female patients. There were no differences between the groups regarding fatal or nonfatal infarction or required revascularization procedures. Overall, the results for female patients were worse irrespective of their membership in intervention or control group than was observed for male patients. Mortality was also greater as a function of higher age and nicotine consumption; however, these parameters did not significantly moderate the other observed treatment outcomes. The effect of treatment on depression and anxiety in surviving patients was marginal and nonsignificant.

9.6.3. Commentary

Frasure-Smith et al. (1997) compared these results with the previous, similarly structured study in which only male patients had been treated (Frasure-Smith & Prince, 1989). There was no ready explanation for the negative results of the more recent study. The researchers first noted that the difference might have been related to the much better medical treatment of heart patients in the last decade, which has reduced mortality rates overall. Instead of an expected mortality rate of 10.0% for the observation period, only 2.5% of the men had died. To use mortality as a sensitive endpoint, a much larger number of male patients would have had to be included to show advantage or disadvantage of any intervention. The treatment of female patients was considerably more difficult and cumbersome than the treatment of male patients, and there was no reduction in the self-reported distress of female patients. These results reveal that for female patients, there is a risk that active intervention may actually decrease a patient's health. Frasure-Smith et al. speculated that the higher death rate from arrhythmia in treated women might be due to an increase in distress that is attributable to the intervention. They hypothesized that monthly screening and home visits may have created a psychological demand situation that is not part of the normal cardiological rehabilitation. During the observation period of 1 year, more than three quarters of the treatment group displayed elevated distress values at least once. This might be related to the frequent contact via telephone. Maybe low-risk female patients were reminded of their poor cardiac health, and this unintended refreshing of memories of a potentially fatal prognosis could have translated into elevated distress. If, indeed, systematic intervention led to even small increases in distress, it may have interfered with adaptive coping mechanisms that could have occurred otherwise, such as denial that might have effectively dealt with the distressing response. To clarify such a hypothesis, a control condition would have been needed in which informa-

tion about distress was assessed but where no intervention would have been offered. Repeated home visits could also have revealed latent familial or social tensions and could have created the expectation of a solution for long-standing problems not possible within the framework of this program. Finally, the participating nurses did not possess diagnostic or therapeutic skills for the role of psychotherapist. In this context, Frasure-Smith et al. emphasized that the objective of the study was not to provide standard treatment of clinical depression but to address psychological distress responses to a supportive environment. Given the design of the study, however, even this expectation might not have been realistic. Lastly, the participating nurses were laypeople as far as psychological treatment was concerned in that they had not received any particular training for this role. For patients in the study, the nurses' training background and what could be expected of them were not obvious. It is possible, or even likely, that these nurses were perceived as experts because of their role in the study and that the study participants anticipated receiving professional help from them. Given this hypothesized constellation of beliefs and expectations, the patients may have expected expertise that these nurses could not have delivered. Given that it was not clear to patients what treatment was supposed to have been provided and why, treatment integrity is in question, and this is apparent in the lack of manualization. Consistent with this observation, there is no evidence that psychological distress, as measured by anxiety or depression, had been reduced for the group as a whole by the intervention. Since publishing the original study, there have been presentations of secondary analyses from Frasure-Smith et al. that provide further conclusions and interpretations for the pessimistic results (Cossette, Frasure-Smith, & Lespérance, 2001). Cossette et al. (2001) showed that when anxiety and depression had been effectively reduced in a subgroup, then the reduction in distress could also be directly related to the reduction and risk for morbidity. Patients whose distress had been reduced also showed a lower mortality rate ($p = .043$) and needed to be hospitalized less often ($p = .001$). This applied equally for male and female patients. In addition, Cossette, Frasure-Smith, and Lespérance (2002) showed a relationship between the actually applied techniques and the specific therapy results. On the basis of analyses of the written therapy protocols, Cossette et al. (2002) concluded that women and men had different preferences for interventions and showed differential benefits from a variety of intervention methods. Male cardiac patients profited the most from methods that were direct and based on the provision of factual information. They were more open to direct advice and instructions than were the women in the study. When women were given such direct advice and concrete instructions, no positive results or even worsening results were shown. When women were offered factual information about blood pressure control or smoking, this had a negative effect on distress reduction. On the other hand, women responded positively to supportive expressions about responsibilities and household chores, whereas this had no effect on male patients. In addition, female patients profited from simply being listened to. Given these facts, Frasure-Smith et al.'s conclusion that psychological treatment of cardiac patients may not be effective appears overly pessimistic. These comments should be read with an open mind insofar as the treatment needs of female cardiac patients are not fully understood (Jackson, Leclerc, Erskine, & Linden, 2005), whereas it is clear at this point only that they are less likely to benefit from therapy, or may even be harmed by it. Frasure-Smith et al. did not comment on the finding that the control condition participants showed quantitatively small but otherwise systematic psychological changes via the two preannounced follow-up interviews at 3 and 12 months when they were contacted by the research assistants. These additional contacts violated the claim of standard care because in a standard care situation, patients are not directly approached by mental health care professionals.

9.7. STUDY BY D. A. JONES AND WEST (1996)

The second large empirical intervention that failed to show effects of psychological intervention is the one by D. A. Jones and West (1996), who investigated the question of whether psychological counseling without contamination through exercise

therapy or other risk factor modification could beneficially impact cardiac rehabilitation. The study was a multicenter, randomized, controlled trial, and patients were invited to participate within 4 weeks after release from the hospital following documented cardiac infarction. The only exclusion criteria were a hospital stay of more than 4 weeks or the transfer into an institution for long-term care. The sample consisted of 2,328 individuals who had been referred via 26 physicians from six different clinics, and these patients were then randomized into intervention ($n = 1,168$) and control ($n = 1,160$) groups. Randomization was undertaken in a coordination center.

Patients in the active treatment condition were invited to participate in a 7-week rehabilitation program that began between 2 and 6 weeks postrelease from the acute care hospital. Patients were invited to participate in the first two sessions. Treatment and control group participants received the usual cardiac care through their general practitioner, at a regional hospital, or through cardiac specialists depending on cardiac need. The intervention consisted of seven 2-hour sessions under the direction of clinical psychologists or "health visitors" (the latter term was not defined). The goals were education about the cardiovascular system, cardiovascular disease, infarction, treatment, and aftercare for the purpose of reduction of fear; they also included improved stress perception, teaching of relaxation skills, improved response to stress source and development of coping skills, support and a positive adaptation to the disease, as well as reconstruction of confidence and optimism in patients and their family members. The methods included education, practical exercises with patient participation, group discussions, and some individual sessions. The importance of training between sessions was highlighted, and patients were encouraged to keep diaries regarding activities, stress, and relaxation. Patients and their partners had opportunities to discuss problems, fears, experiences, and coping strategies. Additional components that were explicitly excluded were efforts at reducing smoking, changing diet, controlling weight, and increasing exercise (D. A. Jones & West, 1996, p. 1517). The control group patients did not participate in any formal rehabilitation, although there was no systematic assessment of potential confounding treatments. The initial chart information was supplemented with data obtained through interviews that were conducted by trained interviewers separately for patients and their partners using a structured set of guidelines. The interviewers were blind to group membership. Validated questionnaires were used to determine angina pectoris, leisure activity, diet, functional restrictions, smoking, drinking, social support, anxiety, depression, basic attitudes toward the infarct, and expectations for the future. Results were determined again via a second structured interview at 6 months and 12 months posttreatment in an ambulatory section of the hospital. Of the total of 2,328 patients, 1,168 were randomized to active treatment and 1,160 to the control group. Complete clinical data were available for 2,255 (97%) patients. Clinical interviews after release from the hospital were conducted with 2,314 patients (99%). Within 6 months, there were 53 deaths (4.5%), of which 19 occurred during the 1st month, and in the control group there were 58 deaths (5.0%), of which 11 occurred during the 1st month. After 1 year, 79 patients (6.8%) in the active treatment group had died, and in the control group, 84 (7.2%) had died. Among surviving patients, complete data were available for the 6-month and 1-year follow-up for 96.8% and 94.5% of the active treatment condition, respectively, and 97.9% and 94.1% of the control group, respectively. There were no reports about the composition of the groups regarding age and gender.

Six months following the intervention, the prevalence rates of anxiety and depression as well as mean scores were unchanged. The percentage of patients with clinically relevant anxiety in the intervention group had changed from 33% to 34%, and in the control group, it had changed from 31% to 32%. The prevalence of clinical depression was 19% in both groups and was the same at 6 months. Patients and their relatives, nevertheless, judged the program in retrospect as very useful. Regarding the prevalence of angina pectoris, the degree of functional impairment and medication use were not different between groups. Twelve months following completion of the intervention, there were no differences regarding mortality or morbidity between the two groups; the mortality rate was 6%. D. A. Jones and West (1996) concluded that a rehabilitation program consisting of psychological therapy, "counseling psychology education," relaxation training, and stress management offered little objective benefit for patients after myocardial infarction.

This conclusion has been soundly criticized on multiple grounds. For example, Ernst (1997) drew the following conclusion in studying the work of W. Linden et al. (1996) and D. A. Jones and West (1996):

> First of all, the final value of psychological treatment in the rehabilitation of infarction patients is at this time not fully supported. Secondly, the fact that patients value a particular intervention does not mean that this is also associated with positive outcomes, even regarding the quality of life. (Ernst, 1997, p. 1, transl. by W. Linden)

Other authors have doubts about the trustworthiness of D. A. Jones and West's (1996) data. Pither and Williams (1997) raised the question of whether the absence of positive effects can be attributed to the failure of reducing the intermediary target of distress reduction. A strong hypothesis is that treatment failed to affect hard endpoints, because anxiety had not changed as a function of the treatment. Furthermore, Pither and Williams speculated that another reason for the lack of effects of this multicenter study can be derived from differential qualifications of therapists in various centers, given that training and competence as well as a variety of protocol features may be critical determinants of outcomes. In a response to these criticisms, D. A. Jones and West noted that the program execution in the six centers was largely standardized and that the qualifications of therapists were comparable. No manual is mentioned as having been used; however, the authors noted that in the reality of clinical practice, therapists are naturally variable in their experience, qualification, and commitment (D. A. Jones & West, 1997). Pither and Williams (1997, p. 979) also raised the question of why a generic stress reduction model has been used as a premise when the interests of patients are largely directed at health-specific anxieties. It is unknown to what degree patients were able to connect subjective stress and illness symptoms with one another and to what degree individual treatments responded to these individual patient experiences. Next, Pither and Williams criticized the fact that the use of relaxation techniques had not been quantitatively determined even though relaxation was considered important. They also questioned whether the control group might have obtained psychologically relevant information in the context of their usual care rehabilitation. This would have created a confounding effect that would have made it difficult to see differences between active treatments and controls. A further criticism related to the dose–response problem: That is, a sufficient dose has to be demonstrated in order to expect a measurable effect. A final criticism was the broadly defined multiple-component application of treatments for individuals with a variety of different problems. The target population of the study by D. A. Jones and West indeed included all patients who had myocardial infarction, irrespective of whether or not there was any evidence of psychological stress. W. Linden (2000) referred to the possibility of floor effects, given that it would be difficult to show a treatment benefit if only 20% to 30% of treated patients actually had problems for which psychological therapy was considered indicated. It was considered surprising that all patients in the six centers had participated in either the treatment or control group, which means that nobody had refused participation. We find this claim to consolidate with our own research and clinical experience. It is also surprising and regrettable that D. A. Jones and West, despite their remarkably large sample, did not report differential analyses of men versus women, nor did they provide information about dropouts. However, it appears that 7.6% of the treatment group and 7.0% of the control group did not provide data for the follow-up investigation after 6 months, and 8.0% and 9.2%, respectively, did not provide data for the 1-year follow-up.

If one focuses exclusively on the prevalence of anxiety and depression at the beginning and after the intervention by D. A. Jones and West (1996), one does not see intervention effects. However, there are numerous possibilities for this observation. It is possible that in a portion of patients posttest, the psychological distress had indeed been reduced, whereas in the larger group, this had not happened. Such differential changes and the possibility of mortality benefits for patients in whom distress had in fact been reduced were not described by D. A. Jones and West, although this would have been possible and of considerable interest.

9.8. STUDY BY BLUMENTHAL ET AL. (1997)

In contrast to the work by D. A. Jones and West (1996), the investigation by Blumenthal et al. (1997), published in a similar time frame, showed numerous statistically and clinically relevant, positive results of a stress management intervention in a population of cardiac rehabilitation patients. Blumenthal et al. investigated to what degree reduction in mental stress can have an impact on rehabilitation and what role physical training plays in this context. They were especially interested in the sensitivity of a variety of different clinical endpoints in this respect. The question was investigated via use of a control group design with a nonrandomized assignment to control; the experimental conditions will be discussed in more detail below. Inclusion criteria were men and women with documented cardiac disease as seen via earlier myocardial infarction, bypass surgery, percutaneous transluminal coronary angioplasty (PTCA), or stenosis in a major coronary artery of more than 75% and recent documentation for stress-induced myocardial ischemia. Inclusion criteria also included relative short distance to the study center, where the participants needed to participate in three sessions per week. Exclusion criteria were cardiomyopathy, ventricular dysfunction, congestive heart failure, severe arrhythmia, left branch block, Wolf-Parkinson-White syndrome, resting blood pressure greater than 220/120 mmHg, ejection fraction less than 30%, and/or stenosis of the left aorta of 50% or more. The sample consisted initially of 136 patients, of which 15 (11%) were women. Of the original sample of 136, 107 showed signs of ischemia on mental stress testing or during ambulatory long-term electrocardiogram. Following initial assessments, the groups were randomized into either a stress management condition or an exercise condition. The first group comprised 33 patients, the second 34 patients. Those who could not be randomized to either condition were assigned to the usual care group (n = 40).

Blumenthal et al.'s (1997) stress management program was based on a social cognitive learning model of behavior. At its center was the interaction of the social environment with personality traits, which in turn were presumed to predispose the patient to react in particular patterns of behavior. This approach has the premise that emotion and behavior are largely determined by cognitive perceptions of the individual. The program was composed of sixteen 90-minute sessions in a group format with 8 participants per group. The first sessions were more educational and included transfer of information about CHD and the anatomy and function of the heart as well as risk factors and stress. In the next sessions, the focus was teaching of specific skills for the reduction of affective, cognitive–behavioral, and physiological stress components. The therapeutic techniques included execution of graded task assignments, observation and control of irrational automatic cognitions for unrealistic thinking patterns, and development of alternative coping skills for a given situation. Patients were taught progressive musculoskeletal training and also had a minimum of two sessions in electromyographic biofeedback training. The exercise condition consisted of three training units in 16 sequential weeks and began with a 10-minute warm-up phase, each including stretching and bicycle ergonometric exercises with a target heart frequency of between 50% and 70% of the maximum heart rate reserve. Thereafter, participants engaged in 35 minutes of jogging or walking with an intended target intensity of 70% to 85% of heart frequency reserve. The participants registered heart rate activity in 10-minute intervals for each training unit and also noted the subjective effort required. Those patients who were not able to participate in these experimental studies for geographic reasons had been assigned to the usual care condition.

They were monitored on a monthly basis regarding participation and questioned about whether they had participated in exercise or stress management programs that could have served as confounds. They were encouraged to maintain the prescribed medication and to consult cardiologists as needed. There was no attempt to influence the treatment offered by their physician. After 4 months; 10 months; and, thereafter, yearly intervals, patients were assessed for cardiac and noncardiac morbidity and mortality using telephone and mail for completion of questionnaires. At this time, information was collected regarding the medical status quo of patients, cardiac symptoms, physician visits, and/or hospitalizations, including need for revascularization. The information was verified using physicians or medical charts. When a patient had died in the meantime, the death certificate was used for determination of the cause of mortality. The follow-up period extended over a period of 2 years with a mean of 37 months (SD = ±18). All participants in the training group could be reached for follow-up. One patient in the stress management group was no longer available. Two people who participated in the exercise training were not available for follow-up because they could not be contacted: 1 could not be contacted after 1 year, and the other could not be contacted after 4 years. Between the two groups, there were no significant differences regarding age, left ventricular dysfunction, angina frequency, previous infarction, previous PTCA or bypass surgery, number of occluded vessels, medical therapy, hypertension, diabetes, smoking, education, income, and occupational status. The number of female participants in the exercise group was higher than the number of men (p = .04; 23.5% of exercise therapy participants were female; in the stress management group, 6.1% were female, and in standard treatment this figure was 7.5%). The distance of people in the standard treatment relative to the study location was significantly greater than that in the other two groups. Their relative distance to the study center did not vary. Ninety-five percent of treated patients completed the intervention. Nobody in the stress management condition dropped out, but 2 participants in the exercise group did not complete the program because of cardiac events, whereas in the standard treatment group, 2 did not complete because of cardiac events, and 1 did not complete because of a back operation. The relative rate of participation in the sessions was 90.5% in the exercise group treatment and 83.0% in the stress management group. Of the total group, 21.0% had an adverse cardiac event during the observation period. The relative proportions were 9.1% (n = 3) in the stress management group, 20.6% (n = 7) in the exercise group, and 30.0% (n = 12) in the standard treatment condition. The relative risk for an adverse event for the stress management group was not comparable with the standard treatment. The relative effect, even after adjustment for initial ejection fraction, previous infarction, and age was 0.26 (95% confidence interval 0.70–0.93, p = .04). The relative risk for the exercise group was less than that of the standard treatment condition but not significantly different (0.68; 95% confidence interval 0.27–1.73, p = .41). The stress management and exercise conditions did not differ in relative risk.

Because the number of women was very low (they represented about 10%) in the study by Blumenthal et al. (1997), the results can only generalize to male patient populations. For good reason—namely, the relatively lower base rate—the authors chose morbidity and not mortality as the critical endpoint. Although the study had relatively low statistical power, the results are clear, given that the usual care group had a rate of new events 3 times higher than the psychological treatment condition, and the intensive exercise group had a risk ratio of 1:2, which fell in between the other two results. The length of treatment for both active treatments was comparable. The monitoring of potentially confounding treatments for the usual group had been diligent. Given the total number of 26 contact hours for all participants, the treatment length was relatively high. Treatment itself largely followed a "garden hose" principle in which all participants were exposed to a large number of different treatment interventions without any attempt to individually tailor therapy plans. The protocol itself represents a mixture of randomization and convenience assignments, given that the usual care

condition was not included in the randomization because of the large distance to the study center. The authors admitted that this was a methodological weakness. In light of the fact that the groups were comparable at the beginning of treatments, this weakness should not interfere with the trustworthiness of results. Given the relatively small sample size, cardiac events could only be assessed in their aggregated form, that is, the frequency of nonfatal infarctions, bypass surgery, and PTCA were aggregated into a single number. Otherwise, statistical power would have been insufficient to show any differences. It is interesting that the different treatments also had very specific patterns of results. Only the participants in exercise therapy showed a reduced minute volume and lowered blood pressure values during the physical exercise test. Both active treatment groups showed a significant reduction in distress. However, only the stress management group showed reduced frequency of ischemic events during the 48-hour measurement, and they showed lower anger scores. The authors were careful to show that the improvement of the critical medical and psychological variables was related to initial values. In the group with low ischemia frequency at the beginning of treatment, the treatment had no effect on ischemia. The 5-year follow-up length is impressive and speaks for the generalizability and trustworthiness of findings. Given that in the United States, only about 1 out of 10 eligible cardiac patients participates in cardiac rehabilitation, it is unclear what the results would be if all eligible patients had been offered such a rich therapy program. Blumenthal et al. (1997) reported honestly that the length of the study and the intensity of the measurement presented a considerable burden for patients and that only a motivated and, therefore, possibly not representative subgroup of patients is likely to complete such a program.

9.9. THE ENHANCING RECOVERY IN CORONARY HEART DISEASE TRIAL

The largest psychological intervention to date, the Enhancing Recovery in Coronary Heart Disease (ENRICHD) Patients trial (Writing Committee for the ENRICHD Investigators, 2003) was designed to test the modifiability of risk that has been associated with the presence of depression in postinfarction patients. On the basis of a series of studies showing that depression is a highly significant prognostic factor for new cardiac events in post–myocardial infarction patients, the trial tested whether reduction of depression and social isolation would lead to better quality of life and reduced mortality and morbidity. Previous criticisms of the literature regarding underrepresentation of women were countered by setting a target of 50% female participation.

9.9.1. Method

Using a randomized clinical trial methodology, 2,481 post–myocardial infarction patients (1,084 women, 1,397 men) were enrolled in eight participating centers. Major or minor depression was diagnosed by modified *Diagnostic and Statistical Manual of Mental Disorders* (4th ed.; American Psychiatric Association, 1994) criteria determined via interview and by severity on the 17-item Hamilton Rating Scale for Depression (HRSD; Hamilton, 1960). Low perceived support was assessed by the ENRICHD Social Support Instrument (ESSI; Vaglio et al., 2004).

Cognitive–behavioral therapy was initiated at a median of 17 days after the index myocardial infarction for a median of 11 individual sessions throughout 6 months, plus group therapy when feasible, with selective serotonin reuptake inhibitors prescribed for patients scoring higher than 24 on the HRSD or having less than 50% reduction in Beck Depression Inventory (A. T. Beck, Ward, Mendelson, Mock, & Erbaugh, 1961) scores after 5 weeks. Primary endpoints were death or recurrent myocardial infarction; secondary endpoints were change in depression or social support perception at 6 months. Of note for the later interpretation of results is that patients with more severe levels of depression could receive antidepressant medication over and above the psychological intervention. The psychological interventions were offered in group and individual form, and some patients participated in both. Treatment was extended until criteria for success were met, but it is not clear whether just one criterion or multiple criteria had to be met for a decision of therapy termination.

9.9.2. Results

Analyses were conducted for three subgroups—depression, depression and social isolation, or social isolation only—that had received psychological therapy or usual care. Improvement in psychosocial outcomes at 6 months favored treatment: Mean changes in HRSD score were −10.1 in the psychosocial treatment versus −8.4 in the usual care group ($p < .001$). Corresponding changes in the ESSI scores were 5.1 and 3.4 ($p < .001$). After an average follow-up of 29 months, there was no significant difference in event-free survival between the two treatment arms (75.9% vs. 75.8%), nor did mortality and morbidity outcomes vary as a function of depression or social isolation subgroupings. At baseline, 9.1% of intervention patients were on antidepressant drugs, and this figure steadily increased to reach 21.0% at time of follow-up.

9.9.3. Commentary

The ENRICHD study results were a big disappointment for a research community that wanted to see clarification and affirmation of the usefulness of psychological treatment of depression for cardiac patients. The high cost of the study translated into a great deal of pressure on the field, because a negative outcome would likely be interpreted as evidence that no future funds should be directed at psychological treatment of depression in cardiac patients. For this reason, it is critical that interpretation of the results be made with utmost objectivity and an open mind. There are many protocol features that deserve careful attention in this regard.

1. The usual care group received health education materials that can be considered a minimal but nevertheless active treatment, which makes it more difficult to find a difference between an active psychological therapy and a true untreated wait-list control. The ENRICHD authors specifically reported that even the usual care group reported considerable improvement in distress relative to their own baseline (about

80% of the effect seen in the active treatment was also seen in the usual care, nonspecific controls; The Writing Committee for the ENRICHD Investigators, 2003).

2. The treatment was initiated very swiftly (i.e., 2 to 3 weeks post–myocardial infarction) and may have been made available to a potentially large subgroup of patients who were depressed at that time but who already possessed good resilience and coping skills and who may have recovered on their own if given sufficient time.

3. The most depressed patients were also given drugs, thus creating a floor effect problem for the psychotherapy-only group, because initial levels of depression also allow little improvement.

4. Throughout the planning process and in the resulting publication of the ENRICHD results, it was not made clear how the therapists would affect social isolation. It appears that the obtained improvements in perceived social support are more likely a byproduct of successful treatment of depression than a direct change in the social network size or network quality of study participants. This is consistent with observations made elsewhere (Hogan, Linden, & Najarian, 2002) that social isolation is not readily modifiable by psychological intervention.

5. The researchers repeated a previous observation that men benefited slightly more from the intervention than did women. This in turn sends an important message to treatment researchers and care providers that psychological treatment of cardiac patients needs gender-specific tailoring that varies according to the degree to which directives and advice are welcomed (found beneficial for men) versus the need for emotion processing (true for women; see Cossette et al., 2002).

6. The therapists in the ENRICHD trial were trained by the Beck Institute, which is recognized as providing excellent training in cognitive therapy for psychiatric depression. This training and treatment model is based on a theory that irrational thought patterns mark psychiatric depression. Clinical observation, however, suggests that irrational thought is not particularly prevalent among cardiac patients

and that the behavioral inactivity thought characteristic of psychiatric depression is at least to some degree confounded with behavioral sequelae of heart disease itself for the case of seemingly depressed cardiac patients. This raises the question whether depression in cardiac patients would not be better conceived as distinct from psychiatric depression; its associated thought patterns may be negative in valence but still rational, and therapy should be correspondingly modified to focus on adaptive thought rather than to emphasize rationality or lack thereof.

9.10. THE ORNISH APPROACH

9.10.1. San Francisco Lifestyle Heart Trial

Although not meeting our a priori inclusion criterion of being a randomized controlled trial of only a psychological intervention, we nevertheless discuss the Ornish approach to lifestyle change because of its overall importance to the field. This approach was specifically developed for cardiac patients (Ornish, 1991, 1999) and has also been referred to as the San Francisco Lifestyle Heart Trial. The objective of the San Francisco Lifestyle Heart Trial was to show that regression of cardiac disease was possible if risk factors were systematically reduced. The question was approached via a nonrandomized prospective control group design. Inclusion criteria were as follows: patient age between 35 and 75 years; living in the larger San Francisco, California area; no other life-threatening illnesses; no myocardial infarct within the last 6 weeks; no earlier therapy with streptokinase or alteplase; no ongoing treatment with cholesterol-lowering drugs; documented one-, two-, or three-vessel disease; left ventricular ejection fraction greater than 25%; nonsmoking status; no planned bypass surgery; and agreement of the cardiologist for patient participation.

Initially, 94 eligible participants had been randomized to intervention or control group. Fifty-three percent ($n = 28$) agreed to be in the intervention group, and 43% ($n = 20$) were in the control group. The primary, most important characteristics of the intervention were related to nutrition, regular stress management, and intensive exercise (Ornish et al., 1990, 1998; Scherwitz, 1996). Treatment began with a 1-week stay in a local hotel, where patients and their partners were familiarized with the lifestyle change program. They participated in daily seminars on the scientific backdrop and also participated in two 1-hour daily sessions to learn stress management and do aerobics, and they had additional group sessions in the evenings. Subsequent to this 1-week training program, patients met twice weekly for about 4 hours each time. One hour was spent on each of the following: aerobics, stress management practices, a common dinner, and a group session.

At the end of core treatment, patients were urged to follow a vegetarian and low-fat nutrition habit for at least 1 year, with emphasis on fruit, vegetables, and soy products without any additional calorie restrictions. The nutrition recommendation did not include any animal products other than egg whites and low-fat milk or low-fat yogurt. About 10% of the daily calorie intake was derived from fat, 15% to 25% from protein, and 70% to 75% from high fiber carbohydrates. Patients also took vitamin B_{12} supplements. The daily cholesterol intake was no more than 5 milligrams. Reduced salt intake was only recommended for patients with hypertension, and caffeine and alcohol consumption was discouraged. For those dependent on alcohol, it was completely forbidden; for all others, the maximum dosage of alcoholic beverages was limited to two drinks per day (equivalent to 45 grams of alcohol). Meals were prepared by the patients and their partners.

The stress management techniques were to be practiced for about 1 hour per day. They were largely yoga based and included stretching, breathing techniques, meditation, progressive muscular relaxation, and visualization. The goal was a greater sense of relaxation, an enhanced self-awareness, and the ability to concentrate. After the initial stretch phase, participants practiced 15 minutes of progressive muscular relaxation, concentration on particular body parts with relaxation imagery, and stretching and breathing meditation with subsequent meditation on the image of peace (Scherwitz,

1996). Afterward, breathing techniques were additionally practiced in a seated position. Following this, participants focused for 5 minutes on an object, a process like breathing a word, or the feeling of freedom. This was followed by visualization that included the heart and an image of arterial expansion and good blood flow through the heart muscle.

Following the guidelines of the American College of Sports Medicine, a mild to moderate endurance training of 3 hours per week was recommended. The training level was based on individual assessment of treadmill performance ability and was regularly tested over a 4-year period. The participants were asked to practice in intervals of at least 30 minutes, and the heart frequency for the practice was determined using the Karvonen formula, with 50% to 80% of maximal heart rate during the treadmill measurement. Patients were strongly encouraged to monitor exactly their level of effort on the treadmill. They were asked to keep their scores between 6 and 20 while training and to spend most of the time between 11 and 14. Patients preferred walking as regular exercise; many also swam or used a bicycle.

The group sessions continued for 1 year, twice a week, and the goal was to create a perception of social support, which was to enhance the program gains. At these twice-weekly meetings, there was a common dinner, after which patients and the group leader sat together in groups of 8 to 14. A session began with a brief meditation, and participants were encouraged to recall recent events that had given them joy or anger and then to contemplate the accurate meaning of this emotional recognition. Following this, participants attempted to refine their recognition ability and accuracy for emotions. The largest portion of the sessions was spent using this type of exchange such that most patients had a chance to participate. Scherwitz (1996) reported that this type of communication about emotion recognition was very unfamiliar to most patients and was considered difficult. They were not used to talking about their feelings and behaving empathetically toward others. In his opinion, this is part of a cluster of behaviors at which cardiac patients are often particularly inept. Differences between patients were acknowledged and highlighted.

Adherence to the program was determined with three diet diaries, protocols for exercise and stress management, and measurement of plasma cotinine concentrations. The researchers created a compliance score in which a value of 1 indicated 100% adherence, and a score of 0 indicated no adherence. A value of 1 indicated that a person did more than expected.

9.10.1.1. Results.
After 1 year as well as after 4 years, participants had maintained most of the lifestyle changes, and this was particularly true for nutrition. Physical training was continued by both groups after 4 years to a similar degree. Persons in the intervention group exercised an average of 3.2 times per day and spent 43.7 minutes engaged in stress management; persons in the control group exercised 6.3 times per day and spent 9.8 minutes on stress management. Regarding vascular stenosis, the following observations could be made: After 1 year, a regression was apparent in 82% of patients in the intervention group, and a progression was observed in 53% of patients in the control group. Controlling for adherence to the nutrition recommendations, those who were also particularly invested in stress management showed the strongest relationship to a regress. The frequency of required practices correlated significantly with reduction in low-density lipoprotein (LDL) and a reduction in negative affect (Scherwitz, 1996). After 4 years, stenosis in the intervention group had further regressed, but not at the same rate as was seen in the 1st year. In the control group, however, the stenosis had continued to get worse. These results were determined via measurement of cardiac circulation using positron emission tomography (Gould et al., 1995). An improvement of blood flow in the treated group was in contrast to the worsening in the control group. During the 4-year follow-up, cardiac morbidity was higher in the control group than the intervention group, with a risk ratio of 2.47:1. Control group participants needed coronary artery bypass graft (CABG) or a vascular dilatation more often than patients in the intervention group. In the intervention group, there were two myocardial infarcts where in the control group there were four (Ornish et al., 1998).

9.10.1.2. Commentary.
The most important basic research finding of the San Francisco Lifestyle Heart Trial was that regression of cardiac disease itself was possible via lifestyle changes. Furthermore, it showed that differences between treated and untreated patients did not disappear over time but actually increased. A major problem is that the study did not have a randomized control group, and this will be discussed later. Despite the important observation that regression of cardiac disease could be achieved, this does not mean that the Ornish approach is easy to translate into standard clinical care. This quality could only be assigned to an approach where one could also ensure that a large number of patients are able to execute and maintain the program.

9.10.2. The Multicenter Lifestyle Demonstration Project
The Multicenter Lifestyle Demonstration Project (Ornish et al., 1998) was a continuation of the earlier intervention effort. It was pursued to test the question of whether lifestyle changes for particular patients with cardiac disease could be considered an immediate alternative to revascularization surgery without increasing the number of cardiac events. It was to be determined whether or not cardiac patients were motivated for substantial and maintained lifestyle changes, with appropriate supports, and this was to parallel cost analyses. This question was assessed using a multicenter, nonrandomized comparison study with matched pairs. The primary inclusion criterion was ideographically documented cardiac disease with a severity that would have justified revascularization. Health insurance paid for treatment of both groups. Exclusion criteria were stenosis greater than 50% in the left main coronary artery, CABG in the past 6 weeks or angioplasty in the past 6 months, chronic nonresponsive congestive heart failure, malignant uncontrolled arrhythmia, a myocardial infarct during the past month, a homozygotic hypercholesterolemia psychosis, a hypertensive reaction to physical exercise training, alcohol or

drug misuse, and/or a life-threatening comorbid condition.

The intervention group was composed of 194 patients; no information was provided about the total number of patients who had been approached for participation. It is not known whether the patients who did participate showed systematic differences from those who refused. Mean age of the study sample was 58 years; 79.0% were men, 77.0% were married, and 63.5% were in the workforce. Regarding classic risk factors, 50.0% were hypertensive, 62.0% had elevated lipid levels, 19.6% had diabetes, 66.0% were cigarette smokers, and 58.0% showed a family history of cardiac disease. For the constitution of the control group, the participating centers forwarded data about other patients who had been admitted at the same time but were not participating in the acute treatment. Using a retrospective matching procedure, the data bank of the health insurance company (Mutual of Omaha) was used to create pairs that were matched on age, gender, left ventricular function, and a "cardiac score." The cardiac score was formed by adding severity scores for the three coronaries such that stenosis of less than 50% was given a value of 0, 50% to 75% a value of 0.5, and greater than 75% was given a value of 1. All 139 patients in the control group had undergone revascularization in the past month, 73 had had CABG, and 66 had had a PTCA. There were no significant differences between intervention and control groups regarding age, gender, marital status, occupational status, hypertension, elevated lipid levels, diabetes, smoking, or family history. The angiographically determined severity of cardiac disease was comparable in both groups; however, 55% of the intervention group compared with 28% of the control group had suffered a myocardial infarct. The mean illness length of the control group had been longer than the one of the control group. Fifty-four percent of the treatment group and 32% of the control group were also taking lipid-lowering medications.

The program began in 1993 at eight different sites, and training was provided by specially trained teams consisting of cardiologists, nutritionists, exercise specialists, psychologists, chefs, stress management specialists, and administrative person-

nel. The program was followed over a period of 1 year (see Ornish et al., 1998). In the first 12 weeks of the intervention, participants met three times per week, and in the remaining 9 months, they met once per week. The individual sessions lasted 4 hours and consisted of physical training, stress management practice, supportive group participation, and a common meal. Each of these components took 1 hour. The total cost per person (based on a total length of 288 hours of program exposure with a total of 72 meetings) was $7,000. No information was provided about the care given to the control group.

The data provided by Ornish et al. (1998) referred to the status at baseline and at 3 months, 1 year, 2 years, and 3 years following program beginning. There were no data recording stress management for baseline. Also, no baseline data were provided regarding cholesterol and fat consumption. Over the 3-year observation period, adherence to the program recommendations decreased. The degree of physical training and the amount of time spent on stress management decreased noticeably over the observation period; however, even after 3 years, it was substantially higher than at baseline. The average consumption of fat and cholesterol had also increased over time but was still relatively low even after 3 years. The mean serum cholesterol and LDL levels decreased from baseline to the first measurement after 3 months 9% and 14%, respectively, and remained at this level for the subsequent measurement periods. High-density lipoprotein values dropped on average between the first two measurement points from 36.7 mg/dl to 32.8 mg/dl. Afterward, these values increased, and at the 3-year measurement point they averaged 42.2 mg/dl. Triglyceride values increased, but not significantly, between baseline and 3-month follow-up, and then dropped, also not significantly, at later measurement. Mean body weight was substantially reduced after 3 months, and even after 3 years, it was substantially lower than at baseline. The physical endurance tolerance measured as metabolic equivalence increased in the first 3 months from 9.59 metabolic equivalents to 11.15 metabolic equivalents and remained at this level for 3 years. Angina pectoris prevalence decreased in the treated group just as much as would have been expected following revascularization surgery. Patients in the treatment group indicated an angina frequency with prevalence of 49% at 3-month follow-up. After 3 years, this percentage was 61%. Throughout the observation period, there were no differences in the frequency of infarct, apoplex, and noncardiac or cardiac death in either group. The 194 female and male patients of the intervention group had met all the necessary conditions for needed revascularization. In a sample of 150, 70.7% therefore avoided revascularization over the 3-year period. Among participants of the intervention group, a total of 31 dilatations (0.06 per patient/year) and 26 bypass surgeries (0.05 per patient/year) were seen during follow-up. The 139 participants in the control group had been chosen because all of them had gone through some form of revascularization during the preceding 4 weeks. Sixty-six had had a PTCA, and 73 had had CABG. During the observation period, these patients required another 23 dilatations and 11 bypass surgeries.

9.10.2.1. Commentary.

The Multicenter Lifestyle Demonstration Project, with 194 patients, included people who all met the criteria for revascularization. In more than three quarters of them, however, none required revascularization during the 3 years after the beginning of the program. It would be interesting to determine how many patients would have been able to avoid revascularization even if they had not participated in the program. This would have required the use of a matched-pair control group who had not yet received revascularization. One has to presume that not all 194 participants actually would have received a revascularization procedure. Ornish himself noted that this type of intervention is not only a function of the cardiac status quo, it is also affected by local values and practices, individual preferences of treating cardiologists and cardiac surgeons, and the funding situation of the patient. In support of this claim, he noted that in one of the centers there had been more angioplasties than in all of the seven other centers together (Ornish et al., 1998). From the perspective of cost effectiveness, it could be

shown that the Ornish program would have been cost effective if only 18% of the patients eligible for revascularization had been revascularized without participating in the program. This estimate is based on Ornish's calculation of total program cost of $7,000 for the 1-year program compared with costs of $31,000 for each PTCA and $46,000 for each CABG. In the control group, consumption of fat and cholesterol rose over time; however, they did remain relatively low overall. The reported values are substantially below the recommended values of the American Heart Association of 20% of daily caloric intake via fat and are less than 200 mg/dl of cholesterol, which had been the target in the Heidelberg study for the regression of cardiac disease by Schuler, Hambrecht, and Schlierf (1991). Mean serum cholesterol, LDL, and triglyceride levels decreased as did mean body weight between baseline and 3-month follow-up, and they did not rise again after 1, 2, and 3 years. This is in contrast to a variety of more recent studies in the German-language countries, which also showed an improvement in risk factors following cardiac rehabilitation, but follow-up assessments after 6 months to 3 years showed large increases in risk factors, at times even exceeding those observed at baseline (Badura, Grande, Janssen, & Schott, 1995; Grande, Schott, & Badura, 1999). This comparison of follow-up success across different studies shows that there is an apparent failure of transfer from Phase 2 of cardiac rehabilitation, which in Germany is predominantly inpatient care, to Phase 3, when the patient returns home. Rugulies and Siegrist (1999) described a mismatch between a short-term intensive treatment outside of the traditional learning environment and then a lack of long-term professional support after return to the patient's natural environment (Rugulies & Siegrist, 1999, p. 228). It is not known whether successful transfer as shown by Ornish et al. (1998) is due to the specific form or length of the intervention or whether it is primarily due to the selection of particularly motivated patients. Lack of randomized controlled trials of this approach is problematic. Furthermore, the demands on patients that are characteristic of the Ornish approach are not viable in daily practice for a large number of patients. As has been shown above, patients must be informed about treatment alternatives prior to randomization and must agree to accept randomization to different treatment arms. In this particular example, they must agree to treatment arms of revascularization or lifestyle change. Ornish et al. (1998) noted that the decision to revascularize corresponded more with patients who approached their physicians with a "wish for repair," whereas a decision for a consequently applied comprehensive lifestyle change requires engagement, discipline, and a desire to accept responsibility for one's health. It is therefore considered very difficult to recruit patients for whom the discussed alternatives are equally attractive and who would allow the assignment to be based on a randomization principle.

9.10.3. Rugulies and Siegrist (1999) Study

Rugulies and Siegrist (1999) wanted to establish whether the Ornish approach could be equally appealing in Germany. To test the question, the researchers used a nonrandomized treatment protocol with an intervention and a control group. Inclusion–exclusion criteria were documented cardiac disease, age between 35 and 77 years, ability to speak German well enough to participate, willingness to not smoke or to quit smoking during the study, and living within the regional catchment area of the clinic. The initial treatment group of 31 patients was composed of 18 patients who had followed a 4-week inpatient cardiac rehabilitation between January and April 1994 and 13 outpatient participants who lived close to the clinic and had heard about the program. Control group participants were recruited from a cardiac rehabilitation program and a clinic that also participated in the study. At the posttreatment assessment, 27 participants of the treatment group, including 1 woman, and 36 participants of the control group, including 6 women, participated. Four of the treatment and 7 of the control group participants were no longer available.

The intervention began with a 2-week program in which participants were familiarized with the program itself. The training comprised daily seminars about the scientific bases of the program and

its components, nutrition consultation, cooking courses, daily stress management and relaxation training, and support groups with psychological leadership. Following this, patients continued with training in an outpatient setting. In this context, patients were required to eat a low-fat, vegetarian, low-cholesterol diet; exercise regularly; practice yoga daily for relaxation and stress management; abstain from smoking; and participate in one group meeting per week. Each group meeting lasted 4.5 hours. The components of all interventions were practiced together. The final 1.5-hour group meeting focused on the exchange of problems with program adherence and also included a component of social and emotional support. The control group patients completed a 1-week inpatient cardiac rehabilitation program and were then referred for continuing usual care to their family physician or a cardiologist.

9.10.3.1. Results. Statistically significant differences were observed in the intervention group, whose members reduced their fat content and caloric intake from 36.2% to 12.1%, whereas the control group reduced them from 39.4% to 34.9%. The program participants increased the length of time spent on relaxation and stress management from 9 to 53 minutes per day, whereas in the control group, the corresponding length of time changed from 4 to 5 minutes. Both groups increased the amount of physical activity per day from 37 to 53 minutes in the intervention group and a roughly comparable 27 to 41 minutes in the control group. The serum cholesterol levels in the intervention group remained essentially the same after 1 year, with 195 mg/dl compared with 192 mg/dl, whereas in the control group, they became significantly worse, moving from 188 mg/dl to 211 mg/dl. At the beginning of the study, 11 patients in the intervention group had been taking a lipid-lowering medication, and this was reduced to only 4 patients after 1 year. The change in the lipid-lowering medication in the control group was minimal: 42.0% were still taking the medication after 1 year, whereas 55.6% had been taking the medication at baseline. The ergometrically determined maximum exercise tolerance was corrected for age and gender. In the intervention group, the maximal electrocardiogram performance improved from 95.5% of the norm to 217.2% of the norm, whereas in the control group there was a much less noticeable improvement of 87.2% to 92.9%. Cardiac symptoms were much less frequent in the intervention group than in the control group. Indicators of quality of life showed improvements in both groups; however, negative affect was reduced only in the intervention group. There were no reports of the program's effect on mortality and morbidity.

9.10.3.2. Commentary. The purpose of this study was to show whether the Ornish approach could be transferred to Germany and to an environment with a different structure of cardiac rehabilitation. The authors noted that the data resulting from the study could not readily be transferred to the entire population of cardiac patients and that given the lack of randomization, results should be interpreted cautiously (Rugulies & Siegrist, 1999, p. 235).

9.10.4 Commentary on the Ornish Approach Overall

The Ornish approach has vitalized the field of nonmedical cardiac rehabilitation because this research group has been able to show that an actual disease regression, defined by change in stenosis, is possible. Furthermore, full adherence to the program recommendations paid off for participants, and although demanding, adherence was found to be possible. Aside from the small sample sizes, the additional limitations of the Ornish approach are that the participants in the trial were a highly motivated subgroup unlikely to be representative of the total cardiac population. A particular challenge for everyday clinical use of this approach is to identify patients who are willing to invest and commit to this demanding program.

9.11. DISCUSSION AND CONCLUSION

This review focused on the question of whether the addition of psychological therapy can have a positive impact on morbidity and mortality of cardiac patients following a first event. Numerous large, well-controlled sample trials and meta-analyses of outcomes were available to help answer the question. These studies did not lead to simple, categorical conclusions, and this is likely due to the following factors:

- Large improvements in the quality of usual cardiological care have been made in the past 2 decades, and it is now exceedingly difficult to show a further reduction in the already low mortality rates attributable to usual care.
- Methodological variations in the protocols of the largest and best studies make interpretations difficult because interventions themselves varied, treatment was initiated at different time points in the rehabilitation trajectory, some patients received confounding treatments, comparison groups varied in the degree to which they were exposed to neutral versus active intervention, some studies had no female participants or only very small subsamples of women (too small to analyze separately), therapist qualifications varied, and studies also showed variability in who was treated (i.e., all cardiac patients vs. only those with demonstrated elevations in distress).

Despite these interpretive difficulties, we conclude here that psychological interventions, when added to usual care, can be of benefit if they are provided by well-trained professionals, offered to individuals in actually demonstrated distress, tailored to patient needs, and not confounded by additional pharmacotherapy. Unfortunately, female patients clearly benefit less than male patients, and one cannot rule out that they are actually harmed by psychological intervention; this may be particularly true for elderly female patients.

It has become exceedingly difficult to show the additional benefits of psychological therapy on mortality and event recurrence because of the high quality of current cardiological care in the treatment centers described in the above studies. Nevertheless, there is consistent evidence that existing psychological distress can be effectively reduced and that this may also have a positive generalizing effect on adherence to modification of other risk factors.

On the whole, there is a continuing lack of knowledge about what the right therapy dosage is and which patient benefits most from which type of intervention. Typically, the largest benefits were seen in studies with more intense interventions (e.g., the RCPP or the Blumenthal et al. [1997] study). An unresolved question of considerable urgency is the need for identification of treatments that are maximally beneficial to female patients; they appear to require an approach with an emotional processing focus and tend not to respond well to factual education and behavior prescriptions.

The creation of a sound knowledge base for defining effective psychotherapy frequently is handicapped by poor descriptions of interventions and confusing terminology. In particular, the concept of stress management is so poorly described and unevenly applied that comparisons of the effects of stress management across different studies are highly problematic and difficult to interpret (Ong, Linden, & Young, 2004). Similarly, there is no clear conclusion possible at this time as to what professional psychotherapeutic qualifications are needed for treatment success. Providers involved in cardiac care encompass a broad range of professions that vary greatly in the degree to which they have training and experience in psychological therapy, and there is evidence that psychotherapeutic competence cannot be readily taught in a few weeks as a trial of cognitive–behavioral therapy outcome offered by hastily trained family physicians has shown. It is suggested that mental health care providers who work with cardiac patients should have extensive training in diagnosis, multiple treatment approaches, and tailoring of programs to individual needs and comorbid conditions.

In conclusion, the clinical practice recommendations arising from this review are as follows:

1. Offer all cardiac patients some support and factual guidance for risk factor modification.
2. Closely follow all patients' rehabilitation processes in a standardized fashion for at least 1 year, preferably longer.
3. Identify those patients who do not cope well and who show clear signs of distress and offer them additional psychological supports.
4. Pay close attention to individual patients' needs and allow for gender-specific program tailoring.
5. When psychological treatment is offered, it should be provided by a trained professional who understands basic psychotherapy processes as well as the cardiac context, and this professional needs to continue the intervention until the desired target (i.e., significant distress reduction) is demonstrably reached.
6. Consider aggressive plans to attract all cardiac patients to comprehensive cardiac rehabilitation programs, which in turn will facilitate identification of those patients in greatest need of psychological support.
7. In some health care environments, like Germany's, there is a dichotomized system of care where relatively high-quality programming can be offered in inpatient rehabilitation settings (often far away from patients' home communities) that cannot be readily matched with continuous outpatient care once patients return home. Providing such continuity of care will likely continue to be a great challenge to health care systems.

CHAPTER 10

CARDIAC REHABILITATION FROM A HEALTH SYSTEMS ANALYSIS PERSPECTIVE

Gesine Grande and Bernhard Badura

10.1. INTRODUCTION

Within the developed Western industrialized countries, the importance of cardiac rehabilitation (CR) as part of the long-term medical care for heart patients is continuously increasing. Historically, the myocardial infarction (MI) represented the most important indication for CR. Meanwhile, the number of patients with chronic coronary heart disease (CHD) who must be treated repeatedly because of cardiac or cardiosurgical interventions is considerably more significant. On top of that, there are other interventions—for example, valvular heart surgery, implantation of pacemakers or cardioverter–defibrillators, and heart transplants—after which CR appears to be an appropriate service to support the processes of recovery and coping with the illness as well as lifestyle modification.

The prevalence of CHD in Western industrialized countries is very high. According to the data of the Framingham Heart Study, the lifetime risk of being affected by CHD from age 40 is 49% for men and 32% for women (American Heart Association [AHA], 2005). For the United States, prevalence rates of 18% (men) and 11% (women) have been reported for the 65-to-74 age group and 19% and 16% for older men and women (≥75 years), respectively. At present in the United States, about 13 million people are suffering from CHD (among them a higher proportion of men than women; AHA, 2005). Approximately 1 million MI survivors each year in the United States are potential candidates for CR (S. J. Glassman, Rashbaum, & Walker,

2001). In Germany in 2003, more than 820,000 hospital treatments were carried out because of a CHD diagnosis (for women, $n = 292,269$; for men, $n = 528,603$), of which just under 23% were performed because of an acute MI (AMI; for women, $n = 71,267$; for men, $n = 79,732$; Bruckenberger, 2004; Statistisches Bundesamt, 2005). The risk of falling ill increases with age in both women and men. The relationship between MI rates in men and women varies significantly between countries; however, the incidence rate in men is higher (World Health Organization [WHO], 2003).

The economic costs of medical care as well as of social protection (e.g., pension guarantee) are extremely high, even if they vary considerably internationally. For the United States, the direct (medical treatment including medication, etc.) and indirect costs of CHD amount to an estimated total of $142.1 billion (AHA, 2005). In Germany, approximately €2.8 billion were spent on coronary angiography, percutaneous transluminal coronary angioplasty (PTCA), and heart surgery in 2003 alone (Bruckenberger, 2004).

Quality of life is impaired by CHD and the consequences of coronary events to a varying extent. CR services are supposed to help patients in recovering as far as possible or in preserving their physical, mental, and social capability and quality of life as well as, by implementing long-term strategies of secondary prevention, to slow down the progression of the illness process and to decrease the probability of (further) coronary events. It is estimated that within 6 years after a coronary event has been diagnosed ("heart attack"), 18% of men and 35% of women experience another coronary event; 7% of men and 6% of women die of sudden heart failure; and for about 22% of men and 46% of women, life will be disabled by heart failure (AHA, 2005). Therefore, the need for rehabilitation services cannot be overestimated.

Little is known, however, about the practice of rehabilitating heart patients. Many evaluation studies are available (see, e.g., N. K. Wenger et al., 1995), but the results mostly reveal little about the usual practice of CR and practically nothing about the conditions of delivery—that is, health care structures (staff, qualification, equipment, etc.) and processes (therapy process, cooperation, communication, etc.).

The present analyses focus particularly on psychosocial aspects, their consideration in guidelines for CR, and the practice of rehabilitation in everyday life. The chapter is organized by important analytical categories of health systems analysis: aims of CR, care process, international recommendations concerning the program structure, service components, and personnel structure. The chapter also includes descriptions of CR practices in different countries in Europe (Germany, Great Britain, Ireland, Portugal, Switzerland) and North America (United States, Canada). We conclude with a short overview of the available scientific evidence on the effectiveness of training-based CR.

10.2. METHOD

For the present report, no particular survey was conducted—that is, all data, facts, and information were taken from publications, documents, and statistics accessible to the public. Literature research was carried out in the databases PubMed, PsycINFO, and REHADAT. For the search, the keywords *cardiac rehabilitation*, *rehabilitation*, *heart disorders*, and *coronary heart disease* were entered as well as combinations. Among the references, 247 reviews were found on CR. Evaluation studies that looked only at the effectiveness of CR programs were excluded. Editorials, reviews, and articles on health policy were obtained if they provided references to information on rehabilitation policy, on

aims and objectives of rehabilitation, and on rehabilitation structure and practice. The lists of references of current reviews and of articles on aspects of the national rehabilitation system were checked for further references to literature that could not be researched through databases (statistics, guidelines, online publications). All relevant teaching books and anthologies on CR were looked through, and relevant articles were considered. Furthermore, research was carried out on the Internet through the Web sites of relevant national and international scientific and medical societies, of the National Institutes of Health, and of the Cochrane Library. This made it possible to record the current guidelines for CR.

10.3. AIMS OF CARDIAC REHABILITATION

From a historical point of view, the conception and practice of CR were shaped by three illness models: the biomedical illness model of cardiology–cardiosurgery, the epidemiological risk factor model of CHD, and the biopsychosocial model of the WHO. All three illness models make certain assumptions about the etiology of CHD. In CR oriented toward secondary prevention, the risk factor model has a particular significance in being used as a conceptual frame, whereas the biomedical model defines the care concept of acute cardiology and consumes the largest part of financial and structural resources. This has a direct influence on the number of patients leaving acute hospital care with a definite need for rehabilitative services as well as on the clinical picture of CHD. For long-term and comprehensive CR, the biomedical approach does not provide an adequate conceptual basis.

At the beginning, CR was a service that had been provided exclusively for post-MI patients. The past approximately 50 years have seen radical changes with regard to the CR of MI. Even up until the 1960s, MI was treated with strict bed rest for at least 6 weeks (Kavanagh, 1996). S. A. Levine and Lown (1952) introduced their new method of "armchair treatment" in 1952, which initiated the beginning of modern CR. Following the concept of "early mobilization" and later "early rehabilitation," efforts have since been made to mobilize patients earlier and earlier after MI to reduce the negative consequences of long periods of inactivity on circulation, the heart, and the muscular system as well as to minimize the traumatization of patients due to lack of activity. CR in the strict sense has existed since the late 1950s. In Israel, V. Gottheiner introduced a training method for heart patients in 1955. He compiled the findings of his experiences with over 1,000 patients until 1968 (Gottheiner, 1968). Hellerstein and Ford (1957) published guidelines for exercise training in CR. In 1969, a first, normative definition of CR was adopted by the WHO (1969). According to this definition, the purpose of CR was to eliminate or alleviate negative consequences of the illness (functional, mental, and social restrictions) in patients after discharge from acute hospital care. In the following years, the concept was broadened by the aspect of secondary prevention to form a holistic approach to CR:

> The rehabilitation of cardiac patients is the sum of activities required to influence favourably the underlying cause of the disease, as well as to ensure the patients the best possible physical, mental and social conditions so that they may, by their own efforts, preserve, or resume when lost, as normal a place as possible in the life of the community. (WHO, 1993, p. 5)

The definition of the European Society of Cardiology reads nearly identically (Tavazzi et al. for the Task Force of the Working Group on Cardiac Rehabilitation of the European Society of Cardiology, 1992). Core elements of the WHO definition are the demand for modification of the causes of the disease, the biopsychosocial approach, as well as the central position of the patient in terms of being responsible for overcoming the illness and social reintegration.

The WHO concept differentiates between three targeted areas:

- Medical aims (prevention of cardiac mortality, reduction of cardiac morbidity, of the rate of MI and embolisms, decrease of angina pectoris and dyspnea);

- Psychological aims (restoring the patients' self-confidence, reducing anxiety and depression, improving stress management, regaining a satisfying sexuality); and

- Socioeconomic aims (return to work, if appropriate; independence in everyday life activities; reduction of direct medical costs through, e.g., early discharge from the hospital; less medication; fewer rehospitalizations). (WHO, 1993, p. 6)

The official formulations of the aims of CR in Germany fall behind the recommendations of the WHO with regard to the comprehensive nature of CR and the central role of the patient in the rehabilitation process. In Germany, the official targets of CR closely follow the legal requirements of the pension scheme. Therefore, the avoidance of a significant risk for patients' fitness for work ("rehab before pension") as well as their reintegration into working life and their social environment are considered to be the urgent goals for CR in Germany. In older patients, the focal point is the avoidance or reduction of the need for nursing (Schliehe & Haaf, 1996; Weidemann et al., 1991). Secondary prevention aims are not explicitly mentioned, although they are of central importance in CR practice.

To sum up, there is international agreement about the aims and tasks of CR: secondary prevention and reduction of somatic, psychological, and social consequences of the disease. The emphasis on the interests of the funding providers in the official formulation of targets and—in opposition to that—the lack of emphasis on the patient's autonomy and independence are aspects of the specific situation of rehabilitation in Germany.

10.4. THE REHABILITATION PROCESS

The process of CR is usually divided into three phases according to the criteria of the WHO (Denolin, 1985). Phase I is the *acute phase* (treatment in the hospital), Phase II is *convalescence* (after the acute cardiac event), and Phase III involves long-term rehabilitation at home.

In the United States, a "Phase IV" is occasionally added with the idea of targeting the aspect of lifelong and autonomous efforts of the patients (e.g., self-help groups, cardiac groups without medical presence, medical control by the general practitioner [GP]). Phase III is characterized as a transition to everyday life, whereas the stabilization of lifestyle modification and achievement of physical fitness are at the center of Phase IV. The guidelines of Great Britain and Scotland also work with a definition of four phases: the inpatient stage (Phase I), early postdischarge period (Phase II), late postdischarge period (structured exercise program; Phase III), and long-term maintenance (Phase IV; Bethell, 2000; Scottish Intercollegiate Guidelines Network, 2002; D. R. Thompson, Bowman, Kitson, de Bono, & Hopkins, 1996). In many countries, however, Phase III has been defined as lifelong rehabilitation at home, in which GPs or health centers carry out the tasks of medical care both in cases of cardiac crisis and regular checks on risk factors and cardiac condition, and has the same meaning and aims as Phase III when only three phases are defined.

Discussion about the adequacy of these defined phases is increasing. The individual phases and their contents overlap because of varying lengths of stay in the hospital and CR programs (McCall Comoss, 1999). In the meantime, the current guidelines of Canada and the American Association of Cardiovascular and Pulmonary Rehabilitation (AACVPR) for the United States distinguish only between inpatient and outpatient programs (AACVPR, 1999; J. A. Stone et al., 2001).

There are significant differences internationally in the shaping of the rehabilitation process (see Table W10.1 on the accompanying Web site: http://www.apa.org/books/resources/jordan/). They relate to, among other things, the length of Phases I and II. Nowadays, the mean duration of a stay in the hospital (e.g., after an MI) varies between 13 days in Germany and 6 days in the United States. The length of the CR programs in Phase II in the various industrialized nations either depends on individual peculiarities (medical, psychosocial, and insurance-related and financial conditions) or is generally regulated, as in Germany (see section 10.6 in this chapter).

Differences also exist with regard to the delivery and implementation of rehabilitation services. Only a few countries (e.g., the United States and Great Britain) have formalized CR programs of Phase I for the hospital and specially qualified personnel (usually nurses; see section 10.6). CR programs of Phase II are (a) nearly exclusively offered as outpatient treatment (e.g., United States, Great Britain), (b) completed on outpatient or inpatient bases of varying length and intensity (e.g., France, the Netherlands, Switzerland), or (c) carried out nearly exclusively in specialized rehabilitation hospitals (Germany, Austria).

In a report on 20 years of CR in Europe, Mulcahy (1991) summed up the position of the WHO Working Group on Cardiac Rehabilitation:

> It is accepted that rehabilitation programs can be organized and can be successful despite the many different forms they may take. Formal institutional rehabilitation is valuable, particularly in problem cases and for research purposes but, for logistic and financial reasons, it is not applicable to most patients and to many countries. Informal outpatient rehabilitation programs have been shown to be successful and are more cost-effective for the great majority. Many cultural, political and economic factors play a part in determining the type of rehabilitation programs that are most suitable in each community. (p. 92)

10.5. RECOMMENDATIONS AND GUIDELINES FOR THE SERVICE COMPONENTS OF CARDIAC REHABILITATION PROGRAMS

The existing recommendations of institutions and scientific and medical societies for the delivery of CR programs vary internationally with regard to the service components. The requirements refer to the elements of the program, the allocation of patients to these services, and the composition and qualification of the personnel who should ideally be available. There are also regulations regarding access, that is, for the definition of a medical or social need for CR.

10.5.1. Service Components

Recommendations for the service components of CR by various scientific and medical societies and institutions exist in nearly all developed industrialized countries. Some essential guidelines were considered for this overview: a WHO consensus paper on cardiac rehabilitation (WHO, 1993); recommendations of the Working Group on Cardiac Rehabilitation of the European Society of Cardiology (Tavazzi et al., 1992); guidelines for CR for Great Britain (D. R. Thompson et al., 1996); recommendations for Germany (Weidemann, 1996; Weidemann et al., 1991); guidelines of the AACVPR, the Agency for Health Care Policy and Research, and the National Heart, Lung and Blood Institute (N. K. Wenger et al., 1995); recommendations of the AHA (Balady et al., 1994); and the common recommendations of the AHA and the AACVPR (Balady et al., 2000) for the United States.

The WHO consensus paper distinguished between three service components as the main elements of a comprehensive CR:

- Exercise training (at 70% to 85% of the maximum heart rate in the exercise test, 30 to 45 minutes, 3 to 5 sessions/week);
- Secondary prevention and risk factor control for cholesterol, high blood pressure, smoking, diabetes, and stress (health education, exercise training, stress management, social support, drug therapy); and
- Return to work (evaluation of the patient's functional capacity and of the patient's motivation and attitude toward return to work, of the employer's attitude, and of the physical strains of work; WHO, 1993).

Recommendations and requirements of other countries have deviated from the WHO requirements only in certain aspects. All of them have named exercise training and modification of risk factors/secondary prevention as cornerstones of the CR programs offered. More recent works have assessed both components as being of equal importance, and it is pointed out explicitly that the term *rehabilitation* is no longer applicable to exercise training only (e.g., Ades, Balady, & Berra, 2001; Balady et al., 2000; McCall Comoss, 1999). The

Working Group on Cardiac Rehabilitation of the European Society of Cardiology (Tavazzi et al., 1992) assigned the aims of rehabilitation to risk stratification and interventions to decrease the risk of cardiac events and reduced quality of life. Medical and psychosocial assessments and interventions here follow a stricter comprehension of secondary prevention.

Concrete details for the delivery of exercise training are given (e.g., regarding length and frequency of training sessions, exercise levels, forms of training [walking, jogging, bicycle ergometer training, strength training, etc.], and supervision and electrocardiogram [ECG] monitoring; e.g., AACVPR, 1999; Tavazzi et al. 1992; WHO, 1993). Many guidelines have explicitly referred to the necessity for medical diagnostics, especially of cardiopulmonary fitness, before starting exercise training and as a basis for an individual training schedule (AACVPR, 1999; Balady et al., 2000; Tavazzi et al., 1992; D. R. Thompson et al., 1996; Weidemann et al., 1991; WHO, 1993).

There is a standard demand for the modification of risk factors to be based on the intake assessment (e.g., AACVPR, 1999; Balady et al., 2000; Tavazzi et al., 1992, D. R. Thompson et al., 1996). A multifactorial approach is considered necessary for a successful modification of risk factors; there is a distinction between measures of health education, behavior modification, and stress management. These three approaches are regarded as standard, with the exception of the guideline from Great Britain, which only mentions health education (Thompson et al., 1996). There are no details on how to combine these approaches effectively or which protocol and strategies they should be based on. An exception worth mentioning is the guidelines of the AACVPR: In the chapter "Education and Behavior Modification," detailed theories and principles of learning were outlined (adult learning, behavior modification, social learning theory, "readiness for change" theory; AACVPR, 1999). Pharmacological treatment of medical risk factors has been explicitly mentioned as an option in some recommendations, though behavior modification has been given priority (AACVPR, 1999; Balady et al., 2000; WHO, 1993).

Psychosocial counseling and intervention are mainly or exclusively mentioned in the context of secondary prevention aims, for example, in the WHO consensus paper (relaxation, stress management; WHO, 1993), in the recommendations of the European Society of Cardiology (health education, modification of risk factors, relaxation; Tavazzi et al., 1992), in the German recommendations (information, behavior therapy, health education, relaxation training/stress management; Weidemann et al., 1991), and recently also in the common statement of the AHA and AACVPR (Balady et al., 2000). Only the second edition of the AACVPR guidelines (AACVPR, 1995) explicitly distinguished between psychosocial interventions to support the process of coping with the illness and interventions in the context of risk factor modification. The requirements for CR in Great Britain comprise, besides health education, the area of psychosocial care, with the aim of improving quality of life and supporting secondary prevention. For the practice of CR, however, only screening for anxiety and depression is required (excluding other relevant aspects such as self-esteem, social support, coping efforts, etc.) as well as, in some cases, referral to external psychosocial services.

According to the guidelines of the AACVPR (1999), psychosocial evaluation in outpatient CR should investigate the following aspects: evidence of posttraumatic stress syndrome; significant negative affect, particularly depression; substance abuse; patient's and family's perceptions of health status; patient's goals with regard to sexual adjustment and problem behavior; level of social support; and effectiveness of social support.

Interventions should be tailored as much as possible to the needs of the individual, but there is no single definition of an appropriate psychological intervention, nor is it known which type of psychological treatment is best for which type of cardiac patient (W. Linden, 2000). The expectations of psychological interventions are rather low: "Assessment of psychosocial status including depression is recommended at entry although implementation of the practice of appropriate and acceptable techniques for management is sometimes difficult" (AACVPR, 1999, p. 48).

Return to work has always been, aside from improvement of exercise tolerance, a central goal of CR. The idea has remained the same in principle, even if other goals are relevant for the increasing number of older patients with CHD, such as maintaining autonomy in everyday life. Most guidelines continue to list return to work as an important aim of CR and demand vocational counseling as a standard part of their programs (Tavazzi et al., 1992; WHO, 1993), at least in terms of a medical assessment of physical fitness according to work demands (D. R. Thompson et al., 1996; Weidemann et al., 1991).

The allocation of rehabilitation services according to patients' needs is considered significant, with a demand for a consequent individualization of the therapy schedule (McCall Comoss, 1999; N. K. Wenger et al., 1995). At the social and psychological level, however, there is still a lack of diagnostic standards governing allocation of individual treatment in CR (see AACVPR, 1995; Badura, Grande, Janßen, & Schott, 1995; McGee, 1999; Wenger et al., 1995).

Table W10.2 (see the accompanying Web site) shows that international recommendations with regard to essential service components of programs on CR work very much along the same lines. Therefore, ideas about which services should be offered essentially coincide. What remains unclear, however, especially in view of health education, behavior modification, and psychosocial intervention, is how these services are to be shaped in concrete terms and which models, methods, and procedures in the context of rehabilitation represent efficient strategies for achieving the long-term aims of care. The requirements and guidelines are not specific concerning this point. Only the guidelines of the AACVPR provide, for example, concrete references to theoretical models and principles according to which health education should be offered as part of CR (AACVPR, 1999, p. 77).

Most recommendations do not refer to technical equipment, personnel, or questions of organization and delivery of CR programs. Two exceptions could be found regarding the recommended mode of organizing programs: In the United States, the

AHA recommends comprehensive supervised programs or, alternatively, rehabilitation programs that can be carried out at home with monitoring or as training programs without supervision, respectively (Balady et al., 1994). In Germany, there is a demand for inpatient programs in specialized hospitals (Weidemann et al., 1991). Both recommendations can probably be seen as justification for existing delivery modes rooted in history rather than in empirical evidence.

10.5.2. Indications

From a medical point of view, there are hardly any differences internationally with regard to the indication ranges (see AACVPR, 1995; Balady et al., 1994; Franz, 1998; Lear & Ignaszewski, 2001; WHO, 1993). If at first patients were referred only after an uncomplicated MI, the spectrum has strongly expanded as a consequence of quickly developing cardiac and cardiosurgical interventions for the treatment of CHD (e.g., PTCA, coronary artery bypass grafting [CABG], heart transplant). For patients with other forms of acute and chronic heart disease (e.g., stable angina, chronic heart failure, cardiomyopathy, valvular heart surgery, implanted cardioverter–defibrillator/pacemaker), participation in a CR program also has been recommended in recent years (e.g., AACVPR, 1995; Lear & Ignaszewski, 2001; Tavazzi et al., 1992; WHO, 1993). The number of cardiac or cardiosurgical interventions in older patients is increasing, and the proportion of the elderly in CR will continue to rise (Köhler, 1995; Pashkow, 1995; L. A. Richardson et al., 2000; Schott, Iseringhausen, & vom Orde, 2002).

In principle, there is international agreement on contraindications for CR. These generally relate to the exercise-training component of CR programs. Criteria for exclusion, for example, are unstable angina, blood pressure higher than 200/110 mmHg, uncontrolled dysrhythmias, and orthopedic problems that forbid physical exercise (AACVPR, 1995; Tavazzi et al., 1992; Weidemann & Meyer, 1991).

Indications and contraindications, however, are only preconditions for participation in CR programs. Many programs have admission restrictions that influence the makeup of the participants independent of basically existing medical diagnosis and recommendations. So in the early 1990s, approximately 75% of persons undergoing CR in Great Britain were patients after MI. One fifth of the programs took on no patients after CABG, and 44% took no patients after PTCA. Nearly 70% of the programs had an age limit for participation (the cutoff ranging between 60 and 75 years of age; Davidson, Reval, Chamberlain, Pentecost, & Parker, 1995). A survey in England and Wales in 1994 confirmed that participation was generally restricted to younger male patients after uncomplicated MI (D. R. Thompson, Bowman, Kitson, de Bono, & Hopkins, 1997).

10.5.3. Personnel

Rehabilitation personnel are required to have multidisciplinary competencies. Recommended staff–patient ratios are closely connected to the recommendations for rehabilitation services and the program structure.

The WHO demands that all health professionals participating in CR possess clinical competence in their own disciplines as well as special skills for motivating patients toward long-term lifestyle modification. They further specify that the rehabilitation team be composed of a cardiologist as medical director, nursing staff, physiotherapists, dieticians, and clinical psychologists. In larger rehabilitation facilities, other medical disciplines, occupational therapists, and social workers also can be included (WHO, 1993).

In Germany, the recommendations of the Reha-Commission of the Federation of German Pension Insurance Institutes (VDR) have provided important standards for CR programs. Here, the status quo is reflected more strongly than in the recommendations of other societies and working groups (Gabanyi & Schneider, 1993): The VDR emphasizes occupation groups with medicosomatic qualifications compared with psychosocial ones as well as nursing staff, although nurses generally have neither rehabilitation-specific training nor carry out rehabilitation-specific tasks (see Table W10.3 on the accompanying Web site).

In Great Britain, the British Cardiac Society has only some general recommendations for the personnel structure of the CR team. A work report from 1992 stated that "the cardiologist will remain the most appropriate individual to co-ordinate the activities involved in CR in most district hospitals" (J. Horgan et al., 1992, p. 417). More recent recommendations have involved a cardiologist or physician to support programs in terms of resource allocation, patient selection, knowledge transfer, and medical presence (for the latter, once a month is considered to be sufficient—it seems there is an ongoing decrease in the role and importance of physicians in Great Britain in CR; Davidson, 1996); program coordination should be performed by nurses with experience in cardiac care (Davidson, 1996; Davidson et al., 1995).

For the United States, the AACVPR (1995) defined minimal standards regarding personnel structure as a staff–patient ratio of 1:5 in Phase II and 1:15 in Phases III and IV. Different competencies should be represented in the team as a minimum: CHD, cardiovascular nursing, emergency procedures, diet, training physiology, health psychology, and medical and pedagogic strategies for the management of risk factors. Cardiac core competencies are recommended for the areas of assessment, goal setting, intervention, and evaluation (e.g., communication and advice, psychosocial diagnostics, health education) for nurses and physical therapists, independent of the respective academic discipline (Southard et al., 1994).

To sum up, recommendations for personnel competencies and qualifications were available only from the WHO, the United States, and Germany and are difficult to compare. It becomes evident in the U.S. guidelines of the AACVPR (1995) that the acquisition of specific rehabilitation-related competencies is credited with more importance than the academic professional basic education. Recommendations for personnel competencies in CR in Germany focus on the occupation groups to which members of staff belong, independent of (additional) rehabilitation-specific qualifications. The high number of nursing staff in all recommendations in Germany can only be explained by the fact that patients are nearly exclusively treated in specialized rehabilitation hospitals.

10.6. REHABILITATION MODELS

The practice of CR in Phases I, II, and III will be presented for different countries: Germany, Great Britain, Ireland, Switzerland, the United States, and Canada. The selection of these countries is based solely on the availability of reports that allow insight into their respective national rehabilitation practices. The description of the rehabilitation models is preceded by an overview of the utilization of CR.

10.6.1. Utilization of Cardiac Rehabilitation

Table W10.4 (see the accompanying Web site) shows available data on participation rates of CHD patients in CR programs of Phase II. The percentages refer to the proportion of rehabilitation participants in relation to the (estimated) incidence of CHD (treatments in the hospital and discharges with an ischemic heart disease diagnosis).

In nearly all countries, CR has experienced a significant growth over the past 20 years. In 1970, no more than 3% of CHD patients participated in CR programs in the United States; the number in Great Britain was between 6% and 8% (N. K. Wenger, 1976). In Great Britain, most programs were established in the 1980s and later because of a health policy initiative. In Australia, where CR has been established only recently, a 30% increase of participation rates was registered within 2 years' time, between 1996 and 1998 (from 24% to 53%; I. A. Scott, Eyeson-Annan, Huxley, & West, 2000). Causes for the tentative introduction of CR programs in most countries are likely to be found in their low acceptance by clinical medicine, a lack of appropriate health care facilities for long-term cardiac care, and problems of financing.

In Germany, the situation is fundamentally different. The rehabilitation of chronically ill persons developed within the tradition of the spa, which was already well established there by the beginning of the 20th century. With the drop in infectious diseases, German rehabilitation institutions were troubled by the problem of underuse of facilities; existing facilities (spa clinics, sanatoria) were transformed into specialist hospitals for medical rehabilitation. In 1975, 3 times more rehabilitation measures for patients after MI were supplied in Germany than in 1995 (32,765 vs. 11,329; Statistisches Bundesamt, 1976, 1998). Despite this fall in numbers, Germany still has the highest participation rates compared with the other countries whose data we examined. Presumably, the legal entitlement to rehabilitation services and the guarantee of costs being covered by statutory pension insurance or compulsory health insurance are of importance here.

Participation rates vary depending on medical problems; a preceding CABG, especially, leads to higher participation rates in Germany and the United States (Rost, Hartmann, Horstmann, Koll, & Bjarnason-Wehrens, 1999, R. J. Thomas et al., 1996). Independent of medical diagnosis, references were found that pointed to differences between hospitals concerning patient referral: The participation rates of MI patients varied, according to the respective hospital, from 49% to 65% in Cologne, Germany (Rost et al., 1999), and from 34% to 72% in the United States (Evenson, Rosamond, & Luepker, 1998). In the study by Pell, Pell, Morrison, Blatchford, and Dargie (1996), the participation rate was best predicted by the hospital in charge of the treatment. The significance of sociodemographic characteristics like age, sex, occupation, and socioeconomic status for the utilization of CR services cannot be discussed in more detail within the bounds of this report. In general, the pathways and determinants of referral to CR programs are largely unknown (K. M. King & Theo, 1998).

10.6.2. Care Models

10.6.2.1. Germany. Following is a description of the typical CR process in Germany: its organization, funding, services, and involved personnel.

10.6.2.1.1. Phase I. There are no formal CR programs for Phase I in acute care hospitals in Germany. The length of stay in the hospital is still long in Germany compared with other countries. Badura et al. (1987) reported an average hospital stay of 32 days after an AMI; in 1994 this period had decreased to 18 days, and in 2001, to 13 days (Statistisches Bundesamt, 2005). Because of a longer stay in the hospital, Phase I in Germany comprises a longer period than is common internationally. Early mobilization and control of medical risk factors are seen as integral parts of acute medical care. Providing psychosocial care is considered equally desirable but too difficult to implement because of the lack of psychosocial qualified personnel in hospitals and insufficient psychosocial competence of the doctors employed.

10.6.2.1.2. Phase II. In 1995, approximately 130,000 rehabilitation measures were provided because of heart disease. Rehabilitation in Germany is funded by pension schemes or health insurance, depending on who is bearing the financial risk of rehabilitation failure. Health insurance pays for all persons who are receiving a pension already or who have no pension scheme (e.g., housewives). In 1995, 48% of rehabilitation measures were financed by health insurance and 45% by pension schemes. Thirty percent of CR measures were taken up by women, and the gender differences in participation rates reflect the sex-specific differences in prevalence fairly well.

The rehabilitation landscape in Germany has undergone some changes over the past few years (see Figure W10.1 on the accompanying Web site). This is due to new legal regulations, which were supposed to limit the costs of rehabilitation services. Since January 1, 1997, the length of CR has been reduced to 3 weeks, although CR services have been reduced only to a small extent.

As discussed earlier, CR during Phase II in Germany has been traditionally carried out nearly exclusively in rehabilitation hospitals. The first rehabilitation hospital was established in 1968. At present, 142 rehabilitation facilities are run in Germany, with which funding providers have established contracts to provide follow-up rehabilitation services relating to heart and circulation diseases (Bruckenberger, 2004; Deutsche Gesellschaft für Prävention und Rehabilitation [DGPR], 2004). Only a small fraction of CR programs are delivered in an outpatient mode—either hospital based or organized by specialized physicians or rehabilitation centers. Pension schemes and health insurance do not, as a general rule, undertake to pay the costs of outpatient rehabilitation supplied by cardiologists in their own practices. Differences were found in staff, equipment, and other resources between inpatient and outpatient facilities but not with regard to the outcomes (Iseringhausen, Schott, & vom Orde, 2002; vom Orde, Schott, & Iseringhausen, 2002).

The standard is very high with regard to diagnostic procedures. All hospitals carry out stress tests, resting and long-term ECGs, and echocardiography; more than half of the hospitals work with telemetry ECG monitoring. Evaluation of pulmonary function can be carried out in more than 80% of the hospitals.

There is no representative overview on program structure and individual offerings in rehabilitation facilities in Germany. In a current evaluation study on a total of more than 1,000 patients undergoing CR in seven rehabilitation facilities, patients took advantage of 4.1 to 4.7 services per day (Iseringhausen et al., 2002).

Programs are structured in a comprehensive way (see Table W10.5 on the accompanying Web site). Services like hydrotherapy or massage are surely unique in comparison with other countries; here too, the spa tradition of German rehabilitation may have an influence. As shown already for the 1980s and 1992–1993 (Badura et al., 1995; Lehmann, 1987), interventions aiming at the restoration or improvement of exercise tolerance and physical fitness followed by measures of health education also predominate. Psychological services in the stricter sense are offered to only a small number of patients (Grande, Leppin, Romppel, Altenhöner, & Mannebach, 2002; Iseringhausen et al., 2002).

The different weighting of service components in CR is reflected in the staffing ratio in CR programs (see Table W10.6 on the accompanying Web site). After the nursing staff, whose specific tasks in the context of rehabilitation have not yet been defined, physicians and physiotherapists or physical education teachers are the best-represented occupation groups. On the other hand, psychosocial professionals, including dieticians, are of quantitatively minute importance. This ratio is in agreement with the official recommendations (VDR, 1992). Under these conditions, individual psychotherapy is offered to a very small number of patients. The tasks

of psychological professionals in the data we reviewed covered a broad range, from supervision in the wards to professional training for employees and patient care, which took the form of lessons on health education. Psychological services (content and scope) varied significantly between individual facilities (Badura et al., 1995; see Table W10.6).

The entire process of health care delivery in Germany is fragmented because of the variety of funding providers and institutions. One characteristic of the situation is the legal and institutional separation of CR from, on the one hand, acute care and, on the other hand, long-term treatment by GPs or medical specialists (Schott et al., 2002). Individual providers take on parts of the health problems of persons with heart conditions in phases but without sufficient liaison with preceding or following care facilities and without mutual cooperation. The responsibility of a facility starts with admission and ends with discharge of patients.

The short program duration of just 3 weeks as well as problems in coordination and transition between the rehabilitation hospitals and the GP or medical specialist at home are probably partly responsible for the poor medium- and long-term effects in everyday life conditions (e.g., Badura et al., 1995; Grande, Schott, & Badura, 1996; Niebauer et al., 1994; Nüssel, Scheuermann, & Halhuber, 1992; Völler et al., 1999; Weidemann et al., 1999).

10.6.2.1.3. Phase III. In Phase III, CR in Germany is carried out by medical specialists or GPs and outpatient cardiac groups. In 1971, the first organized outpatient cardiac groups came into being. In 1977, there were 77 such groups; in 1985, there were 1,000; and in 1992, around 3,000. Currently, about 6,000 outpatient cardiac groups exist, used by an estimated 100,000 patients (DGPR, 2005). The figure is considered much too low compared with the annual rate of newly affected persons. According to various studies, between 13% and 35% of the participants in CR programs of Phase II take part in outpatient cardiac groups afterward (Badura et al., 1995; Budde & Keck, 1998; Lehmann, 1987). Exercise training and sports are essential components of outpatient cardiac groups, usually occurring once a week for over 60 minutes (Unverdorben, Brusis, & Rost, 1995). The exercise trainers are in charge of carrying out physiotherapy and sports, but a doctor must always be present (Ilker, Brusis, & Unverdorben, 1995).

10.6.2.2. Great Britain. In Great Britain, the first outpatient CR programs were established in the late 1960s. The focus was on Phases II and III. The program structure was determined by regular exercise sessions over 4 to 12 weeks, complemented by information on secondary prevention. In 1970, the British Cardiac Society did a survey of all members in active practice in adult cardiology and found that 90 of 113 replies reported no special CR facilities; an advisory pamphlet was used in 11 hospitals, and 9 hospitals reported some form of exercise program (from early mobilization to organized exercise regimens; Groden, Semple, & Shaw, 1971). In reaction to a report of the British Cardiac Society on the status of CR in Britain in 1989 and on future tasks for development, funding was supplied that increased the number of CR programs significantly in the following years. For 1996, 273 programs were reported, and for 1998, approximately 300 rehabilitation programs were reported (Dinnes, 1998; see also National Health Service [NHS] Centre for Reviews and Dissemination, 1998). Many programs were initiated by physiotherapists or nurses rather than physicians:

> Cardiac rehabilitation has developed through the enthusiasm of local nurses, physiotherapists, and sometimes occupational therapists, but rarely doctors. These unsupported individuals have seen the need and set up programs in a haphazard way depending upon their own resources and skills, usually with little or no clinical backing from physicians or cardiologists. (Bethell, 2000, p. 93)

It is assumed that the delayed development of CR in Great Britain is due to the lack of support and the critical attitude of physicians, especially cardiologists, toward CR supply and its benefits (Davidson et al., 1995; J. Horgan et al., 1992). Yet, there has always been a strong emphasis in Great Britain on the importance of integrating cardiologi-

cal specialist competence into the rehabilitation process of heart patients, because acute medical care after MI in district hospitals is mostly carried out not by cardiologists but by doctors of other medical disciplines (Bethell, 1997).

10.6.2.2.1. Organization. Nearly all district hospitals taking care of cardiac patients have cardiac CR programs for Phase I (inpatient) and Phases II and III (outpatient). The programs for Phases II and III are organized as hospital-based or community-based services. In England and Wales, hospital-based programs are predominant; in Scotland, half of the CR programs are community based but supply services for only 20% of persons undergoing CR (see Table W10.7 on the accompanying Web site).

10.6.2.2.2. Services. Table W10.8 (see the accompanying Web site) gives an overview of the services supplied in CR programs in Great Britain. It is striking that the programs display an extremely large variation with regard to frequency and length of services, and the services at the lower end of the spectrum are inadequate to meet the formulated standards and aims. In summary, note the following:

- Assessment of cardiopulmonary function and risk stratification is not routinely supplied. Intake assessment and outcome evaluation have been introduced only recently and only for single parameters and in less than half of the facilities.
- Exercise training is a basic element of all programs. The delivery, however, seems to vary significantly between individual facilities. A mean frequency of one to two sessions per week of about 1 hour in length is inadequate for achieving positive training effects.
- Health education constitutes the main component of CR programs besides exercise training and is offered in 70% to 80% of all facilities in the form of individual or group counseling. There is no information available on content or quality. Special training programs such as smoking cessation were not mentioned. The frequency of services offered varies between facilities as with exercise training. Nurses and dieticians are mainly responsible for delivering health education, but doctors, pharmacists, and

physiotherapists also provide some education on a casual basis.

- Psychosocial assessment and interventions are generally not carried out by psychologists. The use of validated psychological questionnaires is an exception, as is the provision of formal psychotherapy. Approximately 60% of the programs offer relaxation training, and only four programs included any other psychological therapy (there were no details on content or methods; Campbell, Grimshaw, Ritchie, & Rawles, 1996). In England and Wales, as many facilities reported the prescription of psychoactive drugs for patients with mental problems (44%) as offered psychological advice (40%).

> There is a wide variation in practice and in the organisation and management of cardiac rehabilitation services: there is evidence that current service provision fails to meet the national guidelines for cardiac rehabilitation and that secondary prevention measures are underapplied. (NHS Centre for Reviews and Dissemination, 1998, p. 2)

In Great Britain, there has been no supervised long-term rehabilitation—only some patient support groups who meet regularly for exercise training (Davidson, 1996). Therefore, the continuity of cardiac care cannot be guaranteed. Secondary prevention—a key component of a comprehensive rehabilitation of patients with CHD—is insufficient, and it remains doubtful whether GPs can influence the current situation, especially in terms of the modification of health-relevant behavior (Campbell et al., 1998; see Table W10.8).

10.6.2.2.3. Personnel. The personnel structures in CR programs and their changes since 1989 are summed up in Table W10.9 (see the accompanying Web site). Doctors are not integrated into CR programs or are given only advisory status. In comparison with the situation in 1989 and 1992, there is a strong increase in later surveys of the predominance of nurses both on rehabilitation teams as well as providing services. Nurses are largely responsible for organizing, coordinating, and delivering programs. In addition, most rehabilitation facilities employ physiotherapists on their teams. Psychosocial services are mainly performed by non-psychologically qualified health professionals. This corresponds to the recommendations and guidelines, which recommend a nurse therapist with training in cognitive behavioral therapy rather than a clinical psychologist for the first contact with patients with mental problems. Nurse therapists provide advice and treatment (Scottish Intercollegiate Guidelines Network, 2002). Health education, information, counseling, and modifying inappropriate illness concepts should ideally be taken on by the medical staff. In the context of risk factor modification, psychological knowledge is considered to be necessary; the importance of involving psychologists, however, is less acknowledged for the provision itself than for the development and evaluation of such behavior modification programs. That is, psychologists are not required as counselors or face-to-face psychotherapists; their main competencies and responsibilities are in conceptualization and evaluation of behavior modification programs. Instead, nurses are seen as the ideal professional group to offer counseling and behavior modification (B. Lewin, 1996).

10.6.2.3. Ireland. In 1998, a survey of all hospitals with coronary or intensive care units in the Republic of Ireland ($N = 41$) and Northern Ireland ($N = 12$) was carried out regarding CR service availability (McGee, Hevey, & Horgan, 2001). One third of the hospitals in the Republic of Ireland offered CR programs, and another third were planning implementation of a program. In Northern Ireland, 75% of the hospitals had a program. All but two programs in the Republic of Ireland had been established within the past 5 years. There were no details available on participation rates. Five programs had upper age restrictions between 66 and 75 years. In an earlier survey of nine CR programs in Northern Ireland, participation was limited to patients after MI or CABG (J. M. Bradley, Wallace, McCoy, & Dalzell, 1997). In 18 centers, there was no cost to the patients for services.

10.6.2.3.1. Services. All programs had facilities for groups, with a mean of 8.3 persons (range

2–20). Number of weekly sessions ranged from one to four ($M = 1.7$), and program duration was 8 weeks (range 3–12; see also J. M. Bradley et al., 1997). The most frequent intervention by far was exercise, with a mean of 13.7 sessions ($SD = 10.3$) per program, followed by relaxation training ($M = 3.1$), cardiac education ($M = 2.5$), stress management ($M = 1.9$), diet ($M = 1.6$), general psychological advice ($M = 1.3$), medication advice ($M = 0.9$), smoking cessation ($M = 0.7$), sexual counseling ($M = 0.6$), and vocational counseling ($M = 0.4$). Variation between programs was, however, significant. The same applies to the length of individual sessions. A mean of approximately 50 minutes is reported for training, relaxation, stress management, diet, and medication advice; 40 minutes for psychological advice; and 18 minutes for vocational counseling.

10.6.2.3.2. Personnel. All programs worked with a multidisciplinary team, and most had designated CR coordinators (most with formal training). Coordinators provided most time to the programs ($M = 28.2$ hours/week, range 0–40.0), followed by nurses ($M = 7.5$ hours/week, range 0–40.0), dieticians ($M = 3.1$ hours/week, range 0–37.5), physiotherapists ($M = 2.8$ hours/week, range 0–35.0), and ECG technicians ($M = 2.7$ hours/week, range 0–37.5). Other occupation groups with quantitatively lower participation were psychologists ($M = 1.7$ hours/week, range 0–17.5), social workers ($M = 1.3$ hours/week, range 0–20.0), occupational therapists ($M = 0.7$ hours/week, range 0–10.0), and medical consultants ($M = 0.3$ hours/week, range 0–2.0). Concerning the program and personnel structure, the extremely high variation does not allow us to draw general conclusions for CR in Ireland.

10.6.2.4. Switzerland. In Switzerland, there is a distinction between outpatient and inpatient rehabilitation centers as well as outpatient cardiac groups (Schweizerische Arbeitsgruppe für Kardiale Rehabilitation, 1998). Health insurance provides funding for both outpatient and inpatient rehabilitation programs. Centers are accepted by the Schweizerische Arbeitsgruppe für Kardiale Rehabilitation if they provide a comprehensive, structured rehabilitation program with minimum requirements regarding the course of the program, personnel, and infrastructure: (a) a minimum of 200 (inpatient) or 50 (outpatient) patients per year, two thirds after an acute cardiac event; (b) medical management by a cardiologist or an internist with experience in cardiology (or in cooperation with an experienced cardiologist); (c) equipped for emergencies (including complete resuscitation equipment); (d) multichannel ECG; (e) ergometry facility with bicycle or treadmill ergometer; (f) Doppler echocardiography; (g) telemetry or long-term ECG; (h) intake assessment (exercise test, risk factor profile) and evaluation of outcomes; (i) a minimum of three (inpatient) or two (outpatient) exercise levels, respectively, in exercise training (Schweizerische Arbeitsgruppe für Kardiale Rehabilitation, 1998).

In 1989, 39 rehabilitation centers were registered in Switzerland out of a total of 42 CR programs, of which 21 each worked in outpatient and inpatient mode, respectively. In 1998, 21 outpatient and 13 inpatient rehabilitation centers for cardiac patients met the quality standards described previously and were listed in the official register (Schweizerische Arbeitsgruppe für kardiale Rehabilitation, 1998)—in other words, there were 8 inpatient facilities fewer than there were 10 years earlier (Pfiffner & Saner, 1990; Saner & Pfiffner, 1995). During that 10 years, between 60% (Naegeli et al., 1998) and 75% (Saner, 2000) of persons undergoing CR took advantage of an outpatient program. Outpatient rehabilitation centers are not spread extensively throughout the entire country (Saner, 2000); they are mainly associated with acute care hospitals or organized by local physician groups (Schweizerische Arbeitsgruppe für Kardiale Rehabilitation, 1998).

CR programs are provided for patients after MI, PTCA, CABG, or other interventions of the heart or large vessels, but they are also provided for those with chronic heart disease and multiple risk factors or low ventricle function. The duration of the programs differs according to the setting (outpatient vs. inpatient) and between facilities. In the "Cardiac Rehabilitation" register, a program duration of between 4 and 36 weeks (most are 12 weeks) is indicated for outpatient rehabilitation centers, a standard program duration of between 3 and 4 weeks for inpatient rehabilitation centers. The duration of CR programs is determined individually (Schweizerische Arbeitsgruppe für Kardiale Rehabilitation, 1998).

In 1989, the extent of the training program varied between 9 and 32 hours per week in specialist rehabilitation hospitals and lasted 3 to 4 weeks. In other hospitals, a maximum of 29 hours of exercise training was prescribed. In outpatient centers, CR took place one to three times weekly and comprised approximately 36 hours over 12 to 36 weeks, depending on frequency per week. The time needed for health education was between 7 and 25 hours in inpatient programs. In outpatient facilities, the focus was on individual patient advice by the doctor or physiotherapist (Pfiffner & Saner, 1990). Cardiologists or internists are generally the types of professionals entrusted with the management of the rehabilitation centers. In inpatient facilities, exercise training was mostly carried out by physiotherapists ($N = 14$) or physical education teachers ($N = 7$); two institutions also used a nurse for this training. In 25% of outpatient and 50% of inpatient CR programs, a psychotherapist was part of the team. A social worker was employed only in inpatient facilities, and only in half of these (Pfiffner & Saner, 1990).

10.6.2.5. United States. Following is a description of the typical rehabilitation services in all phases of CR in the United States.

10.6.2.5.1. Phase I. For many patients, the application of a CR program begins after MI, CABG, and heart transplant while they are still in the hospital. From there, a referral can take place to an outpatient CR program that begins after discharge. The length of inpatient CR programs depends on the length of the stay in the hospital, which shows a trend toward extreme shortening (Franklin, Hall, & Timmis, 1997; Froelicher, Herbert, Myers, & Ribisl, 1996). Therefore, little time remains for rehabilitative interventions, so the focus is more frequently on risk stratification as well as on motivating patients to participate in outpatient CR programs (Pashkow, 1995, 1996). A study of 5,204 Worcester, Massachusetts residents hospitalized

with AMI between 1986 and 1997 established a participation rate of 68% for CR programs in Phase I (Spencer et al., 2001).

10.6.2.5.2. Phases II and III. The duration and services of outpatient CR in Phases II and III vary depending on the care models, insurance coverage, and treatment protocols. Because there is no standard for cardiac care delivery during convalescence in the United States, care models are characterized by large variation in frequency and extent of services (N. K. Wenger, 1989). CR programs after discharge from the hospital are offered exclusively as an outpatient service. The GP takes the role of gatekeeper; GP recommendations for participation are the strongest single predictor of later utilization of such programs by patients (Ades, Waldmann, McCann, & Weaver, 1992). The focus is on exercise training; many insurance companies do not cover other rehabilitation services (Gutin, Prince, & Stein, 1990).

There are three different program modes: (a) CR programs organized by the cardiac departments of hospitals (*hospital-based*); (b) programs organized in local health centers by GPs, communities, or universities (*community-based*); and (c) programs carried out by patients at home (*home-based*).

A survey of the program directors of 163 CR programs in the United States in 1990 established that all facilities offered Phase II CR programs, and more than 70% offered programs of Phases I (inpatient), II, and III (long-term, outpatient). Most programs were hospital-based (85%); others were community-based. A mean of 88 cardiac patients each were rehabilitated per facility per year (R. J. Thomas et al., 1996). An earlier study reported annual patient figures (Phases I, II, and III) of between 50 and 950 for the early 1980s in hospitals in Virginia, with approximately 75% of the patients having participated in inpatient Phase I CR programs (Wolfe, Herbert, Miller, & Miller, 1987).

Not all insurance companies cover outpatient supervised CR in a rehabilitation center. The length of the program, too, depends not only on individual medical requirements but also on financing possibilities. It is suspected that a significant number of patients could be persuaded to participate in exercise training tailored to their needs[1] in a home setting (with or without telephone ECG monitoring; Fletcher, 1998; N. K. Wenger et al., 1995). Therefore, more and more models of home-based rehabilitation are implemented in the care of CHD patients in the United States. Rehabilitation programs at home are considered to be more economical, practicable, and convenient as well as having a higher potential for supporting independence and autonomy. They are seen as being particularly suitable for low-risk patients (e.g., Fletcher, 1998) and are recommended for all rehabilitation phases (Rogutski, Berra, & Haskell, 1999). The results of home-based rehabilitation are considered to be comparable—at least with regard to the improvement of physical fitness—to the outcome of supervised rehabilitation programs in rehabilitation centers (DeBusk et al., 1994; NHS Centre for Reviews and Dissemination, 1998; N. K. Wenger et al., 1995). Home-based rehabilitation is commonly organized by a nurse with complementary training in cardiology who contacts patients, introduces the program, allocates patients to the respective interventions (exercise training, diet counseling, drug therapy for lipid reduction, smoking cessation, etc.), arranges diagnostics and outcome evaluation, and continuously keeps in contact with patients (by phone or in person). He or she essentially carries out health education, supervises the exercise training, and is responsible for the coordination with other care providers (GP, cardiological department in the hospital; K. Green & Lydon, 1995; Imich, 1997; Salisbury, 1996).

There is no representative survey of the program and personnel structure of CR facilities in the United States; the few published surveys have been mostly limited to individual areas and were often not up to date. Exercise training was the most important program element, according to the data available. Health education and psychosocial services often were not financed by insurance (DeBusk, 1992). A survey of 672 of all 1,027 operating centers determined in the late 1980s that most of the programs provided diet counseling and patient–family education (94% and 88%, respectively; Byl, Reed, Franklin, & Gordon, 1988). Seventy-five percent of the programs offered stress management, 69% weight reduction, and 59% smoking cessation. In contrast, only 1 in 4 programs addressed vocational counseling or work evaluation.

In New England, an evaluation was carried out in the mid-1990s that analyzed the personnel structure in outpatient (Phases II, III, and IV) and inpatient (Phase I) CR programs that employed a program director and at least one other health professional (S. B. Bennett & Pescatello, 1997). Compared with the guidelines of the AACVPR, the minimum requirements concerning the provision of staff were met by about 40% and the preferred requirements by only 7% of the programs. Nurses and physiotherapists had the best qualifications, fulfilling 90% and 84% of the minimum requirements, respectively, whereas only 11% of the program directors had at least the minimum qualifications. In New England, 70% of the program directors belonged to the occupation group of nursing (D. R. Thompson & Bowman, 1998).

Regarding the question to what extent psychosocial services were provided in CR programs, results are only available from the 1980s. Sikes and Rodenhauser (1987) did a survey of representatives of hospital-based programs. Thirteen percent of the facilities included in the survey did not offer any form of counseling for patients. Psychosocial counseling services in the hospital (Phase I) were carried out by nurses in 95%, by social workers in 50%, by doctors in 30%, by dieticians in 23%, and by psychologists in only 12% of the programs. In outpatient settings (Phase II), nurses were involved in psychosocial counseling in 80%, social workers in 43%, psychologists in 27%, and dieticians in 22% of the facilities (Sikes & Rodenhauser, 1987). A survey of rehabilitation programs in Virginia that was carried out during the same period of time showed that approximately 40% of the programs in

---

[1] "Tailored to their needs" mainly refers to establishing individual levels for exercise training (maximum heart rate, duration of training sessions) as well as recommendations for the modification of risk factor profiles. The patients have to carry out the training alone at home; its course is discussed with a nurse over the phone. Some programs also offer the possibility of telephone ECG monitoring.

that state provided psychological counseling, 63% offered stress management, and only one program offered vocational counseling; exercise training was part of all programs (Wolfe et al., 1987). A survey of 20 CR programs in New York showed that there was a lack of psychosocial services in particular, or these services were provided only as complementary services and were usually not covered by insurance (Gutin et al., 1990). More up-to-date studies are not available.

The low participation rates in the United States are attributed to, among other things, the lack of support from doctors, especially cardiologists: "It is much more practical and realistic to teach cardiology and exercise physiology to physical medicine rehabilitation physicians and to family practitioners than to expect cardiologists to perform cardiac rehabilitation" (Morris & Froelicher, 1991, p. 76). Especially in low-risk patients, the lack of a positive attitude toward CR is also important (DeBusk, 1992). DeBusk (1992) concluded that even if insurance reimbursement was not an issue, it was unlikely that the proportion of patients participating in CR programs would more than double.

10.6.2.6. Canada. According to the results of a nationwide survey, 94 CR units (CRUs) existed between 1987 and 1990 in Canada (Armstrong, Wolfe, & Amey, 1994). Around 17,000 patients were treated in these facilities per year. Fifty-three percent received rehabilitation after MI (less than 20% of the yearly survivors after MI), 32% were postcardiac surgery patients, and 9% were angina patients. Other indications (heart transplant, pacemakers, valve defects, etc.) were possible but rare. Most patients were referred by cardiologists (44%) and personal physicians (38%); self-referral was allowed occasionally in CRUs that included Phase III components (8%). In combined models of Phases I and II, the referral from I to II could take place automatically (Armstrong et al., 1994).

10.6.2.6.1. Care models. There is a distinction between models of Phase I (closely supervised inpatient therapeutic units), Phase II (outpatient therapeutic units), and Phase III (outpatient maintenance units) and combined models. The most common type was a freestanding Phase III unit

($n = 40$). Some CRUs offered both inpatient and outpatient services ($n = 28$); only 7 facilities provided exclusively inpatient rehabilitation and a further 4 exclusively outpatient rehabilitation of Phase II. Half of the CRUs were sponsored by hospitals. Programs of Phase III (or Phases II and III) were sponsored by YMCAs and YWCAs, community centers, universities, and private hospitals (Armstrong et al., 1994).

10.6.2.6.2. Services. All programs offered formal exercise training. Other services varied according to the respective care model, the CRUs of Phase II providing the largest number of services, followed by inpatient programs (Phase I) and the Phase III models. Inpatient units offered nutritional counseling, psychological counseling, and stress management more frequently than outpatient maintenance units. Across all facilities, smoking cessation and vocational counseling were offered less frequently. There is no detailed information on how many patients take advantage of these services, how frequently individual services are offered as part of the programs, or supervised exercise.

Most programs required a graded exercise test before program entry ($n = 79$). Exercise training in the hospital was supervised by physiotherapists (51%) or nurses (43%). In other rehabilitation facilities, noncardiologist physicians (61%), physical educators (55%), and nurses (36%) supervised sessions. The most common modes of exercise were walking or jogging (99%), warm-up exercises (89%), stationary cycling (71%), and aerobic calisthenics (47%). Continuous telemetry was used most often during Phase I (86%) and Phase II (83%) exercise training. Across all unit types, manual pulse monitoring was most commonly used (Armstrong et al., 1994).

10.6.2.6.3. Staffing and technical equipment. In an earlier survey of 37 of the 43 CR programs across Ontario, Canada, data were collected on management and personnel structure (Wolfe, Dafoe, Hendren-Roberge, & Goodman, 1990). One third of the program directors were physicians; another third were physiatrists, exercise physiologists, or physical therapists; and 8% were nurses. Additionally, physicians were employed in 60% to 70%; nurses in 60%; and physical therapists, exercise physiologists, or kinesiologists in 20% to 40% of CRUs (Wolfe et al., 1990). In inpatient facilities, the patient–staff ratio was less than 5:1; in Phase II units and combined Phase II and III units, the ratio was between 30:1 and 5:1 (Armstrong et al., 1994). Seventy-seven percent of the units had access to stress test facilities, and on-site exercise testing laboratories were available in 52% and included treadmills (88%), 12-lead electrocardiographs (83%), and cycle ergometers (67%). Seventy-six percent of CRUs had access to blood biochemistry laboratories, 61% to echocardiography, and 54% to thallium imaging. Exercise equipment used in CRUs included stationary cycle ergometers (80%), treadmills (46%), and arm ergometers (28%; Armstrong et al., 1994).

10.6.3. Summary

There are some methodological limitations regarding representativeness and quality of data used here. At this time, there are no public quality assurance reports on CR internationally available. The reports that were considered here vary significantly with regard to the databases; the extent to which the information is representative of the national rehabilitation system; the range of information; and the goals for collecting, selecting, and presenting data on CR (e.g., to provide more transparency, promote CR programs, justify the national rehabilitation system). A recently published article on CR in Europe tried to overcome the significant lack of information by an international comparative survey (Vanhees, McGee, Dugmore, Schepers, & van Daele, 2002). Methodological problems of such a demanding enterprise become apparent, however: Some statements were based on information from single experts who used estimates because of a lack of valid data sources in individual countries (e.g., for Germany). The extremely low response rates to some of the questionnaires and even the mean response rate of 57% are too small to make the results representative, especially in view of the wide variation of services provided in individual countries (e.g., Bethell, Turner, Evans, & Rose, 2001, also refer to inaccurate estimates for Great Britain).

It is possible, however, to draw some conclusions from the data surveyed here. There is inter-

national agreement on the definition of the CR process and the differentiation of three or four progressive phases. International differences lie in the delivery of CR in Phase II (outpatient, partially inpatient, or inpatient), connecting with preceding and following providers, the services offered, the length of programs, and the staff involved in the rehabilitation team as well as its leadership. These fundamental differences arise from different historical roots of the rehabilitation systems and reflect the variety of existing health care systems in different countries. They are based structurally on different financing models and funding providers for CR as well as on differences in the way rehabilitative services are linked to existing health care structures (acute sector, GPs, rehabilitation centers, spas, and rehabilitation hospitals). Although the organization of CR (Phase II) in Germany is highly standardized, in other countries and especially in the United States, a large number of different modes exist concerning the setting, services, and length and whether they work in parallel or in competition with each other.

In the United States and in Great Britain, nurses are of crucial importance as coordinators and providers of rehabilitative services. In contrast to the situation in Germany, for example, the definition of their tasks in CR are located exclusively outside of traditional nursing (e.g., Thompson & Webster, 1992). The rare presence or the absence of physicians in CR programs has been discussed, however (Davidson et al., 1995; J. Horgan et al., 1992; Kellermann, 1993), and various (medical) rehabilitation experts (e.g., Barnwell, 1979; Kellermann, 1993) have demanded repeatedly that the pivotal role in CR programs ought to be played by a well-trained cardiologist because of the severity of the medical problems involved in rehabilitating specific groups of patients (Kellermann, 1993).

In all countries, services offered on exercise training predominate. Psychosocial services are provided less frequently and are usually limited to secondary prevention aims of risk factor modification (patient education, stress management). In contrast mostly with Great Britain and the United States, an especially great distance seems to exist in Germany between acute cardiac care, CR, and long-term care by GPs and specialists. The individual rehabilitation phases are formally connected neither in regard to location or health care facility nor personnel or immediate transfer. Continuous cardiac care can therefore not be guaranteed. In the United States and in Great Britain, for instance, the transition between CR programs of the acute phase and Phases II and III can be carried out often continuously in the same hospital under the responsibility of the same health professionals (nurses). On the other hand, there are no formalized services provided for long-term rehabilitation (Phases III and IV) in Great Britain, apart from some self-help groups. The fragmentation of health care processes through insufficient integration of the various service providers who are involved in CR and long-term care of cardiac patients is also criticized in the United States (e.g., Tate Unger & Warren, 1999).

There is practically no information on CR from less developed industrialized countries. CR in Asia, Africa, and Latin America, if implemented at all, seems to play a quantitatively marginal role and is not or only in part covered by insurance because other more important health care services are needed to deal with problems such as high infant mortality and infectious disease (Guzman, Lopez-Grillo, Dorossiev, & Feher, 1986).

10.7. EFFECTIVENESS

In 1998, the NHS Centre for Reviews and Dissemination counted 215 systematic reviews on CR. The quality of these reviews, however, was considered to be so poor that only 7 were included in an up-to-date overview article (NHS, 1998; see also Dinnes, Kleijnen, Leitner, & Thompson, 1999). The present report cannot be concerned with providing another review of evaluation studies of CR programs. The following summarizing statements are based on the four meta-analyses published so far and a review on the effectiveness of training-based CR. The review was also considered for the description of the latest developments in research, because it represents the most comprehensive compilation of empirical findings on the effectiveness of CR to date and because it includes randomized as well as nonrandomized controlled studies and

observational studies if they were published in English. The effectiveness of purely psychosocial interventions with CHD patients was not considered here (see Table W10.10 on the accompanying Web site).

The meta-analyses by Bobbio (1989); O'Connor et al. (1989); and Oldridge, Guyatt, Fischer, and Rimm (1988) were frequently discussed with regard to methodological aspects of the studies on which they are based: The sample size was often small, the dropout rates high, the interventions not specified, and the studies themselves were restricted to middle-aged men after MI with a low cardiac risk. A selection bias caused by insufficient or incomplete literature research is often suspected (NHS, 1998).

The meta-analysis by Jolliffe et al. (2001) considered 32 randomized studies until the end of 1998 and doubled the number of patients included. The preceding meta-analyses were complemented by randomized controlled trials that were published in the 1990s. Only comparisons between CR programs and usual care were included. Jolliffe et al. also questioned the methodological quality of the studies considered: Only 16% of the studies gave a clear description of an adequate randomization, and 29% of the studies had a dropout rate of more than 20% on the follow-up. A publication bias was statistically excluded.

In October 1995, the clinical guideline *Cardiac Rehabilitation* was published in the United States (N. K. Wenger et al., 1995). On behalf of the Agency for Health Care Policy and Research (1995) and the National Heart, Lung, and Blood Institute, an expert group of the AACVPR carried out a very extensive literature review on the effectiveness of CR. In total, 344 randomized and nonrandomized controlled studies were considered as well as observational studies that had been published in English in a peer-reviewed journal since 1966.

The selection of studies for the review was based on the following criteria.

- *Indication*: CHD (angina, silent ischemia, AMI, revascularization) and heart failure (including patients prior to or after heart transplantation).
- *Components of cardiac rehabilitation*: exercise, patient education, counseling, risk factor modi-

fication, intake assessment, risk stratification, adherence, and costs.

- *Outcomes*: exercise tolerance, exercise habits, symptoms, smoking, lipids, weight, blood pressure, psychological status, social adjustment and functioning, return to work, morbidity, mortality.

Methodological criteria for inclusion and exclusion respectively were not formulated.

In the following summary, only the findings on the effects of exercise training (as the only intervention or in combination with other psychosocial interventions or health education) are considered. In addition, pathophysiological outcomes were not included because these specific aspects are beyond the bounds of this summary.

Exercise-based CR has a consistent effect on the improvement of exercise tolerance (see Table W10.11 on the accompanying Web site). Cardiovascular morbidity could be influenced in terms of symptom reduction (angina), not concerning a reduction of the rate of nonfatal MI. Some evidence suggests that CR leads to a reduction in mortality, including cardiovascular and total mortality as well as "sudden death." The meta-analyses refer to a reduction of mortality rates of between 20% and 30%, whereas the included studies on their own do not produce significant effects of CR on mortality. Effects of training-based CR on other outcomes and particularly on psychosocial well-being are comparatively difficult to interpret. Only the meta-analysis by Jolliffe et al. (2001) considered outcomes other than morbidity and mortality.

Only a small number of studies were included in an analysis of the effects of CR on the risk factor profile. Multifactorial CR programs resulted in improved levels of total cholesterol and high-density lipoprotein; no effect for cigarette smoking and reduction in blood pressure could be proven (because of completely heterogeneous measuring instruments, no meta-analysis was calculated for the outcome area of quality of life). Similarly, no consistent results arose from the review by N. K. Wenger et al. (1995; see Table W10.12 on the accompanying Web site), according to which exercise training seems to have no effect on cigarette smok-

ing, body weight, or blood pressure, especially when not combined with other interventions. Slightly more than 50% of the studies reported positive effects of CR programs on the blood lipid levels. Approximately two thirds of exercise-only programs and multifactorial interventions had positive effects on psychosocial well-being.

O'Connor et al. (1989) as well as Jolliffe et al. (2001) compared the effects for studies with exercise only with multifactorial programs in their meta-analyses. O'Connor et al. determined significant effects for cardiovascular mortality and sudden death only for multifactorial interventions; this, however, could be due to the small number of exercise-only programs in the analyses (between two and five). Jolliffe et al. found different effects for exercise-only versus multifactorial interventions with respect to total mortality; only the exercise-only programs were linked to a significant reduction of the mortality rate. The authors suggested caution in the interpretation of these results because of the inadequate data quality. There were no differences between both types of programs for cardiovascular mortality and nonfatal MI as well as cardiac events altogether.

No definitive statements can be made on the effectiveness or on additional effects of psychosocial interventions as complements of exercise-based CR from the selected meta-analyses and the review. When interpreting the results, it should be taken into account that in most, especially older, studies, so-called "psychosocial" or "multifactorial" interventions included no more than unstructured interventions on information or advice on risk factors, respectively (e.g., the so-called "WHO studies" included in the meta-analyses by Jolliffe et al., 2001; O'Connor et al., 1989; Oldridge et al., 1988). Quantity and quality of these "additional" services offered are usually low. What is more, the idea cannot be excluded that relevant information was communicated to the patients as well, as part of usual care in exercise-only programs. Other meta-analyses aiming at the specific effectiveness of health education, stress management, or psychosocial interventions in cardiac patients (Dusseldorp, van Elderen, Maes, Meulman, & Kraaij, 1999; W. Linden, Stossel, & Maurice, 1996; Mullen,

Mains, & Velez, 1992) found significant effects for the considered structured psychosocial intervention programs on risk factors, mortality, and morbidity. The psychosocial interventions are very heterogeneous with regard to patients, type of service providers, group-based or individual services, and type of intervention (behavioral interventions for lifestyle modification, relaxation strategies, stress management, cognitive–behavioral therapies, etc.), which makes it more difficult to come to final conclusions (W. Linden, 2000).

It is not possible to draw conclusions from the available data regarding differences in effectiveness depending on rehabilitation settings or systems, such as between outpatient and inpatient services or between different countries. There is no single international comparative study to date on the effectiveness of CR in different rehabilitation systems. The randomized and nonrandomized controlled studies chosen in the meta-analyses and the review were carried out nearly exclusively in an outpatient setting. All evidence for the effectiveness of training-based CR applies to programs carried out in an outpatient setting (usually hospital-based or community-based). Comparative evaluation studies in the United States suggest a comparable effectiveness of supervised outpatient programs in rehabilitation centers, at hospitals, or as home-based CR programs (N. K. Wenger et al., 1995). The same applies to Germany: The data show no important differences in effectiveness between outpatient and inpatient services despite their different structural and process qualities (Badura et al., 1995; vom Orde et al., 2002).

The various studies were published between 1972 and 1999, a period of time in which rehabilitation concepts and services provided changed significantly, as did the need for CR arising from cardiac diagnoses, medical problems, secondary prevention strategies, and changing coping tasks. However, aside from changes over time, programs in different settings or rehabilitation systems evaluated at the same time often varied significantly with regard to service components and program structure, so that an actual comparability of effectiveness was not given. Finally, an aggressive pharmacological therapy in secondary prevention (aspirin, beta-blockers, statines, angiotensin converting enzyme blockers) has become established over the past few years that questioned the capacity for additional effects of multifactorial CR programs on mortality, morbidity, and risk factor profile.

The meta-analyses and the review cannot be considered representative for all cardiac patients. The effectiveness of CR reported here was determined mainly for groups of men under the age of 65 after MI and with low cardiovascular risk. There is not enough evidence to prove whether comparable (or, as suspected, more significant) effects of CR can be achieved for the elderly, for women, or for patients who are more seriously affected by their disease.

10.8. SUMMARY AND FUTURE PERSPECTIVES

Because of the chosen approach, the present report cannot claim to be complete. International publications on the structure, quality, services, and results of CR are almost exclusively limited to English-speaking countries (above all the United States and Great Britain). Furthermore, health systems are subject to significant changes and restructuring as a consequence of rapidly developing medicotechnical progress and the dynamic increases in the costs of modern health care. This also has an impact on financing and (consequently) the delivery of rehabilitation services.

10.8.1. Need for Cardiac Rehabilitation

CR programs in all developed industrialized countries have seen significant changes in their patient samples over the past few years regarding an increase in medical complexity and illness severity in patients with CHD as well as an increase in the proportion of the elderly. One cause of this development is seen in the opening of CR programs to patients with poor health status or at high cardiac risk because of greater experience in the delivery of cardiac exercise training and very low complication rates. Demographic changes (an overproportional increase in old and very old parts of the population) that are linked to an overall rise in the number of CHD patients and especially in the elderly, women, and patients from different ethnic groups influence the sample of CR patients. These changes also refer to changes in the demography of cardiovascular diseases. Already a polarization has become visible between CHD patient groups, one at low cardiac risk and with minimal functional impairments after cardiac events because of early and invasive cardiological and cardiosurgical interventions (thrombolysis, PTCA, CABG) and the other chronically ill after recurrent MIs or revascularization, who have reached the final stage of the disease (heart failure, cardiomyopathy) in their old age (N. K. Wenger, 1999; see also Saner, 1993). Improvements in acute cardiac care have produced an extended spectrum of cardiac clinical pictures (e.g., patients after revascularization, valvular heart surgery, or heart transplant; implantation of pacemakers or cardioverter defibrillators; N. K. Wenger, 1999). Participation rates have been particularly low, however, among patients with a higher cardiac risk and more serious cardiac conditions and in general among the elderly, although it is assumed that patients with severe functional restrictions, pronounced risk factor profiles, and/or psychosocial problems could benefit most of all from CR (Hotta, 1991; NHS, 1998).

10.8.2. Services

As the patient structure has changed, the aims and services of CR have had to be modified. Two areas representing these changes are the focus of discussion: altered significance of service components in CR and individualization of intervention.

10.8.2.1. Service components. The importance of exercise training for the improvement in exercise tolerance and functional capacity for patients after uncomplicated MI decreases with the possibilities of thrombolysis and the avoided deconditioning of the cardiovascular system because of shorter immobilization and bed rest after MI. Meanwhile, patients with high cardiac risk, heart failure, multimorbidity, or old age are considered to be the candidates who can benefit most from exercise training, whereas exercise training cannot contribute more to an improvement of the prognosis in patients with a low or medium cardiac risk

(DeBusk, 1992; Froelicher et al., 1996; Köhler & Held, 1996; Pashkow, 1996; Tavazzi et al., 1992; N. K. Wenger, 1992). Drugs of effectiveness comparable to exercise programs, like beta blockers, are less costly, and the costs are covered by usual care (DeBusk, 1992). In the context of secondary prevention, exercise training is only one aspect; it does not contribute—or not considerably—to the modification of other risk factors like smoking, overweight, and cholesterol level (Dinnes et al., 1999; Moore, 1997). A CR program based primarily on exercise training, applied after uncomplicated MI treated with contemporary therapies, including coronary thrombolysis and acute angioplasty, can only result in a small (additional) effect on return to work by improving functional capacity, apart from the fact that functional capacity is not a consistent predictor for return to work under current labor market and workplace conditions (DeBusk, 1992). In the future, important fields of CR will be psychosocial and lifestyle counseling, training of health-related skills, and long-term motivation of patients to adhere to secondary prevention strategies (Froelicher et al., 1996, Pashkow, 1996; see also Tavazzi et al., 1992). The WHO Expert Committee stated in 1993 that the components of health education and counseling in CR deserve more attention and that health education alone is not sufficient but must be complemented by cognitive–behavioral interventions (WHO, 1993; Sivarajan Froelicher, 1999).

There is a significant lack of psychosocial aspects of CR, however, when it comes to actual delivery. In the current practice of CR, psychosocial services are of no importance or play an insignificant role, as can be observed in the absence of formal psychosocial services as well as of psychosocial health professionals from CR programs. If counseling and education are part of CR programs, they are usually provided by persons without special psychological qualifications. In most programs, psychosocial services only deal with the area of health education. Emotional support and support in coping efforts are not even mentioned as important goals in guidelines and recommendations. Many psychosocial aspects of CHD are not well described by commonly used screening instruments for serious mental health problems (see, e.g., McGee, Hevey, & Horgan, 1999). The meaning of psychosocial aspects such as anxiety and depression are often reduced to their instrumental function for lifestyle modification and long-term adherence; depression, especially, is considered a risk factor for adherence and long-term outcomes. There is currently neither a coherent theory regarding the relevance of psychological and social factors for the etiology and progression of CHD nor a standard intervention model or consensus on psychosocial screening in practice. Interventions relating to changes in the social environment are not even part of guidelines and rehabilitation care.

10.8.2.2. Individualization.

In the early 1990s, the WHO observed a trend toward a more individual tailoring of CR services according to the severity of illness and patients' needs and preferences (WHO, 1993). Although an emphasis on prevention or secondary prevention components seems adequate for low-risk patients, exercise training could be more suitable for patients with chronic and advanced CHD to attain goals like maintaining functional independence in everyday life and the regaining of a personally satisfying lifestyle.

With strict individualization, CR programs could be designed not as a maximum service for each participant but such that each patient would receive only services he or she needed according to intake assessment (Ades et al., 2001, McCall Comoss, 1999). This referral should be based on medical recommendations and patients' preferences. This would help to include various patient groups (medical problems, age, comorbidity, seriousness of CHD) in CR and to reduce costs (Dafoe & Huston, 1997; N. K. Wenger, 1993).

No one doubts the necessity and appropriateness of a more individualized CR. But to what extent can an extremely individualized CR, focusing exclusively on single parameters according to intake evaluation, continue to represent a comprehensive approach? Even more than at present, CR will probably become a range of coexisting intervention goals and isolated services whose integration in the perspective of a comprehensive approach to coping with and adapting to illness is left to the patient alone.

10.8.3. Comparative Evaluation of Rehabilitation Systems

Cardiac rehabilitation: one term; many goals, services, and approaches. With regard to concepts and aims, there are no significant differences to point out. Important differences do exist between the examined countries in terms of rehabilitation structures and resources like financing, personnel, diagnostic and therapeutic equipment, services provided, and therapy schedule, but also within the facilities of one country, as shown, for example, by the evaluation studies in Great Britain. With regard to the goals and guidelines of CR—especially in view of psychosocial aspects of rehabilitation—the structural conditions of practically all rehabilitation models presented must be considered insufficient, though with clear gradual differences.

There is no empirical evidence suggesting which structural conditions characterize high-quality CR or which ones are linked to the best results. International comparative studies of different rehabilitation systems are lacking. The large number of available evaluation studies has proved the effectiveness of CR for the improvement of cardiopulmonary capacity and for the reduction of mortality. Even so, these studies contribute little to a comparative evaluation of different rehabilitation systems and models of usual care in CR. They prove the efficacy and effectiveness under model circumstances but rarely under everyday circumstances. In addition, the outcome of the individual studies can hardly be compared because they were generated on different rehabilitation systems and settings and on the basis of different services provided (Dinnes et al., 1999). A comparative rating of the presented care models of CR with regard to the ideal system conditions is therefore not possible at the present time.

10.8.4. Perspectives

In many countries, the current (and future) delivery of CR is determined by lasting changes in contemporary medical therapies and in insurance company policies, that is, primarily by financing possibilities. It has been reported for the United States (DeBusk, 1992; N. K. Wenger, 1999) that intensity and frequency of professional integration in CR programs are on the decrease; an early independence is pushed forward, and home-based rehabilitation is becoming an economical alternative available for a larger number of cardiac patients. Already-low participation rates in rehabilitation centers, the decreasing significance of exercise training in general, and the growing number of home-based services could result in the centers' losing a large part of their previous tasks and functions. They would remain important for high-risk patients and patients with a greater need for integration into a structured program and a social group (Moore, 1997). On the other hand, the GP could play a much more important role in the context of CR, which, however, would also require better and more specific qualifications. GPs could act as comprehensive consultants, and should the occasion arise, they could supervise exercise training at home and above all support and further secondary prevention and lifestyle modification (Moore, 1997; Froelicher et al., 1996). Previous experience shows, however, that physicians in clinical practice have not been particularly effective in secondary prevention. CR programs and preventive cardiology clinics could therefore play a particularly important role in secondary prevention in the future (Ades et al., 2001).

There is a growing emphasis on multidisciplinary care and individualized services, and the criteria of cost-effectiveness could lead to a greater variety of CR models, which should be specifically tailor-made for different patient groups (e.g., age, seriousness of illness, symptoms, comorbidity, and expected outcomes; N. K. Wenger, 1999). The following questions will be essential: Is a specific aspect of CR really needed? Are there better and

more cost-effective ways of providing this service? Which patients have a need for and predictable benefit from individual service components? (See Froelicher et al., 1996.) Case management is seen as an adequate strategy for multiple risk reduction and could provide a structural framework for the organization of CR programs. It should involve the coordination of risk reduction for groups of patients by a single professional, commonly a nurse or exercise physiologist, with appropriate medical supervision (Ades et al., 2001).

This book is dedicated to the attempt to compile systematically the scientific evidence for the impact of psychosocial factors on CHD incidence, progression, and mortality as well as on the success of illness adjustment and patients' and their relatives' quality of life. Solid evidence has shown an urgent need to establish psychosocial intervention as a third main focus—in addition to exercise and risk factor modification—in CR programs. Aside from the problem of how to provide sufficient financing for psychosocial services, many unresolved questions remain. Future tasks involve development of an adequate working definition of the need for psychosocial interventions (e.g., which are the relevant parameters, what should the cutoffs be, how should transient and longer lasting dysfunctions be differentiated) and the development or adaptation of methods of counseling and psychotherapy to the CR program setting. Finally, we are confronted with the challenge of improving evaluation methods and strategies so that we can gain a deeper insight into the mode of action and the effectiveness of individual psychosocial intervention strategies. This could undoubtedly be an important step to an individualized referral of certain patient groups (e.g., by gender, age, or stage of disease) to certain psychosocial programs tailored to their needs within a CR program.

References

*References marked with an asterisk are cited only in materials on the accompanying Web site.

Aaronson, N. K., Acquadro, C., Alonso, J., Apolone, G., Bucquet, D., Bullinger, M., et al. (1992). International Quality of Life Assessment (IQOLA) Project. *Quality of Life Research, 1*, 349–351.

Abbot, N. C., Stead, L. F., White, A. R., Barnes, J., & Ernst, E. (1998). Hypnotherapy for smoking cessation. *The Cochrane Library*. Available at http://www.cochrane.org/reviews/clibintro.htm

Abbott, E. C. (1993). Endothelial dysfunction in microvascular angina [Letter; comment]. *New England Journal of Medicine, 329*, 1740.

Abel, T. (1991). Measuring health lifestyles in a comparative analysis: Theoretical issues and empirical findings. *Social Science & Medicine, 32*, 899–908.

Aberg, A., Bergstrand, R., Johansson, S., Ulvenstam, G., Vedin, A., Wedel, H., et al. (1983). Cessation of smoking after myocardial infarction: Effects on mortality after 10 years. *British Heart Journal, 49*, 416–422.

Ades, P. A. (2001). Cardiac rehabilitation and secondary prevention of coronary heart disease. *New England Journal of Medicine, 345*, 892–902.

Ades, P. A., Balady, G. J., & Berra, K. (2001). Transforming exercise-based cardiac rehabilitation programs into secondary prevention centers: A national imperative. *Journal of Cardiopulmonary Rehabilitation, 21*, 263–272.

Ades, P. A., Waldmann, M. L., McCann, W. J., & Weaver, S. O. (1992). Predictors of cardiac rehabilitation participation in older coronary patients. *Archives of Internal Medicine, 152*, 1033–1035.

Adler, N. E., Boyce, T., Chesney, M. A., Cohen, S., Folkman, S., Kahn, R. L., et al. (1994). Socioeconomic status and health: The challenge of the gradient. *American Psychologist, 49*, 15–24.

Adsett, C. A., & Bruhn, J. (1968). Short-term group psychotherapy for post–myocardial infarction patients and their wives. *Canadian Medical Association Journal, 99*, 577–584.

Agency for Health Care Research and Quality. (1995). *AHCPR supported clinical practice guidelines: 17. Cardiac rehabilitation.* Retrieved September 15, 2005, from http://www.ncbi.nlm.nih.gov/books/bv.fcgi?rid=hstat2.chapter.6677

Agmon, Y. (1993). Endothelial dysfunction in microvascular angina [Letter, comment]. *New England Journal of Medicine, 329*, 1739–1740.

Ahern, D. K., Gorkin, L., Anderson, J. L., Tierney, C., Hallstrom, A., Ewart, C., et al. (1990). Biobehavioral variables and mortality for cardiac arrest in the Cardiac Arrhythmia Pilot Study (CAPS). *American Journal of Cardiology, 66*, 59–62.

Ahto, M., Isoaho, R., Puolijoki, H., Laippala, P., Romo, M., & Kivelä, S. L. (1997). Coronary heart disease and depression in the elderly: A population-based study. *Family Practice, 14*, 436–445.

Ainsworth, B. E., Haskell, W. L., Whitt, M. C., Irwin, M. L., Swartz, A. M., Strath, S. J., et al. (2000). Compendium of physical activities: An update of activity codes and MET intensities. *Medicine and Science in Sports and Exercise, 32*(Suppl.), 498–516.

Ajzen, I. (1991). The theory of planned behavior. *Organizational Behavior and Human Decision Processes, 50*, 179–211.

Ajzen, I., & Madden, T. J. (1986). Prediction of goal directed behaviour: Attitudes, intentions, and perceived behavioral control. *Journal of Experimental and Social Psychology, 22*, 453–474.

Albrecht, D., Ostermann, R., Franzen, D., & Höpp, H. W. (1995). Wiedereingliederung in das Arbeitsleben nach perkutaner transluminaler Koronarangioplastie (PTCA) [Reentry into the workforce after percutaneous transluminal coronary angioplasty (PTCA)]. *Zeitschrift für Kardiologie, 84,* 885–891.

Alexander, F. (1950). *Psychosomatic medicine: Its principles and applications.* New York: Norton.

Alexander, F., & French, T. M. (Eds.). (1948). *Studies in psychosomatic medicine: An approach to the cause and treatment of vegetative disturbances.* Oxford, England: Ronald Press.

*Alexander, P. J., Prabhu, S. G., Krishnamoorthy, E. S., & Halkatti, P. C. (1994). Mental disorders in patients with noncardiac chest pain. *Acta Psychiatrica Scandinavica, 89,* 291–293.

Alfredsson, L., Spetz, C. L., & Theorell, T. (1985). Type of occupation and near-future hospitalization for myocardial infarction and some other diagnoses. *International Journal of Epidemiology, 14,* 378–388.

Allan, R., & Scheidt, S. E. (1996). *Heart and mind: The practice of cardiac psychology.* Washington, DC: American Psychological Association.

Allan, R., & Scheidt, S. E. (1998). Group psychotherapy for patients with coronary heart disease. *International Journal of Group Psychotherapy, 48,* 187–214.

Allen, J. K. (1996). Coronary risk factor modification in women after coronary artery bypass surgery. *Nursing Research, 45,* 260–265.

Allen, J. K., Fitzgerald, S. T., Swank, R. T., & Becker, D. M. (1990). Functional status after coronary artery bypass grafting and percutaneous transluminal coronary angioplasty. *American Journal of Cardiology, 66,* 921–925.

Alonzo, A. A. (1999). Acute myocardial infarction and posttraumatic stress disorder: The consequences of cumulative adversity. *Journal of Cardiovascular Nursing, 13,* 33–45.

Alonzo, A. A. (2000). The experience of chronic illness and post-traumatic stress disorder: The consequences of cumulative adversity. *Social Science & Medicine, 50,* 1475–1484.

Alonzo, A. A., & Reynolds, N. R. (1998). The structure of emotions during acute myocardial infarction: A model of coping. *Social Science & Medicine, 46,* 1099–1110.

Alter, C. L., Pelcovitz, D., Axlerod, A., Goldenberg, B., Harris, A., Meyers, B., et al. (1996). Identification of PTSD in cancer survivors. *Psychosomatics, 37,* 137–143.

Alterman, T., Shekelle, R. B., Vernon, S. W., & Burau, K. D. (1994). Decision latitude, psychological demand, job strain, and coronary heart disease in the Western Electric Study. *American Journal of Epidemiology, 139,* 620–627.

Altmann-Herz, U., Reindell, A., Petzold, E., & Ferner, H. (1983). Zur psychosomatischen Differe-

nzierung von Patienten nach Herzinfarkt [Psychosomatic differentiation of patients after a heart attack]. *Zeitschrift für Psychosomatische Medizin und Psychoanalyse, 29,* 234–252.

American Association of Cardiovascular and Pulmonary Rehabilitation. (1995). *Guidelines for cardiac rehabilitation programs* (2nd ed.). Champaign, IL: Human Kinetics.

American Association of Cardiovascular and Pulmonary Rehabilitation. (1999). *Guidelines for cardiac rehabilitation and secondary prevention* (3rd ed.). Champaign, IL: Human Kinetics.

American College of Cardiology and the American Heart Association. (2002). *ACC/AHA guideline update for the management of patients with unstable angina and non–ST-segment elevation myocardial infarction: A report of the American College of Cardiology/American Heart Association Task Force on Practice Guidelines (Committee on the Management of Patients With Unstable Angina).* Retrieved July 28, 2006, from http://www.americanheart.org/downloadable/heart/1016214837537 UANSTEMI2002Web.pdf

American College of Sports Medicine. (1995). *Guidelines for exercise testing and exercise prescription.* Philadelphia: Lea & Febiger.

American Heart Association. (1990). Statement on exercise. *Circulation, 81,* 396.

American Heart Association. (2005). *Heart disease and stroke statistics—2005 update.* Retrieved September 10, 2005, from http://www.americanheart.org/downloadable/heart/110539091811hdsstats2005update.pdf

American Heart Association. (2002). *Heart and stroke statistical update.* Dallas, TX: American Heart Association.

*American Heart Association, Medical/Scientific Statement. (1994). Cardiac rehabilitation programs: A statement for healthcare professionals from the AHA. *Circulation, 90,* 1602–1610.

American Psychiatric Association. (1980). *Diagnostic and statistical manual of mental disorders* (3rd ed.). Washington, DC: Author.

American Psychiatric Association. (1994). *Diagnostic and statistical manual of mental disorders* (4th ed.). Washington, DC: Author.

American Psychiatric Association. (1998). Practice guideline for the treatment of patients with panic disorder. *American Journal of Psychiatry, 155,* 1–34.

American Psychiatric Association. (2000). Practice guideline for the treatment of patients with major depressive disorder (revision). *American Journal of Psychiatry, 157*(4 Suppl.), 1–45.

Amick, B. C., 3rd, McDonough, P., Chang, H., Rogers, W. H., Pieper, C. F., & Duncan, G. (2002). Relationship between all-cause mortality and cumulative working life course psychosocial and physical exposures in the United States labor market from 1968 to 1992. *Psychosomatic Medicine, 64,* 370–381.

*Anderson, E. A. (1987). Preoperative preparation for cardiac surgery facilitates recovery, reduces psychological distress, and reduces the incidence of acute postoperative hypertension. *Journal of Consulting and Clinical Psychology, 55,* 513–520.

Anderson, K. O., & Masur, F. T., 3rd. (1983). Psychological preparation for invasive medical and dental procedures. *Journal of Behavioral Medicine, 6,* 1–40.

Anderson, K. O., & Masur, F. T., 3rd. (1989). Psychological preparation for cardiac catheterization. *Heart & Lung, 18,* 154–163.

Andrew, M. J., Baker, R. A., Kneebone, A. C., & Knight, J. L. (2000). Mood state as a predictor of neuropsychological deficits following cardiac surgery. *Journal of Psychosomatic Research, 48,* 537–546.

Andrykowski, M. A., Cordova, M. J., McGrath, P. C., Sloan, D. A., & Kenady, D. E. (2000). Stability and change in posttraumatic stress disorder symptoms following breast cancer treatment: A 1-year follow-up. *Psychooncology, 9,* 69–78.

Antonovsky, A. (1967). Social class, life expectancy and overall mortality. *Milbank Memorial Fund Quarterly, 45*(2), 31–73.

Appels, A. (1979). Myocardial infarction and depression: A crossvalidation of Dreyfuss' findings. *Activitas Nervosa Superior, 21,* 65–66.

*Appels, A. (1980). Psychological prodromata of myocardial infarction and sudden death. *Psychotherapy and Psychosomatics, 34,* 187–195.

Appels, A., Bär, F., Bär, J., Bruggeman, C., & de Baets, M. (2000). Inflammation, depressive symptomatology, and coronary artery disease. *Psychosomatic Medicine, 62,* 601–605.

Appels, A., Bär, F., Lasker, J., Flamm, U., & Kop, W. (1997). The effect of a psychological intervention program on the risk of a new coronary event after angioplasty: A feasibility study. *Journal of Psychosomatic Research, 43,* 209–217.

*Appels, A., Falger, P. R., & Schouten, E. G. (1993). Vital exhaustion as risk factor for myocardial infarction in women. *Journal of Psychosomatic Research, 37,* 881–890.

Appels, A., Höppener, P., & Mulder, P. (1987). A questionnaire to assess premonitory symptoms of myocardial infarction. *International Journal of Cardiology, 17,* 15–24.

Appels, A., Kop, W., Bär, F., de Swart, H., & Mendes de Leon, C. (1995). Vital exhaustion, extent of atherosclerosis, and the clinical course after successful

percutaneous transluminal coronary angioplasty. *European Heart Journal, 16,* 1880–1885.

Appels, A., Kop, W., Meesters, C., Markusse, R., Golombeck, B., & Falger, P. R. (1994). Vital exhaustion and the acute coronary syndromes. *International Review of Health Psychology, 3,* 65–95.

*Appels, A., & Mulder, P. (1984). Imminent myocardial infarction: A psychological study. *Journal of Human Stress, 10,* 129–134.

Appels, A., & Mulder, P. (1985). Type A behavior and myocardial infarction: A 9.5-year follow-up of a small cohort. *International Journal of Cardiology, 8,* 465–473.

*Appels, A., & Mulder, P. (1989). Fatigue and heart disease: The association between "vital exhaustion" and past, present and future coronary heart disease. *Journal of Psychosomatic Research, 33,* 727–738.

Appels, A., Mulder, P., van't Hof, M., Jenkins, C. D., van Houtem, J., & Tan, F. (1987). A prospective study of the Jenkins Activity Survey as a risk indicator for coronary heart disease in the Netherlands. *Journal of Chronic Diseases, 40,* 959–965.

*Appels, A., & Schouten, E. (1993). Erschöpftes Erwachen als Risikofaktor der koronaren Herzkrankheit [Waking exhausted as a risk factor for coronary heart disease]. *Psychotherapie, Psychosomatik, Medizinische Psychologie, 43,* 166–170.

Appels, A., Siegrist, J., & De Vos, Y. (1997). "Chronic workload," "need for control," and "vital exhaustion" in patients with myocardial infarction and controls: A comparative test of cardiovascular risk profiles. *Stress Medicine, 13,* 117–121.

Applebaum, I. L., Bernstein, A., Levine, B., Shoshkes, M., Becker, M., Carrol, W., et al. (1955). Myocardial infarction: A clinical review of 888 cases. *Journal of the Newark Beth Israel Hospital, 6,* 305.

Aresin, L. (1960). *Über Korrelationen zwischen Lebensgeschichte und Herzkrankheit* [Correlations between life history and heart disease]. Jena, Germany: G. Fischer.

Arlow, J. A. (1945). Identification mechanisms in coronary occlusion. *Psychosomatic Medicine, 7,* 195–209.

Armstrong, K. L., Wolfe, L. A., & Amey, M. C. (1994). Cardiovascular rehabilitation in Canada: A national survey. *Journal of Cardiopulmonary Rehabilitation, 14,* 262–272.

Arnaot, M. R. (1995). Nicotine patches may not be safe. *British Medical Journal, 310,* 663–664.

Arntz, A., & de Jong, P. (1993). Anxiety, attention and pain. *Journal of Psychosomatic Research, 37,* 423–431.

*Aromaa, A., Raitasalo, R., Reunanen, A., Impivaara, O., Heliovaara, M., Knekt, P., et al. (1994). Depression and cardiovascular diseases. *Acta Psychiatrica Scandinavica, 377*(Suppl.), 77–82.

Aronow, E. (1999). *The Rorschach: An integrative approach* [Book review]. Retrieved September 27, 2005, from http://www.psycinfo.com/psyccritiques/

Atchison, M., & Condon, J. (1993). Hostility and anger measures in coronary heart disease. *Australian and New Zealand Journal of Psychiatry, 27,* 436–442.

Aust, B. (1999). *Gesundheitsförderung in der Arbeitswelt: Umsetzung streßtheoretischer Erkenntnisse in eine Intervention bei Busfahrern* [Work site health promotion: Application of knowledge from stress research to an intervention study with bus drivers]. Münster, Germany: LIT.

Aust, B., Peter, R., & Siegrist, J. (1997). Stress management in bus drivers: A pilot study based on the model of effort–reward imbalance. *International Journal of Stress Management, 4,* 297–305.

Badura, B., Grande, G., Janßen, H., & Schott, T. (1995). *Qualitätsforschung im Gesundheitswesen: Ein Vergleich ambulanter und stationärer kardiologischer Rehabilitation* [Quality research in health care: A comparison of outpatient and inpatient cardiac rehabilitation]. Weinheim, Germany: Juventa.

Badura, B., Kaufhold, G., Lehmann, H., Pfaff, H., Schott, T., & Waltz, M. (1987). *Leben mit dem Herzinfarkt: Eine sozialepidemiologische Studie* [Living with a heart attack: A socioepidemiological study]. Berlin, Germany: Springer.

Bahnson, C. B., & Wardwell, W. I. (1962). Parent constellation and psychosexual identification in male patients with myocardial infarction. *Psychological Reports, 10,* 831–852.

Baillie, A. J., Mattick, R. P., Hall, W., & Webster, P. (1994). Meta-analytic review of the efficacy of smoking cessation interventions. *Drug & Alcohol Review, 13,* 157–170.

*Baker, R. A., Andrew, M. J., Schrader, G., & Knight, J. L. (2001). Preoperative depression and mortality in coronary artery bypass surgery: Preliminary findings. *Australian and New Zealand Journal of Surgery, 71,* 139–142.

Balady, G. J., Ades, P. A., Comoss, P., Limacher, M., Pina, I. L., Southard, D., et al. (2000). Core components of cardiac rehabilitation/secondary prevention programs: A statement for healthcare professionals from the American Heart Association and the American Association of Cardiovascular and Pulmonary Rehabilitation Writing Group. *Circulation, 102,* 1069–1073.

Balady, G. J., Fletcher, B. J., Froelicher, E. S., Hartley, H., Krauss, R. M., Oberman, A., et al. (1994). Cardiac rehabilitation programs. *Circulation, 90,* 1602–1610.

Balint, M. (1973). *Therapeutische Aspekte der Regression* [Therapeutic aspects of relapse]. Reinbek, Germany: Rowohlt.

Balmer, H., Eicke, D., Kindler, N., Kraiker, C., Stolze, H., & Zeier, H. (Eds.). (1976–1981). *Die Psychologie des 20. Jahrhunderts* [The psychology of the 20th century] (16 vols.). Zürich, Switzerland: Kindler.

Bandura, A. (1977). Self-efficacy: Toward a unifying theory of behavioral change. *Psychological Review, 84,* 191–215.

Bandura, A. (1986). *Social foundations of thought and action.* Englewood Cliffs, NJ: Prentice Hall.

*Bandura, A. (1999). Self efficacy: Toward a unifying theory of behaviour change. In R. F. Baumeister (Ed.), *The self in social psychology* (pp. 285–298). Philadelphia: Psychological Press/Taylor & Francis.

Bardé, B. (1997). Leben nach dem Herzinfarkt: Eine Einzelfallstudie [Life after a heart attack: A single case study]. In P. Kutter (Ed.), *Psychoanalyse interdisziplinär* [Interdisciplinary psychoanalysis] (pp. 19–49). Frankfurt, Germany: Suhrkamp.

Bardé, B., & Kutter, P. (1996). Biographische Integration als Krankheitsbewältigung: Psychoanalytische Kurztherapie in der Anschlußheilbehandlung von Herzinfarktpatienten [Biographic integration as a way of overcoming illness: Short-term psychoanalytic therapy as a complementary treatment with heart attack patients]. In *Forschung Frankfurt, 3. Sammelband Medizin* (pp. 90–96). Frankfurt, Germany: University of Frankfurt.

Barefoot, J. C., Beckham, J. C., Peterson, B. L., Haney, T. L., & Williams, R. B. (1992). Measures of neuroticism and disease status in coronary angiography patients. *Journal of Consulting and Clinical Psychology, 60,* 127–132.

Barefoot, J. C., Brummett, B. H., Helms, M. J., Mark, D. B., Siegler, I. C., & Williams, R. B. (2000). Depressive symptoms and survival of patients with coronary artery disease. *Psychosomatic Medicine, 62,* 790–795.

Barefoot, J. C., Dahlstrom, W. G., & Williams, R. B. (1983). Hostility, CHD incidence, and total mortality: A 25-year follow-up study of 255 physicians. *Psychosomatic Medicine, 45,* 59–63.

Barefoot, J. C., Dodge, K. A., Peterson, B. L., Dahlstrom, W. G., & Williams, R. B. (1989). The Cook–Medley Hostility Scale: Item content and ability to predict survival. *Psychosomatic Medicine, 51,* 46–57.

Barefoot, J. C., Helms, M. J., Mark, D. B., Blumenthal, J. A., Califf, R. M., Haney, T. L., et al. (1996). Depression and long-term mortality risk in patients with coronary artery disease. *American Journal of Cardiology, 78,* 613–617.

Barefoot, J. C., Larsen, S., von der Lieth, L., & Schroll, M. (1995). Hostility, incidence of acute myocardial infarction, and mortality in a sample of older Danish men and women. *American Journal of Epidemiology, 142,* 477–484.

Barefoot, J. C., Patterson, J. C., Haney, T. L., Cayton, T. G., Hickman, J. R., Jr., & Williams, R. B. (1994). Hostility in asymptomatic men with angiographically confirmed coronary artery disease. *American Journal of Cardiology, 74,* 439–442.

Barefoot, J. C., Peterson, B. L., Dahlstrom, W. G., & Siegler, I. C. (1991). Hostility patterns and health implications: Correlates of Cook–Medley Hostility Scale scores in a national survey. *Health Psychology, 10,* 18–24.

Barefoot, J. C., Peterson, B. L., Harrell, F. E., Hlatky, M. A., Pryor, D. B., Haney, T. L., et al. (1989). Type A behavior and survival: A follow-up study of 1,467 patients with coronary artery disease. *American Journal of Cardiology, 64,* 427–432.

Barendregt, J. J., Bonneux, L., & Maas, P. J. (1997). The health care costs of smoking. *New England Journal of Medicine, 337,* 1052–1057.

Barker, D. (1994). *Mothers, babies, and disease in later life.* London: BMJ Publishing.

Barnwell, W. H. (1979). Cardiac rehabilitation. *Journal of the South Carolina Medical Association, 142,* 420–422.

Barr-Taylor, C., Houston-Miller, N., Ahn, D. K., Haskell, W., & DeBusk, R. F. (1997). The effects of exercise training programs on psychosocial improvement in uncomplicated myocardial infarction patients. *Journal of Psychosomatic Research, 30,* 581–587.

Bartels, R. (2002). Körperliche Aktivität und plötzlicher Herztod [Physical activity and sudden cardiac arrest]. In G. Samitz & G. Mensink (Eds.), *Körperliche Aktivität in Prävention und Therapie* [Physical activity in prevention and therapy] (pp. 227–230). Munich, Germany: Hans Marseille.

Barth, J., & Bengel, J. (1997). Die Rezeption und Verarbeitung von gesundheitsbezogenen Warnhinweisen bei Alkohol und Zigaretten [Response to and internalization of health-related warnings about alcohol and tobacco use]. *Zeitschrift für Medizinische Psychologie, 6,* 5–14.

Barth, J., & Bengel, J. (1998). *Prevention through fear? The state of fear appeal research.* Cologne, Germany: Bundeszentrale für Gesundheitliche Aufklärung.

Barth, M., & Sender, I. (1991). Hilfe, ich darf wieder arbeiten: Analyse des Wiedereingliederungsprozesses ins Erwerbsleben eines chronisch Kranken nach ueberstandenem Herzinfarkt [Help, I want to work again: An analysis of the process of reintegration into the workplace of a chronically ill survivor of a heart attack]. *Psychotherapie, Psychosomatik, Medizinische Psychologie, 41,* 437–445.

Barth, J., Schumacher, M., & Herrmann-Lingen, C. (2004). Depression as a risk factor for mortality in patients with coronary heart disease: A meta-analysis. *Psychosomatic Medicine, 66,* 802–813.

*Basha, I., Mukerji, V., Langevin, P., Kushner, M., Alpert, M., & Beitman, B. D. (1989). Atypical angina in patients with coronary artery disease suggests panic disorder. *International Journal of Psychiatric Medicine, 19,* 3341–3346.

Basler, H.-D., Brinkmeier, U., Buser, K., & Gluth, G. (1992). Nicotine gum assisted group therapy in smokers with an increased risk of coronary disease: Evaluation in a primary care setting format. *Health Education Research: Theory and Practice, 7,* 87–95.

Bass, C. (1989). Non-cardiac chest pain. *Practitioner, 233,* 355–357.

Bass, C., Cawley, R., Wade, C., Ryan, K. C., Gardner, W. N., Hutchison, D. C., et al. (1983). Unexplained breathlessness and psychiatric morbidity in patients with normal and abnormal coronary arteries. *Lancet, 1,* 605–609.

Bass, C., Chambers, J. B., Kiff, P., Cooper, D., & Gardner, W. N. (1988). Panic anxiety and hyperventilation in patients with chest pain: A controlled study. *Quarterly Journal of Medicine, 69,* 949–959.

Bass, C., & Wade, C. (1984). Chest pain with normal coronary arteries: A comparative study of psychiatric and social morbidity. *Psychological Medicine, 14,* 51–61.

Bass, C., Wade, C., Hand, D., & Jackson, G. (1983). Patients with angina with normal and near normal coronary arteries: Clinical and psychosocial state 12 months after angiography. *British Medical Journal (Clinical Research Edition), 287,* 1505–1508.

Bassan, M. (2002). Cardiac syndrome X. *New England Journal of Medicine, 347,* 1377–1379.

Bastiaans, J. (1968). Psychoanalytic investigations on the psychic aspects of acute myocardial infarction. *Psychotherapy and Psychosomatics, 16,* 202–209.

Bastiaans, J. (1969). The role of aggression in the genesis of psychosomatic disease. *Journal of Psychosomatic Research, 13,* 307–314.

Bastiaans, J. (1982). On freedom and induction. *Psychotherapy and Psychosomatics, 38,* 24–31.

Beattie, S., & Geden, E. (1990). Reducing pain and discomfort following percutaneous transluminal coronary angioplasty. *Dimensions in Critical Care Nursing, 9,* 150–155.

Beck, A. T., & Steer, R. A. (1987). *Beck Depression Inventory—Manual.* San Antonio, TX: Psychological Corporation.

Beck, A. T., Steer, R. A., & Brown, G. K. (1988). Psychometric properties of the Beck Depression Inventory:

Twenty-five years of evaluation. *Clinical Psychology Review, 8,* 77–100.

Beck, A. T., Ward, C., Mendelson, M., Mock, J., & Erbaugh, J. (1961). An inventory for measuring depression. *Archives of General Psychiatry, 4,* 561–571.

Beck, J. G., Berisford, M. A., Taegtmeyer, H., & Bennett, A. (1990). Panic symptoms in chest pain without coronary artery disease: A comparison with panic disorder. *Behavior Therapy, 21,* 241–252.

Beck, J. G., Berisford, M. A., & Taegtmeyer, H. (1991). The effects of voluntary hyperventilation on patients with chest pain without coronary artery disease. *Behaviour Research and Therapy, 29,* 611–621.

Beck, J. G., Taegtmeyer, H., Berisford, M. A., & Bennett, A. (1989). Chest pain without coronary artery disease: An exploratory comparison with panic disorder. *Journal of Psychopathology and Behavioral Assessment, 11,* 209–220.

Becker, M. H. (1974). *The health belief model and personal health behavior.* Thorofare, NJ: Slack.

Beckermann, A., Grossmann, D., & Marquez, L. (1995). Cardiac catheterization: The patient's perspective. *Heart & Lung, 24,* 213–219.

Beitman, B. D., Basha, I., Flaker, G., DeRosear, L., Mukerji, V., Trombka, L., & Katon, W. (1987). Atypical or nonanginal chest pain. *Archives of Internal Medicine, 147,* 1548–1552.

Beitman, B. D., DeRosear, L., Basha, I. M., & Flaker, G. (1987). Panic disorder in cardiology patients with atypical or non-anginal chest pain: A pilot study. *Journal of Anxiety Disorders, 1,* 277–282.

Beitman, B. D., Mukerji, V., Flaker, G., & Basha, I. M. (1988). Panic disorder, cardiology patients, and atypical chest pain. *Psychiatric Clinics of North America, 11,* 387–397.

Beitman, B. D., Mukerji, V., Kushner, M., Thomas, A. M., Russell, J. L., & Logue, M. B. (1991). Validating studies for panic disorder in patients with angiographically normal coronary arteries. *Medical Clinics of North America, 75,* 1143–1155.

Beitman, B. D., Mukerji, V., Lamberti, J. W., Schmid, L., DeRosear, L., & Kushner, M. (1989). Panic disorder in patients with chest pain and angiographically normal coronary arteries. *American Journal of Cardiology, 63,* 1399–1403.

Beitman, B. D., Mukerji, V., Russell, J. L., & Grafting, M. (1993). Panic disorder in cardiology patients: A review of the Missouri Panic/Cardiology Project. *Journal of Psychiatric Research, 27*(Suppl. 1), 35–46.

Beitman, B. D., Thomas, A. M., & Kushner, M. G. (1992). Panic disorder in the families of patients with normal coronary arteries and non-fear panic disorder. *Behaviour Research and Therapy, 30,* 403–406.

Belkić, K., Savic, C., Theorell, T., Rakic, L., Ercegovac, D., & Djordjevic, M. (1994). Mechanisms of cardiac risk among professional drivers. *Scandinavian Journal of Work, Environment and Health, 20,* 73–86.

Bengtson, A., Herlitz, J., Karlsson, T., & Hjalmarson, A. (1994). The epidemiology of a coronary waiting list: A description of all of the patients. *Journal of Internal Medicine, 235,* 263–269.

Bengtson, A., Herlitz, J., Karlsson, T., & Hjalmarson, A. (1996). Distress correlates with the degree of chest pain: A description of patients awaiting revascularisation. *Heart, 75,* 257–260.

Bengtson, A., Karlsson, T., & Herlitz, J. (2000). Differences between men and women on the waiting list for coronary revascularization. *Journal of Advanced Nursing, 31,* 1362–1367.

Bennett, P., & Brooke, S. (1999). Intrusive memories, post-traumatic stress disorder and myocardial infarction. *British Journal of Clinical Psychology, 38,* 411–416.

Bennett, P., Conway, M., Clatworthy, J., Brooke, S., & Owen, R. (2001). Predicting post-traumatic symptoms in cardiac patients. *Heart & Lung, 30,* 458–465.

Bennett, P., Owen, R. L., Koutsakis, S., & Bisson, J. (2002). Personality, social context and cognitive predictors of post-traumatic stress disorder in myocardial infarction patients. *Psychology and Health, 17,* 489–500.

Bennett, S. B., & Pescatello, L. S. (1997). A regional comparison of cardiac rehabilitation personnel. *Journal of Cardiopulmonary Rehabilitation, 17,* 92–102.

Benowitz, N. L., & Gourlay, S. G. (1997). Cardiovascular toxicity of nicotine: Implication for nicotine replacement therapy. *Journal of the American College of Cardiology, 29,* 1422–1431.

Berkman, L. F., Blumenthal, J., Burg, M., Carney, R. M., Catellier, D., Cowan, M. J., et al. (2003). Effects of treating depression and low perceived social support on clinical events after myocardial infarction: The Enhancing Recovery in Coronary Heart Disease Patients (ENRICHD) Randomized Trial. *JAMA, 289,* 3106–3116.

Berkman, L. F., & Kawachi, I. (Eds.). (2000). *Social epidemiology.* New York: Oxford University Press.

Bernet, A., Drivet-Perrin, J., Blanc, M. M., Ebagosti, A., & Jouve, A. (1982). Type A behavior pattern in a screened female population. *Advances in Cardiology, 29,* 96–105.

Bethell, H. (1997). Coronary patients need cardiologists. *Heart, 77,* 389.

Bethell, H. (2000). Cardiac rehabilitation: From Hellerstein to the millennium. *International Journal of Clinical Practice, 54,* 92–97.

Bethell, H., Turner, S., Evans, J., & Rose, L. (2001). Cardiac rehabilitation in the United Kingdom: How complete is the provision? *Journal of Cardiopulmonary Rehabilitation, 21,* 111–115.

Billing, E., Hjemdahl, P., & Rehnqvist, N. (1997). Psychosocial variables in female vs male patients with stable angina pectoris and matched healthy controls. *European Heart Journal, 18,* 911–918.

*Billing, E., Lindell, B., Sederholm, M., & Theorell, T. (1980). Denial, anxiety, and depression following myocardial infarction. *Psychosomatics, 21,* 639–645.

Biostat. (2002). Comprehensive meta-analysis program [Computer software]. Englewood, NJ: Author.

Birdwell, B., Herbers, J., & Kroenke, K. (1993). Evaluating chest pain: The patient's presentation style alters the physician's diagnostic approach. *Archives of Internal Medicine, 153,* 1991–1995.

*Bittner, V., Breland, J., & Green, D. (1999). Referral patterns to a university-based cardiac rehabilitation program. *American Journal of Cardiology, 83,* 252–255.

Bjarnason-Wehrens, B., Kretschmann, E., Lang, M., & Rost, R. (1998). Ist die Ambulante Herzgruppe der "Königsweg" der kardialen Rehabilitation der Phase III [Is the ambulent heart group the silver bullet of cardiac rehabilitation in Phase III]? *Herz-Kreislauf, 30,* 400–411.

Black, J. L., Allison, T. G., Williams, D. E., Rummans, T. A., & Gau, G. T. (1998). Effects of intervention for psychological distress on rehospitalization rates in cardiac rehabilitation patients. *Psychosomatics, 39,* 134–143.

*Blackburn, G. G., Foody, J. M., Sprecher, D. L., Park, E., Apperson-Hansen, C., & Pashkow, F. J. (2000). Cardiac rehabilitation participation patterns in a large, tertiary care center: Evidence for selection bias. *Journal of Cardiopulmonary Rehabilitation, 20,* 189–195.

Blair, S. N., Kohl, H. W., Barlow, C. E., Pfaffenbarger, R. S., Gibbons, L. W., & Macera, C. A. (1995). Changes in physical fitness and all-cause mortality. *JAMA, 273,* 1093–1098.

*Blanchard, E. B., & Miller, S. T. (1977). Psychological treatment of cardiovascular disease. *Archives of General Psychiatry, 34,* 1402–1413.

Blane, D., Brunner, E., & Wilkinson, R. (Eds.). (1996). *Health and social organization.* London: Routledge.

Bliley, A. V., & Ferrans, C. E. (1993). Quality of life after coronary angioplasty. *Heart & Lung, 22,* 193–199.

Bloch, A., & Bersier, A. L. (1979). *Die Psychologie des Koronarpatienten* [The psychology of the coronary patient] (Folia Psychopractica Nr. 8 ed.). Basel, Switzerland: Hoffmann-LaRoche.

Blumenthal, J. A., & Emery, C. F. (1988). Rehabilitation of patients following myocardial infarction. *Journal of Consulting and Clinical Psychology, 56,* 374–381.

Blumenthal, J. A., Jiang, W., Babyak, M. A., Krantz, D. S., Frie, D. J., Coleman, R. E., et al. (1997). Stress management and exercise training in cardiac patients with myocardial ischemia. *Archives of Internal Medicine, 157,* 2213–2223.

Blumenthal, J. A., Madden, D. J., Burker, E., Croughwell, N., Schniebolk, S., Smith, R., et al. (1991). A preliminary study of the effects of cardiac procedures on cognitive performance. *International Journal of Psychosomatics, 38,* 13–16.

Blumenthal, J. A., Williams, R. S., Wallace, A. G., Williams, R. B., & Needles, T. L. (1982). Physiological and psychological variables predict compliance to prescribed exercise therapy in patients recovering from myocardial infarction. *Psychosomatic Medicine, 44,* 519–527.

Blumlein, S. L., Anderson, A. J., Barboriak, J. J., & Rimm, A. A. (1977). Changes in occupation after coronary arteriography. *Scandinavian Journal of Rehabilitation Medicine, 9,* 79–83.

Bobbio, M. (1989). Does post myocardial infarction rehabilitation prolong survival? *Giornale Italiano di Cardiologia, 19,* 1059–1067.

Bock, B. C., Albrecht, A. E., Traficante, R. M., Clark, M. M., Pinto, B. M., Tilkemeier, P., & Marcus, B. H. (1997). Predictors of exercise adherence following participation in a cardiac rehabilitation program. *International Journal of Behavioral Medicine, 4,* 60–75.

*Bohachick, P. (1984). Progressive relaxation training in cardiac rehabilitation: Effect on psychologic variables. *Nursing Research, 33,* 283–287.

Bonami, M., & Rime, B. (1972). Approche exploratoire de la personnalite pre-coronarienne par analyse standardisee de donnes projectives thematiques [A study of the personality of pre-coronaries by standardized analysis of thematic projective data]. *Journal of Psychosomatic Research, 16,* 103–113.

Bongers, P. M., de Winter, C. R., Kompier, M. A., & Hildebrandt, V. H. (1993). Psychosocial factors at work and musculoskeletal disease. *Scandinavian Journal of Work, Environment and Health, 19,* 297–312.

Bongers, P. M., Kremer, A. M., & ter Laak, J. (2002). Are psychosocial factors risk factors for symptoms and signs of the shoulder, elbow, or hand/wrist? A review of the epidemiological literature. *American Journal of Industrial Medicine, 41,* 315–342.

Booth-Kewley, S., & Friedman, H. S. (1987). Psychological predictors of heart disease: A quantitative review. *Psychological Bulletin, 101,* 343–362.

Bormann, C. (1994). Are self-reported diseases reliable and plausible? Problems in the estimation of the prevalence of heart infarct using questionnaire data from the National Health Survey. *Sozial- und Praventivmedizin, 39,* 67–74.

Bortner, R. W. (1969). A short rating scale as a potential measure of Pattern A behavior. *Journal of Chronic Diseases, 22,* 87–91.

Bory, M., Pierron, F., Panagides, D., Bonnet, J. L., Yvorra, S., & Desfossez, L. (1996). Coronary artery spasm in patients with normal or near normal coronary arteries: Long-term follow-up of 277 patients. *European Heart Journal, 17,* 1015–1021.

Bös, K., Woll, A., Bösing, L., & Huber, G. (Eds.). (1994). *Gesundheitsförderung in der Gemeinde* [Health promotion in the community]. Schorndorf, Germany: Hofmann.

Bosma, H., Marmot, M. G., Hemingway, H., Nicholson, A. C., Brunner, E., & Stansfeld, S. A. (1997). Low job control and risk of coronary heart disease in Whitehall II (prospective cohort) study. *British Medical Journal, 314,* 558–565.

Bosma, H., Peter, R., Siegrist, J., & Marmot, M. (1998). Two alternative job stress models and the risk of coronary heart disease. *American Journal of Public Health, 88,* 68–74.

Botker, H. E., Moller, N., Ovesen, P., Mengel, A., Schmitz, O., & Orskov, H. (1993). Insulin resistance in microvascular angina (syndrome X). *Lancet, 342,* 136–140.

Botker, H. E., Sonne, H. S., Frøbert, O., & Andreasen, F. (1999). Enhanced exercise-induced hyperkalemia in patients with syndrome X. *Journal of the American College of Cardiology, 33,* 1056–1061.

Bouchard, C., Shephard, R. J., Stephens, T., Sutton, J. R., & McPherson, B. D. (Eds.). (1994). *Physical activity, fitness, and health.* Champaign, IL: Human Kinetics.

Boudrez, H., & De Backer, G. (2001). Psychological status and the role of coping style after coronary artery bypass graft surgery: Results of a prospective study. *Quality of Life Research, 10,* 37–47.

Bouman, C. C. (1984). Intracoronary thrombolysis and percutaneous transluminal coronary angioplasty: Nursing implications. *Nursing Clinics of North America, 19,* 397–409.

Bowlby, J. (1958). The nature of the child's tie to his mother. *International Journal of Psychoanalysis, 39,* 350–373.

Brackett, C. D., & Powell, L. H. (1988). Psychosocial and physiological predictors of sudden cardiac death after healing of acute myocardial infarction. *American Journal of Cardiology, 61,* 979–983.

Bradley, J. M., Wallace, E. S., McCoy, P. M., & Dalzell, G. W. N. (1997). A survey of exercise based cardiac rehabilitation services in Northern Ireland. *Ulster Medical Journal, 66,* 100–106.

Bradley, L. A., Richter, J. E., Scarinci, I. C., Haile, J. M., & Schan, C. A. (1992). Psychosocial and psychophysical assessments of patients with unexplained chest pain. *American Journal of Medicine, 92*(5A), 65S–73S.

*Brägelmann, F., Eisenriegler, E., Jokiel, R., Jetté, M., & Blümchen, G. (1990). Eine Befragung zur medizinischen und psychosozialen Situation von 140 Arbeiterinnen 32 Monate nach Myokardinfarkt [A survey of the medical and psychosocial situations of 140 female workers 32 months after myocardial infarction]. *Zeitschrift fur Kardiologie, 79,* 268–272.

Braun, L. (1920). *Herz und Psyche in ihren Wirkungen auf einander* [The interplay of heart and mind]. Leipzig, Germany: Franz Deuticke.

Braun, L. (1932). *Herz und Angst: Eine ärztlich-psychologische Studie* [The heart and fear: A medical–psychological study]. Vienna, Austria: Franz Deuticke.

Braunwald, E. (1988). *Heart disease* (3rd ed.). Philadelphia: W. B. Saunders.

Breier, A., Charney, D. S., & Heninger, G. R. (1984). Major depression in patients with agoraphobia and panic disorder. *Archives of General Psychiatry, 41,* 1129–1135.

Breitkopf, L. (1983). Das Phänomen "Verleugnung" aus sozialpsychologischer Sicht [Denial from the social–psychological point of view]. *Medizin, Mensch, Gesellschaft, 8,* 159–165.

*Bremer-Schulte, M., Pluym, B., & Van-Schendel, G. (1986). Reintegration with Duos: A self-care program following myocardial infarction. *Patient Education and Counseling, 8,* 233–244.

Brezynskie, H., Pendon, E., Lindsay, P., & Adam, M. (1998). Identification of the perceived learning needs of balloon angioplasty patients. *Canadian Journal of Cardiovascular Nursing, 9,* 8–14.

Brodman, K., Erdmann, A. J., & Wolff, H. G. (1949). *The Cornell Medical Index Health Questionnaire manual.* New York: Cornell University.

Brody, M. (1968). Depression and somatic illness (the neuropathoneuroses). *Psychosomatics, 9,* 245–247.

Brown, G. W., & Harris, T. O. (1978). *Social origins of depression: A study of psychiatric disorder in women.* London: Tavistock.

Brown, G. W., & Harris, T. O. (Eds.). (1989). *Life events and illness.* New York: Guilford Press.

Brown, M. A., & Munford, A. (1984). Rehabilitation of post MI depression and psychological invalidism:

A pilot study. *International Journal of Psychiatry and Medicine, 13,* 291–298.

Brown, T. M., & Fee, E. (2003). Friedrich Engels: Businessman and revolutionary. *American Journal of Public Health, 93,* 1248–1249.

*Bruce, E. M., Frederick, R., Bruce, R. A., & Fischer, L. D. (1976). Comparison of active participants and dropouts in CAPRI cardiopulmonary rehabilitation programs. *American Journal of Cardiology, 37,* 53–60.

Bruce, J. M. J., & Thomas, C. B. (1953). A method of rating certain personality factors as determined by the Rorschach test for use in a study of the precursors of hypertension and coronary artery disease. *Psychiatric Quarterly Supplement, 27,* 207–238.

Bruckenberger, E. (2004). *Herzbericht 2003 mit Transplantationschirurgie. 16. Bericht des Krankenhausausschusses der Arbeitsgemeinschaft der obersten Landesgesundheitsbehörden der Länder* [2003 Cardiology Report with discussion of transplant surgery. 16th report of the Hospital Committee of the Executive Health Authorities' Working Group for the German States]. Hannover, Germany: Author.

Bruhn, M., & Tilmes, J. (1994) *Social marketing: Einsatz des Marketing für nichtkommerzielle Organisationen* (12. Aufl.) [Social marketing: Introducing marketing to nonprofit organizations (12th ed.). Stuttgart, Germany: Kohlhammer.

Brummett, B. H., Babyak, M. A., Barefoot, J. C., Bosworth, H. B., Clapp-Channing, N. E., Siegler, I. C., et al. (1998). Social support and hostility as predictors of depressive symptoms in cardiac patients one month after hospitalization: A prospective study. *Psychosomatic Medicine, 60,* 707–713.

Brusis, O. A., & Weber-Falkensammer, H. (1999). *Handbuch der Herzgruppenbetreuung* [Caretakers' handbook for cardiac rehabilitation group leaders]. Ballingen, Germany: Spitta Verlag.

*Bryant, B., & Mayou, R. (1989). Prediction of outcome after coronary artery surgery. *Journal of Psychosomatic Research, 33,* 419–427.

Budde, H.-G. (1999). Motivation zur ambulanten Herzgruppe [Motivating outpatient cardiac rehabilitation groups]. *Prävention und Rehabilitation, 11,* 53–55.

Budde, H.-G. (2000). Psychische Faktoren oder Verhaltenseinflüsse bei andernorts klassifizierten Erkrankungen in der Kardiologie [Mental factors and behavioral influences in "otherwise-specified" cardiac illnesses]. In W. Beiglböck, S. Feselmayer, & E. Honemann (Eds.), *Handbuch der klinisch-psychologischen Behandlung* [Manual of clinical–psychological treatment] (pp. 329–343). Vienna: Springer.

Budde, H.-G., Grün, O., & Keck, M. (1988). Motivation von Patienten der Arbeiterrentenversicherung zur Teilnahme an der ambulanten Herzgruppe (AHG) [Retired pensioners' motivation to participate in an outpatient cardiac rehabilitation group]. *Deutsche Rentenversicherung, 4–5,* 184–191.

Budde, H.-G., Grün, O., & Keck, M. (1993). Regelmäßige Teilnahme an der ambulanten Herzgruppe—Welche Hindernisse gibt es? [Regular participation in an outpatient cardiac rehabilitation group: What are the obstacles?]. *Herz-Kreislauf, 25,* 392–396.

Budde, H.-G., & Keck, M. (1996). Zusammenhänge zwischen beruflicher Perspektive und Gesundheitsverhalten nach stationär kardiologischer Rehabilitation [The relationship between work philosophy and health-related behaviors after inpatient cardiac rehabilitation]. *Herz-Kreislauf, 28,* 169–172.

Budde, H.-G., & Keck, M. (1998). Vier-Jahres-Teilnahmepersistenz in der Ambulanten Herzgruppe [Commitment to attending an outpatient cardiac rehabilitation group over a 4-year period]. *Prävention und Rehabilitation, 10,* 56.

Budde, H.-G., & Keck, M. (1999). Vier-Jahresteilnahmepersistenz in einer ambulanten Herzgruppe [Four-year attendance in an outpatient exercise heart group]. *Prävention und Rehabilitation, 11,* 55–60.

Budde, H.-G., & Keck, M. (2001). Prädiktoren der beruflichen Wiedereingliederung nach stationärer kardiologischer Rehabilitation im Rahmen der Arbeiterrentenversicherung [Predictors of reintegration into work life in the framework of social security insurance after inpatient cardiac rehabilitation]. *Rehabilitation, 40,* 208–216.

Burell, G. (1996). Group psychotherapy in Project New Life: Treatment of coronary-prone behaviors for patients who have had coronary artery bypass graft surgery. In R. Allan & S. Scheidt (Eds.), *Heart and mind: The practice of cardiac psychology* (pp. 291–310). Washington, DC: American Psychological Association.

*Burgess, A. W., Lerner, D. J., D'Agostino, R. B., Vokonas, P. S., Hartman, C. R., & Gaccione, P. (1987). A randomized control trial of cardiac rehabilitation. *Social Science & Medicine, 24,* 359–370.

*Burker, E. J., Blumenthal, J. A., Feldman, M., Burnett, R., White, W., Smith, L. R., et al. (1995). Depression in male and female patients undergoing cardiac surgery. *British Journal of Clinical Psychology, 34,* 119–128.

Burling, T. A., Singleton, E. G., & Bigelow, G. E. (1984). Smoking following myocardial infarction: A critical review of the literature. *Health Psychology, 3,* 83–96.

Burns, K. J., Camaione, D. N., Froman, R. D., & Clark, B. A. (1998). Predictors of referral to cardiac rehabilitation and cardiac exercise self-efficacy. *Clinical Nursing Research, 7,* 147–163.

Burt, A., Thornley, P., Illingworth, D., White, P., Shaw, T. D. R., & Turner, R. (1974). Stopping smoking after myocardial infarction. *Lancet, 23,* 304–306.

Bush, D. E., Ziegelstein, R. C., Tayback, M., Richter, D., Stevens, S., Zahalsky, H., & Fauerbach, J. A. (2001). Even minimal symptoms of depression increase mortality risk after acute myocardial infarction. *American Journal of Cardiology, 88,* 337–341.

Buss, U. (1999). *Zur Diskrepanz zwischen subjektiven Beschwerden und objektivem Koronarstatus: Eine vergleichende Untersuchung kardiologischer Patienten in Hinsicht auf Beschwerdeverlauf und Krankheitsverhalten* [On the discrepancy between subjective experience of pain and objective coronary status: A comparative study of cardiac patients with respect to pain trajectory and illness]. Unpublished doctoral dissertation, University of Göttingen, Göttingen, Germany.

Buss, U., & Herrmann, C. (2000). The course of illness behavior in silent myocardial ischemia. *Psychosomatic Medicine, 62,* 131.

Buss, U., Wydra, P., & Herrmann-Lingen, C. (2001a). Effects of depressed mood on chronotropic response and heart rate recovery in patients undergoing an exercise test. *Psychosomatic Medicine, 63,* 98.

*Buss, U., Wydra, P., & Herrmann-Lingen, C. (2001b). Interactive effects of depression, chronotropic response, and heart rate recovery on five-year mortality in patients with coronary heart disease (CHD). *Psychosomatic Medicine, 63,* 105.

Byl, N., Reed, P., Franklin, B., & Gordon, S. (1988). Cardiac rehabilitation program services: A national survey. *Journal of Cardiopulmonary Rehabilitation, 8,* 401.

*Byrne, D. G. (1982). Psychological responses to illness and outcome after survived myocardial infarction: A long term follow-up. *Journal of Psychosomatic Research, 26,* 105–112.

*Byrne, D. G., & Whyte, H. M. (1983). State and trait anxiety correlates of illness behavior in survivors of myocardial infarction. *International Journal of Psychiatric Medicine, 13,* 1–9.

Caffray, C. M., & Schneider, S. L. (2000). Why do they do it? Active motivators in adolescents' decisions to participate in risk behaviours. *Cognition and Emotion, 14,* 543–576.

Cahill, D. (1993). No thank you kindly. *Catheterization and Cardiovascular Diagnosis, 28,* 95–98.

Calfas, K. J., Long, B. J., Sallis, J. F., Wooten, W. J., Pratt, M., & Patrick, K. (1996). A controlled trial of physician counselling to promote the adoption of physical activity. *Preventive Medicine, 25,* 225–233.

Cameron, P. M. (1989). Psychodynamic psychotherapy for the depressive syndrome. *Psychiatric Journal of the University of Ottawa, 14,* 397–402.

Camici, P. G., Marraccini, P., Lorenzoni, R., Buzzigoli, G., Pecori, N., & Perissinotto, A. (1991). Coronary hemodynamics and myocardial metabolism in patients with Syndrome X: Response to pacing stress. *Journal of the American College of Cardiology, 17,* 1461–1470.

*Campbell, N. C., Grimshaw, M. J., Rawles, J. M., & Ritchie, L. D. (1996). Cardiac rehabilitation in Scotland: Is current provision satisfactory? *Journal of Public Health Medicine, 18,* 478–480.

*Campbell, N. C., Grimshaw, J. M., Ritchie, L. D., & Rawles, J. M. (1996). Outpatient cardiac rehabilitation: Are the potential benefits being realised? *Journal of the Royal College of Physicians of London, 30,* 514–519.

Campbell, N. C., Ritchie, L. D., Thain, J., Deans, H. G., Rawles, J. M., & Squair, J. L. (1998). Secondary prevention in coronary heart disease: A randomised trial of nurse led clinics in primary care. *Heart, 80,* 447–452.

Campbell, N. C., Thain, J., Deans, H. G., Ritchie, L. D., & Rawles, J. M. (1998). Secondary prevention in coronary heart disease: Baseline survey of provision in general practice. *British Medical Journal, 316,* 1430–1434.

Canadian Task Force on the Periodic Health Examination. (1979). The Periodic Health Examination. *Canadian Medical Association Journal, 121,* 1193–1254.

Cannon, R. O., III. (1991). Microvascular angina: Cardiovascular investigations regarding pathophysiology and management. *Medical Clinics of North America, 75,* 1097–1118.

Cannon, R. O., III. (1995). Chest pain and the sensitive heart. *European Journal of Gastroenterology and Hepatology, 7,* 1161–1171.

Cannon, R. O., III. (1997). Does coronary endothelial dysfunction cause myocardial ischemia in the absence of obstructive coronary artery disease? *Circulation, 96,* 3251–3254.

Cannon, R. O., III. (1998). The conundrum of cardiovascular syndrome X. *Cardiology Review, 6,* 213–220.

Cannon, R. O., III, Camici, P. G., & Epstein, S. E. (1992). Pathophysiological dilemma of syndrome X. *Circulation, 85,* 883–892.

Caplan, R. D., & Van Harrison, R. (1993). Person–environment fit theory: Some history, recent developments, and future directions. *Journal of Social Issues, 49,* 253–275.

Carey, M. P., Snel, D. L., Carey, K. B., & Richards, C. S. (1989). Self-initiated smoking cessation: A review of the empirical literature from a stress and coping perspective. *Cognitive Therapy and Research, 13,* 323–341.

Carinci, F., Nicolucci, A., Ciampi, A., Labbrozzi, D., Bettinardi, O., Zotti, A. M., et al. (1997). Role of interactions between psychological and clinical factors in determining 6-month mortality among patients with acute myocardial infarction. *European Heart Journal, 18,* 835–845.

Carlson, J. J., Norman, G. J., Feltz, D. L., Franklin, B. A., Johnson, J. A., & Locke, S. K. (2001). Self-efficacy, psychosocial factors, and exercise behavior in traditional versus modified cardiac rehabilitation. *Journal of Cardiopulmonary Rehabilitation, 21,* 363–373.

Carlsson, R., Lindberg, G., Westin, L., & Israelsson, B. (1997). Influence of coronary nursing management follow up on lifestyle after acute myocardial infarction. *Heart, 77,* 256–259.

Carney, R. M., Blumenthal, J. A., Stein, P. K., Watkins, L., Catellier, D., Berkman, L., et al. (2001). Depression, heart rate variability, and acute myocardial infarction. *Circulation, 104,* 2024–2028.

*Carney, R. M., Freedland, K. E., Clark, K. A., Skala, J. A., Smith, L. J., Delamater, A., et al. (1992). Psychosocial adjustment of patients arriving early at the emergency department after acute myocardial infarction. *American Journal of Cardiology, 69,* 160–162.

*Carney, R. M., Freedland, K. E., Eisen, S. A., Rich, M. W., & Jaffe, A. S. (1995). Major depression and medication adherence in elderly patients with coronary artery disease. *Health Psychology, 14,* 88–90.

*Carney, R. M., Freedland, K. E., Eisen, S. A., Rich, M. W., Skala, J. A., & Jaffe, A. S. (1998). Adherence to a prophylactic medication regimen in patients with symptomatic versus asymptomatic ischemic heart disease. *Behavioral Medicine, 24,* 35–39.

*Carney, R. M., Freedland, K. E., & Jaffe, A. S. (1990). Insomnia and depression prior to myocardial infarction. *Psychosomatic Medicine, 52,* 603–609.

*Carney, R. M., Freedland, K. E., Rich, M. W., Smith, L. J., & Jaffe, A. S. (1993). Ventricular tachycardia and psychiatric depression in patients with coronary artery disease. *American Journal of Medicine, 95,* 23–28.

Carney, R. M., Freedland, K. E., Stein, P. K., Skala, J. A., Hoffman, P., & Jaffe, A. S. (2000). Change in heart rate and heart rate variability during treatment for depression in patients with coronary heart disease. *Psychosomatic Medicine, 62,* 639–647.

*Carney, R. M., Rich, M. W., Freedland, K. E., Saini, J., teVelde, A., Simeone, C., & Clark, K. (1988). Major depressive disorder predicts cardiac events in patients with coronary artery disease. *Psychosomatic Medicine, 50,* 627–633.

*Carney, R. M., Rich, M. W., teVelde, A., Saini, J., Clark, K., & Freedland, K. E. (1988). The relationship between heart rate, heart rate variability and depression in patients with coronary artery disease. *Journal of Psychosomatic Research, 32,* 159–164.

*Carney, R. M., Rich, M. W., teVelde, A., Saini, J., Clark, K., & Jaffe, A. S. (1987). Major depressive disorder in coronary artery disease. *American Journal of Cardiology, 60,* 1273–1275.

*Carney, R. M., Saunders, R. D., Freedland, K. E., Stein, P., Rich, M. W., & Jaffe, A. S. (1995). Association of depression with reduced heart rate variability in coronary artery disease. *American Journal of Cardiology, 76,* 562–564.

*Carroll, K. M. (1997). Relapse prevention as a psychosocial treatment: A review of controlled clinical trials. In G. Marlatt & T. Vanden Bos (Eds.), *Addictive behaviors: Readings on aetiology, prevention, and treatment* (pp. 697–717). Washington, DC: American Psychological Association.

*Carson, M. A., Hathaway, A., Tuohey, J. P., & McKay, B. M. (1988). The effect of a relaxation technique on coronary risk factors. *Behavioral Medicine, 14,* 71–77.

Carter, C. S., & Maddock, R. J. (1992). Chest pain in generalized anxiety disorder. *International Journal of Psychiatry in Medicine, 22,* 291–298.

*Carter, C., Maddock, R., Amsterdam, E., McCormick, S., Waters, C., & Billett, J. (1992). Panic disorder and chest pain in the coronary care unit. *Psychosomatics, 33,* 302–309.

Carter, C. S., Servan-Schreiber, D., & Perlstein, W. M. (1997). Anxiety disorders and the syndrome of chest pain with normal coronary arteries: Prevalence and pathophysiology. *Journal of Clinical Psychiatry, 58*(Suppl. 3), 70–73; discussion 74–75.

Carvalho, M., & Carrageta, M. (1990). X syndrome: Review of concepts. *Revista Portuguesa de Cardiologia, 9,* 915–921.

Case, R. B., Heller, S. S., Case, N. B., & Moss, A. J. (1985). Type A behavior and survival after acute myocardial infarction. *New England Journal of Medicine, 312,* 737–741.

Case, R. B., Moss, A. J., Case, N., McDermott, M., & Eberly, S. (1992) Living alone after myocardial infarction—Impact on prognosis. *JAMA, 267,* 515–519.

Cason, C., Russell, D., & Fincher, S. (1992). Preparatory sensory information for cardiac catheterization. *Cardiovascular Nursing, 28,* 41–45.

Cassem, N. H., & Hackett, T. P. (1971). Psychiatric consultation in a coronary care unit. *Annals of Internal Medicine, 75,* 9.

Cassell, S. (1965). Effect of brief puppet therapy upon the emotional responses of children undergoing cardiac catheterization. *Journal of Consulting and Clinical Psychology, 29,* 1–8.

Castell, D. O. (1992). Chest pain of undetermined origin: Overview of pathophysiology. *American Journal of Medicine, 92*(5A), 2S–4S.

Castro, C. M., King, A. C., & Brassington, G. S. (2001). Telephone versus mail interventions for maintenance of physical activity in older adults. *Health Psychology, 20,* 438–444.

Cavender, J. B., Rogers, W. J., Fisher, L. D., Gershi, B. J., & Coggin, C. J. (1992). Effects of smoking on survival and morbidity in patients randomized to medical or surgical therapy in the Coronary Artery Surgery Study (CASS): 10-year follow-up. *Journal of the American College of Cardiology, 20,* 287–294.

Chaiken, S. (1980). Heuristic versus systematic information processing and the use of source versus message cues in persuasion. *Journal of Personality and Social Psychology, 39,* 752–766.

Chandra, V., Szklo, M., Goldberg, R., & Tonascia, J. (1983). The impact of marital status on survival after an acute myocardial infarction: a population based study. *American Journal of Epidemiology, 117,* 320–325.

*Channer, K. S., Papouchado, M., James, M. A., & Rees, J. R. (1985). Anxiety and depression in patients with chest pain referred for exercise testing. *Lancet, 2,* 820–823.

Chapman, C., Casey, K., Dubner, R., Foley, K., Gracely, R., & Reading, A. (1985). Pain measurement: An overview. *Pain, 22,* 1–31.

Chauhan, A., Mullins, P. A., Thuraisingham, S. I., Taylor, G., Petch, M. C., & Schofield, P. M. (1994). Abnormal cardiac pain perception in syndrome X. *Journal of the American College of Cardiology, 24,* 329–335.

Chen, J., Hsu, N., Ting, C., Lin, S., & Chang, M. (2000). Differential coronary hemodynamics and left ventricular contractility in patients with syndrome X. *International Journal of Cardiology, 75,* 49–57.

Chen, J. W., Ting, C. T., Chen, Y. H., Wu, T. C., Hsu, N. W., Lin, S. J., et al. (1999). Differential coronary microvascular function in patients with left ventricular dysfunction of unknown cause—Implication for possible mechanism of myocardial ischemia in early stage of cardiomyopathy. *International Journal of Cardiology, 69,* 251–261.

*Chernen, L., Friedman, S., Goldberg, N., Feit, A., Kwan, T., & Stein, R. (1995). Cardiac disease and nonorganic chest pain: Factors leading to disability. *Cardiology, 86,* 15–21.

Chessick, R. D. (1977). The coronary-prone personality. *Medikon International, 6,* 17–20.

Chessick, R. D. (1987a). Coronary artery disease as a narcissistic psychosomatic disorder: Part 1. *Dynamic Psychotherapy, 5,* 16–29.

Chessick, R. D. (1987b). Coronary heart disease as a narcissistic psychosomatic disorder: Part 2. Case presentation. *Dynamic Psychotherapy, 5,* 131–143.

Chierchia, S. L., & Fragasso, G. (1996). Angina with normal coronary arteries: Diagnosis, pathophysiology and treatment. *European Heart Journal, 17*(Suppl. G), 14–19.

*Chignon, J. M., Lepine, J. P., & Ades, J. (1993). Panic disorders in cardiac outpatients. *American Journal of Psychiatry, 150,* 780–785.

*Chorot, P., & Sandín, B. (1994). Life events and stress reactivity as predictors of cancer, coronary heart disease and anxiety disorders. *International Journal of Psychosomatics, 41,* 34–40.

Christian, P. (1966). Risikofaktoren und Risikopersönlichkeit beim Herzinfarkt [Risk factors for heart attack and personality-based risk factors]. In R. Thauer & C. Albers (Eds.), *Verhandlungen der Deutschen Gesellschaft für Kreislaufforschung* [Proceedings of the German Society for Research Into Circulatory Diseases] (pp. 97–107). Darmstadt, Germany: Steinkopff.

Clancy, C. M. (1997). Ensuring health care quality: An AHCPR perspective. *Clinical Therapeutics, 19,* 1564–1571.

Clancy, J., & Noyes, R., Jr. (1996). Anxiety neurosis: A disease for the medical model. *Psychosomatics, 17,* 90–93.

Cleary, P. D., Epstein, A. M., Oster, G., Morrissey, G. S., Stason, W. B., Debussey, S., et al. (1991). Health-related quality of life among patients undergoing percutaneous transluminal coronary angioplasty. *Medical Care, 29,* 939–950. [Erratum published in Volume 30, p. 76]

Cleveland, S., & Johnson, D. L. (1962). Personality patterns in young males with coronary disease. *Psychosomatic Medicine, 24,* 600–610.

Cochrane Collaboration. (2004). Review manager [Computer software]. Retrieved April 27, 2004, from http://www.cc-ims.net/revman

The Cochrane Society. (2002). *Handbook.* Retrieved from http://www.cochrane.dk/cochrane/handbook/handbook.htm

Cohen, H. W., Gibson, G., & Alderman, M. H. (2000). Excess risk of myocardial infarction in patients treated with antidepressant medications: Association with use of tricyclic agents. *American Journal of Medicine, 108,* 2–8.

Cohen, H. W., Madhavan, S., & Alderman, M. H. (2001). History of treatment for depression: Risk factor for myocardial infarction in hypertensive patients. *Psychosomatic Medicine, 63,* 203–209.

Cohen, J. (1977). *Statistical power analysis for the behavior sciences* (2nd ed.). New York: Academic Press.

Cohen, J., & Hasler, M. (1987). Sensory preparation for patients undergoing cardiac catheterization. *Critical Care Nurse, 7,* 68–73.

Cohen, J. B., & Reed, D. (1985). The Type A behavior pattern and coronary heart disease among Japanese men in Hawaii. *Journal of Behavioral Medicine, 8,* 343–352.

*Cohen, L., Stokhof, L. H., & van der Ploeg, H. M. (1996). Identifying patients recovering from a recent myocardial infarction who require and accept psychological care. *Psychological Reports, 79,* 1371–1377.

Cohen, S., & Herbert, T. B. (1996). Health psychology: Psychological factors and physical disease from the perspective of human psychoneuroimmunology. *Annual Review of Psychology, 47,* 113–142.

Colligan, R. C., & Offord, K. P. (1988). The risky use of the MMPI Hostility Scale in assessing risk for coronary heart disease. *Psychosomatics, 29,* 188–196.

Collins, A. (2002). Cardiac syndrome X. *New England Journal of Medicine, 347,* 1377–1379.

Condon, J. T. (1987). Type A coronary-prone behaviour pattern and pathological narcissism. *Australian and New Zealand Journal of Psychiatry, 21*(2), 16–23.

Condrau, G., & Gassmann, M. (1989). *Das verletzte Herz: Zur Psychosomatik von Herz-Kreislauf-Erkrankungen* [The wounded heart: Psychosomatic aspects of heart and circulatory disease]. Zurich, Switzerland: Kreuz.

*Conn, V. S., Taylor, S. G., & Casey, B. (1992). Cardiac rehabilitation program participation and outcomes after myocardial infarction. *Rehabilitation Nursing, 23,* 58–62.

Cook, D. G., Shaper, A. G., Pocock, S. J., & Kussick, S. J. (1986). Giving up smoking and the risk of heart attacks: A report from the British Regional Heart Study. *Lancet, 2,* 1376–1379.

Cook, D. J., Guyatt, G. H., Laupacis, A., Sackett, D. L., & Goldberg, R. J. (1995). Clinical recommendations using levels of evidence for antithrombotic agents. *Chest, 108*(4 Suppl.), 227S–230S.

Cook, W., & Medley, D. (1954). Proposed hostility and pharisaic-virtue scales for the MMPI. *Journal of Applied Psychology, 38,* 414–418.

Cooper, A., Lloyd, G., Weinman, J., & Jackson, G. (1999). Why patients do not attend cardiac rehabilitation: Role of intentions and illness beliefs. *Heart, 82,* 234–236.

Cordova, M. J., Andrykowski, M. A., Kenady, D. E., McGrath, P. C., Sloan, D. A., & Redd, W. H. (1995). Frequencies and correlates of posttraumatic-stress-disorder-like symptoms after treatment for breast cancer. *Journal of Consulting and Clinical Psychology, 63,* 981–986.

Cormier, L. E., Katon, W., Russo, J., & Hollifield, M. (1988). Chest pain with negative cardiac diagnostic studies: Relationship to psychiatric illness. *Journal of Nervous and Mental Disease, 176,* 351–358.

*Corone, S., de Vernejoul, N., Gomont, A. M., & Sellier, P. (2002). Readaption cardiaque en Ile-de-France: Etat de l'organisation actuelle et propositions d'amenagement [Cardiac rehabilitation in Ile-de-France: State of the current organization and proposals for an installation]. *Archives des Maladies du Coeur et des Vaisseaux, 95,* 581–588.

Corruble, E., & Guelfi, J. D. (2000). Pain complaints in depressed inpatients. *Psychopathology, 33,* 307–309.

Cossette, S., Frasure-Smith, N., & Lespérance, F. (2001). Clinical implications of a reduction in psychological distress on cardiac prognosis in patients participating in a psychosocial intervention program. *Psychosomatic Medicine, 63,* 257–266.

Cossette, S., Frasure-Smith, N., & Lespérance, F. (2002). Nursing approaches to reducing psychological distress in men and women recovering from myocardial infarction. *International Journal of Nursing Studies, 39,* 479–494.

Costa, P. T., Jr. (1987). Influence of the normal personality dimension of neuroticism on chest pain symptoms and coronary artery disease. *American Journal of Cardiology, 60,* 20J–26J.

Costa, P. T., Fleg, J. L., McCrae, R. R., & Lakatta, E. G. (1982). Neuroticism, coronary artery disease, and chest pain complaints: Cross-sectional and longitudinal studies. *Experimental Aging Research, 8,* 37–44.

Costa, P. T., Krantz, D. S., Blumenthal, J. A., Furberg, C. D., Rosenman, R. H., & Shekelle, R. B. (1987). Task force 2: Psychological risk factors in coronary artery disease. *Circulation, 76*(Suppl. I), I-145–I-149.

Costa, P. T., & McCrae, R. R. (1985). Hypochondriasis, neuroticism, and aging: When are somatic complaints unfounded? *American Psychologist, 40,* 19–28.

Costa, P. T., Zonderman, A. B., Engel, B. T., Baile, W. F., Brimlow, D. L., & Brinker, J. (1985). The relationship of chest pain symptoms to angiographic findings of coronary artery stenosis and neuroticism. *Psychosomatic Medicine, 47,* 285–293.

Costa, P. T., Zonderman, A. B., McCrae, R. R., & Williams, R. B. (1986). Cynicism and paranoid alienation in the Cook and Medley HO Scale. *Psychosomatic Medicine, 48,* 283–285.

Coupland, N., Wilson, S., & Nutt, D. (1997). Antidepressant drugs and the cardiovascular system: A comparison of tricyclics and selective serotonin reuptake inhibitors and their relevance for the treatment of psychiatric patients with cardiovascular problems. *Journal of Psychopharmacology, 11,* 83–92.

Cox, B. J. (1996). The nature and assessment of catastrophic thoughts in panic disorder. *Behavioral Research and Therapy, 34,* 363–374.

Cramer, P. (2000). Thematic Apperception Test. In A. E. Kazdin (Ed.), *Encylopedia of psychology* (Vol. 8, pp. 56–57). Washington, DC: American Psychological Association.

Crea, F., Gaspardone, A., Kaski, J. C., Davies, G., & Maseri, A. (1992). Relation between stimulation site of cardiac afferent nerves by adenosine and distribution of cardiac pain: Results of a study in patients with stable angina. *Journal of the American College of Cardiology, 20,* 1498–1502.

*Crisp, A. H., Queenan, M., & D'Souza, M. F. (1984). Myocardial infarction and the emotional climate. *Lancet, 1*(8377), 616–619.

Critchley, J. A., & Capewell, S. (2003). Mortality risk reduction associated with coronary heart disease: A systematic review. *JAMA, 290,* 86–97.

Crow, R., Blackburn, H., Jacobs, D., Hannan, P., Pirie, P., Mittelmark, M., et al. (1986). Population strategies to enhance physical activity: The Minnesota Heart Health Program. *Acta Medica Scandinavica, 711*(Suppl.), 93–112.

Crowe, J. M., Runions, J., Ebbesen, L. S., Oldridge, N. B., & Streiner, D. L. (1996). Anxiety and depression after acute myocardial infarction. *Heart & Lung, 25,* 98–107.

Cullen, P., Schulte, H., & Assmann, G. (1997). The Münster Heart Study. *Circulation, 96,* 2128–2136.

Cunningham, J., Strassberg, D., & Roback, H. (1978). Group psychotherapy for medical patients. *Comprehensive Psychiatry, 19,* 135–140.

*Czajkowski, S. M., Terrin, M., Lindquist, R., Hoogwerf, B., Dupuis, G., Shumaker, S. A., et al. (1997). Comparison of preoperative characteristics of men and women undergoing coronary artery bypass grafting [The post coronary artery bypass graft (CABG) biobehavioral study]. *American Journal of Cardiology, 79,* 1017–1024.

Dacosta, A., Guy, J. M., Tardy, B., Gonthier, R., Denis, L., Lamaud, M., et al. (1993). Myocardial infarction and nicotine patch: A contributing or causative factor? *European Heart Journal, 14,* 1709–1711.

Dafoe, W., & Huston, P. (1997). Current trends in cardiac rehabilitation. *Canadian Medical Association Journal, 156,* 527–532.

Dath, N. N. S., Mishra, H., Kumaraiah, V., & Yavagal, S. T. (1997). Behavioural approach to coronary heart disease. *Journal of Personality and Clinical Studies, 13,* 29–33.

Dault, L., Groene, J., & Herick, R. (1992). Helping your patient through cardiac catheterization. *Nursing, 22,* 52–55.

Davey Smith, G. (1997). Is control at work the key to socioeconomic gradients in mortality? [Letter]. *Lancet, 350,* 1369.

Davidson, C. (1996). Cardiac rehabilitation in the district hospital. In D. Jones & R. West (Eds.), *Cardiac rehabilitation* (pp. 144–166). London: BMJ Publishing.

Davidson, C., Reval, K., Chamberlain, D. A., Pentecost, B., & Parker, J. (1995). A report of a working group of the British Cardiac Society: Cardiac rehabilitation services in the United Kingdom 1992. *British Heart Journal, 73,* 201–202.

Davies, R. F., Linden, W., Habibi, H., Klinke, W. P., Nadeau, C., Phaneuf, D. C., et al. (1993). Relative importance of psychologic traits and severity of ischemia in causing angina during treadmill exercise: Canadian Amlodipine/Atenolol in Silent Ischemia Study (CASIS) investigators. *Journal of the American College of Cardiology, 21,* 331–336.

Davies Osterkamp, S., & Salm, A. (1980). Ansaetze zur Erfassung psychischer Adaptationsprozesse in medizinischen Belastungssituationen [Assessment of coping mechanisms in medical stress situations]. *Medizinische Psychologie, 6,* 66–80.

Davis, T., Maguire, T., Haraphongse, M., & Schaumberger, M. (1994a). Preparing adult patients for cardiac catheterization: Informational treatment and coping style interactions. *Heart & Lung, 23,* 130–139.

Davis, T., Maguire, T., Haraphongse, M., & Schaumberger, M. (1994b). Undergoing cardiac catheterization: The effects of informational preparation and coping style on patient anxiety during the procedure. *Heart & Lung, 23,* 140–150.

Dean, G. (1993). What is it like to have an angioplasty? *Journal of the Royal College of Physicians (London), 27,* 73–74.

de Bruijn, N. (1989). General anesthesia during percutaneous transluminal coronary angioplasty for acute myocardial infarction. *Anesthesia and Analgesia, 68,* 201–207.

DeBusk, R. F. (1992). Why is cardiac rehabilitation not widely used? *Western Journal of Medicine, 156,* 206–208.

DeBusk, R. F., Miller, N. H., Superko, R., Dennis, C. A., Thomas, R. J., Lew, H. T., et al. (1994). A case-management system for coronary risk factor modification after acute myocardial infarction. *Annals of Internal Medicine, 120,* 721–729.

de Dowiakowski, M. L., & Luminet, D. (1969). Psychosomatic study of 32 cases of myocardial infarct. *Acta Neurologica et Psychiatrica Belgica, 69,* 78–89.

Defontaine-Catteau, M.-C., Pedinielle, J.-L., & Bertagne, P. (1992). L'alexithymie: Défence contre le stress ou de-métaphorisation selective [Alexithymia: Defence against stress or selective de-metaphorization?]. *Psychologie Médicale, 24,* 1562–1566.

Defourny, M., & Frankignoul, M. (1973). A propos du comportement predisposant aux coronaropathies (overt pattern A) [Concerning behavior predisposing coronary disease (Type A behavior)]. *Journal of Psychosomatic Research, 17,* 219–230.

Defourny, M., Hubin, P., & Luminet, D. (1976). Alexithymia, "pensee operatoire" and predisposition to coronopathy. *Psychotherapy and Psychosomatics, 27,* 106–114.

Defourny, M., Timsit, M., & Dongier, M. (1972). Etude comparée de 15 sujets atteints d'angor coronarien et de 30 sujets victimes d'un infarctus du myocarde au moyen du test de Rorschach [Comparative study of 15 victims of coronary angina and 30 victims of myocardial infarction using the Rorschach test]. *Revue de Medecine Psychosomatique et de Psychologie Medicale, 14,* 157–169.

de Jong, M., Erdman, R. A. M., van den Brand, M. J. B. M., Verhage, F., Trijsburg, R. W., & Passchier, J. (1994). Home measures of anxiety, avoidant coping and defense as predictors of anxiety, heart rate and skin conductance level just before invasive cardiovascular procedures. *Journal of Psychosomatic Research, 38,* 315–322.

de Jonge, J., Mulder, M. J., & Nijhuis, F. J. (1999). The incorporation of different demand concepts in the job demand–control model: Effects on health care professionals. *Social Science & Medicine, 48,* 1149–1160.

De Leo, D., Caracciolo, S., Berto, F., & Mauro, P. (1986). Type A behavior pattern and mortality after recurrent myocardial infarction: Preliminary results from a follow-up study of 5 years. *Psychotherapy and Psychosomatics, 46,* 132–137.

Dembroski, T. M. (1978). Reliability and validity of methods used to assess coronary prone behavior. In T. M. Dembroski, S. M. Weiss, J. L. Shields, S. G. Haynes, & M. Feinlieb (Eds.), *Coronary-prone behavior* (pp. 95–106). New York: Springer-Verlag.

Dembroski, T. M, & Costa, P. T. (1987). Coronary prone behavior: Components of the Type A pattern and hostility. *Journal of Personality, 55,* 211–235.

Dembroski, T. M., MacDougall, J. M., Costa, P. T., & Grandits, G. A. (1989). Components of hostility as predictors of sudden death and myocardial infarction in the Multiple Risk Factor Intervention Trial. *Psychosomatic Medicine, 51,* 514–522.

Dembroski, T. M., Schmidt, T. H., & Blümchen, G. (Eds.). (1983). *Biobehavioral bases of coronary heart disease.* Basel, Germany: Karger.

Dembroski, T. M., Weiss, S. M., Shields, J. L., Haynes, S. G., & Feinlieb, M. (Eds.). (1978). *Coronary-prone behavior.* New York: Springer-Verlag.

Denolin, H. (1985). Rehabilitation as part of comprehensive care. In V. Kallio & E. Cay (Eds.), *Rehabilitation after myocardial infarction* (pp. 1–8). Copenhagen, Denmark: World Health Organization.

Denollet, J. (1998a). Personality and coronary heart disease: The type-D scale-16 (DS16). *Annals of Behavioral Medicine, 20,* 209–215.

Denollet, J. (1998b). Personality and risk of cancer in men with coronary heart disease. *Psychological Medicine, 28,* 991–995.

Denollet, J. (2000). Type D personality: A potential risk factor refined. *Journal of Psychosomatic Research, 49,* 255–266.

*Denollet, J., & Brutsaert, D. L. (1995). Enhancing emotional well-being by comprehensive rehabilitation in patients with coronary heart disease. *European Heart Journal, 16,* 1070–1078.

Denollet, J., & Brutsaert, D. L. (1998). Personality, disease severity, and the risk of long-term cardiac events in patients with a decreased ejection fraction after myocardial infarction. *Circulation, 97,* 167–173.

Denollet, J., & de Potter, B. (1992). Coping subtypes for men with coronary heart disease: Relationship to well-being, stress and Type-A behaviour. *Psychological Medicine, 22,* 667–684.

*Denollet, J., Sys, S. U., & Brutsaert, D. L. (1995). Personality and mortality after myocardial infarction. *Psychosomatic Medicine, 57,* 582–591.

Denollet, J., Sys, S. U., Stroobant, N., Rombouts, H., Gillebert, T. C., & Brutsaert, D. L. (1996). Personality as independent predictor of long-term mortality in patients with coronary heart disease. *Lancet, 347,* 417–421.

Denollet, J., Vaes, J., & Brutsaert, D. L. (2000). Inadequate response to treatment in coronary heart disease: Adverse effects of Type D personality and younger age on 5-year prognosis and quality of life. *Circulation, 102,* 630–635.

Derogatis, L. R. (2000). SCL-90-R. In K. A. Alan (Ed.), *Encyclopedia of psychology* (Vol. 7, pp. 192–193). Washington, DC: American Psychological Association.

Deter, H. C., Hahn, P., & Petzold, E. (1987). Krankheitsorientierte Gruppentherapie—Ein tiefenpsychologisch orientiertes Behandlungsverfahren fuer koerperlich Kranke (psychosomatische und somatopsychische Patienten) [Illness-oriented group therapy: A depth-psychology oriented treatment model for the physically ill (psychosomatic and somatoform patients)]. In H. Quint & P. L. Janssen (Eds.), *Psychotherapie in der psychosomatischen Medizin: Erfahrungen, Konzepte, Ergebnisse* [Psychotherapy in psychosomatic medicine: Experiences, concepts, and results] (pp. 12–19). Berlin, Germany: Springer.

Deutsch, F., & Kauf, E. (1923). Psycho-physische Kreislaufstudien: II. Mitteilung. Über die Ursachen der Kreislaufstörungen bei Herzneurosen [Psycho-physiological circulatory studies: Second report. On the causes of circulatory problems in cardiac neuroses]. *Zeitschrift für die Gesamte Experimentelle Medizin, 34,* 71–81.

Deutsche Gesellschaft für Prävention und Rehabilitation. (2002). *Entwicklung der Herzgruppen in Deutschland* [Development of outpatient cardiac exercise groups in Germany]. Koblenz, Germany: Peter Ritter.

Deutsche Gesellschaft für Prävention und Rehabilitation. (2004). *Verzeichnis von zertifizierten Herzkreislaufrehabilitationkliniken und ambulanten kardiologischen Rehabilitationszentren in Deutschland, die dem Qualitätsstandard der DGPR entsprechen* [Listing of certified heart cycle rehabilitation hospitals and ambulatory cardiological rehabilitation centers in Germany that meet the quality standard of the DGPR]. Koblenz, Germany: Author.

Deutsche Gesellschaft für Prävention und Rehabilitation. (2005). *Die ambulanten Herzgruppen Deutschlands* [German outpatient cardiac rehabilitation groups]. Retrieved September 10, 2005, from http://www/dgpr.de/l.html

*Deutsche Herzstiftung. (1996). *Herz-Kreislauf-Reha-Kliniken* [Cardiovascular rehabilitation hospitals]. Frankfurt, Germany: Author.

Devaul, R. B. (2000). Posttraumatic stress disorder in Vietnam veterans following an acute myocardial infarction. *Dissertation Abstracts International, 60B,* 4215.

Dimsdale, J. E., & Hackett, T. P. (1982). Effect of denial on cardiac health and psychological assessment. *American Journal of Psychiatry, 139,* 1477–1480.

Dimsdale, J. E., Hackett, T. P., Hutter, A. M., Jr., & Block, P. C. (1980). The risk of Type A mediated coronary artery disease in different populations. *Psychosomatic Medicine, 42,* 55–62.

Dimsdale, J. E., Hackett, T. P., Hutter, A. M., Jr., & Block, P. C. (1982). The association of clinical, psychosocial, and angiographic variables with work status in patients with coronary artery disease. *Journal of Psychosomatic Research, 26,* 215–221.

Dinnes, J. (1998). Cardiac rehabilitation. *Nursing Times, 94*(38), 60–62.

Dinnes, J., Kleijnen, J., Leitner, M., & Thompson, D. (1999). Cardiac rehabilitation. *Quality in Health Care, 8,* 65–71.

Dishman, R. K. (1993). Exercise adherence. In R. N. Singer, M. Murphy, & L. K. Tenant (Eds.), *Handbook of research on sport psychology* (pp. 770–778). New York: MacMillan.

Doerfler, L. A., Pbert, L., & DeCosimo, D. (1994). Symptoms of posttraumatic stress disorder following myocardial infarction and coronary artery bypass surgery. *General Hospital Psychiatry, 16,* 193–199.

*Doerfler, L. A., Pbert, L., & DeCosimo, D. (1997). Self-reported depression in patients with coronary heart disease. *Journal of Cardiopulmonary Rehabilitation, 17,* 163–170.

Dolman, S. (1994). PTCA: The role of the angioplasty program nurse. *Canadian Journal of Cardiovascular Nursing, 5,* 25–28.

Döring, S., Mumelter, C., Bonatti, J., Oturanlar, D., Gaggl, S., Pachinger, O., et al. (2001). Zur Variabilitat des Coping bei Patienten mit aortokoronarer Bypass-Operation [Variability of coping strategies in patients recovering from coronary artery bypass surgery]. *Zeitschrift für Psychosomatische Medizin und Psychotherapie, 47,* 262–276.

Dorn, J., Naughton, J., Imamura, D., & Trevisan, M. (2001). Correlates of compliance in a randomized exercise trial in myocardial infarction patients. *Medicine and Science in Sports and Exercise, 33,* 1081–1089.

Dornelas, E. A., Sampson, R. A., Gray, J. F., Waters, D., & Thompson, P. D. (2000). A randomized controlled trial of smoking cessation counselling after myocardial infarction. *Preventive Medicine, 30,* 261–268.

Dotson, R. (1997). Clinical neurophysiology laboratory tests to assess the nociceptive system in humans. *Journal of Clinical Neurophysiology, 14,* 32–45.

*Dracup, K., Moser, D. K., Marsden, C., Taylor, S. E., & Guzy, P. M. (1991). Effects of a multidimensional cardiopulmonary rehabilitation program on psychosocial function. *American Journal of Cardiology, 68,* 31–34.

Dreyfuss, F. (1953). Role of emotional stress preceding coronary occlusion. *American Journal of Cardiology, 3,* 590–596.

Dreyfuss, F., Dasberg, H., & Assael, M. (1969). The relationship of myocardial infarction to depressive illness. *Psychotherapy and Psychosomatics, 17,* 73–81.

Dreyfuss, F., Shanan, J., & Sharon, M. (1966). Some personality characteristics of middle-aged men with coronary artery disease. *Psychotherapy and Psychosomatics, 14,* 1–16.

*Droste, C., & Roskamm, H. (1983). Experimental pain measurement in patients with asymptomatic myocardial ischemia. *Journal of the American College of Cardiology, 1,* 940–945.

Druss, B. G., Bradford, D. W., Rosenheck, R. A., Radford, M. J., & Krumholz, H. M. (2000). Mental disorders and use of cardiovascular procedures after myocardial infarction. *JAMA, 283,* 506–511.

Dubbert, P. M., Rappaport, N. B., & Martin, J. E. (1987). Exercise in cardiovascular disease. *Behavior Modification, 11,* 329–347.

*Duits, A. A., Boeke, S., Duivenvoorden, H. J., & Passchier, J. (1996). Depression in patients undergoing cardiac surgery: A comment. *British Journal of Health Psychology, 1,* 283–286.

Duits, A. A., Duivenvoorden, H. J., Boeke, S., Taams, M. A., Mochtar, B., Krauss, X. H., et al. (1998). The course of anxiety and depression in patients undergoing coronary artery bypass surgery. *Journal of Psychosomatic Research, 45,* 127–138.

Duits, A. A., Duivenvoorden, H. J., Boeke, S., Taams, M. A., Mochtar, B., Krauss, X. H., et al. (1999). A structural modeling analysis of anxiety and depression in patients undergoing coronary artery bypass graft surgery: A model generating approach. *Journal of Psychosomatic Research, 46,* 187–200.

Duivenvoorden, H. J., & van Dixhoorn, J. (1991). Predictability of psychic outcome for exercise training and exercise training including relaxation therapy after myocardial infarction. *Journal of Psychosomatic Research, 35,* 569–578.

Dunbar, F. (1936). Psychic factors in cardiovascular disease. *New York State Journal of Medicine, 36,* 423–429.

Dunbar, F. (1939). Character and symptom formation. *Psychoanalytic Quarterly, 8,* 18–47.

Dunbar, F. (1940). Emotions and bodily changes: A report of some recent psychosomatic studies. *Annals of Internal Medicine, 14,* 837–853.

Dunbar, F. (1942). The relationship between anxiety states and organic disease. *Clinics, 1,* 879–908.

Dunbar, F. (1943). *Psychosomatic diagnosis.* New York: Harper.

Dunbar, F. (1954). *Emotions and bodily changes—A survey of literature on psychosomatic interrelationships 1910–1953* (4th ed.). New York: Columbia University Press.

Dunbar, F., Wolfe, T., & Rioch, J. (1936). Psychiatric aspects of medical problems: The psychic component of the disease process (including convalescence) in cardiac, diabetic and fracture patients. *American Journal of Psychiatry, 93,* 649–679.

Dunbar, F., Wolfe, T. P., Tauber, E. S., & Brush, A. L. (1939). The psychic component of the disease process (including convalescence) in cardiac, diabetic and fracture patients (Part 2). *American Journal of Psychiatry, 95,* 1319–1342.

Durkheim, É. (1951). *Suicide: A study in sociology.* Glencoe, IL: Free Press. (Original work published 1897)

Dusseldorp, E., van Elderen, T., Maes, S., Meulman, J., & Kraaij, V. (1999) A meta-analysis of psychoeducational programs for coronary heart disease patients. *Health Psychology, 18,* 506–519.

Eaker, E. D., Abbott, R. D., & Kannel, W. B. (1989). Frequency of uncomplicated angina pectoris in Type A compared with Type B persons (the Framingham Study). *American Journal of Cardiology, 63,* 1042–1045.

*Ebert, A., & Moehler, A. (1997). Integrative Therapie bei Patienten mit koronarer Herzkrankheit: Aspekte der Foerderung von Integritaet, Wohlbefinden und Sinnerleben [Integrative therapy with patients suffering from coronary heart disease: Aspects of promoting integrity, well-being, and meaningfulness]. *Integrative Therapie, 23,* 289–315.

*Ebrahim, S., & Smith, G. D. (1997). Systematic review of randomised controlled trials of multiple risk factor interventions for preventing coronary heart disease. *British Medical Journal, 314,* 1666–1674.

Echtheld, M., van der Kamp, L., & van Elderen, T. (2001). How goal disturbance, coping and chest pain relate to quality of life: A study among patients waiting for PTCA. *Quality of Life Research, 10,* 487–501.

*Edéll-Gustafsson, U. M., & Hetta, J. E. (1999). Anxiety, depression and sleep in male patients undergoing coronary artery bypass surgery. *Scandinavian Journal of Caring Sciences, 13,* 137–143.

Edwards, J. C., & White, P. D. (1934). A note on the incidence of neurocirculatory asthenia with and without organic heart disease. *New England Journal of Medicine, 211,* 53.

Edwards, M., & Payton, V. (1976). Cardiac catheterization. *Nursing Clinics of North America, 11,* 271–280.

Egashira, K., Hirooka, Y., Kuga, T., Mohri, M., & Takeshita, A. (1996). Effects of L-arginine supplementation on endothelium-dependent coronary vasodilatation in patients with angina pectoris and normal coronary arteriograms. *Circulation, 94,* 130–134.

Egashira, K., Inou, T., Hirooka, Y., Yamada, A., Urabe, Y., & Takeshita, A. (1993). Evidence of impaired endothelium-dependent coronary vasodilatation in patients with angina pectoris and normal coronary angiograms. *New England Journal of Medicine, 328,* 1659–1664.

Eichenberger, E. (1929). Somatisch bedingte Angstträume: Ein Beitrag zur Pathogenese des Angstgefühls [Somatically derived anxiety dreams: On the pathogenesis of anxiety]. *Archiv für Psychiatrie, 87,* 640–664.

Eifert, G. H. (1992). Cardiophobia: A paradigmatic behavioural model of heart-focused anxiety and nonanginal chest pain. *Behavioral Research and Therapy, 30,* 329–345.

Eifert, G. H., Hodson, S. E., Tracey, D. R., & Seville, J. L. (1996). Heart-focused anxiety, illness beliefs, and behavioral impairment: Comparing healthy heart-anxious patients with cardiac and surgical inpatients. *Journal of Behavioral Medicine, 19,* 385–399.

Eifert, G. H., Zvolensky, M. J., & Lejuez, C. W. (2000). Heart-focused anxiety and chest pain: A conceptual and clinical review. *Clinical Psychology: Science and Practice, 7,* 403–417.

Elder, J. P., McGraw, S. A., Abrams, D. B., Ferreira, A., Lasater, T. M., Longpre, H., et al. (1986). Organizational and community approaches to communitywide prevention of heart disease: The first two years of the Pawtucket Heart Health Program. *Preventive Medicine, 15,* 107–117.

Elias, M. F., Robbins, M. A., Blow, F. C., Rice, A. P., & Edgecomb, J. L. (1982). A behavioral study of middle-aged chest pain patients: Physical symptom reporting, anxiety, and depression. *Experimental Aging Research, 8,* 45–51.

*Elliott, D. (1993). Comparison of three instruments for measuring patient anxiety in a coronary care unit. *International Critical Care Nursing, 9,* 195–200.

*Elliott, D. (1994). The effects of music and muscle relaxation on patient anxiety in a coronary care unit. *Heart & Lung, 23,* 27–35.

Elliott, P. M., Krzyowska-Dickinson, K., Calvino, R., Hann, C., & Kaski, J. C. (1997). Effect of oral aminophylline in patients with angina and normal coronary arteriograms (cardiac syndrome X). *Heart, 77,* 523–526.

Emery, C. F. (1995). Psychosocial issues: Adherence in cardiac pulmonary rehabilitation. *Journal of Cardiopulmonary Rehabilitation, 15,* 420–423.

Engblom, E., Rönnemaa, T., Hämäläinen, H., & Kallio, V. (1992). Coronary heart disease risk factors before and after bypass surgery: Results of a controlled trial on multifactorial rehabilitation. *European Heart Journal, 13,* 232–237.

*Engebretson, T. O., Clark, M. M., Niaura, R. S., Phillips, T., Albrecht, A., & Tilkemeier, P. (1999). Quality of life and anxiety in a phase II cardiac rehabilitation program. *Medicine and Science in Sports and Exercise, 31,* 216–223.

Engel, G. L. (1975). The death of a twin: Mourning and anniversary reactions: Fragments of 10 years of self-analysis. *International Journal of Psycho-Analysis, 56,* 23–40.

Engel, P. A. (2001). George L. Engel, M.D., 1913–1999: Remembering his life and work; rediscovering his soul. *Psychosomatics, 42,* 94–95.

Engels, F. (1987). *The condition of the working class in England.* Harmondsworth, England: Penguin Classics. (Original work published 1845)

Engels, F. (2003). The condition of the working class in England: 1845. *American Journal of Public Health, 93,* 1246–1249. (Original work published 1845)

Englehart, R. (1993). Quality of life of people six months post percutaneous transluminal coronary angioplasty. *Canadian Journal of Cardiovascular Nursing, 4,* 7–14. [Erratum published in Volume 5, p. 3]

ENRICHD Investigators. (2000). Enhancing Recovery in Coronary Heart Disease Patients (ENRICHD): Study design and methods. *American Heart Journal, 139,* 1–9.

ENRICHD Investigators. (2001). Enhancing Recovery in Coronary Heart Disease Patients (ENRICHD) study intervention: Rationale and design. *Psychosomatic Medicine, 63,* 747–755.

Epstein, F. H. (1979). Predicting, explaining, and preventing coronary heart disease. *Modern Concepts in Cardiovascular Disease, 48,* 7–12.

Erdman, R. A. M., & Duivenvoorden, H. J. (1983). Psychologic evaluation of a cardiac rehabilitation program: A randomized clinical trial in patients with myocardial infarction. *Journal of Cardiac Rehabilitation, 3,* 696–704.

Erickson, M. H., Rossi, E. L., & Rossi, S. I. (1976). *Hypnotic realities: The induction of clinical hypnosis and forms of indirect suggestion.* Oxford, England: Irvington.

Erikson, E. H. (1959). *Identity and the life cycle: Selected papers.* Oxford, England: International Universities Press.

Eriksson, B. E., Jansson, E., Kaijser, L., & Sylvén, C. (1999). Impaired exercise performance but normal skeletal muscle characteristics in female syndrome X patients. *American Journal of Cardiology, 84,* 176–180.

Ernst, E. (1997). Editorial: Psychologische Herzinfarktrehabilitation [Editorial: Psychological recovery from a heart attack]. *Perfusion, 10,* 1.

Escobar, J. I., Swartz, M., Rubio-Stipec, M., & Manu, P. (1991). Medically unexplained symptoms: Distribution, risk factors, and comorbidity. In L. J. Kirmayer & J. M. Robbins (Eds.), *Current concepts of somatization: Research and clinical perspectives* (pp. 63–78). Washington, DC: American Psychiatric Press.

*Espnes, G. A. (1996). The Type 2 construct and personality traits: Aggression, hostility, anxiety and depression. *Personality and Individual Differences, 20,* 641–648.

Esser, P. (1987). Erfahrungen und Ueberlegungen zur Situation des Therapeuten in der stationaeren Gruppenarbeit mit Herzinfarkt-Patienten: Eine persoenliche Darstellung [Experiences and reflections on the situation of the therapist who works with inpatient groups of cardiac rehabilitation patients: A personal description]. In P. Esser (Ed.), *Psychologische Gruppenarbeit im Rahmen der Rehabilitation von Herzpatienten: Erfahrungen, Praxismodelle, Entwicklungen* [Psychological group work in the rehabilitation of heart patients: Experiences, practice models, and developments] (pp. 12–26). Stuttgart, Germany: Enke.

Esteve, L. G., Valdes, M., Riesco, N., & Jodar, I. (1992). Denial mechanisms in myocardial infarction: Their relations with psychological variables and short-term outcome. *Journal of Psychosomatic Research, 36,* 491–496.

Ettin, M. F., Vaughan, E., & Fiedler, N. (1987). Managing group process in nonprocess groups: Working with the theme-centered psychoeducational group. *Group, 11,* 177–192.

European Science Foundation. (2000). *Social variations in health expectancy in Europe.* Retrieved June 9, 2002, from http://www.uni-duesseldorf.de/health

Evans, R. G., Barer, M. L., & Marmor, T. R. (Eds.). (1994). *Why are some people healthy and others not? The determinants of health of populations.* New York: Aldine de Gruyter.

Evenson, K. R., Rosamond, W. D., & Luepker, R. V. (1998). Predictors of outpatient cardiac rehabilitation utilization: The Minnesota Heart Survey Registry. *Journal of Cardiopulmonary Rehabilitation, 18,* 192–198.

Everson, S. A., Kauhanen, J., Kaplan, G. A., Goldberg, D. E., Julkunen, J., Tuomilehto, J., et al. (1997). Hostility and increased risk of mortality and acute myocardial infarction: The mediating role of behavioral risk factors. *American Journal of Epidemiology, 146,* 142–152.

Ewart, C. K., Taylor, C. B., Reese, L. B., & DeBusk, R. F. (1983). Effects of early postmyocardial infarction exercise testing on self-perception and subsequent physical activity. *American Journal of Cardiology, 51,* 1076–1080.

Eysenck, S. B. G., & Eysenck, H. J. (1978). Impulsiveness and venturesomeness: Their position in a dimensional system of personality description. *Psychological Reports, 43,* 1247–1255.

Fahrenkamp, K. (1929). Psychosomatische Beziehungen beim Herzkranken [Psychosomatic factors in the cardiac patient]. *Der Nervenarzt, 2,* 697–710.

Fahrenkamp, K. (1941). *Der Herzkranke* (2., erneuerte Aufl. ed.) [The heart patient (2nd and rev. ed.)]. Stuttgart, Germany: Hippokrates-Verlag.

*Falger, P. R. (1983). Psychosoziale Belastung, Krisen, Vitalitätsverlust und Depression im Lebenslauf von Herzinfarktpatienten [Psychosocial stress, crises, loss of vitality, and depression in the life experiences of heart attack patients]. *Zeitschrift für Gerontologie, 16,* 121–129.

*Falger, P. R., Appels, A., & Bekkers, J. (1986). Biographische Analyse und Herzinfarkt: Eine Untersuchung an Herzinfarktpatienten und zwei Referenzgruppen [Biographical analyses and heart attack: Investigations of heart attack patients and two control groups]. *Zeitschrift für Gerontologie, 19,* 276–285.

Faller, H. (1989). Subjektive Krankheitstheorie des Herzinfarktes [Subjective theories of heart attack as a disease]. In C. Bischoff & H. Zenz (Eds.), *Patientenkonzepte von Koerper und Krankheit* [Patients' concepts of body and disease] (pp. 49–59). Bern, Switzerland: Huber.

Faris, J. A., & Stotts, N. A. (1990). The effect of percutaneous transluminal coronary angioplasty on quality of life. *Progress in Cardiovascular Nursing, 5,* 132–140.

Farquhar, J. W., Fortmann, S. P., Flora, J. A., Taylor, C. B., Haskell, W. L., Williams, P. T., et al. (1990). The Stanford Five City Project: Effects of community-wide education on cardiovascular disease risk factors. *JAMA, 264,* 359–365.

Fassbender, C. F., Cziepluch, W., & Nippe, W. (1984). Psychotherapeutische Arbeit mit Herzinfarktpatienten [Psychotherapeutic work with heart attack patients]. In Berufsverband Deutscher Psychologen (Ed.), *Psychologische Hilfen für Behinderte* [Psychological aids for the disabled] (pp. 73–76). Weinsberg, Germany: Weissenhof.

*Fauerbach, J. A., Bush, D. E., Sordo, S. S., & Ziegelstein, R. C. (1997). Post-MI depression predicts poor compliance with risk modifying recommendations. *Circulation, 96,* 1351.

Fenichel, O. (1977). *Psychoanalytische Neurosenlehre* [Psychoanalytic theory of neuroses] (Vol. 1). Olten, Switzerland: Walter.

Ferrans, C., & Powers, M. J. (1985). Quality of Life Index: Development and psychometric properties. *Advances in Nursing Science, 8,* 15–24.

Fields, W. L. (1991). Description of indicator development for a percutaneous transluminal coronary angioplasty monitor. *Journal of Nursing Care Quality, 6,* 6–19.

Finesilver, C. (1978). Preparation of adult patients for cardiac catheterization and coronary cineangiography. *International Journal of Nursing Studies, 15,* 211–221.

Finesilver, C. (1980). Reducing stress in patients having cardiac catheterization. *American Journal of Nursing, 80,* 1807.

Fiore, M. C., Jorenby, D. E., & Baker, T. B. (1997). Smoking cessation: Principles and practice based upon the AHCPR Guideline, 1996. Agency for Health Care Policy and Research. *Annals of Behavioral Medicine, 19,* 213–219.

Fiore, M. C., Novotny, T. F., Pierce, J. P., Giovino, G. A., & Davis, R. M. (1990). Methods used to quit smoking in the United States: Do cessation programs help? *JAMA, 263,* 2760–2765.

Fiore, M. C., Smith, S., Jorenby, D., & Baker, T. (1994). The effectiveness of the nicotine patch for smoking cessation: A meta-analysis. *JAMA, 271,* 1940–1947.

Fischer, G., & Riedesser, P. (1998). *Lehrbuch der Psychotraumatologie* [Textbook of psychotraumatology]. Munich, Germany: Reinhardt.

Fischer, H. K. (1977). Management of emotional factors in coronary disease. *Psychosomatics, 18,* 10–13.

Fischer, W. (1984). *Soziale und biographische Konstitution chronischer Krankheiten. Verhandlungen der deutschen Soziologentag* [The social and biographical components of chronic illnesses. Proceedings of the German Sociologists' Congress]. Frankfurt, Germany: Campus Verlag.

Fitzgerald, S. T. (1996). Factors related to functional status after percutaneous transluminal coronary angioplasty. *Heart & Lung, 25,* 24–30.

Flagle, C. D., & Cahn, M. A. (1992). AHCPR-NLM joint initiative for health services research information: 1992 update on OHSRI. *Quality Review Bulletin, 18,* 410–412.

Flatten, G., Gast, U., Hoffmann, A., Liebermann, P., Reddemann, L., Siol, T., et al. (2004). *Posttraumatische Belastungsstörungen. Leitlinie und Quellentext* [Posttraumatic stress disorder. Guidelines and source text]. Stuttgart, Germany: Schattauer.

Fleet, R. P., Dupuis, G., Kaczorowski, J., Marchand, A., & Beitman, B. D. (1997). Suicidal ideation in emergency department chest pain patients: Panic disorder a risk factor. *American Journal of Emergency Medicine, 15,* 345–349.

Fleet, R. P., Dupuis, G., Marchand, A., Burelle, D., Arsenault, A., & Beitman, B. D. (1996). Panic disorder in emergency department chest pain patients: Prevalence, comorbidity, suicidal ideation, and physician recognition. *American Journal of Medicine, 101,* 371–380.

Fleet, R. P., Dupuis, G., Marchand, A., Burelle, D., & Beitman, B. D. (1994). Panic disorder, chest pain and coronary artery disease: Literature review. *Canadian Journal of Cardiology, 10,* 827–834.

Fleet, R. P., Dupuis, G., Marchand, A., Kaczorowski, J., Burelle, D., Arsenault, A., & Beitman, B. D. (1998). Panic disorder in coronary artery disease patients with noncardiac chest pain. *Journal of Psychosomatic Research, 44,* 81–90.

Fletcher, G. F. (1998). Current status of cardiac rehabilitation. *American Family Physician, 58,* 1778–1782.

Flugelman, M. Y., Weisstub, E., Galun, E., Weiss, A. T., Fischer, D., Kaplan De-Nour, A., et al. (1991). Clinical, psychological and thallium stress studies in patients with chest pain and normal coronary arteries. *International Journal of Cardiology, 33,* 401–408.

Follick, M. J., Ahern, D. K., Gorkin, L., Niaura, R. S., Herd, J. A., Ewart, C., et al. (1990). Relation of psychosocial and stress reactivity variables to ventricular arrhythmias in the Cardiac Arrhythmia Pilot Study (CAPS). *American Journal of Cardiology, 66,* 63–67.

*Forrester, A. W., Lipsey, J. R., Teitelbaum, M. L., DePaulo, J. R., & Andrzejewski, P. L. (1992). Depression following myocardial infarction. *International Journal of Psychiatric Medicine, 22,* 33–46.

Fraenkel, Y. M., Kindler, S., & Melmed, R. N. (1996). Differences in cognitions during chest pain of patients with panic disorder and ischemic heart disease. *Depression and Anxiety, 4,* 217–222.

Fraguas Junior, R., Ramadan, Z. B., Pereira, A. N., & Wajngarten, M. (2000). Depression with irritability in patients undergoing coronary artery bypass graft surgery: The cardiologist's role. *General Hospital Psychiatry, 22,* 365–374.

Frank, U. (2000). Subjektive Gesundheitsvorstellungen und gesundheitsförderlicher Lebensstil von Herzinfarktpatienten und -patientinnen [Subjective notions of health and health-promoting lifestyles in male and female heart-attack patients]. *Zeitschrift für Gesundheitspsychologie, 8,* 155–167.

Frankignoul, M., & Melon, J. (1971). Methodological problems in psychosomatic research. *Feuillets Psychiatriques de Liege, 4,* 5–47.

Franklin, B. A., Bonzheim, K., Gordon, S., & Timmis, G. C. (1998). Rehabilitation of cardiac in the twenty-first century: Changing paradigms and perceptions. *Journal of Sports Sciences, 16,* 57–70.

Franklin, B. A., Hall, L., & Timmis, G. C. (1997). Contemporary cardiac rehabilitation services. *American Journal of Cardiology, 79,* 1075–1077.

Franz, I. -W. (1998). Rehabilitation bei Herz-Kreislauf-Erkrankungen [Rehabilitation in cases of heart and circulatory disease]. In H. Delbrück & E. Haupt (Eds.), *Rehabilitationsmedizin* [Rehabilitation medicine] (2nd ed., pp. 136–185). Munich, Germany: Urban & Schwarzenberg.

Franzen, D., Nicolai, C., Schannwell, M., Albrecht, D., & Höpp, H. (1993). Functional health status in male patients without restenosis following successful PTCA. *Clinical Cardiology, 16,* 199–203.

Fraser, A. (1984). Do patients want to be informed? *British Heart Journal, 52,* 468–470.

Frasure-Smith, N., & Lespérance, F. (1998). Depression and anxiety increase physician costs during the first post-MI year. *Psychosomatic Medicine, 60,* 99.

Frasure-Smith, N., Lespérance, F., Gravel, G., Masson, A., Juneau, M., Talajic, M., & Bourassa, M. G. (2000a). Depression and health-care costs during the first year following myocardial infarction. *Journal of Psychosomatic Research, 48,* 471–478.

Frasure-Smith, N., Lespérance, F., Gravel, G., Masson, A., Juneau, M., Talajic, M., & Bourassa, M. G. (2000b). Social support, depression, and mortality during the first year after myocardial infarction. *Circulation, 101,* 1919–1924.

Frasure-Smith, N., Lespérance, F., Juneau, M., Talajic, M., & Bourassa, M. G. (1999). Gender, depression, and one-year prognosis after myocardial infarction. *Psychosomatic Medicine, 61,* 26–37.

Frasure-Smith, N., Lespérance, F., Prince, R. H., Verrier, P., Garber, R. A., Juneau, M., et al. (1997). Randomised trial of home-based psychosocial nursing intervention for patients recovering from myocardial infarction. *Lancet, 350,* 473–479.

Frasure-Smith, N., Lespérance, F., & Talajic, M. (1993). Depression following myocardial infarction: Impact on 6-month survival. *JAMA, 270,* 1819–1825.

Frasure-Smith, N., Lespérance, F., & Talajic, M. (1995a). Depression and 18-month prognosis after myocardial infarction. *Circulation, 91,* 999–1005.

Frasure-Smith, N., Lespérance, F., & Talajic, M. (1995b). The impact of negative emotions on prognosis following myocardial infarction: Is it more than depression? *Health Psychology, 14,* 388–398.

Frasure-Smith, N., & Prince, R. H. (1985). The Ischemic Heart Disease Life Stress Monitoring Program: Impact on mortality. *Psychosomatic Medicine, 47,* 431–445.

Frasure-Smith, N., & Prince, R. H. (1986). The Ischemic Heart Disease Life Stress Monitoring Program: 18-month mortality results. *Canadian Journal of Public Health, 77*(Suppl. 1), 46–50.

Frasure-Smith, N., & Prince, R. H. (1989). Long-term follow-up of the Ischemic Heart Disease Life Stress Monitoring Program. *Psychosomatic Medicine, 51,* 431–445.

*Frederickson, K. (1989). Anxiety transmission in the patient with myocardial infarction. *Heart & Lung, 18,* 17–22.

Frederickson, P. A., Hurt, R. D., Lee, G. M., Wingender, L., Coghan, I. T., Lauger, G., et al.

(1995). High dose transdermal nicotine therapy for heavy smokers: Safety, tolerability and measurement of nicotine and cotinine levels. *Psychopharmacology, 122,* 215–222.

Freedland, K. E., Carney, R. M., Krone, R. J., Case, N. B., & Case, R. B. (1996). Psychological determinants of anginal pain perception during exercise testing of stable patients after recovery from acute infarction or unstable angina pectoris. *American Journal of Cardiology, 77,* 1–4.

*Freedland, K. E., Carney, R. M., Krone, R. J., Smith, L. J., Rich, M. W., Eisenkramer, G., & Fischer, K. C. (1991). Psychological factors in silent myocardial ischemia. *Psychosomatic Medicine, 53,* 13–24.

*Freedland, K. E., Carney, R. M., Lustman, P. J., Rich, M. W., & Jaffe, A. S. (1992). Major depression in coronary artery disease with vs. without a prior history of depression. *Psychosomatic Medicine, 54,* 416–421.

*Freeman, L. J., Nixon, P. G., Sallabank, P., & Reaveley, D. (1987). Psychological stress and silent myocardial ischemia. *American Heart Journal, 114,* 477–482.

Freeman, W., Pichard, A., & Smith, H. (1981). Effect of informed consent and educational background on patient knowledge, anxiety, and subjective responses to cardiac catheterization. *Catheterization and Cardiovascular Diagnosis, 7,* 119–134.

Frenn, M., Fehring, R., & Kartes, S. (1986). Reducing the stress of cardiac catheterization by teaching relaxation. *Dimensions in Critical Care Nursing, 5,* 108–116.

Freud, S. (1915). Bemerkungen über die Übertragungsliebe [Remarks on projective love]. *Internationale Zeitschrift für ärztliche Psychoanalyse, 3,* 1–34.

Freund, U. (1987). Vom Umgang mit dem Widerstand in der Herzgruppe—Eine Orientierung an der Psychotherapie Milton H. Ericksons [How to handle resistance in cardiac rehabilitation groups: An introduction to the psychotherapy of Milton Erickson]. In P. Esser (Ed.), *Psychologische Gruppenarbeit im Rahmen der Rehabilitation von Herzpatienten* [Psychological group work in the rehabilitation of heart patients] (pp. 89–100). Stuttgart, Germany: Enke.

Fridlund, B., Hogstedt, B., Lidell, E., & Larsson, P. A. (1991). Recovery after myocardial infarction: Effects of a caring rehabilitation programme. *Scandinavian Journal of Caring Sciences, 5,* 23–32.

*Friedman, H. S., & Booth-Kewley, S. (1987). Personality, Type A behavior, and coronary heart disease: The role of emotional expression. *Journal of Personality and Social Psychology, 53,* 783–792.

Friedman, M. (1986). Type A behavior and myocardial infarction. *American Heart Journal, 111,* 1216.

Friedman, M., & Rosenman, R. H. (1959). Association of specific overt behavior pattern with blood and cardiovascular findings. *JAMA, 169,* 1286–1296.

Friedman, M., & Rosenman, R. H. (1974). *Type A behavior and your heart.* New York: Alfred A. Knopf.

Friedman, M., & Rosenman, R. H. (1975). *Der A-Typ und der B-Typ* [The A-type and the B-type]. Reinbek, Germany: Rowohlt.

Friedman, M., Rosenman, R. H., & Carroll, V. (1958). Changes in serum cholesterol and blood clotting time in men subjected to cyclic variation of occupational stress. *Circulation, 17,* 852–861.

Friedman, M., Thoresen, C. E., Gill, J. J., Powell, L. H., Ulmer, D., Thompson, L., et al. (1984). Alteration of Type A behavior and reduction in cardiac recurrences in postmyocardial infarction patients. *American Heart Journal, 108,* 237–248.

Fritz, H. L. (2000). Gender-linked personality traits predict mental health and functional status following a first coronary event. *Health Psychology, 19,* 420–428.

Frøbert, O., Arendt-Nielsen, L., Bak, P., Funch-Jensen, P., & Peder Bagger, J. (1996). Pain perception and brain evoked potentials in patients with angina despite normal coronary angiograms. *Heart, 75,* 436–441.

Frøbert, O., Molgaard, H., Botker, H. E., & Bagger, J. P. (1995). Autonomic balance in patients with angina and a normal coronary angiogram. *European Heart Journal, 16,* 1356–1360.

Froelicher, V. F., Herbert, W., Myers, J., & Ribisl, P. (1996). How cardiac rehabilitation is being influenced by changes in health care delivery. *Journal of Cardiopulmonary Rehabilitation, 16,* 151–159.

Froese, A., Hackett, T. P., Cassem, N. H., & Silverberg, E. L. (1974). Trajectories of anxiety and depression in denying and nondenying acute myocardial infarction patients during hospitalization. *Journal of Psychosomatic Research, 18,* 413–420.

Froese, A., Vasquez, E., Cassem, N. H., & Hackett, T. P. (1974). Validation of anxiety depression and denial scales in a coronary care unit. *Journal of Psychosomatic Research, 18,* 137–141.

Fuchs, R. (1997). *Psychologie und körperliche Bewegung* [Pyschology and physical exercise]. Göttingen, Germany: Hogrefe.

Fuchs, R. (2001). Entwicklungsstadien des Sporttreibens [Stages in developing sports and physical activity as a habit]. *Sportwissenschaft, 31,* 255–281.

Fuchs, R., & Schwarzer, R. (1994). Selbstwirksamkeit zur sportlichen Aktivität: Reliabilität und Validität eines neuen Messinstruments [Self-efficacy in sports and physical activity: Reliability and validity of a new measurement instrument]. *Zeitschrift für Differentielle und Diagnostische Psychologie, 15,* 141–154.

Fuchs, R., & Schwarzer, R. (1997). Tabakkonsum: Erklärungsmodelle und Interventionsansätze [Tobacco consumption: Explanatory models and intervention strategies]. In R. Schwarzer (Ed.), *Gesundheitspsychologie* [Health psychology] (pp. 209–244). Göttingen, Germany: Hogrefe.

*Fukunishi, I., & Hattori, M. (1997). Mood states and Type A behavior in Japanese male patients with myocardial infarction. *Psychotherapeutics and Psychosomatics, 66,* 314–318.

*Fukunishi, I., Hattori, M., Hattori, H., Imai, Y., Miyake, Y., Miguchi, M., & Yoshimatsu, K. (1992). Japanese Type A behavior pattern is associated with "typus melancholicus": A study from the sociocultural viewpoint. *International Journal of Social Psychiatry, 38,* 251–256.

Fulton, J. E., & Shekelle, R. B. (1997). Cigarette smoking, weight gain, and coronary mortality: Results from the Chicago Western Electric Study. *Circulation, 96,* 1438–1444.

Fuster, V., & Pearson, T. A. (1999). Matching the intensity of risk factor modification with the hazard for coronary disease events. In N. K. Wenger, L. K. Smith, E. S. Froelicher, & P. McCall Comoss (Eds.), *Cardiac rehabilitation: A guide to practice in the 21st century* (pp. 193–199). New York: Marcel Dekker.

Gabanyi, M., & Schneider, M. (1993). *Herzinfarkt-Rehabilitation in Europa* [Heart attack rehabilitation in Europe]. Augsburg, Germany: BASYS.

Galan, K. M., Deligonul, U., Kern, M. J., Chaitman, B. R., & Vandormael, M. G. (1988). Increased frequency of restenosis in patients continuing to smoke cigarettes after percutaneous transluminal coronary angioplasty. *American Journal of Cardiology, 61,* 260–263.

Garachemani, A., Kipfer, B., Fleisch, M., Kaufmann, U., Luscher, T. F., Althaus, U., & Meier, B. (1997). Myokardrevaskularisation bei geriatrischen Patienten [Myocardial revascularization in geriatric patients]. *Schweizerische medizinische Wochenschrift, 127,* 425–429.

Garamoni, G. L., & Schwartz, R. M. (1986). Type A behavior pattern and compulsive personality: Toward a psychodynamic–behavioral integration. *Clinical Psychology Review, 6,* 311–336.

Garma, A. (1969). The displacement of psychosomatic illness: From obesity to migraine, to gastric ulcer, and to myocardial infarction in a manifest homosexual. *Revista de Psicoanalisis, 26,* 39–96.

Gaw-Ens, B., & Laing, G. P. (1994). Risk factor reduction behaviours in coronary angioplasty and myocardial infarction patients. *Canadian Journal of Cardiovascular Nursing, 5,* 4–12.

Gentz, C. A. (2000). Perceived learning needs of the patient undergoing coronary angioplasty: An integrative review of the literature. *Heart & Lung, 29,* 161–172.

Gerhardt, U. (1984). Typenkonstruktion bei Patientenkarrieren [Type construction with patient careers]. In M. Kohli & G. Robert (Eds.), *Biographie und soziale Wirklichkeit* [Biography and social reality] (pp. 53–77). Stuttgart, Germany: Metzler.

Gerstenkorn, A. (1990). The phenomenon of nonutilization of medical services by persons suffering from angina pectoris. *Sozial- und Praeventivmedizin, 35,* 206–208.

Gibbons, R. J., Balady, G. J., Beasley, J. W., Bricker, J. T., Duvernoy, W. F., & Froelicher, V. F. (1997). ACC/AHA guidelines for exercise testing: A report of the American College of Cardiology/American Heart Association Task Force on Practice Guidelines (Committee on Exercise Testing). *Journal of the American College of Cardiology, 30,* 260–311.

Gidron, Y., & Davidson, K. (1996). Development and preliminary testing of a brief intervention for modifying CHD-predictive hostility components. *Journal of Behavioral Medicine, 91,* 203–220.

Gildea, E. F. (1949). Special features of personality which are common to certain psychosomatic disorders. *Psychosomatic Medicine, 11,* 273–281.

*Gilliss, C. L., Gortner, S. R., Hauck, W. W., Shinn, J. A., Sparacino, P. A., & Tompkins, C. (1993). A randomized clinical trial of nursing care for recovery from cardiac surgery. *Heart & Lung, 22,* 125–133.

Glassman, A. H. (1998a). Cardiovascular effects of antidepressant drugs: Updated. *Journal of Clinical Psychiatry, 59*(Suppl. 15), 13–18.

Glassman, A. H. (1998b). Depression, cardiac death, and the central nervous system. *Neuropsychobiology, 37,* 80–83.

Glassman, A. H., O'Connor, C. M., Calif, R. M., Swedberg, K., Schwartz, P., Bigger, J. T., Jr., et al. (2002). Sertraline treatment of major depression in patients with acute MI or unstable angina. *JAMA, 288,* 701–709.

Glassman, A. H., Rodriguez, A. I., & Shapiro, P. A. (1998). The use of antidepressant drugs in patients with heart disease. *Journal of Clinical Psychiatry, 59*(Suppl. 10), 16–21.

Glassman, S. J., Rashbaum, I. G., & Walker, W. C. (2001). Cardiopulmonary rehabilitation and cancer rehabilitation: 1. Cardiac rehabilitation. *Archives of Physical Medicine and Rehabilitation, 82*(Suppl. 1), S47–S51.

Goel, P. K., Gupta, S. K., Agarwal, A., & Kapoor, A. (2001). Slow coronary flow: A distinct angiographic subgroup in Syndrome X. *Angiology, 52,* 507–514.

Goldberg, D. (1978). *Manual of the General Health Questionnaire.* Manchester, England: Nfer-Nelson.

Goldberg, D., & Williams, P. (1988). *A user's guide to the General Health Questionnaire.* Windsor, England: NFER-Nelson.

Gonzáles, M., Artalejo, F., & del Rey Calero, J. (1998). Relationship between socioeconomic status and ischaemic heart disease in cohort and case-control studies: 1960–1993. *International Journal of Epidemiology, 27,* 350–358.

*Gonzales, M. B., Snyderman, T. B., Colket, J. T., Arias, R. M., Jiang, J. W., O'Connor, C. M., & Krishnan, K. R. (1996). Depression in patients with coronary artery disease. *Depression, 4,* 57–62.

Goodman, M., Quigley, J., Moran, G., Meilman, H., & Sherman, M. (1996). Hostility predicts restenosis after percutaneous transluminal coronary angioplasty. *Mayo Clinic Proceedings, 71,* 729–734.

Gorlin, R. (1993). Endothelial dysfunction in microvascular angina [Letter, comment]. *New England Journal of Medicine, 329,* 1739–1740.

Gottheiner, V. (1968). Long strenuous sports training for cardiac reconditioning and rehabilitation. *American Journal of Cardiology, 22,* 426–435.

Gould, K. L., Ornish, D., Scherwitz, L., Brown, S., Edens, R. P., Hess, M. J., et al. (1995). Changes in myocardial perfusion abnormalities by positron emission tomography after long-term, intense risk factor modification. *JAMA, 274,* 894–901.

*Graff Low, K., Fleisher, C., Colman, R., Dionne, A., & Casey, G. (1998). Psychosocial variables, age, and angiographically determined coronary artery disease in women. *Annals of Behavioral Medicine, 20,* 221–226.

Grande, G., & Badura, B. (2001). *Die Rehabilitation der KHK aus gesundheitssystemanalytischer Perspektive* [Rehabilitating patients with CHD from a health systems analysis perspective]. Frankfurt, Germany: VAS.

Grande, G., Leppin, A., Romppel, M., Altenhöner, T., & Mannebach, H. (2002). Frauen und Männer nach Herzinfarkt: Gibt es in Deutschland geschlechtsspezifische Unterschiede in der Inanspruchnahme rehabilitativer Leistungen? [Men and women after a heart attack: In Germany are there gender-specific differences in the utilization of rehabilitative options?]. *Die Rehabilitation, 41,* 320–328.

Grande, G., Schott, T., & Badura, B. (1996). Ergebnisorientierte Evaluation kardiologischer Rehabiliation [A results-oriented evaluation of cardiac rehabilitation]. *Zeitschrift für Gesundheitswissenschaften, 4,* 335–348.

Grande, G., Schott, T., & Badura, B. (1999). Ergebnisevaluation kardiologischer Rehabilitation: Ein Langzeitvergleich über 3 Jahre zwischen stationären und ambulanten Versorgungsformen [Evaluation of the results of cardiac rehabilitation: A 3-year longitudinal comparison of outpatient and inpatients systems of care]. In B. Badura & J. Siegrist (Eds.), *Evaluation im Gesundheitswesen* [Evaluation in health care systems] (pp. 203–225). Weinheim and Munich, Germany: Juventa.

*Gray, A. M., Bowman, G. S., & Thompson, D. R. (1997). The cost of cardiac rehabilitation services in England and Wales. *Journal of the Royal College of Physicians of London, 31,* 57–61.

Green, B. L., Lindy, J. D., & Grace, M. C. (1994). Psychological effects of toxic contamination. In R. J. Ursano, B. G. McCaughey, & C. S. Fullerton (Eds.), *Individual and community responses to trauma and disaster* (pp. 154–176). Cambridge, England: Cambridge University Press.

Green, K., & Lydon, S. (1995). Home health cardiac rehabilitation. *Home Healthcare Nurse, 13*(2), 29–39.

Greiner, B. A., Krause, N., Ragland, D. R., & Fisher, J. M. (1998). Objective stress factors, accidents, and absenteeism in transit operators: A theoretical framework and empirical evidence. *Journal of Occupational Health Psychology, 3,* 130–146.

*Griego, L. C. (1993). Physiologic and psychologic factors related to depression in patients after myocardial infarction: A pilot study. *Heart & Lung, 22,* 392–400.

Groden, B. M., Semple, T., & Shaw, G. B. (1971). Cardiac rehabilitation in Britain. *British Heart Journal, 33,* 756–758.

Groen, J. J. (1951). Emotional factors in the etiology of internal diseases. *Journal of the Mt. Sinai Hospital, 18,* 71–88.

Groen, J. J. (1964). *Psychosomatic research: A collection of papers.* Oxford, England: Pergamon Press.

Groen, J., van der Valk, J. M., Treurniet, N., van Heyningen, K. H., Pelser, H. E., & Wilde, G. J. S. (1965). *Acute myocardial infarction: A psychosomatic study.* Haarlem, the Netherlands: De Erven F. Bohn.

Groen, J. J., Welner, A., & Ishay, D. B. (1970). Exploration and aggressive behavior in rats with and without experimental hypertension. *Psychotherapy and Psychosomatics, 18,* 326–331.

Guiry, E., Conroy, R. M., Hickey, N., & Mulcahy, R. (1987). Psychological response to an acute coronary event and its effect on subsequent rehabilitation and lifestyle change. *Clinical Cardiology, 10,* 256–260.

Gulanick, M., Bliley, A., Perino, B., & Keough, V. (1997). Patients' responses to the angioplasty experience: A qualitative study. *American Journal of Critical Care, 6,* 25–32.

Gulanick, M., Bliley, A., Perino, B., & Keough, V. (1998). Recovery patterns and lifestyle changes after coronary angioplasty: The patient's perspective. *Heart & Lung, 27,* 253–262.

Gulanick, M., & Naito, A. (1994). Patients' reactions to angioplasty: Realistic or not? *American Journal of Critical Care, 3,* 368–373.

Gulli, G., Cemin, R., Pancera, P., Menegatti, G., Vassanelli, C., & Cevese, A. (2001). Evidence of parasympathetic impairment in some patients with cardiac Syndrome X. *Cardiovascular Research, 52,* 208–216.

*Gundle, M. J., Reeves, B. R., Tate, S., Raft, D., & McLaurin, L. P. (1980). Psychosocial outcome after coronary artery surgery. *American Journal of Psychiatry, 137,* 1591–1594.

Gutin, B., Prince, L., & Stein, R. (1990). Survey of cardiac rehabilitation centers in New York City. *Journal of Community Health, 15,* 227–238.

Gutzwiller, F. (1980). The National Research Program 1A: A community-oriented intervention study. Methodological considerations on various types of studies. *Sozial- und Praeventivmedizin, 25,* 244–249.

Gutzwiller, F., Junod, B., Epstein, F., Jeanneret, O., & Schweizer, W. (1980). Community-oriented prevention: The National Research Program 1A "Prevention of cardiovascular diseases in Switzerland." *Sozial- und Praeventivmedizin, 25,* 239–234.

Guzman, S. V., Lopez-Grillo, L., Dorossiev, D. L., & Feher, J. (1986). Cardiac rehabilitation in different geographic areas. *Advances in Cardiac Surgery, 33,* 142–151.

Haan, M. N. (1988). Job strain and ischaemic heart disease: An epidemiologic study of metal workers. *Annals of Clinical Research, 20,* 143–145.

Hacker, W. (1994). Action regulation theory and occupational psychology: Review of German empirical research since 1987. *German Journal of Psychology, 18,* 91–120.

Hackett, T. P., & Cassem, N. H. (1970). Psychological reactions to life-threatening illness: Acute myocardial infarction. In H. S. Abram (Ed.), *Psychological aspects of stress* (pp. 29–43). Springfield: Charles C Thomas.

Hackett, T. P., & Cassem, N. H. (1974). Development of a quantitative rating scale to assess denial. *Journal of Psychosomatic Research, 18,* 93–100.

Hackett, T. P., Cassem, N. H., & Wishnie, H. A. (1968). The coronary-care unit: An appraisal of its psychologic hazards. *New England Journal of Medicine, 279,* 1365–1370.

Hadorn, D. C., Baker, D., Hodges, J. S., & Hicks, N. (1996). Rating the quality of evidence for clinical practice guidelines. *Journal of Clinical Epidemiology, 49,* 749–754.

Hahn, P. (1968a). Gruppenpsychotherapie bei Herzinfarktpatienten [Group psychotherapy with heart attack patients]. In R. Schindler, H. Gestager, & T. Lindner (Eds.), *Gruppe und Somatotherapie und*

Technik der Gruppenpsychotherapie [Group- and somatotherapy and group psychotherapy techniques] (Vol. 1, pp. 101–104). Vienna, Austria: Verlag der Wiener Medizinischen Akademie.

Hahn, P. (1968b). Psychosomatische Aspekte des Infarktprofiles [Psychosomatic aspects of heart attack profiles]. *Psychotherapeutics and Psychosomatics, 16,* 224–232.

Hahn, P. (1969). Über den psychotherapeutischen Umgang mit Herzinfarktpatienten [Psychotherapeutic work with heart attack patients]. In A. Schelkopf & S. Elhardt (Eds.), *Aspekte der Psychoanalyse: Festschrift für F. Riemann* [Aspects of psychoanalysis: A festschrift for F. Riemann] (pp. 79–102). Göttingen, Germany: Vandenhoeck & Ruprecht.

Hahn, P. (1971). *Der Herzinfarkt in psychosomatischer Sicht: Analyse und Darstellung der Grundlagen mit psychosozialen Untersuchungen an 50 männlichen Herzinfarktpatienten* [Psychosomatic aspects of heart attack: Analysis and description of the fundamentals, based on psychosocial examinations of 50 male heart attack patients]. Göttingen, Germany: Vandenhoeck & Ruprecht.

Hahn, P. (1987). Zur Psychosomatik des Kranken mit Herzinfarkt. In D. Matthes & H. Stegemann (Eds.), *Praevention und Rehabilitation in der Inneren Medizin, Psychosomatik, Psychiatrie und Psychotherapie: Symposium Bad Schwalbach, Juli 1986* [Prevention and rehabilitation in internal medicine: Somatization, psychiatry, and psychotherapy. Bad Schwalbach Symposium, July 1986] (pp. 19–30). Passau, Germany: Passavia.

Hahn, P. (1988). Aus den Anfängen der klinisch psychosomatischen Gruppentherapie am Beispiel der Herzinfarktforschung [Early stages of clinical psychosomatic group therapy, drawing on heart attack research]. In H. C. Deter & W. Schüffel (Eds.), *Gruppen mit körperlich Kranken* [Group work with the physically ill] (pp. 29–38). Berlin and Heidelberg, Germany: Springer.

Hahn, P., & Hüllemann, K. D. (1972). Ambulante gruppentherapeutische Rehabilitation von Herzinfarktpatienten: Psychodynamische und bewegungstherapeutishce Ansätze [Ambulatory group-therapeutic rehabilitation of cardiac infarct patients: The beginning of psychodynamic and motion therapy]. *Praxis Psychotherapie, 17,* 96–103.

Hahn, P., & Kämmerer, W. (1985). Die Risikopersoenlichkeit bei koronaren Herzerkrankungen: Rueckblick und Ausblick [Risk-prone personality in heart patients: Retrospect and future prospects]. *Praxis der Psychotherapie und Psychosomatik, 30,* 104–113.

Hahn, P., Nüssel, E., & Stiehler, M. (1966). Psychosomatik und Epidemiologie des Herzinfarktes [Somatic and epidemiological aspects of heart attack]. *Psychosomatic Medicine, 12,* 229–253.

Hajek, P., & Stead, L. F. (1997). Aversive smoking for smoking cessation. *The Cochrane Library.* Available at http://www.cochrane.org/reviews/clibintro.htm

Halhuber, C. (1984). *Ambulante Herzgruppen: Interdisziplinäre Aspekte einer umfassenden Betreuung* [Outpatient cardiac rehabilitation groups: Interdisciplinary aspects of comprehensive care]. Erlangen, Germany: Perimed.

Halhuber, M. J. (1985). Leserbrief zum Beitrag von M. Myrtek: Streß und Typ-A-Verhalten, Risikofaktoren der koronaren Herzkrankheit? Eine Kritische Bestandsaufnahme [A reader's response to a contribution by M. Myrtek: Stress and Type A behavior—risk factors for coronary heart disease? A critical review]. *Psychotherapie, Psychosomatik, Medizinische Psychologie, 35,* 247–248.

Hall, E. M., Johnson, J. V., & Tsou, T. S. (1993). Women, occupation, and risk of cardiovascular morbidity and mortality. *Occupational Medicine, 8,* 709–719.

Hämäläinen, H., Smith, R., Puukka, P., Lind, J., Kallio, V., Kuttila, K., et al. (2000). Social support and physical and psychological recovery one year after myocardial infarction or coronary artery bypass surgery. *Scandinavian Journal of Public Health, 28,* 62–70.

Hamilton, M. (1960). A rating scale for depression. *Journal of Neurology, Neurosurgery, and Psychiatry, 23,* 56–62.

Hamlin, C. (1995). Could you starve to death in England in 1839? The Chadwick–Farr controversy and the loss of the "social" in public health. *American Journal of Public Health, 85,* 856–866.

Hamner, M. B. (1994). Exacerbation of posttraumatic stress disorder symptoms with medical illness. *General Hospital Psychiatry, 16,* 135–137.

Hance, M., Carney, R. M., Freedland, K. E., & Skala, J. (1996). Depression in patients with coronary heart disease: A 12-month follow-up. *General Hospital Psychiatry, 18,* 61–65.

Haney, T. L., Maynard, K. E., Houseworth, S. J., Scherwitz, L. W., Williams, R. B., & Barefoot, J. C. (1996). Interpersonal Hostility Assessment Technique: Description and validation against the criterion of coronary artery disease. *Journal of Personality Assessment, 66,* 386–401.

Hartmann, F. (1984). *Patient, Arzt und Medizin—Beiträge zur ärztlichen Anthropologie* [Patient, physician, and medicine: Contributions to medical anthropology]. Göttingen, Germany: Verlag für Medizinische Psychologie im Verlag Vandenhoeck & Ruprecht.

Hasdai, D., Garratt, K. N., Grill, D. E., Lerman, A., & Holmes, D. R. (1997). Effect of smoking status on the long-term outcome after successful percutaneous coronary revascularization. *New England Journal of Medicine, 336,* 755–761.

Hathaway, S. H., & McKinley, J. C. (1943). *The Minnesota Multiphasic Personality Inventory.* Minneapolis: University of Minnesota Press.

Hattingberg, I. (1967). Erfahrungen mit Gruppenbehandlungen und Einzelaussprachen bei der Rehabilitation von Infarktpatienten [Experiences with group treatment and individual reports during the rehabilitation of heart attack patients]. *Psychotherapy and Psychosomatics, 15,* 27.

Hattingberg, I. (1968). Psychologische Probleme und Erfahrungen bei der Rehabilitationsbehandlung von Arbeitern mit Herzinfarkt [Psychological problems and experiences in rehabilitative treatment of workers recovering from a heart attack]. *Zeitschrift für Psychotherapie und Psychosomatik, 16,* 233–248.

Hattingberg, I., & Mensen, H. (1963). Systematische Langzeitbehandlung nach Herzinfarkt [Systematic long-term treatment after a heart attack]. *Münchner Medizinische Wochenschrift, 103,* 2534–2536.

Hauss, W. H. (1954). *Angina pectoris.* Stuttgart, Germany: Thieme.

Havik, O. E., & Maeland, J. G. (1988). Changes in smoking behavior after a myocardial infarction. *Health Psychology, 7,* 403–420.

*Havik, O. E., & Maeland, J. G. (1990). Patterns of emotional reactions after a myocardial infarction. *Journal of Psychosomatic Research, 34,* 271–285.

Hayano, J., Kimura, K., Hosaka, T., Shibata, N., Fukunishi, I., Yamasaki, K., et al. (1997). Coronary disease-prone behavior among Japanese men: Job-centered lifestyle and social dominance. *American Heart Journal, 134,* 1029–1036.

Haynes, S. G., Feinleib, M., & Kannel, W. B. (1980). The relationship of psychosocial factors to coronary heart disease in the Framingham study: III. Eight-year incidence of coronary heart disease. *American Journal of Epidemiology, 111,* 37–58.

Haynes, S., Levine, S., Scotch, N., Feinleib, M., & Kannel, W. (1978). The relationship of psychosocial factors to coronary heart disease in the Framingham study: I. Methods and risk factors. *American Journal of Epidemiology, 107,* 362–383.

He, J., Vupputuri, S., Allen, K., Prerost, M. R., Hughes, J., & Whelton, P. K. (1999). Passive smoking and the risk of coronary heart disease—A meta-analysis of epidemiologic studies. *New England Journal of Medicine, 340,* 920–926.

Hearn, M. D., Murray, D. M., & Luepker, R. V. (1989). Hostility, coronary heart disease, and total mortality: A 33-year follow-up study of university students. *Journal of Behavioral Medicine, 12,* 105–121.

Hecker, M. H., Chesney, M. A., Black, G. W., & Frautschi, N. (1988). Coronary-prone behaviors in the Western Collaborative Group Study. *Psychosomatic Medicine, 50,* 153–164.

Hedbäck, B., & Perk, J. (1987). 5-year results of a comprehensive rehabilitation program after myocardial infarction. *European Heart Journal, 8,* 234–242.

Hegglin, R. (1975). *Differentialdiagnose innerer Krankheiten* (13. Auflage ed.). [Differential diagnosis of internal disease (13th ed.)] Stuttgart, Germany: Thieme Verlag.

Heijningen, H. K., & Treurniet, N. (1966). Psychodynamic factors in acute myocardial infarction. *International Journal of Psychoanalysis, 47,* 370–374.

Heikkila, J., Paunonen, M., Laippala, P., & Virtanen, V. (1998). Nurses' ability to perceive patients' fears related to coronary arteriography. *Journal of Advanced Nursing, 28,* 1225–1235.

Heikkila, J., Paunonen, M., Laippala, P., & Virtanen, V. (1999). Patients' fears in coronary arteriography. *Scandinavian Journal of Caring Sciences, 13,* 3–10.

Heikkila, J., Paunonen, M., Virtanen, V., & Laippala, P. (1998). Fear of patients related to coronary arteriography. *Journal of Advanced Nursing, 28,* 54–62.

Heikkila, J., Paunonen, M., Virtanen, V., & Laippala, P. (1999). Gender differences in fears related to coronary arteriography. *Heart & Lung, 28,* 20–30.

Heller, R. F., Knapp, C., Valenti, L. A., & Dobson, A. J. (1993). Secondary prevention after acute myocardial infarction. *American Journal of Cardiology, 72,* 759–762.

Hellerstein, H., & Ford, A. B. (1957). Rehabilitation of the cardiac patient. *JAMA, 164,* 225–231.

Hellmann, E. A. (1997). Use of the stage of change in exercise adherence model among older adults with a cardiac diagnosis. *Journal of Cardiopulmonary Rehabilitation, 17,* 145–156.

Helmer, D. C., Ragland, D. R., & Syme, S. L. (1991). Hostility and coronary artery disease. *American Journal of Epidemiology, 133,* 112–122.

Helmert, U., Herman, B., Joeckel, K. H., Greiser, E., & Madans, J. (1989). Social class and risk factors for coronary heart disease in the Federal Republic of Germany: Results of the baseline survey of the German Cardiovascular Prevention Study (GCP). *Journal of Epidemiology and Community Health, 43,* 37–42.

Hemingway, H., & Marmot, M. (1999). Evidence based cardiology: Psychosocial factors in the aetiology and prognosis of coronary heart disease. Systematic review of prospective cohort studies. *British Medical Journal, 318,* 1460–1467.

Hermanson, B., Omenn, G. S., Kronmal, R. A., & Gersh, B. J. (1988). Beneficial six-year outcome of smoking cessation in older men and women with coronary artery disease: Results from the CASS Registry. *New England Journal of Medicine, 319,* 1365–1369.

Herrmann, C., Bergmann, G., Drinkmann, A., Dumm, A., Fritzsche, K., Kanwischer, H., et al. (1999). Anxiety and depressed mood predict one-year quality of life and defibrillator shocks in patients receiving an implanted defibrillator. *PACE, 22*(6, Part 2), A73.

Herrmann, C., Brand-Driehorst, S., Buss, U., & Rüger, U. (2000). Effects of anxiety and depression on five-year mortality in 5,057 patients referred for exercise testing. *Journal of Psychosomatic Research, 48,* 455–462.

*Herrmann, C., Breuker, A., Schmidt, T., Gonska, B. D., & Kreuzer, H. (1993). Angina pectoris bei Myokardischämie: Bedeutung psychischer Distressfaktoren [Angina pectoris in myocardial ischemia: The significance of psychological distress factors]. *Zeitschrift für Kardiologie, 82*(Suppl. 3), 41.

Herrmann, C., Buss, U., Breuker, A., Gonska, B. D., & Kreuzer, H. (1994). Beziehungen kardiologischer Befunde und standardisierter psychologischer Skalenwerte zur klinischen Symptomatik bei 3705 ergometrisch untersuchten Patienten [The relationship between cardiological findings and standardized psychological measures of clinical symptomatology in 3,705 ergometrically examined patients]. *Zeitschrift für Kardiologie, 83,* 264–272.

Herrmann, C., Buss, U., Lingen, R., & Kreuzer, H. (1998). Persoenlichkeitsfaktoren und Beschwerdepersistenz bei Patienten mit thorakalen Beschwerden und angiographisch freien Koronarien [Personality factors and pain persistence in patients with chest pain and angiographically clear coronaries]. *Zeitschrift für Psychosomatische Medizin und Psychoanalyse, 44,* 37–53.

Herrmann, C., Scholz, K. H., & Kreuzer, H. (1991). Psychologisches Screening von Patienten einer kardiologischen Akutklinik mit einer deutschen Fassung der "Hospital Anxiety and Depression" (HAD)-Skala [Psychological screening of acute-care cardiac patients using a German version of the "Hospital Anxiety and Depression" (HAD) Scale]. *Psychotherapie, Psychosomatik, Medizinische Psychologie, 41,* 83–92.

Herrmann, K. S., & Kreuzer, H. (1989). A randomized prospective study on anxiety reduction by preparatory disclosure with and without video film show about a planned heart catheterization. *European Heart Journal, 10,* 753–757.

Herrmann-Lingen, C. (1998). *Prävalenz und klinische Relevanz von Angst und Depressivität bei internistischen Patienten* [Prevalence and clinical relevance of anxiety and depression in internal medicine patients]. Göttingen, Germany: Habilitationsschrift.

Herrmann-Lingen, C. (2001). *Angst und Depressivität bei internistischen Patienten—Prävalenz und klinische Relevanz* [Anxiety and depression in internal medicine patients: Prevalence and clinical relevance]. Frankfurt, Germany: VAS.

Herrmann-Lingen, C., & Buss, U. (2002). *Angst und Depressivität im Verlauf der koronaren Herzkrankheit* [Anxiety and depression during coronary illness]. Frankfurt, Germany: VAS.

Herzog, M. (1984). Zu neueren Formen und Konzepten der Gesundheitserziehung in der stationaeren Herzinfarkt-Rehabilitation [Recent models and concepts of health promotion in inpatient rehabilitation of heart attack patients]. In Berufsverband Deutscher Psychologen (Ed.), *Psychologische Hilfen fuer Behinderte: Beitraege vom 11. BDP-Kongress fuer Angewandte Psychologie* [Psychological aids for the disabled: Proceedings of the 11th Federal Republic of Germany Congress of Applied Psychology] (pp. 33–41). Heidelberg, Germany: Weissenhof-Verlag.

Herzog, M., König, K., Maas, A., & Neufert, R. (1982). Gesundheitserziehung und Gruppenarbeit in der Rehabilitation von Patienten mit Herzinfarkt im Rahmen der Anschlussheilbehandlung [Health promotion and group work in the rehabilitation of heart attack patients within an adjunctive care framework]. *Rehabilitation, 21,* 8–12.

Heßlinger, B., Härter, M., Barth, J., Klecha, D., Bode, C., Walden, J., et al. (2002). Komorbidität von depressiven Störungen und Herzerkrankungen—Implikationen für Diagnostik, Pharmako- und Psychotherapie [Comorbidity of depressive symptoms and heart disease: Implications for diagnosis, pharmako- and psychotherapy]. *Der Nervenarzt, 73,* 205–218.

Heyer, G. R. (1925). *Das körperlich–seelische Zusammenwirken in den Lebensvorgängen anhand klinischer und experimenteller Tatsachen dargestellt* [The body–mind connection in significant life events, viewed in the light of clinical and experimental data]. Munich, Germany: J. F. Bergmann.

Hill, N. E., Baker, M., Warner, R. A., & Taub, H. (1988). Evaluating the use of a videotape in teaching the precardiac catheterization patient. *Journal of Cardiovascular Nursing, 2,* 71–78.

Hillebrand, T., Frodermann, H., Lehr, D., & Wirth, A. (1995). Vermehrte Teilnahme an ambulanten Herzgruppen durch poststationäre Nachsorge [Increased participation in outpatient cardiac rehabilitation groups through post-inpatient aftercare]. *Herz-Kreislauf, 27,* 346–349.

Hippisley-Cox, J., Pringle, M., Hammersley, V., Crown, N., Wynn, A., Meal, A., & Coupland, C. (2001). Antidepressants as risk factor for ischaemic heart disease: Case-control study in primary care. *British Medical Journal, 323,* 666–669.

Hlatky, M. A. (1997). Bypass Angioplasty Revascularization Investigation. *New England Journal of Medicine, 336,* 92–99.

*Hlatky, M. A., Haney, T., Barefoot, J. C., Califf, R. M., Mark, D. B., Pryor, D. B., & Williams, R. B. (1986). Medical, psychological and social correlates of work disability among men with coronary artery disease. *American Journal of Cardiology, 58,* 911–915.

Hlatky, M. A., Lam, L. C., Lee, K. L., Clapp-Channing, N. E., Williams, R. B., Pryor, D. B., et al. (1995). Job strain and the prevalence and outcome of coronary artery disease. *Circulation, 92,* 327–333.

Hlatky, M., Rogers, W., Johnstone, I., Boothroyd, D., Brooks, M., Pitt, B., et al. (1997). Medical care costs and quality of life after randomization to coronary angioplasty or coronary bypass surgery. *New England Journal of Medicine, 336,* 92–99.

*Hoffmann, A., Pfiffner, D., Hornung, R., & Niederhauser, H. (1995). Psychosocial factors predict medical outcome following a first myocardial infarction. *Coronary Artery Disease, 6,* 147–152.

Hogan, B., Linden, W., & Najarian, B. (2002). Social support interventions: Do they work? *Clinical Psychology Review, 22,* 381–440.

Hollis, J. F., Connett, J. E., Stevens, V. J., & Greenlick, M. R. (1990). Stressful life events, Type A behavior, and the prediction of cardiovascular and total mortality over six years. MRFIT Group. *Journal of Behavioral Medicine, 13,* 263–280.

Holroyd, J. (1991). The uncertain relationship between hypnotizability and smoking treatment outcome. *International Journal of Clinical and Experimental Hypnosis, 39,* 93–102.

*Honig, A., Lousberg, R., Wojciechowski, F. L., Cheriex, E. C., Wellens, H. J., & van Praag, H. M. (1997). [Depression following a first heart infarct: Similarities with differences from "ordinary" depression]. *Ned Tijdschr Geneeskd, 141,* 196–199.

*Horgan, D., Davies, B., Hunt, D., Westlake, G. W., & Mullerworth, M. (1984). Psychiatric aspects of coronary artery surgery: A prospective study. *Medical Journal of Australia, 141,* 587–590.

Horgan, J., Bethell, H., Carson, P., Davidson, C., Julian, D., Mayou, R. A., & Nagle, R. (1992). Working party report on cardiac rehabilitation. *British Heart Journal, 67,* 412–418.

Horowitz, M. J. (1974). Stress response syndromes: Character style and dynamic psychotherapy. *Archives of General Psychiatry, 31,* 768–781.

Horowitz, M. J., Wilner, N., & Alvarez, W. (1979). Impact of Event Scale: A measure of subjective stress. *Psychosomatic Medicine, 41,* 209–218.

Horsten, M., Mittleman, M. A., Wamala, S. P., Schenck-Gustafsson, K., & Orth-Gomér, K. (2000). Depressive symptoms and lack of social integration in relation to prognosis of CHD in middle-aged women. *European Heart Journal, 21,* 1072–1080.

Hotta, S. S. (1991). Cardiac rehabilitation programs. *Health Technology Assessment Reports, 3,* 1–10.

Houston, B. K., Babyak, M. A., Chesney, M. A., Black, G., & Ragland, D. R. (1997). Social dominance and 22-year all-cause mortality in men. *Psychosomatic Medicine, 59,* 5–12.

Huang, M. H., & Ewy, G. A. (2002). Cardiac Syndrome X. *New England Journal of Medicine, 347,* 1377–1379.

Hübel, M., & Kauderer-Hübel, M. (1987). *Themenzentrierte Gesprächsführung in Herzgruppen: Ein praktischer Leitfaden zur Durchführung von Gruppengesprächen mit Herzpatienten: Vol. 7: Wege der Patientenführung* [Thematically oriented conversations in cardiac rehabilitation groups: Practical tips on leading group explorations with heart patients: Vol. 7. Methods of patient care]. Erlangen, Germany: Perimed.

Hübschmann, H. (1966). Vom Leiden organisch Herzkranker [On the suffering of patients with organic heart disease]. *Der Landarzt, 16,* 677–682.

Hughes, J. R., Stead, L. F., & Lancaster, T. (1999). Anxiolytics for smoking cessation. *The Cochrane Library.* Available at http://www.cochrane.org/reviews/clibintro.htm

Hughes, J. R., Stead, L. F., & Lancaster, T. (2002). Antidepressants for smoking cessation. *The Cochrane Library.* Available at http://www.cochrane.org/reviews/clibintro.htm

Huijbrechts, I. P., Duivenvoorden, H. J., Deckers, J. W., Leenders, I. C., Pop, G. A., Passchier, J., & Erdman, R. A. (1996). Modification of smoking habits five months after myocardial infarction: Relationship with personality characteristics. *Journal of Psychosomatic Research, 40,* 369–378.

Huijbrechts, I. P. A. M., Erdman, R. A. M., Duivenvoorden, H. J., Deckers, J. W., Leenders, I. C. M., Pop, G. A. M., & Passchier, J. (1997). Modification of physical activity 5 months after myocardial infarction: Relevance of biographic and personality characteristics. *International Journal of Behavioral Medicine, 4,* 76–91.

Hulley, S. B., Cohen, R., & Widdowson G. (1977). Plasma high-density lipoprotein cholesterol level. *JAMA, 238,* 2269–2271.

Hummel, G. (1992). *Herzsprache: Eine Psychoanalyse des Herzens* [Heart language: A psychoanalysis of the heart]. Munich, Germany: Quintessenz.

Hunt, S. M., McKenna, S. P., McEwen, J., Williams, J., & Papp, E. (1981). The Nottingham Health Profile:

Subjective health status and medical consultations. *Social Science & Medicine: Part A. Medical Sociology, 15,* 221–229.

Huonker, M. (2002). Körperliche Aktivität und kardiovaskuläre Erkrankungen—Prävention und Rehabilitation [Physical activity and cardiovascular disease—Prevention and rehabilitation]. In G. Samitz & G. Mensink (Eds.), *Körperliche Aktivität in Prävention und Therapie—Evidenzbasierter Leitfaden für Klinik und Praxis* [Physical activity in prevention and therapy—Evidence-based guidelines for hospital and practice] (pp. 107–119). Munich, Germany: Hans Marseille Verlag.

Hupcey, J. E., & Gilchrist, I. C. (1993). A pilot study: Responses to chest pain following coronary angioplasty. *American Journal of Critical Care, 2,* 450–452.

Hussey, L. C. (1997). Strategies for effective patient education material design. *Journal of Cardiovascular Nursing, 11,* 37–46.

Hütter, B. (1994). *Wahrnehmung, Belastungswirkung und Bewältigung von invasiven Eingriffen in Kardiologie und Herzchirurgie* [Perception of negative side-effects, and the process of coming to terms with invasive procedures in cardiology and heart surgery]. Weinheim, Germany: Deutscher Studienverlag.

Ilker, H.-G., Brusis, O. A., & Unverdorben, M. (1995). Die Phasen der Rehabilitation [The phases of rehabilitation]. In M. Unverdorben, O. A. Brusis, & R. Rost (Eds.), *Kardiologische Prävention und Rehabilitation* [Cardiology prevention and rehabilitation] (pp. 152–162). Cologne, Germany: Deutscher Ärzteverlag.

Imich, J. (1997). Home-based cardiac rehabilitation. *Nursing Times, 93*(50), 8–9.

Irvine, J., Baker, B., Smith, J., Jandciu, S., Paquette, M., Cairns, J., et al. (1999). Poor adherence to placebo or amiodarone therapy predicts mortality: Results from the CAMIAT study. *Psychosomatic Medicine, 61,* 566–575.

Irvine, J., Basinski, A., Baker, B., Jandciu, S., Paquette, M., Cairns, J., et al. (1999). Depression and risk of sudden cardiac death after acute myocardial infarction: Testing for the confounding effects of fatigue. *Psychosomatic Medicine, 61,* 729–737.

Iseringhausen, O., Schott, T., & vom Orde, A. (2002). The quality of organization in cardiac rehabilitation: A comparison of inpatient and outpatient forms of service delivery. *Rehabilitation, 41,* 130–139.

Ishihara, T., Seki, I., Yamada, Y., Tamoto, S., Fukai, M., Takada, K., et al. (1990). Coronary circulation, myocardial metabolism and cardiac catecholamine flux in patients with syndrome X. *Journal of Cardiology, 20,* 267–274.

Jackson, L., Leclerc, J., Erskine, Y., & Linden, W. (2005). Getting the most out of cardiac rehabilitation: A review of referral and adherence predictors. *Heart, 91,* 14–19.

Jacobs, D. R., Adachi, H., Mulder, I., Kromhout, S., Menotti, A., Nissinen, A., & Blackburn, H. (1999). Cigarette smoking and mortality risk: Twenty-five-year follow up of the Seven Countries Study. *Archives of Internal Medicine, 159,* 733–740.

*Jacobsen, B. S., & Lowery, B. J. (1992). Further analysis of the psychometric properties of the Levine Denial of Illness Scale. *Psychosomatic Medicine, 54,* 372–381.

Janne, P., Reynaert, C., & Cassiers, L. (1990). Deni et maladie coronarienne: Pour une reconsideration topique du mecanisme de deni dans les maladies psychomatiques et la maladie coronarienne en particulier [Denial and coronary disease: A reconsideration of the subject of the mechanism of denial in psychosomatic diseases and coronary disease in particular]. *Annales Medico Psychologiques, 148,* 165–178.

Jeng, C., & Braun, L. T. (1997). The influence of self-efficacy on exercise intensity, compliance rate and cardiac outcomes among coronary artery disease patients. *Progress in Cardiovascular Nursing, 12,* 13–24.

Jenkins, C. D. (1976). Recent evidence supporting psychologic and social risk factors for coronary disease. *New England Journal of Medicine, 294,* 987–994, 1033–1038.

Jenkins, C. D. (1978a). Behavioral risk factors in coronary artery disease. *Annual Review of Medicine, 29,* 543–562.

Jenkins, C. D. (1978b). A comparative review of the interview and questionnaire methods in the assessment of the coronary-prone behavior pattern. In T. M. Dembroski, S. M. Weiss, J. L. Shields, S. G. Haynes, & M. Feinleib (Eds.), *Coronary-prone behavior* (pp. 71–88). New York: Springer-Verlag.

Jenkins, C. D., Rosenman, R. H., & Zyzanski, S. J. (1974). Prediction of clinical coronary heart disease by a test for the coronary-prone behavior pattern. *New England Journal of Medicine, 290,* 1271–1275.

Jenkins, C. D., Stanton, B. A., & Jono, R. T. (1994). Quantifying and predicting recovery after heart surgery. *Psychosomatic Medicine, 56,* 203–212.

Jenkins, C. D., Stanton, B. A., Savageau, J. A., Denlinger, P., & Klein, M. D. (1983). Coronary artery bypass surgery: Physical, psychological, social, and economic outcomes six months later. *JAMA, 250,* 782–788.

Jenkins, C. D., Zyzanski, S. J., & Rosenman, R. H. (1971). Progress toward validation of a computer-scored test for the Type A coronary-prone behavior pattern. *Psychosomatic Medicine, 33,* 193–202.

Jenkins, N., & Kotrba-Ottoboni, L. (1991). Patient care aspects of PTCA. In D. A. Clark (Ed.), *Coronary angioplasty* (pp. 101–103). New York: Wiley-Liss.

Jenkinson, C. M., Madeley, R. J., Mitchell, J. R., & Turner, I. D. (1993). The influence of psychosocial factors on survival after myocardial infarction. *Public Health, 107,* 305–317.

Jensen, K., Banwart, L., Venhaus, R., Popkess, V. S., & Perkins, S. B. (1993). Advanced rehabilitation nursing care of coronary angioplasty patients using self-efficacy theory. *Journal of Advanced Nursing, 18,* 926–931.

Jette, A. M., Davies, A. R., Cleary, P. D., Calkins, D. R., Rubenstein, L. V., Fink, A., et al. (1986). The Functional Status Questionnaire: Reliability and validity when used in primary care. *Journal of General Internal Medicine, 1,* 143–149.

Johnson, C. C., Hunter, S. M., Amos, C. I., Elder, S. T., & Berenson, G. S. (1989). Cigarette smoking, alcohol, and oral contraceptive use by Type A adolescents: The Bogalusa Heart Study. *Journal of Behavioral Medicine, 12,* 13–24.

*Johnson, J. E., Weinert, C., & Richardson, J. K. (1998). Rural residents' use of cardiac rehabilitation programs. *Public Health Nursing, 15,* 288–296.

Johnson, J. V., & Hall, E. M. (1988). Job strain, workplace social support, and cardiovascular disease: A cross-sectional study of a random sample of the Swedish working population. *American Journal of Public Health, 78,* 1336–1342.

Johnson, J. V., Hall, E. M., & Theorell, T. (1989). Combined effects of job strain and social isolation on cardiovascular disease morbidity and mortality in a random sample of the Swedish male working population. *Scandinavian Journal of Work, Environment and Health, 15,* 271–279.

Johnson, J. V., Stewart, W., Hall, E. M., Fredlund, P., & Theorell, T. (1996). Long-term psychosocial work environment and cardiovascular mortality among Swedish men. *American Journal of Public Health, 86,* 324–331.

Johnson, N. A., & Heller, R. F. (1998). Predictors of patient nonadherence with home-based exercise for cardiac rehabilitation: The role of perceived barriers and perceived benefits. *Preventive Medicine, 27,* 56–64.

Johnston, D. W., Cook, D. G., & Shaper, A. G. (1987). Type A behaviour and ischemic heart disease in middle aged British men. *British Medical Journal, 295,* 86–89.

*Johnston, M., Foulkes, J., Johnston, D. W., Pollard, B., & Gudmundsdottir, H. (1999). Impact on patients and partners of inpatient and extended cardiac counseling and rehabilitation: A controlled trial. *Psychosomatic Medicine, 61,* 225–233.

Joksimović, L., Siegrist, J., Meyer-Hammer, M., Peter, R., Franke, B., Klimek, W. J., et al. (1999). Overcommitment predicts restenosis after coronary angioplasty in cardiac patients. *International Journal of Behavioral Medicine, 6,* 356–369.

Joksimović, L., Starke, D., Knesebeck, O. V. D., & Siegrist, J. (2002). Perceived work stress, overcommitment, and self-reported musculoskeletal pain: A cross-sectional investigation. *International Journal of Behavioral Medicine, 9,* 122–138.

Jolliffe, J. A., Rees, K., Taylor, R. S., Thompson, D., Oldridge, N., & Ebrahim, S. (2001). Exercise-based rehabilitation for coronary heart disease. *The Cochrane Library.* Available at http://www.cochrane.org/reviews/clibintro.htm

Jones, C. A., Valle, M., & Manring, S. (2001). Using survival analysis to explore female cardiac rehabilitation program adherence. *Applied Nursing Research, 14,* 179–186.

Jones, D. A., & West, R. R. (1996). Psychological rehabilitation after myocardial infarction: Multicentre randomised control trial. *British Medical Journal, 313,* 1517–1521.

Jordan, J. (1991). *Zum Erleben und zur psychischen Bewältigung medizinischer Technologie am Beispiel der percutanen transluminalen Coronarangioplastie* [Perception of and psychological coping with medical technology after experiencing percutaneous transluminary coronary angioplasty]. Frankfurt, Germany: VAS.

Jordan, J. (1999). Psychosomatik: Leitdisziplin einer emanzipatorischen Medizin? [Psychosomatics: The primary discipline in an emancipated medicine?]. In N. Schmacke (Ed.), *Gesundheit und Demokratie: Von der Utopie der sozialen Medizin* [Health and democracy: On the utopia of socialized medicine] (pp. 193–211). Frankfurt, Germany: VAS.

Jordan, J., Bardé, B., Stirn, A., & Girth, E. (1997). Der Umgang mit Medizintechnik und die Folgen der iatrogenen Organfixierung am Beispiel der Koronardilatation (PTCA) [Dealing with medical technology and the consequences of iatrogenic organ fixation after experiencing coronary dilation (PTCA)]. In H. Willenberg & S. O. Hoffmann (Eds.), *Handeln— Ausdrucksform psychosomatischer Krankheit und Faktor der Therapie* [The treatment and expression of psychosomatic illness and factors influencing therapy] (pp. 185–196). Frankfurt, Germany: VAS.

Jordan, J., Bardé, B., & Zeiher, A. M. (1998). *Statuskonferenz Psychokardiologie* [Status of Psychocardiology Conference]. Unpublished manuscript, Frankfurt University, Frankfurt, Germany.

Jordan, J., Bardé, B., & Zeiher, A. M. (2001). Psychokardiologie heute [Psychocardiology today]. *Herz, 26,* 335–344.

Jorenby, D. E., Leischow, S. J., Nides, M. A., Rennard, S. I., Johnston, J. A., Hughes, A. R., et al. (1999). A controlled trial of sustained-release bupropion, a nicotine patch, or both for smoking cessation. *New England Journal of Medicine, 340,* 685–691.

Joseph, A. M., Normann, S. M., Ferry, L. H., Prochazka, A. V., Westman, E. C., Steele, B. G., et al. (1996). The safety of transdermal nicotine as an aid to smoking cessation in patients with cardiac disease. *New England Journal of Medicine, 335,* 1792–1798.

Jost, S. (1994). Bedeutung von Nikotinverzicht, körperlichem Training und psychologischen Interventionen in der Sekundärprävention der koronaren Herzkrankheit [The significance of giving up nicotine and of physical training and psychological intervention in the secondary prevention of coronary heart disease]. *Zeitschrift für Kardiologie, 83,* 742–758.

*Jousilahti, P., Toumilehto, J., Vartiainen, E., Korhonen, H. J., Pitkaniemi, J., Nissinen, A., et al. (1995). Importance of risk factor clustering in coronary heart disease mortality and incidence in eastern Finland. *Journal of Cardiovascular Risk, 2,* 63–70.

Jousilahti, P., Vartiainen, E., Korhonen, H. J., Puska, P., & Tuomilehto, J. (1999). Is the effect of smoking on the risk for coronary heart disease even stronger than was previously thought? *Journal of Cardiovascular Risk, 6,* 293–298.

Jouve, A., & Dongier, M. (1962). L'approche psychosomatique en cardiologie: A propos de recherches statistique récentes [The psychosomatic approach in cardiology: Comments on recent statistical studies]. *Revue de Médecine Psychosomatique, 4,* 299–308.

Jouve, A., Dongier, M., & Delaage, M. (1960). Personnalité et stress dans la genèse de l'ischémie cardiaque (angor et infarctus) [Personality and stress in the genesis of cardiac ischemia (angina and infarctus)]. *Archives des Maladies du Coeur, 2,* 154–165.

Jouve, A., Dongier, M., Delaage, M., & Mayaud, R. (1961). Etude comparée de 100 sujets atteints d'anger coronarien ou d'infarctus du myocarde et de 100 sujets témoins [Comparative study of 100 coronary angina or heart attack patients and 100 control patients]. *Presse Medicale, 69,* 2545–2548.

Jouve, A., & Ebagosti, A. (1985). Le comportement de type A dans une population mixte: Sa place parmi les facteurs de risque de cardiopathie ischemique [Type A behavior in a mixed population: Its place among the risk factors for ischemic cardiopathology]. *Bulletin de la Academie Nationale de Médecine, 169,* 471–477.

Jouve, A., Sommer, A., Avierinos, C., & Fondarai, J. (1973). Premiers résultats d'úne enquête prospective sur les maladies cardio-vasculaires dans une grande administration [Preliminary results of a prospective inquiry into cardiovascular diseases in a large-scale study]. *Archives des Maladies du Coeur, 66,* 25–33.

Jouve, A., Sommer, M., Gerard, R., Casanova, P., & Malfroy, P. (1962). Le dépistage de la maladie coronarienne [Derailing coronary heart disease]. *Presse Medicale, 70,* 317.

Jouve, A., & Torresani, J. (1961, September). *Etude expérimentale de l'átherosclerose.* [Experimental study of atherosclerosis]. Paper presented at the Congrès du Société Medicale Français.

Julkunen, J., Idänpään-Heikkilä, U., & Saarinen, T. (1993). Components of Type A behavior and the first-year prognosis of a myocardial infarction. *Journal of Psychosomatic Research, 37,* 11–18.

Junge, B., & Nagel, M. (1998). Das Rauchverhalten in Deutschland [Smoking behavior in Germany]. *Gesundheitswesen, 61*(Suppl. 2), S121–S125.

Kähler, J., Lütke, M., Weckmüller, J., Köster, R., Meinertz, T., & Hamm, C. (1999). Coronary angioplasty in octogenarians. *European Heart Journal, 20,* 1791–1798.

Kallio, V. (1985). *Rehabilitation after myocardial infarction: The European experience.* Copenhagen, Denmark: World Health Organization.

*Kamwendo, K., Hansson, M., & Hjerpe, I. (1998). Relationship between adherence, sense of coherence, and knowledge in cardiac rehabilitation. *Rehabilitation Nursing, 23,* 240–245.

Kannel, W. B., Castelli, W. P., Gordon, T., & McNamara, P. M. (1971). Serum cholesterol, lipoproteins, and the risk of coronary heart disease. *Annals of Internal Medicine, 74,* 1–12.

Kannel, W. B., & Sorlie, P. D. (1978). Remission of clinical angina pectoris: The Framingham Study. *American Journal of Cardiology, 42,* 119–123.

Kaplan, G. A., & Keil, J. E. (1993). Socioeconomic factors and cardiovascular disease: A review of the literature. *Circulation, 88,* 1973–1998.

Kaplan, G. A., & Lynch, J. W. (1997). Whither studies on the socioeconomic foundations of population health? *American Journal of Public Health, 87,* 1409–1411.

Kaplan, G. A., Roberts, R. E., Camacho, T. C., & Coyne, J. C. (1987). Psychosocial predictors of depression: Prospective evidence from the human population laboratory studies. *American Journal of Epidemiology, 125,* 206–220.

Kapp, L. A. (1954). Trauma in relation to coronary thrombosis. *Annals of Internal Medicine, 35,* 1291.

Karasek, R. (1979). Job demands, job decision latitude, and mental strain: Implications for job redesign. *Administration Science Quarterly, 24,* 285–307.

Karasek, R., Baker, D., Marxer, F., Ahlbom, A., & Theorell, T. (1981). Job decision latitude, job demands, and cardiovascular disease: A prospective study of Swedish men. *American Journal of Public Health, 71,* 694–705.

Karasek, R., Brisson, C., Kawakami, N., Houtman, I., Bongers, P., & Amick, B. (1998). The Job Content Questionnaire (JCQ): An instrument of internationally comparative assessments of psychosocial job characteristics. *Journal of Occupational Health Psychology, 3,* 322–355.

Karasek, R., & Theorell, T. (1990). *Healthy work: Stress, productivity, and the reconstruction of working life.* New York: Basic Books.

Karlsson, I., Berglin, E., & Larsson, P. A. (2000). Sense of coherence: Quality of life before and after coronary artery bypass surgery—A longitudinal study. *Journal of Advanced Nursing, 31,* 1383–1392.

Karstens, R., Köhle, K., & Weidlich, S. (1970). A multidisciplinary approach for the assessment of psychodynamic factors in young adults with acute myocardial infarction. *Psychotherapy and Psychosomatics, 18,* 281–285.

Kaski, J. C. (2002). Overview of gender aspects of cardiac syndrome X. *Cardiovascular Research, 53,* 620–626.

Kaski, J. C., & Russo, G. (2000a). Cardiac syndrome X: An overview. *Hospital Practice (Office ed.), 35,* 75–76, 79–82, 85–88.

Kaski, J. C., & Russo, G. (2000b). Microvascular angina in patients with syndrome X. *Zeitschrift für Kardiologie, 89*(Suppl. 9), 121–125.

Katon, W. (1984). Panic disorder and somatization: Review of 55 cases. *American Journal of Medicine, 77,* 101–106.

Katon, W. J. (1990). Chest pain, cardiac disease, and panic disorder. *Journal of Clinical Psychiatry, 51*(Suppl.), 27–30.

Katon, W., Hall, M. L., Russo, J., Cormier, L., Hollifield, M., Vitaliano, P. P., et al. (1988). Chest pain: Relationship of psychiatric illness to coronary arteriographic results. *American Journal of Medicine, 84,* 1–9.

Katon, W., Vitaliano, P. P., Russo, J., Cormier, L., Anderson, K., & Jones, M. (1986). Panic disorder: Epidemiology in primary care. *Journal of Family Practice, 23,* 233–239.

Katzenelbogen, S. (1932). Somatic disorders of functional origin. *Annals of Internal Medicine, 5,* 1017.

Kaufmann, M. W., Fitzgibbons, J. P., Sussman, E. J., Reed, J. F., III, Einfalt, J. M., Rodgers, J. K., & Fricchione, G. L. (1999). Relation between myocardial infarction, depression, hostility, and death. *American Heart Journal, 138,* 549–554.

Kavanagh, T. (1996). The role of exercise training in cardiac rehabilitation. In D. Jones & R. West (Eds.), *Cardiac rehabilitation* (pp. 54–82). London: BMJ Publishing.

Kavanagh, T., Shephard, R. J., Pandit, V., & Doney, H. (1970). Exercise and hypnotherapy in the rehabilitation of coronary patients. *Archives of Physical Medicine and Rehabilitation, 51,* 578–587.

Kawachi, I., Colditz, G. A., Stampfer, M. J., Willett, W. C., Manson, J. E., Rosner, B., et al. (1994). Smoking cessation and time course of decreased risks of coronary heart disease in middle-aged women. *Archives of Internal Medicine, 154,* 169–175.

Kawachi, I., Graham, A. C., Stampfer, M. J., Willett, W. C., Manson, J. E., Rosner, B., et al. (1993). Smoking cessation in relation to total mortality rates in women: A prospective cohort study. *Annals of Internal Medicine, 119,* 992–1000.

Kawachi, I., Sparrow, D., Kubzansky, L. D., Spiro, A., Vokonas, P. S., & Weiss, S. T. (1998). Prospective study of a self-report Type A scale and risk of coronary heart disease: Test of the MMPI–2 Type A scale. *Circulation, 98,* 405–412.

Kazemier, M. (1982). Herzkrankheit und ihre traumatisierende Wirkung auf das Vertrauen des Patienten in den eigenen Koerper [Cardiac disease and its traumatic effect on the patient's trust in his or her own body]. In P. Kielholz, W. Siegenthaler, W. Taggart, & A. Zanchetti (Eds.), *Psychosomatische Herz-Kreislauf-Stoerungen: Wann und wie behandeln?* [Psychosomatic cardiovascular diseases: When and how should they be treated?] (pp. 153–160). Bern, Switzerland: Huber.

Keck, M., & Budde, H.-G. (1999). Ambulante Herzgruppen nach stationärer kardiologischer Rehabilitation [Outpatient cardiac rehabilitation groups after inpatient cardiac rehabilitation]. *Rehabilitation, 38,* 79–87.

Keck, M., Budde, H.-G., & Hamerle, A. (1991). Medizinische und sozialmedizinische Einflussgrößen auf das aktive Nachsorgeverhalten von AHB-Patienten [The extent of medical and sociomedical influences on the active aftercare of AHB patients]. *Herz-Kreislauf, 23,* 163–167.

Keeley, E. C., Pirwitz, M. J., Landau, C., Lange, R. A., Hillis, L. D., Foerster, E. H., et al. (1996). Intranasal nicotine spray does not augment the adverse effects of cigarette smoking on myocardial oxygen demand or coronary arterial dimensions. *American Journal of Medicine, 171,* 357–363.

Keil, U., & Hense, H. -W. (1996). Strategien zur primären Prävention der Herz-Kreislauferkrankungen [Strategies for primary prevention of cardiovascular disease]. In G. Kaiser, J. Siegrist, E. Rosenfeld, & K. Wetzel-Vandai (Eds.), *Die Zukunft der Medizin:*

Neue Wege zur Gesundheit [The future of medicine: New ways to health] (pp. 103–111). Frankfurt, Germany: Campus.

Keil, U., Liese, A. D., Hense, H. W., Filipiak, B., Döring, A., Stieber, J., et al. (1998). Classical risk factors and their impact on incident non-fatal and fatal myocardial infarction and all-cause mortality in southern Germany. *European Heart Journal, 19,* 1197–1207.

Keller, S. (1999). *Motivation zur Verhaltensänderung: Das Transtheoretische Modell in Forschung und Praxis* [Motivation for behavioral change: The transtheoretical model in research and practice]. Freiburg, Germany: Lambertus.

Kellermann, J. J. (1993). Long-term comprehensive cardiac care: The perspectives and tasks of cardiac rehabilitation. *European Heart Journal, 14,* 1441–1444.

*Kelly, R. E., & Fleury, J. (2000). Barriers to outpatient cardiac rehabilitation participation and adherence. *Journal of Cardiopulmonary Rehabilitation, 20,* 241–246.

Kelsey, J. L., & Bernstein, L. (1996). Epidemiology and prevention of breast cancer. *Annual Review of Public Health, 17,* 47–67.

Keltikangas-Järvinen, L. (1992). Emotionale Hilflosigkeit—Ein Risikofaktor für somatische Krankheiten [Emotional helplessness—A risk factor in somatic illness]. *Psychotherapie, Psychosomatik, Medizinische Psychologie, 42,* 409–413.

Kemp, H. G. (1973). Left ventricular function in patients with the anginal syndrome and normal coronary arteriograms. *American Journal of Cardiology, 32,* 375–376.

Kemp, H. G., Elliott, W. C., & Gorlin, R. (1967). The anginal syndrome with normal coronary arteriography. *Transactions of the Association of American Physicians, 80,* 59–70.

Kemper, S. (1997). *Vorhersage von Krankheitsverlauf und Lebensqualität männlicher Postinfarktpatienten mit koronarer 3-Gefäß-Erkrankung* [Prognosis for course of disease and quality of life in male post-infarct patients with coronary 3-vessel-disease]. Unpublished doctoral dissertation, University of Göttingen, Göttingen, Germany.

Kempf, H. -D., Reuß, P., & Brusis, O. (2000). *Praxisbuch Herzgruppen* [The cardiac rehabilitation group practice handbook]. Stuttgart, Germany: Thieme.

Kemple, C. (1945). Rorschach method and psychosomatic diagnosis: Personality traits of patients with rheumatic disease, hypertensive cardiovascular disease, coronary occlusion and fracture. *Psychosomatic Medicine, 7,* 85–89.

Kendall, P. (1983). Stressful medical procedures. In D. Meichenbaum & M. E. Jaremko, *Stress reduction and prevention* (pp. 159–190). New York: Plenum Press.

Kendall, P., & Watson, D. (1982). Psychological preparation for stressful medical procedures. *Medical Psychology, 12,* 197–221.

Kendall, P., Williams, L., Pechacek, T. F., Graham, L. E., Shisslak, C., & Herzoff, N. (1979). Cognitive–behavioral and patient education interventions in cardiac catheterization procedures: The Palo Alto Medical Psychology Project. *Journal of Consulting and Clinical Psychology, 47,* 49–58.

Kerz-Rühling, I. (1980). Psychischer Konflikt [Mental conflict]. *Psyche, 6,* 543–554.

Kessler, R. C., Sonnega, A., Bromet, E., Hughes, M., & Nelson, C. B. (1995). Posttraumatic stress disorder in the national co morbidity survey. *Archives of General Psychiatry, 52,* 1048-1060.

*Ketterer, M. W., Brymer, J., Rhoads, K., Kraft, P., & Lovallo, W. R. (1996). Is aspirin, as used for antithrombosis, an emotion-modulating agent? *Journal of Psychosomatic Research, 40,* 53–58.

*Ketterer, M. W., Fitzgerald, F., Keteyian, S., Ledford, B., Jordon, M., McGowan, C., et al. (1998). Does treatment of emotional distress reduce chest pain in CAD patients? *Psychosomatic Medicine, 60,* 126.

*Ketterer, M. W., Fitzgerald, F., Thayer, B., Moraga, R., Mahr, G., Keteyian, S. J., et al. (2000). Psychosocial and traditional risk factors in early ischaemic heart disease: Cross-sectional correlates. *Journal of Cardiovascular Risk, 7,* 409–413.

*Ketterer, M. W., Huffman, J., Lumley, M. A., Wassef, S., Gray, L., Kenyon, L., et al. (1998). Five-year follow-up for adverse outcomes in males with at least minimally positive angiograms: Importance of "denial" in assessing psychosocial risk factors. *Journal of Psychosomatic Research, 44,* 241–250.

*Ketterer, M. W., Kenyon, L., Foley, B. A., Brymer, J., Rhoads, K., Kraft, P., et al. (1996). Denial of depression as an independent correlate of coronary artery disease. *Journal of Health Psychology, 1,* 93–105.

Khatri, P., Babyak, M., Croughwell, N. D., Davis, R., White, W. D., Newman, M. F., et al. (2001). Temperature during coronary artery bypass surgery affects quality of life. *Annals of Thoracic Surgery, 71,* 110–116.

Kiev, A., Masco, H. L., Wenger, T. L., Johnston, J. A., Batey, S. R., & Holloman, L. (1994). The cardiovascular effects of bupropion and nortriptyline in depressed outpatients. *Annals of Clinical Psychiatry, 6,* 107–115.

Kilgore, E. S. (1929). The nervous heart. *American Heart Journal, 5,* 9.

*Kim, A. K., Moser, D. K., Garvin, B. J., Riegel, B. J., Doering, L. V., Jadack, R. A., et al. (2000). Differences between men and women in anxiety early after acute myocardial infarction. *American Journal of Critical Care, 9,* 245–253.

Kimble, L. P. (1998). Cognitive appraisal and cardiac risk reduction behavior following coronary angioplasty. *Western Journal of Nursing Research, 20,* 733–744.

Kimble, L. P., & King, K. (1998). Perceived side effects and benefits of coronary angioplasty in the early recovery period. *Heart & Lung, 27,* 308–314.

Kindermann, W. (2005). Plötzlicher Herztod beim Sport [Sudden cardiac death in sport]. *Deutsche Zeitschrift für Sportmedizin, 56,* 106–107.

King, A. C., Blair, S. N., Bild, D. E., Dishman, R. K., Dubbert, P. M., Marcus, B. H., et al. (1992). Determinants of physical activity and interventions in adults. *Medicine and Science in Sports and Exercise, 24*(Suppl.), 221–236.

King, K. M., Human, D. P., Smith, H. L., Phan, C. L., & Theo, K. K. (2001). Predicting and explaining cardiac rehabilitation attendance. *Canadian Journal of Cardiology, 17,* 291–296.

King, K. M., & Theo, K. K. (1998). Cardiac rehabilitation referral and attendance: Not one and the same. *Rehabilitation Nursing, 23,* 246–251.

King, S., III. (1998). The development of interventional cardiology. *Journal of the American College of Cardiology, 31,* 64–88.

*Kisely, S. R., Creed, F. H., & Cotter, L. (1992). The course of psychiatric disorder associated with nonspecific chest pain. *Journal of Psychosomatic Research, 36,* 329–335.

Kishi, Y., Robinson, R. G., & Kosier, J. T. (2001). Suicidal ideation among patients during the rehabilitation period after life-threatening physical illness. *Journal of Nervous and Mental Disease, 189,* 623–628.

Kishi, Y., Robinson, R. G., Kosier, J. T., & James, T. (2002). Suicidal ideation among patients with acute life-threatening physical illness: Patients with stroke, traumatic brain injury, myocardial infarction, and spinal cord injury. *Psychosomatics, 42,* 382–390.

Kittel, F. (1986). Type A and other psychosocial factors in relation to CHD. In T. H. Schmidt, T. M. Dembroski, & G. Blümchen (Eds.), *Biological and psychological factors in cardiovascular disease* (pp. 63–84). New York: Springer Verlag.

Kittel, F., Kornitzer, M., De Backer, G., & Dramaix, M. (1982). Metrological study of psychological questionnaires with reference to social variables: The Belgian Heart Disease Prevention Project (BHDPP). *Journal of Behavioral Medicine, 5,* 9–35.

Kivimäki, M., Leino-Arjas, P., Luukkonen, R., Riihimäki, H., Vahtera, J., & Kirjonen, J. (2002). Work stress and risk of cardiovascular mortality: Prospective cohort study of industrial employees. *British Medical Journal, 325,* 857.

Klasmeier, P. (1991). Zum Beziehungsgeschehen mit psychosomatischen Patienten in einer kardiologischen Rehabilitationsklinik [On the dynamics of relationships with psychosomatic patients in a cardiac rehabilitation hospital]. *Zeitschrift für Individualpsychologie, 16,* 274–286.

Klemperer, G. (1929). Gemütsbewegungen und Herzkrankheit [Emotions and heart disease]. *Therapien der Gegenwart, 70,* 1–5.

Klimes, I., Mayou, R. A., Pearce, M. J., Coles, L., & Fagg, J. R. (1990). Psychological treatment for atypical non-cardiac chest pain: A controlled evaluation. *Psychological Medicine, 20,* 605–611.

Knesebeck, O. V. D. (1998). *Subjektive Gesundheit im Alter: Soziale, psychische und somatische Einflüsse* [Subjective health among the elderly: Social, psychological and somatic influences]. Münster, Germany: LIT-Verlag.

Knoll, M. (1997). *Sporttreiben und Gesundheit* [Sports activity and health]. Schorndorf, Germany: Hofmann.

Köhle, K., & Gaus, E. (1986). Psychotherapie von Herzinfarkt-Patienten während der stationären und poststationären Behandlungsphase [Psychotherapy with heart attack patients during the inpatient and postinpatient stages of care]. In T. Uexküll (Ed.), *Psychosomatische Medizin* [Psychosomatic medicine] (pp. 691–714). Munich, Germany: Urban & Schwarzenberg.

Köhle, K., Gaus, E., Karstens, R., & Ohlmeier, D. (1972). Ärztliche Psychotherapie bei Herzinfarktpatienten während der Intensivbehandlungsphase [Psychotherapy with heart attack patients during the intensive care phase]. *Therapiewoche,* 4379–4382.

Köhle, K., Gaus, E., & Wallace, A. G. (1996). Krankheitsverarbeitung und Psychotherapie nach Herzinfarkt—Perspektiven für ein biopsychosoziales Behandlungskonzept [Coming to terms with the illness and psychotherapy after a heart attack: Perspectives on a biopsychosocial treatment model]. In T. Uexküll (Ed.), *Psychosomatische Medizin* [Psychosomatic medicine] (pp. 798–809). Munich, Germany: Urban & Schwarzenberg.

Köhler, E. (1995). Untersuchungen über die Durchführung der stationären und rehabilitativen Behandlung Herzkranker in den Jahren 1982–1993 [Research into the inpatient and rehabilitative treatment of cardiac patients in the years 1982–1993]. *Herz-Kreislauf, 27,* 57–65.

Köhler, E., & Held, K. (1996). Anschlußheilbehandlung nach Myokardinfarkt bzw. nach Herzoperation—

Überlegungen zur verbesserten Integration zwischen akutmedizinischer, rehabilitativer und ambulanter Behandlung [Adjunct rehabilitative treatment of heart patients after myocardial attack or heart surgery—Reflections on improved integration among acute medical, rehabilitative and outpatient care]. *Herz-Kreislauf, 28,* 54–57.

Kollenbaum, V. (1990). *Introzeption kardiovaskulärer Belastung bei Koronarpatienten* [Introception of cardiovascular stress in heart patients]. Frankfurt, Germany: Lang.

Kop, W. J., Appels, A., Mendes de Leon, C. F., & Bär, F. W. (1996). The relationship between severity of coronary artery disease and vital exhaustion. *Journal of Psychosomatic Research, 40,* 397–405.

Kop, W. J., Appels, A. P., Mendes de Leon, C. F., de Swart, H., & Bär, F. W. (1993). The effect of successful coronary angioplasty on feelings of exhaustion. *International Journal of Cardiology, 42,* 269–276.

Kop, W. J., Appels, A. P. W. M., Mendes de Leon, C. F., de Swart, H. B., & Bär, F. W., (1994). Vital exhaustion predicts new cardiac events after successful coronary angioplasty. *Psychosomatic Medicine, 56,* 281–289.

Kop, W. J., Hamulyak, K., Pernot, C., & Appels, A. (1998). Relationship of blood coagulation and fibrinolysis to vital exhaustion. *Psychosomatic Medicine, 60,* 352–358.

Kornitzer, M. D., Dramaix, M., & Gheyssens, H. (1979). Incidence of ischemic heart diseases in two Belgian cohorts followed during 10 years. *European Journal of Cardiology, 9,* 455–472.

Kornitzer, M., Kittel, F., Dramaix, M., & de Backer, G. U. (1982). Job stress and coronary heart disease. *Advances in Cardiology, 29,* 56–61.

Koskenvuo, M., Kaprio, J., Rose, R. J., Kesaeniemi, A., Sarna, S., Heikkila, K., & Langinvainio, H. (1988). Hostility as a risk factor for mortality and ischemic heart disease in men. *Psychosomatic Medicine, 50,* 330–340.

Kostka, M. (1992). Personal experience with "use of hypnosis before and during angioplasty" [Letter]. *American Journal of Clinical Hypnosis, 34,* 281–282.

Kraft, B., & Werner, A. (1994). Subjektive Krankheitstheorien bei Patienten mit funktionellen Herz-Kreislauf-Stoerungen [Subjective theories of illness in patients with functional cardiovascular disorders]. In P. Hahn, A. Werner, G. Bergmann, A. Drinkmann, W. Eich, M. Hayden, & W. Herzog (Eds.), *Modell und Methode in der Psychosomatik* [Model and method in psychosomatics] (pp. 126–130). Weinheim, Germany: Deutscher Studienverlag.

Kramlinger, K. G., Swanson, D. W., & Maruta, T. (1983). Are patients with chronic pain depressed? *American Journal of Psychiatry, 140,* 747–749.

*Krantz, D. S., Hedges, S. M., Gabbay, F. H., Klein, J., Falconer, J. J., Bairey Merz, C. N., et al. (1994). Triggers of angina and ST-segment depression in ambulatory patients with coronary artery disease: Evidence for an uncoupling of angina and ischemia. *American Heart Journal, 128,* 703–712.

Krasemann, E. O. (1990). Koronare Herzkrankheit und Bewegungstherapie—Historische Entwicklung [Coronary heart disease and movement therapy: Historical development]. In O. A. Brusis & H. Weber-Falkensammer (Eds.), *Handbuch der Herzgruppenbetreuung* [Handbook for cardiac rehabilitation group leaders] (3rd ed., pp. 20–22). Erlangen, Germany: Perimed.

Krasemann, E. O., & Traenckner, K. (1989). Herz-Kreislaufkomplikationen und Verletzungen in Herzgruppen [Cardiovascular complications and damage in cardiac rehabilitation groups]. *Herz-Kreislauf, 21,* 421–428.

Krieger, N. (1994). Epidemiology and the web of causation: Has anyone seen the spider? *Social Science & Medicine, 39,* 887–903.

*Krishnan, K. R., George, L. K., Pieper, C. F., Jiang, W., Arias, R., Look, A., & O'Connor, C. (1998). Depression and social support in elderly patients with cardiac disease. *American Heart Journal, 136,* 491–495.

Kristeller, J., Rossi, J., Ockene, J., Goldberg, R., & Prochaska, J. (1992). Processes of change in smoking cessation: A cross-validation study in cardiac patients. *Journal of Substance Abuse, 4,* 263–276.

Kristensen, T. S. (2001). A new tool for assessing psychosocial work environment factors: The Copenhagen Psychosocial Questionnaire. In M. Hagberg, B. Knave, L. Lillienberg, & H. Westberg (Eds.), *X2001—Exposure assessment in epidemiology and practice* (pp. 210–213). Bromma, Sweden: National Institute of Working Life.

*Krittayaphong, R., Cascio, W. E., Light, K. C., Sheffield, D., Golden, R. N., Finkel, J. B., et al. (1997). Heart rate variability in patients with coronary artery disease: Differences in patients with higher and lower depression scores. *Psychosomatic Medicine, 59,* 231–235.

Kroenke, K., & Price, R. (1993). Symptoms in the community: Prevalence, classification, and psychiatric comorbidity. *Archives of Internal Medicine, 153,* 2474–2480.

Krohne, H., & Hock, M. (1993). Coping dispositions, actual anxiety, and the incidental learning of success and failure-related stimuli. *Personality and Individual Differences, 15,* 33–41.

Krumholz, H. M., Cohen, D. J., Williams, C., Baim, D. S., Brinker, J., Cabin, H. S., et al. (1997). Health after coronary stenting or balloon angioplasty: Results from the Stent Restenosis Study. *American Heart Journal, 134,* 337–344.

Krystal, H. (1978). Trauma and affects. *Psychoanalytic Study of the Child, 33,* 81–116.

Kuller, L. H., Ockene, J. K., Meilahn, E., Wentworth, D. N., Svendsen, K. H., & Neaton, J. D. (1991). Cigarette smoking and mortality. *Preventive Medicine, 20,* 638–654.

Kunst, A. E., Groenhof, F., Andersen, O., Borgan, J. K., Costa, G., Desplanques, G., et al. (1999). Occupational class and ischemic heart disease mortality in the United States and 11 European countries. *American Journal of Public Health, 89,* 47–53.

Kunst, A. E., Groenhof, F., Mackenbach, J. P., & EU Working Group on Socioeconomic Inequalities in Health. (1998). Occupational class and cause specific mortality in middle aged men in 11 European countries: Comparison of population based studies. *British Medical Journal, 316,* 1636–1642.

Kuper, H., & Marmot, M. (2003). Job strain, job demands, decision latitude, and risk of coronary heart disease within the Whitehall II study. *Journal of Epidemiology and Community Health, 57,* 147–153.

Kuper, H., Singh-Manoux, A., Siegrist, J., & Marmot, M. (2002). When reciprocity fails: Effort–reward imbalance in relation to coronary heart disease and health functioning within the Whitehall II study. *Occupational and Environmental Medicine, 59,* 777–784.

Kushner, M. G., Thomas, A. M., Bartels, K. M., & Beitman, B. D. (1992). Panic disorder history in the families of patients with angiographically normal coronary arteries. *American Journal of Psychiatry, 149,* 1563–1567.

Kutter, P. (1997). Über eine zeitlich begrenzte Gruppenpsychotherapie bei Patienten nach Herzinfarkt—Erfahrungen und Ergebnisse [A time-limited psychotherapeutic group intervention with post-heart attack patients—Experiences and results]. *Gruppenpychotherapie Gruppendynamik, 33,* 179–193.

Kutz, I., Garb, R., & David, D. (1988). Post-traumatic stress disorder following myocardial infarction. *General Hospital Psychiatry, 10,* 169–176.

Kutz, I., Shabtai, H., Solomon, Z., Neumann, M., & David, D. (1994). Post-traumatic stress disorder in myocardial infarction patients: Prevalence study. *Israeli Journal of Psychiatry and Related Sciences, 31,* 48–56.

Lachauer, R. (1984). Herzinfarktpatienten in einer Rehabilitationsklinik Erfahrungen aus psychoanalytischer Sicht [Heart attack patients in a rehabilitation hospital. A psychoanalytic view of their experi-

ences]. *Psychotherapie, Psychosomatik, Medizinische Psychologie, 34,* 33–40.

LaCroix, A. Z., & Haynes, S. G. (1984). Occupational exposure to high demand/low control work and coronary heart disease incidence in the Framingham cohort. *American Journal of Epidemiology, 120,* 481.

Ladwig, K. H., Erazo, N., & Rugulies, R. (2003). *Vitale Erschöpfung, Depression und Angst vor Ausbruch der koronaren Herzerkrankung.* [Physical exhaustion, depression, and anxiety prior to the manifestation of coronary heart disease]. Frankfurt, Germany: VAS.

Ladwig, K. H., Hoberg, E., & Busch, R. (1998). Psychische Komorbidität bei Patienten mit alarmierender Brust-Schmerzsymptomatik [Comorbidity of psychological symptoms in patients with alarming chest pain symptomatology]. *Psychotherapie, Psychosomatik, Medizinische Psychologie, 48,* 46–54.

Ladwig, K. H., Kieser, M., Konig, J., Breithardt, G., & Borggrefe, M. (1991). Affective disorders and survival after acute myocardial infarction: Results from the Post-Infarction Late Potential study. *European Heart Journal, 12,* 959–964.

Ladwig, K. H., Lehmacher, W., Roth, R., & Breithardt, G. (1992). Factors which provoke post-infarction depression: Results from the Post-Infarction Late Potential Study (PILP). *Journal of Psychosomatic Research, 36,* 723–729.

Ladwig, K. H., Roll, G., Breithardt, G., & Borggrefe, M. (1999). Extracardiac contributions to chest pain perception in patients 6 months after acute myocardial infarction. *American Heart Journal, 137,* 528–535.

Ladwig, K. H., Roll, G., Breithardt, G., Budde, T., & Borggrefe, M. (1994). Post-infarction depression and incomplete recovery 6 months after acute myocardial infarction. *Lancet, 343,* 20–23.

Laederach-Hofmann, K. (1994). Syndrom X, mikrovaskuläre Angina pectoris und Kompanie [Syndrome X, microvascular angina pectoris and friends]. *Sandorama, 2,* 32–38.

Laederach-Hofmann, K., Truniger, C., Mussgay, L., & Jürgensen, R. (2001). Sensorische und affektive Komponenten im Gebrauch von Schmerzwörtern bei Patienten mit Angina pectoris und koronarer Herzkrankheit oder syndrom-X [Sensory and affective components in the use of pain descriptors used by patients with angina pectoris and coronary heart disease or syndrome X.]. *Zeitschrift für Klinische Psychologie und Psychotherapie, 30,* 182–188.

*Laghrissi Thode, F., Wagner, W. R., Pollock, B. G., Johnson, P. C., & Finkel, M. S. (1997). Elevated platelet factor 4 and beta-thromboglobulin plasma levels in depressed patients with ischemic heart disease. *Biology and Psychiatry, 42,* 290–295.

Lahad, A., Heckbert, S. R., Koepsell, T. D., Psaty, B. M., & Patrick, D. L. (1997). Hostility, aggression and the risk of nonfatal myocardial infarction in postmenopausal women. *Journal of Psychosomatic Research, 43,* 183–195.

Lamb, L. S. (1984). Patient understanding of a teaching manual on cardiac catheterization. *Heart & Lung, 13,* 267–271.

Lancaster, T., & Stead, L. F. (1999a). Individual behavioral counselling for smoking cessation. *The Cochrane Library.* Available at http://www.cochrane.org/reviews/clibintro.htm

Lancaster, T., & Stead, L. F. (1999b). Self-help interventions for smoking cessation. *The Cochrane Library.* Available at http://www.cochrane.org/reviews/clibintro.htm

Lancaster, T., Stead, L. F., Silagy, C., & Sowden, A. (2000). Effectiveness of interventions to help people stop smoking: Findings from the Cochrane Library. *British Medical Journal, 321,* 355–358.

*Landreville, P., & Vézina, J. (1994). Differences in appraisal and coping between elderly coronary artery disease patients high and low in depressive symptoms. *Journal of Mental Health, 3,* 79–89.

Landsbergis, P. A., Theorell, T., Schwartz, J., Greiner, B. A., & Krause, N. (2000). Measurement of psychosocial workplace exposure variables. *Occupational Medicine, 15,* 163–188.

Lane, D., Carroll, D., Ring, C., Beevers, D. G., & Lip, G. Y. (2000a). Do depression and anxiety predict recurrent coronary events 12 months after myocardial infarction? *Quarterly Journal of Medicine, 93,* 739–744.

Lane, D., Carroll, D., Ring, C., Beevers, D. G., & Lip, G. Y. (2000b). Effects of depression and anxiety on mortality and quality of life 4 months after myocardial infarction. *Journal of Psychosomatic Research, 49,* 229–238.

Lane, D., Carroll, D., Ring, C., Beevers, D. G., & Lip, G. Y. (2001a). Mortality and quality of life 12 months after myocardial infarction: Effects of depression and anxiety. *Psychosomatic Medicine, 63,* 221–230.

Lane, D., Carroll, D., Ring, C., Beevers, D. G., & Lip, G. Y. (2001b). Predictors of attendance at cardiac rehabilitation after myocardial infarction. *Journal of Psychosomatic Research, 51,* 497–501.

*Langeluddecke, P., Fulcher, G., Baird, D., Hughes, C., & Tennant, C. (1989). A prospective evaluation of the psychosocial effects of coronary artery bypass surgery. *Journal of Psychosomatic Research, 33,* 37–45.

Langosch, W. (1989). *Psychosomatik der koronaren Herzkrankheiten* [Psychosomatic aspects of coronary diseases]. Weinheim, Germany: Edition Medizin.

Langosch, W., Budde, H.-G., & Linden, W. (2003). *Psychologische Interventionen zur KHK* [Psychological intervention for CHD]. Frankfurt, Germany: VAS.

*Lantinga, L. J., Sprafkin, R. P., McCroskery, J. H., Baker, M. T., Warner, R. A., & Hill, N. E. (1988). One-year psychosocial follow-up of patients with chest pain and angiographically normal coronary arteries. *American Journal of Cardiology, 62,* 209–213.

Lanza, G. A., Andreotti, F., Sestito, A., Sciahbasi, A., Crea, F., & Maseri, A. (2001). Platelet aggregability in cardiac syndrome X. *European Heart Journal, 22,* 1924–1930.

Lau, J., Antman, E. M., Jimenez-Silva, J., Kupelnick, B., Mosteller, F., & Chalmers, T. C. (1992). Cumulative meta-analysis of therapeutic trials for myocardial infarction. *New England Journal of Medicine, 327,* 248–254.

Laubinger, G., & Krasemann, E. O. (1995). Zwischenfälle in den Hamburger Herzgruppen 1983–1993 [Episodes and incidents in the Hamburg cardiac rehabilitation groups 1983–1993]. *Münchener Medizinische Wochenschrift, 18,* 301.

*Lawson-Matthew, P. J., Wilson, A. T., Woodmansey, P. A., & Channer, K. S. (1994). Unsatisfactory management of patients with myocardial infarction admitted to general medical wards. *Journal of the Royal College of Physicians of London, 28,* 49–51.

Lazare, A. (1981). Current concepts in psychiatry: Conversion symptoms. *New England Journal of Medicine, 305,* 745–748.

Lear, S. A., & Ignaszewski, A. (2001). Cardiac rehabilitation: A comprehensive review. *Current Controlled Trials in Cardiovascular Medicine, 2,* 221–232.

Lee, D. J., Gomez-Marin, O., & Prineas, R. J. (1996). Type A behavior pattern and change in blood pressure from childhood to adolescence: The Minneapolis Children's Blood Pressure Study. *American Journal of Epidemiology, 143,* 63–72.

Lee, H., Kohlman, G. C., Lee, K., & Schiller, N. B. (2000). Fatigue, mood, and hemodynamic patterns after myocardial infarction. *Applied Nursing Research, 13,* 60–69.

Lee, W. L., Chen, J. W., Lin, S. J., Hsu, N. W., Chang, M. S., & Ting, C. T. (1998). Parasympathetic withdrawal antedates dynamic myocardial ischemia in patients with syndrome X. *International Journal of Cardiology, 66,* 253–260.

*Legault, S. E., Joffe, R. T., & Armstrong, P. W. (1992). Psychiatric morbidity during the early phase of coronary care for myocardial infarction: Association with cardiac diagnosis and outcome. *Canadian Journal of Psychiatry, 37,* 316–325.

Lehmann, H. (1987). Die psychosoziale Dimension im Rehabilitationsverfahren [Psychological dimensions of the rehabilitation process]. In B. Badura, G. Kaufhold, H. Lehmann, H. Pfaff, T. Schott, & M. Waltz (Eds.), *Leben mit dem Herzinfarkt* [Living with a heart attack] (pp. 65–86). Berlin, Germany: Springer.

Lehr, D. (1996). *Hypnotherapie mit Herzpatienten: Erprobung eines psychotherapeutischen Ansatzes in der kardiologischen Rehabilitation* [Hypnotherapy with heart patients: Investigation of a psychotherapeutic intervention in cardiac rehabilitation]. Regensburg, Germany: Roderer.

Lehr, U., & Thomae, H. (1991). *Alltagspsychologie* [Everyday psychology]. Darmstadt, Germany: Wissenschaftliche Buchgesellschaft.

*Lehto, S., Koukkunen, H., Hintikka, J., Viinamaki, H., Laakso, M., & Pyorala, K. (2000). Depression after coronary heart disease events. *Scandinavian Cardiovascular Journal, 34,* 580–583.

Leibing, E., Schünemann, I., Herrmann, C., & Rüger, U. (1998). Psychische Störung oder koronare Herzkrankheit? [Mental disturbance or coronary heart disease?] *Psychotherapie, Psychosomatik, Medizinische Psychologie, 48,* 30–36.

Leiker, M., & Hailey, B. J. (1988). A link between hostility and disease: Poor health habits? *Behavioral Medicine, 14,* 129–133.

Leon, G. R., Finn, S. E., Murray, D., & Bailey, J. M. (1988). Inability to predict cardiovascular disease from hostility scores or MMPI items related to type A behavior. *Journal of Consulting and Clinical Psychology, 56,* 597–600.

Lesage-Desrousseaux, E. (1981). A l'écoute des coronariens rééduqués [Listening to reeducated coronaries]. *Revue de Medicine Psychosomatique et de Psychologie Medicale, 23,* 365–378.

Lespérance, F., Frasure-Smith, N., Juneau, M., & Théroux, P. (2000). Depression and 1-year prognosis in unstable angina. *Archives of Internal Medicine, 160,* 1354–1360.

Lespérance, F., Frasure-Smith, N., & Talajic, M. (1996). Major depression before and after myocardial infarction: Its nature and consequences. *Psychosomatic Medicine, 58,* 99–110.

Leuner, H. (1955). Experimentelles katathymes Bilderleben als ein klinisches Verfahren der Psychotherapie [Experimental catathymic image experiencing as a clinical method of psychotherapy]. *Psychotherapie Psychosomatik Medizinische Psychologie, 5,* 185–203.

Leuner, H. (1994). *Katathym-imaginative Psychotherapie* [Guided affective imagery]. Stuttgart, Germany: Thieme.

*Levine, J., Warrenburg, S., Kerns, R., Schwartz, G., Delaney, R., Fontana, A., et al. (1987). The role of denial in recovery from coronary heart disease. *Psychosomatic Medicine, 49,* 109–117.

Levine, J. B., Covino, N. A., Slack, W. V., Safran, C., Safran, D. B., Boro, J. E., et al. (1996). Psychological predictors of subsequent medical care among patients hospitalized with cardiac disease. *Journal of Cardiopulmonary Rehabilitation, 16,* 109–116.

Levine, S. A., & Lown, B. (1952). "Armchair" treatment of acute coronary thrombosis. *JAMA, 148,* 1365–1369.

Lewin, B. (1996). Psychological factors in cardiac rehabilitation. In D. Jones & R. West (Eds.), *Cardiac rehabilitation* (pp. 83–108). London: BMJ Publishing Group.

*Lewin, B., Robertson, I. H., Cay, E. L., Irving, J. B., & Campbell, M. (1992). Effects of self-help post-myocardial-infarction rehabilitation on psychological adjustment and use of health services. *Lancet, 339,* 1036–1040.

*Lewin, R. J. P., Ingleton, R., Newens, A. J., & Thompson, D. R. (1998). Adherence to cardiac rehabilitation guidelines: A survey of rehabilitation programmes in the United Kingdom. *British Medical Journal, 316,* 1354–1355.

Lewis, S. F., Piasecki, T. M., Fiore, M. C., Anderson, J. E., & Baker, T. B. (1998). Transdermal nicotine replacement for hospitalized patients: A randomized clinical trial. *Preventive Medicine, 27,* 296–303.

Lichtenstein, P., Pedersen, N. L., Plomin, R., & de Faire, U. (1989). Type A behavior pattern, related personality traits and self-reported coronary heart disease. *Personality and Individual Differences, 10,* 419–426.

Light, K. C., Herbst, M. C., Bragdon, E. E., Hinderliter, A. L., Koch, G. G., Davis, M. R., & Sheps, D. S. (1991). Depression and Type A behavior pattern in patients with coronary artery disease: Relationships to painful versus silent myocardial ischemia and β-endorphin responses during exercise. *Psychosomatic Medicine, 53,* 669–683.

Lightwood, J. M., & Glantz, S. A. (1997). Short-term economic and health benefits of smoking cessation: Myocardial infarction and stroke. *Circulation, 96,* 1089–1096.

Likoff, W., Segal, B. L., & Kasparian, H. (1967). Paradox of normal selective coronary arteriograms in patients considered to have unmistakable coronary heart disease. *New England Journal of Medicine, 276,* 1063–1066.

Linden, B. (1995). Evaluation of a home-based rehabilitation programme for patients recovering from acute myocardial infarction. *Intensive and Critical Care Nursing, 11,* 10–19.

Linden, W. (2000). Psychological treatments in cardiac rehabilitation: Review of rationales and outcomes. *Journal of Psychosomatic Research, 48,* 443–454.

Linden, W., Stossel, C., & Maurice, J. (1996). Psychosocial interventions for patients with coronary artery disease. *Archives of Internal Medicine, 156,* 745–752.

Lindy, J. D. (1993). Focal psychoanalytic psychotherapy of posttraumatic stress disorder. In J. P. Wilson & B. Raphael (Eds.), *International handbook of traumatic stress syndromes* (pp. 803–810). New York: Plenum Press.

Lindy, J. D. (1996). Psychoanalytic psychotherapy of posttraumatic stress disorder. In B. A. Van der Kolk, S. McFarlane, & L. Weisaeth (Eds.), *Traumatic stress: The effects of overwhelming experience on mind, body and society* (pp. 525–536). New York: Guilford Press.

Lineberry, M. T. W., Peters, G. E., & Bostwick, J. M. (2001). Bupropion-induced erythema multiforma. *Mayo Clinic Proceedings, 76,* 664–666.

Lipkus, I. M., Barefoot, J. C., Williams, R. B., & Siegler, I. C. (1994). Personality measures as predictors of smoking initiation and cessation in the UNC Alumni Heart Study. *Health Psychology, 13,* 149–155.

*Lisspers, J., Nygren, A., & Söderman, E. (1998). Psychological patterns in patients with coronary heart disease, chronic pain and respiratory disorder. *Scandinavian Journal of Caring Sciences, 12,* 25–31.

Lisspers, J., Sundin, Ö., Hofman-Bang, C., Nordlander, R., Nygren, A., Ryden, L., et al. (1999). Behavioral effects of a comprehensive, multifactorial program for lifestyle change after percutaneous transluminal coronary angioplasty: A prospective, randomized, controlled study. *Journal of Psychosomatic Research, 46,* 143–154.

Little, T., Milner, M. R., Lee, K., Constantine, J., Pichard, A. D., & Lindsay, J. (1993). Late outcome and quality of life following percutaneous transluminal coronary angioplasty. *Catheterization and Cardiovascular Diagnosis, 29,* 261–266.

Lloyd, G., Cooper, A., & Jackson, G. (1997). The provision of written information for patients following coronary angiography and post-discharge management. *International Journal of Clinical Practice, 51,* 387–388.

Long, B. J., Calfas, K. J., Patrick, K., Sallis, J. F., Wooten, W. J., Goldstein, M., et al. (1996). Acceptability, usability and practicality of physician counselling for physical activity promotion: Project PACE. *American Journal of Preventive Medicine, 12,* 164–170.

Lorenz, J., & Bromm, B. (1997). Event-related potential correlates of interference between cognitive performance and tonic experimental pain. *Psychophysiology, 34,* 436–445.

*Löwel, H., Lewis, M., Härtel, U., & Hörmann, A. (1994). Herzinfarkt-Patienten ein Jahr nach dem Ereignis: Ergebnisse des bevölkerungsbezogenen Augsburger Herzinfarktregisters [Heart attack patients one year after the event: Results of the Augsburg population-oriented survey of heart attack patients]. *Münchner Medizinische Wochenschrift, 136,* 29–38.

*Lowery, B. J., Jacobsen, B. S., Cera, M. A., McIndoe, D., Kleman, M., & Menapace, F. (1992). Attention versus avoidance: Attributional search and denial after myocardial infarction. *Heart & Lung, 21,* 523–528.

*Lozano, M., Carcedo, C., Artiago, R., Huertas, D., O'Neill of Tyrone, A., Pelegrin, C., et al. (1989). Psychiatric care of coronary artery disease in a cardiac rehabilitation unit. *Psychotherapy and Psychosomatics, 52,* 80–87.

Lukach, B. M. (1996). Are heart attacks traumatic stressors? *Dissertation Abstracts International, 56,* 6398B.

Luminet, D. (1969). L'infarctus du myocarde et ses aspects psychosomatiques [Myocardial infarction and its psychosomatic aspects]. *Bruxelles-Medicine, 3,* 159–167.

Lumley, M. A., Torosian, T., Ketterer, M. W., & Pickard, S. D. (1997). Psychosocial factors related to noncardiac chest pain during treadmill exercise. *Psychosomatics, 38,* 230–238.

Luoto, R., Prättälä, R., Uutela, A., & Puska, P. (1998). Impact of unhealthy behaviors on cardiovascular mortality in Finland, 1978–1993. *Preventive Medicine, 27,* 93–100.

Lynch, J. W., Davey Smith, G., Kaplan, G. A., & House, J. S. (2000). Income inequality and mortality: Importance to health of individual income, psychosocial environment, or material conditions. *British Medical Journal, 320,* 1200–1204.

Lynch, J. W., Due, P., Muntaner, C., & Davey Smith, G. (2000). Social capital—Is it a good investment strategy for public health? *Journal of Epidemiology and Community Health, 54,* 404–408.

Lynch, J. W., & Kaplan, G. A. (2000). Socioeconomic position. In L. F. Berkman & I. Kawachi (Eds.), *Social epidemiology* (pp. 13–35). New York: Oxford University Press.

Lynch, J. W., Krause, N., Kaplan, G. A., Salonen, R., & Salonen, J. T. (1997). Workplace demands, economic reward, and progression of carotid atherosclerosis. *Circulation, 96,* 302–307.

Lynch, J. W., Krause, N., Kaplan, G. A., Tuomilehto, J., & Salonen, J. T. (1997). Workplace conditions, socioeconomic status, and the risk of mortality and acute myocardial infarction: The Kuopio Ischemic Heart Disease Risk Factor Study. *American Journal of Public Health, 87,* 617–622.

Mackenbach, J. P., Kunst, A. E., Cavelaars, A. E., Groenhof, F., Geurts, J. J., & EU Working Group on Socioeconomic Inequalities in Health. (1997).

Socioeconomic inequalities in morbidity and mortality in western Europe. *Lancet, 349,* 1655–1659.

Mackenbach, J. P., Stronks, K., & Kunst, A. E. (1989). The contribution of medical care to inequalities in health: Differences between socio-economic groups in decline of mortality from conditions amenable to medical intervention. *Social Science & Medicine, 29,* 369–376.

Macleod, J., & Davey Smith, G. (2003). Psychosocial factors and public health: A suitable case for treatment? *Journal of Epidemiology and Community Health, 57,* 565–570.

Macleod, J., Davey Smith, G., Heslop, P., Metcalfe, C., Carroll, D., & Hart, C. (2002). Psychological stress and cardiovascular disease: Empirical demonstration of bias in a prospective observational study of Scottish men. *British Medical Journal, 324,* 1247–1251.

MacWilliam, J. A. (1923). Blood-pressure and heart action in sleep and dreams: Their relation to hemorrhages, angina and sudden death. *British Medical Journal (Clinical Research ed.), 2,* 1196.

Maeland, J. G., & Havik, O. E. (1987). Psychological predictors for return to work after a myocardial infarction. *Journal of Psychosomatic Research, 31,* 471–481.

Maercker, A., & Ehlert, U. (2001). Psychotraumatologie—Eine neue Theorie- und Praxsperspektive für verschiedene medizinische Disziplinen [Psychotraumatology: A new theory and practice perspectives for various medical disciplines]. In A. Maercker & U. Ehlert (Eds.), *Psychotraumatologie* [Psychotraumatology] (pp. 11–23). Göttingen, Germany: Hogrefe.

*Magni, G., Unger, H. P., Valfre, C., Polesel, E., Cesari, F., Rizzardo, R., et al. (1987). Psychosocial outcome one year after heart surgery: A prospective study. *Archives of Internal Medicine, 147,* 473–477.

Malan, D. H. (1962). *Psychoanalytische Kurztherapie* [Short-term psychoanalytic therapy]. Stuttgart, Germany: Klett.

Mandke, R., Mishra, H., Kumaraiah, V., & Yavagal, S. T. (1996). Behavioural intervention in post-operative coronary heart disease patients. *NIMHANS Journal, 14,* 45–50.

Mann, A. H., & Brennan, P. J. (1987). Type A behaviour score and the incidence of cardiovascular disease: A failure to replicate the claimed associations. *Journal of Psychosomatic Research, 31,* 685–692.

Manson, J. E., Hu, F. B., Rich-Edwards, J. W., Colditz, G. A., Stampfer, M. J., Willet, W. C., et al. (1999). A prospective study of walking as compared with vigorous exercise in the prevention of coronary heart disease in women. *New England Journal of Medicine, 341,* 650–658.

Manuck, S. (1994). Cardiovascular reactivity in cardiovascular disease: "Once more unto the breach." *International Journal of Behavioral Medicine, 1,* 4–31.

*Marcus, B. H., Dubbert, P. M., Forsyth, L.-A. H., McKenzie, T. L., Stone, E. J., Dunn, A. L., & Blair, S. N. (2000). Physical activity behavior change: Issues in adoption and maintenance. *Health Psychology, 19,* 32–41.

Marcus, B. H., King, T. K., Bock, B. C., Borrelli, B., & Clark, M. (1998). Adherence to physical activity recommendations and interventions. In S. Shumaker, E. B. Schron, J. K. Ockene, & W. L. McBee (Eds.), *The handbook of health behavior change* (2nd ed., pp. 189–212). New York: Springer Publishing Company.

Marcus, B. H., Rakowski, W., & Rossi, J. S. (1992). Assessing motivational readiness and decision making for exercise. *Health Psychology, 11,* 257–261.

*Margraf, J., DeVries-Wehrhahn, E., & Sonnentag, S. (1991). Myokardinfarkt, funktionelle Herzbeschwerden und Paniksyndrom [Myocardial infarction, functional cardiac symptomatology, and panic syndrome]. *Psychotherapie, Psychosomatik, Medizinische Psychologie, 41,* 31–34.

Marinoni, G., Perotti, R., & Specchia, G. (1987). Ambulatory ECG during screening phase in relation to other technics in patients with precordial pain. *Giornale Italiano di Cardiologia, 17,* 1063–1067.

Markakis, E. (1990). PTCA: A nursing perspective. *Canadian Nurse, 86,* 39–41.

Marmot, M. G. (1994). Social differentials in health within and between populations. *Daedalus, 123,* 197–216.

Marmot, M. G., Bosma, H., Hemingway, H., Brunner, E., & Stansfeld, S. (1997). Contribution of job control and other risk factors to social variations in coronary heart disease incidence. *Lancet, 350,* 235–239.

Marmot, M. G., Davey Smith, G., Stansfeld, S., Patel, C., North, F., Head, J., et al. (1991). Health inequalities among British civil servants: The Whitehall II study. *Lancet, 337,* 1387–1393.

Marmot, M. G., & Feeney, A. (1996). Socioeconomic factors in CHD prevention. In K. Orth-Gomér & N. Schneiderman (Eds.), *Behavioral approaches to cardiovascular disease prevention* (pp. 21–41). Mahwah, NJ: Erlbaum.

Marmot, M. G., Ryff, C. D., Bumpass, L. L., Shipley, M., & Marks, N. F. (1997). Social inequalities in health: Next questions and converging evidence. *Social Science & Medicine, 44,* 901–910.

Marmot, M. G., Shipley, M., & Rose, G. (1984). Inequalities in death—Specific explanation of a general pattern? *Lancet, 1*(8384), 1003–1006.

Marmot, M. G., & Wilkinson, R. G. (1999). *Social determinants of health*. Oxford, England: Oxford, University Press.

Marmot, M. G., & Wilkinson, R. G. (2001). Psychosocial and material pathways in the relation between income and health: A response to Lynch et al. *British Medical Journal, 322*, 1233–1236.

Marra, S., Paolillo, V., Spadaccini, F., & Angelino, P. F. (1985). Long-term follow-up after a controlled randomized post-myocardial infarction rehabilitation programme: Effects on morbidity and mortality. *European Heart Journal, 6*, 656–663.

Marshall, I. A. (1965). The analysis of rage reactions in a case of coronary thrombosis. *Bulletin of the Menninger Clinic, 29*, 131–142.

Marty, P., & de M'Uzan, M. (1962). La pensée opératoire [Operational thinking]. *Revue Française de Psychoanalyse, 27*, 345–356.

Marusic, A., & Gudjonsson, G. H. (1999). Atypical chest pain patients: A comparison with ischaemic heart disease and control patients. *Nordic Journal of Psychiatry, 53*, 191–195.

Maruta, T., Hamburgen, M. E., Jennings, C. A., Offord, K. P., Colligan, R. C., Frye, R. L., & Malinchoc, M. (1993). Keeping hostility in perspective: Coronary heart disease and the Hostility Scale on the Minnesota Multiphasic Personality Inventory. *Mayo Clinic Proceedings, 68*, 109–114.

Matthews, M., & Julian, D. (1985). Angina pectoris: Definition and description. In D. Julian (Ed.), *Angina pectoris* (p. 2). New York: Churchill Livingstone.

Matthews, K. A. (1988). Coronary heart disease and Type A behaviors: Update on and alternative to the Booth-Kewley and Friedman (1987) quantitative review. *Psychological Bulletin, 104*, 373–380.

Matthews, K. A., Kelsey, S. F., Meilahn, E. N., Kuller, L. H., & Wing, R. R. (1989). Educational attainment and behavioral and biologic risk factors for coronary heart disease in middle-aged women. *American Journal of Epidemiology, 129*, 1132–1144.

Maunder, R. G. (1998). Panic disorder associated with gastrointestinal disease: Review and hypotheses. *Journal of Psychosomatic Research, 44*, 91–105.

*Mayou, R., & Bryant, B. (1987). Quality of life after coronary artery surgery. *Quarterly Journal of Medicine, 63*, 405–412.

Mayou, R. A., Gill, D., Thompson, D. R., Day, A., Hicks, N., Volmink, J., et al. (2000). Depression and anxiety as predictors of outcome after myocardial infarction. *Psychosomatic Medicine, 62*, 212–219.

McCall Comoss, P. (1999). The new infrastructure for cardiac rehabilitation practice. In N. K. Wenger, L. K. Smith, E. S. Froelicher, & P. McCall Comoss (Eds.), *Cardiac rehabilitation: A guide to practice in the 21st century* (pp. 315–326). New York: Marcel Dekker.

McCranie, E.W., Watkins, L. O., Brandsma, J. M., & Sisson, B. D. (1986). Hostility, coronary heart disease (CHD) incidence, and total mortality: Lack of association in a 25-year follow-up study of 478 physicians. *Journal of Behavioral Medicine, 9*, 119–125.

McCrone, S., Lenz, E., Tarzian, A., & Perkins, S. (2001). Anxiety and depression: Incidence and patterns in patients after coronary artery bypass graft surgery. *Applied Nursing Research, 14*, 155–164.

McDonough, P., Duncan, G. J., Williams, D., & House, J. (1997). Income dynamics and adult mortality in the United States, 1972 through 1989. *American Journal of Public Health, 87*, 1476–1483.

McDougall, J. (1974). The psychosomatic and the psychoanalytic process. *International Review of Psychoanalysis, 1*, 437–459.

McFarlane, A., Kamath, M. V., Fallen, E. L., Malcolm, V., Cherian, F., & Norman, G. (2001). Effect of sertraline on the recovery rate of cardiac autonomic function in depressed patients after acute myocardial infarction. *American Heart Journal, 142*, 617–623.

McGee, H. M. (1999). Psychosocial issues for cardiac rehabilitation with older individuals. *Coronary Artery Disease, 10*, 47–51.

McGee, H., Graham, T., Crowe, B., & Horgan, J. H. (1993). Return to work following coronary artery bypass surgery or percutaneous transluminal coronary angioplasty. *European Heart Journal, 14*, 623–628.

McGee, H. M., Hevey, D., & Horgan, J. H. (1999). Psychosocial outcome assessments for use in cardiac rehabilitation service evaluation: A 10-year systematic review. *Social Science & Medicine, 48*, 1373–1393.

McGee, H. M., Hevey, D., & Horgan, J. H. (2001). Cardiac rehabilitation service provision in Ireland: The Irish Association of Cardiac Rehabilitation survey. *Irish Journal of Medical Science, 170*, 159–162.

*McGee, H. M., & Horgan, J. H. (1992). Cardiac rehabilitation programmes: Are women less likely to attend? *British Medical Journal, 305*, 283–284.

*McKenna, K. T. (1995). Coronary risk factor status after percutaneous transluminal coronary angioplasty. *Heart & Lung, 24*, 207–212.

McKenna, K. T., McEniery, P. T., Maas, F., Aroney, C. N., Bett, J. H., Cameron, J., et al. (1992). Clinical results and quality of life after percutaneous transluminal coronary angioplasty: A preliminary report. *Catheterization and Cardiovascular Diagnosis, 27*, 89–94.

McKenna, K. T., McEniery, P. T., Maas, F., Aroney, C. N., Bett, J. H., Cameron, J., et al. (1994). Percutaneous transluminal coronary angioplasty: Clinical and quality of life outcomes one year later. *Australian and New Zealand Journal of Medicine, 24,* 15–21.

McNally, R. J. (1990). Psychological approaches to panic disorder: A review. *Psychological Bulletin, 108,* 403–419.

McNally, R. J., & Eke, M. (1996). Anxiety sensitivity, suffocation fear, and breath-holding duration as predictors of response to carbon dioxide challenge. *Journal of Abnormal Psychology, 105,* 146–149.

McPherson, R. W. (1999). Posttraumatic stress disorder as a consequence of myocardial infarction: A study of contributing factors. *Dissertation Abstracts International, 59,* 4473B.

McSweeney, J. C. (1993). Making behavior changes after a myocardial infarction. *Western Journal of Nursing Research, 15,* 441–455.

Mechanic, D. (1962). The concept of illness behavior. *Journal of Chronic Diseases, 15,* 189–194.

Meesters, C. M., & Smulders, J. (1994). Hostility and myocardial infarction in men. *Journal of Psychosomatic Research, 38,* 727–734.

Melon, J. (1971). The Szondi test in psychosomatic research. *Feuillets Psychiatriques de Liege, 4,* 5–47.

Melon, J., Dongier, M., & Bourdouxhe, S. (1971). The psychosomatic profile on the Szondi test: Reflections on the concepts of normality and specificity. *Annales Medico-Psychologiques, 2,* 263–271.

Mendes de Leon, C. F., Kop, W. J., de Swart, H. B., Bar, F. W., & Appels, A. P. (1996). Psychosocial characteristics and recurrent events after percutaneous transluminal coronary angioplasty. *American Journal of Cardiology, 77,* 252–255.

Menninger, K. A., & Menninger, W. C. (1936). Psychoanalytic observations in cardiac disorders. *American Heart Journal, 11,* 10–22.

Mensink, G. B. M. (2002). Körperliches Aktivitätsverhalten in Deutschland [Physical activity in Germany]. In G. B. M. Mensink (Ed.), *Körperliche Aktivität in Prävention und Therapie. Evidenzbasierter Leitfaden für Klinik und Praxis* [Physical activity in prevention and therapy. Evidence-based manual for hospital and practice] (pp. 35–44). Munich, Germany: Hans Marseille.

Mielck, A. (2000). *Soziale Ungleichheit und Gesundheit* [Social inequality and health]. Bern, Switzerland: Huber.

Miles, H. W., Waldfogel, S., Barrabee, E. L., & Cobb, S. (1954). Psychosomatic study of 46 young men with coronary artery disease. *Psychosomatic Medicine, 14,* 455–477.

Miller, C. K. (1965). Psychological correlates of coronary artery disease. *Psychosomatic Medicine, 3,* 257–265.

Miller, M., Hemenway, D., Bell, N. S., Yore, M. M., & Amoroso, P. J. (2000). Cigarette smoking and suicide: A prospective study of 300,000 male active-duty army soldiers. *American Journal of Epidemiology, 151,* 1060–1063.

Miller, T. Q., Markides, K. S., Chiriboga, D. A., & Ray, L. A. (1995). A test of the psychosocial vulnerability and health behavior models of hostility: Results from an 11-year follow-up study of Mexican Americans. *Psychosomatic Medicine, 57,* 572–581.

Miller, T. Q., Smith, T. W., Turner, C. W., Guijarro, M. L., & Hallet, A. J. (1996). A meta-analytic review of research on hostility and physical health. *Psychological Bulletin, 119,* 322–348.

Miller, T. Q., Turner, C. W., Tindale, R. S., Posavac, E. J., & Dugoni, B. L. (1991). Reasons for the trend toward null findings in research on Type A behavior. *Psychological Bulletin, 110,* 469–485.

Miracle, V. A., & Hovekamp, G. (1994). Needs of families of patients undergoing invasive cardiac procedures. *American Journal of Critical Care, 3,* 155–157.

Mitsibounas, D. N., Tsouna-Hadjis, E. D., Rotas, V. R., & Sideris, D. A. (1992). Effects of group psychosocial intervention on coronary risk factors. *Psychotherapy and Psychosomatics, 58,* 97–102.

Mittag, O. (1987). Die Bedeutung psychosomatischer Konzepte für die Rehabilitation von Patienten nach Herzinfarkt: Anmerkungen zu einer Kontroverse [The relevance of psychosomatic concepts for the rehabilitation of post heart-attack patients: Comments on a controversy]. *Psychotherapie, Psychosomatik, Medizinische Psychologie, 37,* 401–406.

Mittag, O., & Ohm, D. (1987). Themenzentrierte Gesprächsgruppen in der Rehabilitation von Patienten nach Herzinfarkt [Topic-oriented conversation groups in the rehabilitation of heart attack patients]. In P. Esser (Ed.), *Psychologische Gruppenarbeit im Rahmen der Rehabilitation von Herzpatienten* [Psychological group work in the context of the rehabilitation of heart patients] (pp. 27–39). Stuttgart, Germany: Enke.

Mittag, O., & Ohm, D. (1992). Raucherentwöhnung durch Hypnose bei 21 Patienten mit koronarer Herzkrankheit oder peripherer Verschlusskrankheit: Ergebnisse nach vier Jahren [Smoking cessation using hypnosis with 21 patients with coronary heart disease or peripheral valve disease: Results after four years]. *Herz-Kreislauf, 24,* 408–411.

Mittag, O., Peschel, U., & Chrosziewski, W. (1997). Zur Reliabilität und Validität einer deutschsprachigen Version der "Cook–Medley Hostility Scale" [On the reliability and validity of a German version of the "Cook–Medley Hostility Scale"]. *Diagnostica, 43,* 255–262.

*Mittleman, M. A., Maclure, M., Sherwood, J. B., Mulry, R. P., Tofler, G. H., Jacobs, S. C., et al. (1995). Triggering of acute myocardial infarction onset by episodes of anger. *Circulation, 92,* 1720–1725.

Mody, F. V., Nademanee, K., Intarachot, V., Josephson, M. A., Robertson, H. A., & Singh, B. N. (1988). Severity of silent myocardial ischemia on ambulatory electrocardiographic monitoring in patients with stable angina pectoris: Relation to prognostic determinants during exercise stress testing and coronary angiography. *Journal of the American College of Cardiology, 12,* 1169–1176.

Moersch, E., Kerz-Rühling, I., Drews, S., Nern, R. D., Kennel, K., Kelleter, R., et al. (1980). Zur Psychopathologie von Herzinfarkt-Patienten [The psychopathology of heart attack patients]. *Psyche, 34,* 493–588.

Moore, G. E. (1997). Secondary prevention: No more exercise? *Journal of Cardiopulmonary Rehabilitation, 17,* 284–285.

Mordkoff, A. M., & Parsons, O. A. (1967). The coronary personality: A critique. *Psychosomatic Medicine, 29,* 1–14.

Morris, C., & Froelicher, V. F. (1991). The current status of cardiac rehabilitation and exercise testing. *Journal of Cardiopulmonary Rehabilitation, 11,* 75–77.

Moser, D. K., & Dracup, K. (1995). Psychosocial recovery from a cardiac event: The influence of perceived control. *Heart & Lung, 24,* 273–280.

*Moser, D. K., & Dracup, K. (1996). Is anxiety early after myocardial infarction associated with subsequent ischemic and arrhythmic events? *Psychosomatic Medicine, 58,* 395–401.

Mott, A. M. (1999). Psychologic preparation to decrease anxiety associated with cardiac catheterization. *Journal of Vascular Nursing, 17,* 41–49.

Motz, W., Vogt, M., Rabenau, O., Scheler, S., Luckhoff, A., & Strauer, B. E. (1991). Evidence of endothelial dysfunction in coronary resistance vessels in patients with angina pectoris and normal coronary angiograms. *American Journal of Cardiology, 68,* 996–1003.

Moustier, J. M., Benichou, S., Giudicelli, S., & Bory, M. (1984). Relation between personality and spastic angina. *Presse Medicale, 13,* 1311–1314.

Mudd, J. (1986). Should coronary angiograms be reviewed with patients? *American Journal of Cardiology, 57,* 501.

Mukerji, V., Beitman, B. D., Alpert, A., & Hewett, J. E. (1987). Panic attack symptoms in patients with chest pain and angiographically normal coronary arteries. *Journal of Anxiety Disorders, 1,* 41–46.

Mulcahy, R. (1991). Twenty years of cardiac rehabilitation in Europe: A reappraisal. *European Heart Journal, 12,* 92–93.

Mulcahy, R., Hickey, N., Graham, I. M., & MacAirt, J. (1977). Factors affecting the 5 year survival rate of men following acute coronary heart disease. *American Heart Journal, 93,* 556–559.

Mullen, P. D., Mains, D. A., & Velez, R. (1992). A metaanalysis of controlled trials of cardiac patient education. *Patient Education and Counseling, 19,* 143–162.

Muntaner, C., & Lynch, J. (1999). Income inequality, social cohesion, and class relations: A critique of Wilkinson's neo-Durkheimian research program. *International Journal of Health Services, 29,* 59–81.

Muntaner, C., Lynch, J., & Oates, G. L. (1999). The social class determinants of income inequality and social cohesion. *International Journal of Health Services, 29,* 699–732.

Murphy, J. M., Olivier, D. C., Monson, R. R., Sobol, A. M., Federman, E. B., & Leighton, A. H. (1991). Depression and anxiety in relation to social status: A prospective epidemiologic study. *Archives of General Psychiatry, 48,* 223–229.

Murphy, M. C., Fishman, J., & Shaw, R. E. (1989). Education of patients undergoing coronary angioplasty: Factors affecting learning during a structured educational program. *Heart & Lung, 18,* 36–45.

Murray, H. A. (1953). Tests of personality: Picture and drawing techniques. A. Thematic Apperception Test. In A. Weider (Ed.), *Contributions toward medical psychology: Theory and psychodiagnostic methods* (pp. 636–649). Oxford, England: Ronald Press.

Myrtek, M. (1983). *Typ-A-Verhalten: Untersuchungen und Literaturanalysen unter besonderer Berücksichtigung der psychophysiologischen Grundlagen* [Type-A behavior: Research and literature analyses with particular reference to psychophysiological bases]. Munich, Germany: Minerva.

Myrtek, M. (1985a). Stellungnahme zum Leserbrief von M. J. Halhuber: Stress und Typ-A-Verhalten, Risikofaktoren der koronaren Herzkrankheit? Eine kritische Bestandsaufnahme [Opinion on a reader's letter by M. J. Halhuber: Stress and Type A behavior, risk factors for coronary heart disease? A critical appraisal]. *Psychotherapie, Psychosomatik, Medizinische Psychologie, 35,* 249–252.

Myrtek, M. (1985b). Stress und Typ-A-Verhalten, Risikofaktoren der koronaren Herzkrankheit? Eine kritische Bestandsaufnahme [Stress and Type A behavior, risk factors of coronary heart disease? A critical review]. *Psychotherapie, Psychosomatik, Medizinische Psychologie, 35,* 54–61.

Myrtek, M. (1986). Type A behavior and myocardial infarction [Letter]. *American Heart Journal, 111,* 1215–1216.

Myrtek, M. (1995). Type A behavior pattern, personality factors, disease, and physiological reactivity: A meta-analytic update. *Personality and Individual Differences, 18,* 491–502.

Myrtek, M. (1997). Streß und Typ-A-Verhalten. In P. Allhoff, G. Flatten, & U. Laaser (Eds.), *Krankheitsverhütung und Früherkennung: Handbuch der Prävention* [Disease prevention and early detection: Handbook of prevention] (pp. 315–336). Berlin, Germany: Springer.

Myrtek, M. (1998a). *Gesunde Kranke—Kranke Gesunde: Psychophysiologie des Krankheitsverhaltens.* [Healthy sick people—Sick healthy people: The psychophysiology of illness behavior]. Bern, Switzerland: Huber.

Myrtek, M. (1998b). Metaanalysen zur Psychophysiologischen Persönlichkeitsforschung [Meta-analyses of psychophysiological personality research studies]. In F. Rösler (Ed.), *Enzyklopädie der Psychologie: Themenbereich C, Theorie und Forschung, Serie I, Biologische Psychologie, Band 5: Ergebnisse und Anwendungen der Psychophysiologie* [Encyclopedia of psychology: Topic area C, Theory and research, Series I Biological psychology, Vol. 5: Results and application of psychophysiology] (pp. 285–344). Göttingen, Germany: Hogrefe.

Myrtek, M. (2000). *Das Typ-A-Verhaltensmuster und Hostility als eigenständige Risikofaktoren der koronaren Herzkrankheit:* [The type-A behavior pattern and hostility as independent risk factors for coronary heart disease]. Frankfurt am Main, Germany: VAS.

Myrtek, M. (2001). Meta-analyses of prospective studies on coronary heart disease, Type A personality, and hostility. *International Journal of Cardiology, 79,* 245–251.

Myrtek, M., Schmidt, T. H., & Schwab, G. (1984). Untersuchungen zur Reliabilität und Validität der deutschen Version des Jenkins Activity Survey (JAS) [Studies of the reliability and validity of the German version of the Jenkins Activity Survey (JAS)]. *Zeitschrift für Klinische Psychologie, 13,* 322–337.

Naegeli, B., Bertel, O., Urban, P., Angehrn, W., Siegrist, P., Stauffer, J.-C., et al. (1998). Der akute Myokardinfarkt in der Schweiz: Resultate aus dem PIMICS-Herzinfarkt-Register [Acute myocardial infarction in Switzerland: Results from the PIMICS heart attack register]. *Schweizerische Medizinische Wochenschrift, 128,* 729–736.

Nagayama, M., Fujita, Y., Kanai, T., Yamada, T., Tozawa, K., & Ushiyama, M. (1996). Changes in myocardial lactate metabolism during ramp exercise in patients with effort angina and microvascular angina. *Japanese Circulation Journal, 60,* 876–888.

*Naidoo, P., & Patel, C. J. (1993). Stress, depression and left-sided psychogenic chest pain. *Acta Psychiatrica Scandinavica, 88,* 12–15.

National Heart, Lung, and Blood Institute. (1998). *Behavioral research in cardiovascular, lung, and blood health and disease (report of the task force).* Washington, DC: U.S. Department of Health and Human Services.

Nelson, F., Zimmerman, L., Barnason, S., Nieveen, J., & Schmaderer, M. (1998). The relationship and influence of anxiety on postoperative pain in the coronary artery bypass graft patient. *Journal of Pain Symptomatology & Management, 15,* 102–109.

Neumann, J. K. (1991). Psychological post-traumatic effects of MI: A comparison study. *Medical Psychotherapy, 4,* 105–110.

*Newton, M., Mutrie, N., & McArthur, J. D. (1991). The effects of exercise in a coronary rehabilitation programme. *Scottish Medical Journal, 36,* 38–41.

New York Heart Association. (1979). *Nomenclature and criteria for diagnoses of diseases of the heart and great vessels.* Boston: Little Brown.

NHS Centre for Reviews and Dissemination. (1998). Cardiac rehabilitation. *Effective Health Care 4,* 1–12.

*Nickel, J. T., Brown, K. J., & Smith, B. A. (1990). Depression and anxiety among chronically ill heart patients: Age differences in risk and predictors. *Research in Nursing and Health, 13,* 87–97.

Niebauer, J., Hambrecht, R., Marburger, C., Schlierf, G., Kübler, W., & Schuler, G. (1994). Fettarme Diät und körperliches Training bei koronarer Herzkrankheit: Langzeitergebnisse der Sekundärprävention [The role of a low-fat diet and physical training in coronary heart disease: Long-term results of secondary prevention]. *Deutsche Medizinische Wochenschrift, 119,* 7–12.

*Niederhauser, H. U. (1991). Die stationäre Rehabilitation nach Herzinfarkt [Inpatient rehabilitation after a heart attack]. *Therapeutische Umschau, 48,* 578–584.

Nielsen, M. L., Kristensen, T. S., & Smith-Hansen, L. (2002). The Intervention Project on Absence and Well-being (IPAW): Design and results from the baseline of a 5-year study. *Work & Stress, 16,* 191–206.

Nielsen, M. L., Rugulies, R., Christensen, K. B., Smith-Hansen, L., Bjorner, J. B., & Kristensen, T. S. (2004). Impact of the psychosocial work environment on registered absence from work: A two-year longitudinal study using the IPAW cohort. *Work & Stress, 18,* 323–335.

Nihoyannopoulos, P., Kaski, J. C., Crake, T., & Maseri, A. (1991). Absence of myocardial dysfunction during stress in patients with Syndrome X. *Journal of the American College of Cardiologists, 18,* 1463–1470.

*Njølstad, I., & Arnesen, E. (1998). Preinfarction blood pressure and smoking are determinants for a fatal outcome of myocardial infarction: A prospective analysis from the Finnmark Study. *Circulation, 158,* 1326–1332.

Njølstad, I., Arnesen, E., & Lund-Larsen, P. G. (1996). Smoking, serum lipids, blood pressure, and sex differences in myocardial infarction: 12 year follow-up of the Finnmark Study. *Circulation, 93,* 450–456.

Noren, J., Frazier, T., Altman, I., & DeLozier, J. (1980). Ambulatory medical care: A comparison of internists and family–general practitioners. *New England Journal of Medicine, 302,* 11–16.

Nuland, W. (1968). The use of hypnotherapy in the treatment of the postmyocardial infarction invalid. *International Journal of Clinical and Experimental Hypnosis, 16,* 139–150.

Numata, Y., Ogata, Y., Oike, Y., Matsumura, T., & Shimada, K. (1998). A psychobehavioral factor, alexithymia, is related to coronary spasm. *Japanese Circulation Journal, 62,* 409–413.

Nunes, E. V., Frank, K. A., & Kornfeld, D. S. (1987). Psychologic treatment for the Type A behavior pattern and for coronary heart disease: A meta-analysis of the literature. *Psychosomatic Medicine, 49,* 159–173.

Nüssel, E., Scheuermann, W., & Halhuber, C. (1992). Werden Risikofaktoren während und nach der stationären kardiologischen Rehabilitation wirklich beeinflußt? [Are risk factors really modified during and after inpatient cardiac rehabilitation?]. *Prävention und Rehabilitation, 4,* 61–67.

Nyboe, J., Jensen, G., Appleyard, M., & Schnohr, P. (1991). Smoking and the risk of first acute myocardial infarction. *American Heart Journal, 2,* 438–447.

Ockene, I. S., Shay, M. J., Alpert, J. S., Weiner, B. H., & Dalen, J. E. (1980). Unexplained chest pain in patients with normal coronary arteriograms: A follow-up study of functional status. *New England Journal of Medicine, 303,* 1249–1252.

Ockene, J. K., Kristeller, J. L., Goldberg, R., Ockene, I., Merriam, P., Barrett, S., et al. (1992). Smoking cessation and severity of disease: The coronary artery smoking intervention study. *Health Psychology, 11,* 119–126.

O'Connell, P. D., & Lundy, R. M. (1961). Level of aspiration in hypertensive cardiac patients compared with non-hypertensive cardiac patients with arteriosclerotic heart disease. *Journal of Consulting Psychology, 25,* 353–358.

O'Connor, G. T., Buring, J. E., Yusuf, S., Goldhaber, S. Z., Olmstead, E. M., Pfaffenbarger, R. S., & Hennekens, C. H. (1989). An overview of randomized trials of rehabilitation with exercise after myocardial infarction. *Circulation, 80,* 234–244.

O'Connor, C., Glassman, A. H., & Harrison, W. M. (for the SADHART Investigators). (2001). A randomized double-blind placebo controlled trial of the selective serotonin reuptake inhibitor (SSRI) sertraline for major depression after acute coronary syndromes (ACS): The SADHART trial. *Circulation, 104,* II-344.

Oevermann, U., Allert, T., Konau, E., & Krambeck, J. (1979). Die Methodologie einer "objective Hermeneutik" und ihre allgemeine forschungslogische Bedeutung in den Sozialwissenschaften [The methodology of "objective hermeneutics" and their general research-logical meaning in the social sciences]. In H. G. Soeffner (Ed.), *Interpretative Verfahren in den Social- und Textwissenschaften* [Interpretive procedures in the social and text sciences] (pp. 352–394). Stuttgart, Germany: Metzler.

Ohlmeier, D. (1980). Gruppenpsychotherapie bei Herzinfarkt-Patienten [Group psychotherapy with heart attack patients]. In C. F. Fassbender & E. Mahler (Eds.), *Der Herzinfarkt als psychosomatische Erkrankung in der Rehabilitation* [The cardiac infarct as psychosomatic illness in rehabilitation] (pp. 169–179). Mannheim, Germany: Mannheimer Morgen.

Ohlmeier, D. (1982). Krise des Individuums—Krise der Gesellschaft: Zur Situation der Psychoanalyse heute [Crisis of the individual—crisis of society: The state of psychoanalysis today]. *Fragmente, 4,* 169–188.

Ohlmeier, D. (1985). Zur psychoanalytischen Gruppentherapie und Persönlichkeitsstruktur von Herzinfarktkranken [Psychoanalytic group therapy and the personality structure of heart attack patients]. In W. Langosch (Ed.), *Psychische Bewältigung der chronischen Herzerkrankung* [Mental mastery of chronic heart disease] (pp. 345–354). Heidelberg, Germany: Springer.

Ohlmeier, D. (1989). Zur Traumaverarbeitung bei schweren Körperkrankheiten—Am Beispiel einer Gruppe von Herzinfarktkranken [Trauma processing in seriously physically ill individuals: The example of a group of heart attack sufferers]. *Gruppenpychotherapie und Gruppendynamik, 25,* 329–342.

Ohlmeier, D. (1999). Die Psychoanalyse in der Gesellschaft [Psychoanalysis in society]. *Psychosozial, 22,* 31–36.

Ohlmeier, D., Karstens, R., & Köhle, K. (1973). Psychoanalytic group interview and short-term group psychotherapy with post-myocardial infarction patients. *Psychiatric Clinics of North America, 6,* 240–249.

Ohm, D. (1987). *Entspannungstraining und Hypnose bei Patienten mit koronarer Herzkrankheit in der stationaeren Rehabilitation Entwicklung, Durchfuehrung und empirische Ueberpruefung eines psychologischen Behandlungsprogramms* [Relaxation training and hypnosis in patients with coronary heart disease in inpatient rehabilitation: Development, implementation and evaluation of a psychological treatment program]. Regensburg, Germany: S. Roderer.

Oldenburg, B., Glanz, K., & French, M. (1999). The application of staging models to the understanding of health behaviour change and the promotion of health. *Psychology and Health, 14,* 503–516.

*Oldenburg, B., Pierce, J., Sicree, R., & Ross, D. (1989). Coronary risk factor outcomes following coronary artery bypass surgery. *Australian and New Zealand Journal of Medicine, 19,* 234–240.

*Oldridge, N. B. (1984). Adherence to adult exercise fitness programs. In J. D. Matarazzo, S. M. Weiss, J. A. Herd, N. E. Miller, & S. M. Weiss (Eds.), *Behavior health: A handbook of health enhancement and disease prevention* (pp. 467–487). New York: Wiley.

Oldridge, N. B., Donner, A. P., Buck, C., Jonas, N. L., Andrew, G. M., Parker, J. P., et al. (1983). Predictors of dropout from cardiac exercise rehabilitation—Ontario Exercise-Heart Collaboration Study. *American Journal of Cardiology, 51,* 70–74.

Oldridge, N. B., Guyatt, G. H., Fischer, M. E., & Rimm, A. A. (1988). Cardiac rehabilitation after myocardial infarction. *JAMA, 260,* 945–950.

Oldridge, N. B., Guyatt, G., Jones, N., Crowe, J., Singer, J., Feeny, D., et al. (1991). Effects on quality of life with comprehensive rehabilitation after acute myocardial infarction. *American Journal of Cardiology, 67,* 1084–1089.

*Oldridge, N. B., & Rogowski, B. L. (1990). Self-efficacy and in-patient cardiac rehabilitation. *American Journal of Cardiology, 66,* 362–365.

Oldridge, N. B., Rogowski, B. L., & Gottlieb, M. (1992). Use of outpatient cardiac rehabilitation services—Factors associated with attendance. *Journal of Cardiopulmonary Rehabilitation, 12,* 25–31.

Oldridge, N. B., & Spencer, J. (1985). Exercise habits and perceptions before and after graduation or dropout from supervised cardiac exercise rehabilitation. *Journal of Cardiopulmonary Rehabilitation, 5,* 313–319.

Oldridge, N. B., Streiner, D., Hoffmann, R., & Guyatt, G. (1995). Profile of mood states and cardiac rehabilitation after acute myocardial infarction. *Medicine and Science in Sports and Exercise, 27,* 900–905.

*O'Malley, P. G., Jones, D. L., Feuerstein, I. M., & Taylor, A. J. (2000). Lack of correlation between psychological factors and subclinical coronary artery disease. *New England Journal of Medicine, 343,* 1298–1304.

O'Neill, R. M. (2000). Heart and unconscious mind: A psychoanalytic examination of cardiovascular psychology. In P. R. Duberstein & J. M. Masling (Eds.), *Psychodynamic perspectives on sickness and health* (pp.

39–71). Washington, DC: American Psychological Association.

Ong, L., Linden, W., & Young, S. (2004). Stress management: What is it? *Journal of Psychosomatic Research, 56,*133–137.

*Organisation for Economic Co-operation and Development. (2004). *OECD Health data 2004.* Paris: Author.

Ornish, D. (1991). *Open your heart.* New York: Random House.

Ornish, D. (1999). *Die revolutionäre Therapie: Heilen mit Liebe.* [The revolutionary therapy: Healing with love]. Munich, Germany: Mosaik-Verlag.

Ornish, D., Brown, S. E., Scherwitz, L. W., Billings, J. H., Armstrong, W. T., Ports, T. A., et al. (1990). Can lifestyle changes reverse coronary heart disease? *Lancet, 336,* 129–133.

Ornish, D., Scherwitz, L. W., Billings, J. H., Gould, K. L., Merritt, T. A., Sparler, S., et al. (1998). Intensive lifestyle changes for reversal of coronary heart disease. *JAMA, 280,* 2001–2007.

Orth-Gomér, K., Eriksson, I., Moser, V., Theorell, T., & Fredlund, P. (1994). Lipid lowering through work stress reduction. *International Journal of Behavioral Medicine, 1,* 204–214.

Orth-Gomér, K., & Unden, A. L. (1990). Type A behavior, social support, and coronary risk: Interaction and significance for mortality in cardiac patients. *Psychosomatic Medicine, 52,* 59–72.

Ott, B. (1982). Percutaneous transluminal coronary angioplasty and nursing implications. *Heart & Lung, 11,* 294–298.

Ottervanger, J. P., Festen, J. M., de Vries, A. G., & Stricker, B. H. C. (1995). Acute myocardial infarction while using the nicotine patch. *Chest, 107,* 1765–1766.

*Oxman, T. E., Barrett, J. E., Freeman, D. H., & Manheimer, E. (1994). Frequency and correlates of adjustment disorder related to cardiac surgery in older patients. *Psychosomatics, 35,* 557–568.

Paffenbarger, R. S., Jr., Hyde, R. T., Wing, A. L., & Hsieh, C. C. (1986). Physical activity, all-cause mortality, and longevity of college alumni. *New England Journal of Medicine, 314,* 605–613.

Pakiz, B., Reinherz, H. Z., & Giaconia, R. M. (1997). Early risk factors for serious antisocial behavior at age 21: A longitudinal community study. *American Journal of Orthopsychiatry, 67,* 92–101.

Palmer, K. J., Langeluddecke, P. M., Jones, M., & Tennant, C. (1992). The relation of the Type A behaviour pattern, factors of the structured interview, and anger to survival after myocardial infarction. *Australian Journal of Psychology, 44,* 13–19.

Panting, J. R., Gatehouse, P. D., Yang, G. Z., Grothues, F., Firmin, D. N., & Collins, P. (2002). Abnormal subendocardial perfusion in cardiac Syndrome X detected by cardiovascular magnetic resonance imaging. *New England Journal of Medicine, 346,* 1948–1953.

Panza, J. A., Laurienzo, J. M., Curiel, R. V., Unger, E. F., Quyyumi, A. A., & Dilsizian, V. (1997). Investigation of the mechanism of chest pain in patients with angiographically normal coronary arteries using transesophageal dobutamine stress echocardiography. *Journal of the American College of Cardiology, 29,* 293–301.

Papadantonaki, A., Stotts, N. A., & Paul, S. M. (1994). Comparison of quality of life before and after coronary artery bypass surgery and percutaneous transluminal angioplasty. *Heart & Lung, 23,* 45–52.

Parent, N., & Fortin, F. (2000). A randomized, controlled trial of vicarious experience through peer support for male first-time cardiac surgery patients: Impact on anxiety, self-efficacy expectation, and self-reported activity. *Heart & Lung, 29,* 389–400.

Pashkow, F. J. (1995). Rehabilitation in the patient after myocardial infarction with or without surgical management. *Seminars in Thoracic and Cardiovascular Surgery, 7,* 240–247.

Pashkow, F. J. (1996). Cardiac rehabilitation and risk factor modification. In V. Fuster, R. Ross, & E. J. Topol (Eds.), *Atherosclerosis and coronary artery disease* (pp. 1267–1282). Philadelphia: Lippincott-Raven.

Pate, R. R., Pratt, M., Blair, S. N., Haskell, W. L., Macera, C. A., Bouchard, C., et al. (1995). Physical activity and public health: A recommendation from the Centers for Disease Control and Prevention and the American College of Sports Medicine. *JAMA, 273,* 402–407.

Paterson, J. C. (1939). Relation of physical exertion and emotion to precipitation of coronary thrombi. *JAMA, 112,* 895.

Patten, C., & Martin, J. E. (1996). Does nicotine withdrawal affect smoking cessation? *Annals of Behavioral Medicine, 18,* 190–200.

Pearce, N. (1993). What does the odds ratio estimate in a case-control study? *International Journal of Epidemiology, 22,* 1189–1192.

Pearson, T. (1994). Optimal risk factor management in the patient after coronary revascularization. *Circulation, 90,* 3125–3133.

Pedersen, S. S. (2001). Post-traumatic stress disorder in patients with coronary artery disease: A review and evaluation of the risk. *Scandinavian Journal of Psychology, 42,* 445–451.

Pederson, K. J., Kuntz, D. H., & Garbe, G. J. (2001). Acute myocardial ischemia associated with ingestion of bupropion and pseudoephedrine in a 21-year-old man. *Canadian Journal of Cardiology, 17,* 599–601.

*Peglar, M., & Borgen, F. H. (1984). The defense mechanisms of coronary patients. *Journal of Clinical Psychology, 40,* 669–679.

Pelcovitz, D., Goldenberg, B., Kaplan, S., Weinblatt, M., Mandel, F., Meyers, B., & Viciguerra, V. (1996). Posttraumatic stress disorder in mothers of pediatric cancer survivors. *Psychosomatics, 37,* 116–126.

Pell, J., Pell, A., Morrison, C., Blatchford, O., & Dargie, H. (1996). Retrospective study of influence of deprivation on uptake of cardiac rehabilitation. *British Medical Journal, 313,* 267–268.

Pelser, H. (1967). Psychological aspects of the treatment of patients with coronary infarct. *Journal of Psychosomatic Research, 11,* 47–49.

Pelser, H. (1988). Gruppengespräche mit Leidensgenossen: Ein Hilfmittel bei der Behandlung chronisch körperlich Kranker [Group discussion with fellow sufferers: A resource in the treatment of the chronically physically ill]. In H. C. Deter & W. Schüffel (Eds.), *Gruppen mit körperlich Kranken* (pp. 21–28). Berlin and Heidelberg, Germany: Springer.

Perkins, K. A. (1988). Maintaining smoking abstinence after myocardial infarction. *Journal of Substance Abuse, 1,* 91–107.

Perkins, S., & Jenkins, L. S. (1998). Self-efficacy expectation, behavior performance, and mood status in early recovery from percutaneous transluminal coronary angioplasty. *Heart & Lung, 27,* 37–46.

Permanyer, M. G., Alonso, J., Brotons, C., Cascant, P., Ribera, A., Moral, I., et al. (1999). Perceived health over 3 years after percutaneous coronary balloon angioplasty. *Journal of Clinical Epidemiology, 52,* 615–623.

Perski, A., Feleke, E., Anderson, G., Samad, B. A., Westerlund, H., Ericsson, C. G., Rehnqvist, N. (1998). Emotional distress before coronary bypass grafting limits the benefits of surgery. *American Heart Journal, 136,* 510–517.

Peter, R., Geissler, H., & Siegrist, J. (1998). Associations of effort–reward imbalance at work and reported symptoms in different groups of male and female public transport workers. *Stress Medicine, 14,* 175–182.

Peterson, M. (1991). Patient anxiety before cardiac catheterization: An intervention study. *Heart & Lung, 20,* 643–647.

Petrie, K. J., Weinman, J., Sharpe, N., & Buckley, J. (1996). Role of patients' view of their illness in predicting return to work and functioning after myocardial infarction: Longitudinal study. *British Medical Journal, 312,* 1191–1194.

Petticrew, M., Gilbody, S., & Sheldon, T. A. (1999). Relation between hostility and coronary heart disease. *British Medical Journal, 319,* 917.

Petty, R. E., & Cacioppo, J. T. (1986). *Communication and persuasion—Central and peripheral routes to attitude change.* New York: Springer-Verlag.

Pfiffner, D., & Saner, H. (1990). Aktuelle Situation der kardialen Rehabilitation in der Schweiz [Actual situation of cardiac rehabilitation in Switzerland]. *Schweizerische Medizinische Wochenschrift, 120,* 1565–1568.

*Philip, A. E., Cay, E. L., Stuckey, N. A., & Vetter, N. J. (1981). Multiple predictors and multiple outcomes after myocardial infarction. *Journal of Psychosomatic Research, 25,* 137–141.

Philpott, S., Boynton, P. M., Feder, G., & Hemingway, H. (2001). Gender differences in descriptions of angina symptoms and health problems immediately prior to angiography: The Appropriateness of Coronary Revascularisation study. *Social Science & Medicine, 52,* 1565–1575.

Piatti, P., Fragasso, G., Monti, L. D., Caumo, A., Van Phan, C., & Valsecchi, G. (1999). Endothelial and metabolic characteristics of patients with angina and angiographically normal coronary arteries: Comparison with subjects with insulin resistance syndrome and normal controls. *Journal of the American College of Cardiology, 34,* 1452–1460.

Piers, G., & Singer, M. B. (1953). *Shame and guilt: A psychoanalytic and a cultural study.* Springfield, IL: Charles C Thomas.

Pichot, P., de Bonis, M. & Somogyi, M. (1977). Etude métrologique d'une batterie de tests destinée à l'étude des facteurs psychologiques en épidémiologie cardio-vasculaire [A measurement study of a test battery designed to study psychological factors in cardiovascular epidemiology]. *International Review of Applied Psychology, 26,* 11–19.

Pickering, T. G. (1985). Should studies of patients undergoing coronary angiography be used to evaluate the role of behavioral risk factors for coronary heart disease? *Journal of Behavioral Medicine, 8,* 203–213.

*Pimm, J., Foote, F., & Feist, J. R. (1986). Depression in coronary bypass patients. In J. H. Lacey & D. A. Sturgeon (Eds.), *Proceedings of the 15th European Conference on Psychosomatic Research.* London: John Libbey.

*Pinna Pintor, P., Torta, R., Bartolozzi, S., Borio, R., Caruzzo, E., Cicolin, A., et al. (1992). Clinical outcome and emotional–behavioural status after isolated coronary surgery. *Quality of Life Research, 1,* 177–185.

Pinsky, J. L., Jette, A. M., Branch, L. G., Kannel, W. B., & Feinleib, M. (1990). The Framingham Disability Study: Relationship of various coronary heart disease manifestations to disability in older persons living in the community. *American Journal of Public Health, 80,* 1363–1367.

Pither, C., & Williams, A. C. (1997). Training of therapists may have influenced usefulness of programme: Comment on Jones & West, 1996. *British Medical Journal, 314,* 978–979.

Pitzalis, M. V., Iacoviello, M., Todarello, O., Fioretti, A., Guida, P., Massari, F., et al. (2001). Depression but not anxiety influences the autonomic control of heart rate after myocardial infarction. *American Heart Journal, 141,* 765–771.

Plevier, C. M., Mooy, J. M., Marang-Van de Mheen, P. J., Stouthard, M. E., Visser, M. C., Grobbee, D. E., & Gunning-Schepers, L. J. (2001). Persistent impaired emotional functioning in survivors of a myocardial infarction? *Quality of Life Research, 10,* 123–132.

*Po, A. L. W. (1993). Transdermal nicotine in smoking cessation: A meta analysis. *European Journal of Clinical Pharmacology, 45,* 519–528.

Pocock, S., Henderson, R., Clayton, T., Lyman, G., & Chamberlain, D. (2000). Quality of life after coronary angioplasty or continued medical treatment for angina: 3 years follow-up in the RITA-2 trial. *Journal of the American College of Cardiology, 35,* 907–914.

Pocock, S. J., Henderson, R. A., Seed, P., Treasure, T., & Hampton, J. R. (1996). Quality of life, employment status, and anginal symptoms after coronary angioplasty or bypass surgery: 3-year follow-up in the Randomized Intervention Treatment of Angina (RITA) Trial. *Circulation, 94,* 135–142.

Poethko-Müller, C. (2002). Regulierung von Bupropion in Deutschland [The regulation of bupropion in Germany]. In WHO-Partnerschaftsprojekt Tabakabhängigkeit (Eds.), *Gemeinsam handeln—Tabakkonsum reduzieren* [Working together—Reducing tobacco consumption] (pp. 68–69). Bonn, Germany: Bundesvereinigung für Gesundheit.

Poettgen, G. (1981). Psychologisch-psychotherapeutische Arbeit in einer Rehabilitationsklinik fuer Herzinfarktpatienten [Psychotherapeutic work in cardiac rehabilitation]. *Rehabilitation, 20,* 114–118.

Popper, K. (1966). *Logik der Forschung* [The logic of scientific discovery]. Tübingen, Germany: Mohr.

Powell, K. E., Thompson, P. D., Caspersen, C. J., & Kendrick, J. S. (1987). Physical activity and the incidence of coronary heart disease. *Annual Review of Public Health, 8,* 253–287.

Powell, L. H. (1996). The hook: A metaphor for gaining control of emotional reactivity. In R. Allan & S. Scheidt (Eds.), *Heart and mind: The practice of cardiac psychology* (pp. 313–327). Washington, DC: American Psychological Association.

*Powell, L. H., Shaker, L. A., Jones, B. A., Vaccarino, L. V., Thoresen, C. E., & Pattillo, J. R. (1993). Psychosocial predictors of mortality in 83 women with premature acute myocardial infarction. *Psychosomatic Medicine, 55,* 426–433.

Pratt, C. M., Francis, M. J., Divine, G. W., & Young, J. B. (1989). Exercise testing in women with chest pain: Are there additional exercise characteristics that predict true positive test results? *Chest, 95,* 139–144.

Prescott, E., Hippe, M., Schnohr, P., Hein, H. O., & Vestbo, J. (1998). Smoking and risk of myocardial infarction in women and men: Longitudinal population study. *British Medical Journal, 316,* 1043–1047.

Price, D. (1984). Roles of psychophysics, neuroscience, and experiential analysis in the study of pain. In L. Kruger & J. Liebeskind (Eds.), *Advances in pain research and therapy* (Vol. 6, pp. 341–355). New York: Raven Press.

Price, V. A. (1982). *Type A behavior pattern: A model for research and practice.* New York: Academic Press.

Priebe, S., & Sinning, U. (2001). Effekte einer kurzen paartherapeutischen Intervention in der Koronarrehabilitation: Eine kontrollierte Studie [The results of a short paired therapeutic intervention during coronary rehabilitation: A controlled study]. *Psychotherapie, Psychosomatik, Medizinische Psychologie, 51,* 276–280.

Procacci, P., Zoppi, M., & Maresca, M. (1986). Clinical approach to visceral sensation. *Progress in Brain Research, 67,* 21–28.

Prochaska, J. O. (1994). Strong and weak principles for progressing from precontemplation to action on the basis of twelve problem behaviors. *Health Psychology, 13,* 47–51.

Prochaska, J. O., & DiClemente, C. C. (1986). Toward a comprehensive model of change. In W. R. Miller & N. Heather (Eds.), *Treating addictive behaviors: Processes of change* (pp. 3–27). New York: Plenum Press.

Prochaska, J. O., Johnson, S., & Lee, P. (1998). The transtheoretical model of behavior change. In S. Shumaker, E. B. Schron, J. K. Ockene, & W. L. McBee (Eds.), *The handbook of health behavior change* (2nd ed., pp. 59–84). New York: Springer Publishing Company.

Racker, H. (1978). *Übertragung und Gegenübertragung: Studien zur psychoanalytischen Technik* [Transference and countertransference: Studies of psychoanalytic technique]. Munich, Germany: Reinhardt.

*Radun, D. (1998). *Erleben der perkutanen transluminalen Koronarangioplastie (PTCA): Einflussgrößen für deren Erfolg und Lebensqualität nach PTCA* [How percutaneous transluminary coronary angioplasty (PTCA) is experienced: The parameters of its success and its influence on subsequent quality of life] Unpublished doctoral dissertation, University of Göttingen, Göttingen, Germany.

Raft, D., McKee, D. C., Popio, K. A., & Haggerty, J. J. (1985). Life adaptation after percutaneous transluminal coronary angioplasty and coronary artery bypass grafting. *American Journal of Cardiology, 56,* 395–398.

Ragland, D. R., & Brand, R. J. (1988a). Coronary heart disease mortality in the Western Collaborative Group Study: Follow-up experience of 22 years. *American Journal of Epidemiology, 127,* 462–475.

Ragland, D. R., & Brand, R. J. (1988b). Type A behavior and mortality from coronary heart disease. *New England Journal of Medicine, 318,* 65–69.

Ragland, D. R., Helmer, D. C., & Seeman, T. E. (1991). Patient selection factors in angiographic studies: A conceptual formulation and empirical test. *Journal of Behavioral Medicine, 14,* 541–553.

Rahe, R. H. (1972). Subjects' recent life changes and their near-future illness susceptibility. *Advances in Psychosomatic Medicine, 8,* 2–19.

Rahe, R. H. (1974). Life change and subsequent illness reports. In E. K. E. Gunderson & R. H. Rahe (Eds.), *Life stress and illness* (pp. 58–78). Springfield, IL: Charles C Thomas.

Rahe, R. H. (1990). Life change, stress responsivity, and captivity research. *Psychosomatic Medicine, 52,* 373–396.

Rahe, R. H. (1994). The more things change . . . . *Psychosomatic Medicine, 56,* 306–307.

Rahe, R. H., & Arthur, R. J. (1978). Life change and illness studies: Past history and future directions. *Journal of Human Stress, 4,* 3–15.

Räikkönen, K., & Keltikangas-Järvinen, L. (1991). Hostility and its association with behaviorally induced and somatic coronary risk indicators in Finnish adolescents and young adults. *Social Science & Medicine, 33,* 1171–1178.

*Raith, L., Hermes, G., Stocksmeier, U., & Natus, W. (1981). Ausprägung depressiver Syndrome bei chronisch Kranken und Gesunden. *Psychotherapie, Psychosomatik, Medizinische Psychologie 31,* 20–29.

Ramm, C., Robinson, S., & Sharpe, N. (2001). Factors determining non-attendance at a cardiac rehabilitation programme following myocardial infarction. *New Zealand Medical Journal, 114,* 227–229.

Ranchor, A. V., Sanderman, R., Bouma, J., Buunk, B. P., & van den Heuvel, W. J. (1997). An exploration of the relation between hostility and disease. *Journal of Behavioral Medicine, 20,* 223–240.

*Rechnitzer, P. A., Cunningham, D. A., Andrew, G. M., Buck, C. W., Jonas, N. L., Kavanagh, T., et al. (1983). Relation of exercise to the recurrence rate of myocardial infarction in men—Ontario Exercise-Heart Collaboration Study. *American Journal of Cardiology, 51,* 65–69.

Reed, D. M., LaCroix, A. Z., Karasek, R. A., Miller, D., & MacLean, C. A. (1989). Occupational strain and the incidence of coronary heart disease. *American Journal of Epidemiology, 129,* 495–502.

Reich, W. (1925). *Der triebhafte Charakter* [The libidinous character]. Leipzig, Germany: International Psychoanalytic Publisher.

Reich, W. (1949). *Character analysis.* New York: Orgone Institute Press.

Reinecker, H., & Lakatos, A. (1999). *Kognitive Verhaltenstherapie bei Zwangsstörungen—Ein Therapiemanual* [Cognitive behavior therapy in obsessive–compulsive disturbances—A therapy manual]. Göttingen, Germany: Hogrefe.

Reiss, S. (1997). Trait anxiety: It's not what you think it is. *Journal of Anxiety Disorders, 11,* 201–214.

Remer, E. (1972). *Ein kasuistischer Beitrag zur Persönlichkeitsforschung des Infarktpatienten* [A casuist contribution to personality research on the heart attack patient]. Unpublished doctoral dissertation, University of Salzburg, Salzburg, Austria.

Revers, W. J., Revers, R., & Widauer, H. (1978). *Herzinfarkt und Psyche* [Heart attack and the mind]. Bern, Switzerland: Verlag Hans Huber.

Review Panel on Coronary-Prone Behavior and Coronary Heart Disease. (1981). Coronary-prone behavior and coronary heart disease: A critical review. *Circulation, 63,* 1199–1215.

Ricci, G., & Angelico, F. (1979). Alcohol consumption and coronary heart-disease. *Lancet, 1,* 404.

Rice, V., Caldwell, M., Butler, S., & Robinson, J. (1986). Relaxation training and response to cardiac catheterization: A pilot study. *Nursing Research, 35,* 39–43.

Rice, V., Sieggreen, M., Mullin, M., & Williams, J. (1988). Development and testing of an arteriography information intervention for stress reduction. *Heart & Lung, 17,* 23–28.

Rice, V. H., & Stead, L. F. (1999). Nursing interventions for smoking cessation. *The Cochrane Library.* Available at http://www.cochrane.org/reviews/clibintro.htm

Richardson, H. E. (1933). Cardiac neurosis. *Minnesota Medicine, 16,* 78.

Richardson, L. A., Buckenmeyer, P. J., Bauman, B. D., Rosneck, J. S., Newman, I., & Josephson, R. A. (2000). Contemporary cardiac rehabilitation: Patient characteristics and temporal trends over the past decade. *Journal of Cardiopulmonary Rehabilitation, 20,* 57–64.

Richmond, R. L. (1997). A comparison of measures used to assess effectiveness of the transdermal nicotine patch at 1 year. *Addictive Behaviors, 22,* 753–757.

Richter, J. E. (1991). Investigation and management of non-cardiac chest pain. *Bailliere's Clinical Gastroenterology, 5,* 281–306.

Richter, J., Richter, G., Leistner, M., & Toellner, H. (1989). Bewaeltigungsverhalten und Kontrollueberzeugungen bei Myokardinfarkt-Patienten und traumatologischen Patienten [Mastering behavior and control convictions with myocardial infarction patients and traumatological patients]. *Zeitschrift für Klinische Medizin, 44,* 2159–2162.

Richter, J. E., & the Working Team for Functional Esophageal Disorders. (1994). *Functional esophageal disorders.* Boston: Little Brown.

*Richter, R., Dahme, B., & Holthusen, R. (1988). Psychophysiologische Untersuchung der subjektiven Belastung vor einer Herzkatheteruntersuchung. In B. F. Klapp & B. Dahme (Eds.), *Psychosoziale Kardiologie* (pp. 161–171). Berlin, Germany: Springer Verlag.

*Riegel, B. J., & Dracup, K. A. (1992). Does overprotection cause cardiac invalidism after acute myocardial infarction? *Heart & Lung, 21,* 529–535.

*Riegel, B., & Gocka, I. (1995). Gender differences in adjustment to acute myocardial infarction. *Heart & Lung, 24,* 457–466.

Riemsma, R. P., Pattenden, J., Bridle, C., Sowden, A., & Mather, L. (2003). Systematic review of the effectiveness of stage based interventions to promote smoking cessation. *British Medical Journal, 326,* 1175–1182.

Rigotti, N. A., McKool, K. M., & Shiffmann, S. (1994). Predictors of smoking cessation after coronary artery bypass graft surgery. *Annals of Internal Medicine, 120,* 287–293.

Rigotti, N. A., & Pasternak, R. C. (1996). Cigarette smoking and coronary heart disease: Risks and management. *Cardiology Clinics, 14,* 51–68.

Rivers, J. T., White, H. D., Cross, D. B., Williams, B. F., & Morris, R. M. (1990). Reinfarction after thrombolytic therapy for acute myocardial infarction followed by conservative management: Incidence and effect of smoking. *Journal of the American College of Cardiology, 16,* 340–348.

Robins, L. N., Helzer, J. E., Croughan, J., & Ratcliff, K. S. (1981). National Institute of Mental Health Diagnostic Interview Schedule: Its history, characteristics, and validity. *Archives of General Psychiatry, 38,* 381–389.

Röckle, N. A. (1999). *Depressivität, Angst und Krankheitsverlauf bei perkutaner transluminaler koronarer Angioplastie (PTCA)* [Depression, anxiety, and course of illness associated with percutaneous coronary angioplasty (PTCA)]. Unpublished doctoral dissertation, University of Würzburg, Würzburg, Germany.

Rodrigues, L., & Kirkwood, B. R. (1990). Case-control designs in the study of common diseases: Updates on the demise of the rare disease assumption and the choice of sampling scheme for controls. *International Journal of Epidemiology, 19,* 205–213.

Roeters van Lennep, J. E., Zwinderman, A. H., & van der Wall, E. E. (2000). Angina pectoris and normal coronary arteries: Prevalence and prognosis in men and women. *Nederlands Tijdschrift voor Geneeskund, 144,* 1139–1140.

Roettger, U. (1982). Gestalttherapie: Möglichkeiten und Grenzen in der Herzinfarktrehabilitation [Gestalt therapy: Possibilities and limitations in patient rehabilitation after heart attack]. *Psychotherapie und Medizinische Psychologie, 32,* 60–63.

Rogers, D. E. (1986). Some observations on having a coronary. *Pharos, 49,* 12–14.

*Rogner, J., Bartram, M., Hardinghaus, W., Lehr, D., & Wirth, A. (1994). "Depressiv getoente Krankheitsbewaeltigung" bei Herzinfarktpatienten—Zusammenhaenge mit dem laengerfristigen Krankheitsverlauf und Veraenderbarkeit durch eine Gruppentherapie auf indirekt-suggestiver Grundlage [Overcoming illness with depressive symptoms in heart attack patients—The relationship between the longer term course of illness and its amenability to change through group work based on indirect suggestion]. In G. Schuessler (Ed.), *Coping: Verlaufs- und Therapiestudien chronischer Krankheit* [Coping: Process and therapy studies of chronic illness] (pp. 95–109). Göttingen, Germany: Hogrefe.

*Rogner, J., Hardinghaus, W., Bartram, M., & Wirth, A. (1993). Konkurrente und prädiktive Zusammenhänge zwischen Emotionen und kardiovaskulären sowie Stoffwechsel-Parametern bei Herzinfarktpatienten [Concurrent and predictive relationships among emotions, cardiovascular parameters and metabolic parameters in heart attack patients]. *Zeitschrift für Psychosomatische Medizin und Psychoanalyse, 39,* 147–159.

Rogutski, S., Berra, K., & Haskell, W. (1999). Home-based cardiac rehabilitation: Variations on a theme. In N. K. Wenger, L. K. Smith, E. S. Froelicher, & P. McCall Comoss (Eds.), *Cardiac rehabilitation: A guide to practice in the 21st century* (pp. 343–360). New York: Marcel Dekker.

Roll, M., & Theorell, T. (1987). Acute chest pain without obvious organic cause before age 40: Personality and recent life events. *Journal of Psychosomatic Research, 31,* 215–221.

Romano, J. M., & Turner, J. A. (1985). Chronic pain and depression: Does the evidence support a relationship? *Psychological Bulletin, 97,* 18–34.

Ronnevik, P., Gundersen, T., & Abrahamsen, A. M. (1985). Effect of smoking habits and timolol treatment on mortality and reinfarction in patients surviving acute myocardial infarction. *British Heart Journal, 54,* 134–139.

Roose, S. P., Dalack, G. W., Glassman, A. H., Woodring, S., Walsh, T., & Giardina, E. G. V. (1991). Cardiovascular effects of bupropion in depressed patients with heart disease. *American Journal of Psychiatry, 148,* 512–516.

Roose, S. P., Devanand, D., & Suthers, K. (1999). Depression: Treating the patient with comorbid cardiac disease. *Geriatrics, 54,* 20–21, 25–26, 29–31.

Roose, S. P., Glassman, A. H., Giardina, E. G. V., Johnson, L. L., Walsh, T., & Bigger, T. (1987). Cardiovascular effects of imipramine and bupropion in depressed patients with congestive heart failure. *Journal of Clinical Psychopharmacology, 7,* 247–251.

Roose, S. P., Laghrissi Thode, F., Kennedy, J. S., Nelson, J. C., Bigger, J. T., Jr., Pollock, B. G., et al. (1998). Comparison of paroxetine and nortriptyline in depressed patients with ischemic heart disease. *JAMA, 279,* 287–291.

Rorschach, H. (1951). *Psychodiagnostics: A diagnostic test based on perception* (5th ed., rev.). Oxford, England: Grune & Stratton.

Rosal, M. C., Ockene, J. K., Hebert, J. R., Ockene, I. S., Merriam, P., & Hurley, T. G. (1998). Coronary Artery Smoking Intervention Study (CASIS): 5-year follow-up. *Health Psychology, 17,* 476–478.

Rose, G., Ahmeteli, M., Checcacci, L., Fidanza, F., Glazunov, I., & De Haas, J. (1968). Ischemic heart disease in middle-aged men: Prevalence comparisons in Europe. *Bulletin of the World Health Organization, 38,* 885–895.

Rosen, C. S. (2000). Is the sequencing of change processes by stage consistent across health problems? A meta-analysis. *Health Psychology, 19,* 593–604.

Rosen, S. D., & Camici, P. G. (1994). Syndrome X: Background, clinical aspects, pathophysiology and treatment. *Giornale Italiano di Cardiologia, 24,* 779–790.

Rosen, S. D., & Camici, P. G. (2000). The brain–heart axis in the perception of cardiac pain: The elusive link between ischaemia and pain. *Annals of Medicine, 32,* 350–364.

Rosenman, R. H. (1978). The interview method of assessment of the coronary-prone behavior pattern. In T. M. Dembroski, S. M. Weiss, J. L. Shields, S. G. Haynes, & M. Feinleib (Eds.), *Coronary-prone behavior* (pp. 55–69). New York: Springer-Verlag.

Rosenman, R. H., Brand, R. J., Jenkins, D., Friedman, M., Straus, R., & Wurm, M. (1975). Coronary heart disease in Western Collaborative Group Study: Final follow-up experience of 8 1/2 years. *JAMA, 233,* 872–877.

Rosenman, R. H., Brand, R. J., Sholtz, R. I., & Friedman, M. (1976). Multivariate prediction of coronary heart disease during 8.5 year follow-up in the Western Collaborative Group Study. *American Journal of Cardiology, 37,* 903–910.

Rosenman, R. H., Friedman, M., Straus, R., Wurm, M., Jenkins, C. D., & Messinger, H. B. (1966). Coronary heart disease in the Western Collaborative Group Study: A follow-up experience of two years. *JAMA, 195,* 130–136.

Rosenman, R. H., Friedman, M., Straus, R., Wurm, M., Kositcheck, R., Hahn, W., & Werthessen, N. (1964). A predictive study of coronary heart disease: The Western Collaborative Group Study. *JAMA, 189,* 103–110.

Rosenstock, I. M. (1966). Why people use health services. *Milbank Memorial Fund Quarterly, 44,* 94.

Rosenthal, R. (1984). *Meta-analytic procedures for social research.* Beverly Hills, CA: Sage.

Rösler, F. (Ed.). (1988). *Enzyklopädie der Psychologie: Themenbereich C, Theorie und Forschung, Serie I, Biologische Psychologie, Band 5: Ergebnisse une Anwendungen der Psychophysiologie* [Encyclopedia of psychology: Topic area C, Theory and research, Series I, Biological psychology, Vol. 5: Results and application of psychophysiology]. Göttingen, Germany: Hogrefe.

Rost, R. (1998). *Sport und Gesundheit* [Sports and health]. Heidelberg, Germany: Springer.

Rost, R., Hartmann, T., Horstmann, G., Koll, U., & Bjarnason-Wehrens, B. (1999). Der Bedarf an ambulanter kardiologischer Anschlussrehabilitation in einem großstädtischen Ballungsgebiet: Ergebnisse des Kölner Modells der ambulanten kardiologischen Rehabilitations—Phase II [The need for adjunct outpatient cardiac rehabilitation in a big-city metro area: Outcomes of the Cologne model of outpatient cardiac rehabilitation—Phase II]. *Zeitschrift für Kardiologie, 88,* 34–43.

Rothman, A. J., & Salovey, P. (1997). Shaping perceptions to motivate healthy behavior: The role of message framing. *Psychological Bulletin, 121,* 3–19.

Rothman, K., & Greenland, S. (1998). Precision and validity in epidemiologic studies. In K. Rothman & S. Greenland (Eds.), *Modern epidemiology* (2nd ed., pp. 115–134). Philadelphia: Lippincott Williams & Wilkins.

Roy-Byrne, P., Uhde, T., Post, R., King, A., & Buchsbaum, M. (1984). Normal pain sensitivity in patients with panic disorder. *Psychiatry Research, 14,* 75–82.

Rozanski, A., Blumenthal, J. A., & Kaplan, J. (1999). Impact of psychological factors on the pathogenesis of cardiovascular disease and implications for therapy. *Circulation, 99,* 2192–2217.

Ruberman, W., Weinblatt, E., Goldberg, J. D., & Chaudhary, B. S. (1984). Psychosocial influences on mortality after myocardial infarction (nonvalidated scale). *New England Journal of Medicine, 311,* 552–559.

Ruggeri, A., Taruschio, G., Loricchio, M., Samory, G., Borghi, A., & Bugiardini, R. (1996). The correlation between the clinical characteristics and psychological status in syndrome X patients. *Cardiologia, 41,* 551–557.

Rugulies, R. (1998). *Die psychosoziale Dimension der koronaren Herzkrankheit und die Chancen multiprofessioneller Intervention* [The psychosocial dimension of coronary heart disease and the chances of multiprofessional intervention]. Lengerich, Germany: Pabst Science Publishers.

Rugulies, R. (2002). Depression as a predictor for coronary heart disease: A review and meta-analysis. *American Journal of Preventive Medicine, 23,* 51–61.

Rugulies, R., Aust, B., & Syme, S. L. (2004). The epidemiology of health and illness: A socio-psychophysiological perspective. In S. Sutton, A. Baum, & M. Johnston (Eds.), *The Sage handbook of health psychology* (pp. 27–68). London: Sage.

Rugulies, R., & Krause, N. (2000, November). *The impact of job stress on musculoskeletal disorders, psychosomatic symptoms and general health in hotel room cleaners.* Paper presented at the Sixth International Congress of Behavioral Medicine, Brisbane, Australia.

Rugulies, R., & Siegrist, J. (1999). Kardiologische Rehabilitation durch umfassende Lebensstiländerung und psychosoziale Betreuung—Evaluation eines verhaltensmedizinischen Modellversuchs [Cardiac rehabilitation through total lifestyle change and psychosocial support—Evaluation of a behavioral-medicine-based trial model]. In B. Badura & J. Siegrist (Eds.), *Evaluation im Gesundheitswesen* [Evaluation of health services] (pp. 227–238). Weinheim, Germany: Juventa.

Rugulies, R., & Siegrist, J. (2002). *Soziologische Aspekte der Entstehung und des Verlaufs der koronaren Herzkrankheit: Soziale Ungleichverteilung der Erkrankung und chronische Distress-Erfahrungen im Erwerbsleben* [Sociological aspects of the development and course of coronary heart disease: Social inequality and chronic emotional stress in the workplace]. Frankfurt, Germany: VAS.

Rumpf, H. -J., Meyer, C., Hapke, U., Dilling, H., & John, U. (1998). Stadien der Änderungsbereitschaft bei Rauchern in der Allgemeinbevölkerung [Stages of change readiness among smokers in the general population]. *Gesundheitswesen, 60,* 592–597.

Rust, M. (1990). Der Riss in der Hauswand—Herzinfarkt und Trigeminusneuralgie im Verlauf einer tiefenpsychologisch fundierten Behandlung mit dem Katathymen Bilderleben [The crack in the wall—Heart attack and trigeminus neuralgia during the course of a depth-psychology based treatment addressing catathymic imagery]. In E. Wilke & H. Leuner (Eds.), *Das Katathyme Bilderleben in der Psychosomatischen Medizin* [The catathymic life picture in psychosomatic medicine] (pp. 258–265). Bern, Switzerland: Huber.

Rutledge, T., Linden, W., & Davies, R. F. (1999). Psychological risk factors may moderate pharmacological treatment effects among ischemic heart disease patients: Canadian Amlodipine/Atenolol in Silent Ischemia Study (CASIS) Investigators. *Psychosomatic Medicine, 61,* 834–841.

*Rutledge, T., Reis, S. E., Olson, M., Owens, J., Kelsey, S. F., Pepine, C. J., et al. (2001). History of anxiety disorders is associated with a decreased likelihood of angiographic coronary artery disease in women with chest pain: The WISE study. *Journal of the American College of Cardiology, 37,* 780–785.

Sackett, D. L. (1986). Rules of evidence and clinical recommendations on use of antithrombotic agents. *Chest, 89*(2 Suppl.), 2S–3S.

Sackett, D. L. (1996). Evidence-based medicine: What it is and what it isn't. *British Medical Journal, 312,* 71–72.

Saha, S., Stettin, G. D., & Redberg, R. F. (1999). Gender and willingness to undergo invasive cardiac procedures. *Journal of General Internal Medicine, 14,* 122–125.

Salisbury, C. (1996). Rehabilitation after myocardial infarction: The role of the community nurse. *Nursing Standard, 10*(23), 49–51.

Sallis, J. F., & Owen, N. (1998). *Physical activity and behavioral medicine.* Thousand Oaks, CA: Sage.

Salm, A. (1982). Der Umgang mit der Angst am Beispiel der Herzkatheteruntersuchung [Handling anxiety with exploratory heart catheterization as an example]. In D. Beckmann, S. Davies-Osterkamp, & J. W. Scheer (Eds.), *Medizinische Psychologie* [Medical psychology] (pp. 275–306). Berlin, Germany: Springer.

Salonen, J. T. (1980). Stopping smoking and long term mortality after acute myocardial infarction. *British Heart Journal, 43,* 463–467.

*Sandler, D. A., Sandler, G., Benison, D., Weatcroft, S., Leakey, P., & Blair, A. (1999). Psychological and physical benefits of an exercise-based cardiac rehabilitation programme for patients recovering from a first MI. *British Journal of Cardiology, 6,* 102–112.

Saner, H. (1993). Stand der kardialen Rehabilitation [The state of cardiac rehabilitation]. In H. Saner (Ed.), *Kardiale Rehabilitation* [Cardiac rehabilitation] (pp. 1–12). Stuttgart, Germany: Thieme.

Saner, H. (2000). Kardiale Rehabilitation—Medizinpolitische und ökonomische Aspekte [Cardiac rehabilitation—Medicopolitical and economic aspects]. *Medizinspiegel, 3,* 47–50.

Saner, H., & Pfiffner, D. (1995). Ambulante Rehabilitation von Herzpatienten in der Schweiz [Outpatient rehabilitation of heart patients in Switzerland]. *Wiener Klinische Wochenschrift, 107,* 771–773.

Sapolsky, R. M. (1995). Social subordinance as a marker of hypercortisolism: Some unexpected subtleties. In G. P. Chrousos, R. McCarty, K. Pacák, E. Sternberg, P. W. Gold. & R. Kvetsnansky (Eds.), *Annals of the New York Academy of Sciences: Vol. 771. Stress: Basic mechanisms and clinical implications* (pp. 626–639). New York: New York Academy of Sciences.

*Sarantidis, D., Thomas, A., Iphantis, K., Katsaros, N., Tripodianakis, J., & Katsabouris, G. (1997). Levels of anxiety, depression and denial in patients with myocardial infarction. *European Psychiatry, 12,* 149–151.

Sargent, H. D., & Hirsch, E. A. (1954). Projective methods. In L. A. Pennington & I. A. Berg (Eds.), *An introduction to clinical psychology* (2nd ed., pp. 188–219). New York: Ronald Press.

Sato, I., Nishida, M., Okita, K., Nishijima, H., Kojima, S., Matsamura, N., & Yasuda, H. (1992). Beneficial effect of stopping smoking on future cardiac events in male smokers with previous myocardial infarction. *Japanese Circulation Journal, 56,* 217–222.

Sauer, W. H., Berlin, J. A., & Kimmel, S. E. (2001). Selective serotonin inhibitors and myocardial infarction. *Circulation, 104,* 1894–1898.

Saur, C. D., Granger, B. B., Muhlbaier, L. H., Forman, L. M., McKenzie, R. J., Taylor, M. C., & Smith, P. K. (2001). Depressive symptoms and outcome of coronary artery bypass grafting. *American Journal of Critical Care, 10,* 4–10.

Scarinci, I. C., McDonald-Haile, J., Bradley, L. A., & Richter, J. E. (1994). Altered pain perception and psychosocial features among women with gastrointestinal disorders and history of abuse: A preliminary model. *American Journal of Medicine, 97,* 108–118.

Schaubroeck, J., Ganster, D. C., & Kemmerer, B. E. (1994). Job complexity, "Type A" behavior, and cardiovascular disorder: A prospective study. *Academy of Management Journal, 37,* 426–439.

Schauenburg, H., Beutel, M., Hautzinger, M., Leichsenring, F., Reimer, C., Rüger, U., et al. (1999). Zur Psychotherapie der Depression [On psychotherapy for depression]. *Psychotherapeut, 44,* 127–136.

Scheidt, C., Koester, B., & Deuschel, G. (1996). Diagnose, Symptomatik und Verlauf des psychogenen Tremor [Diagnosis, symptomatology, and progression of psychogenic tremor]. *Nervenarzt, 67,* 198–204.

Scheier, M. F., Matthews, K. A., Owens, J. F., Schulz, R., Bridges, M. W., Magovern, G. J., Sr., & Carver, C. (1999). Optimism and rehospitalization after coronary artery bypass graft surgery. *Archives of Internal Medicine, 159,* 829–835.

Scherwitz, L. (1996). Lebensweise und Gesundheit— Das Beispiel Herz-Kreislauf-Erkrankungen [Lifelong habits and health: Cardiovascular disease as an example]. In G. Kaiser (Ed.), *Zukunft der Medizin— Neue Wege zur Gesundheit* (pp. 79–93). Frankfurt, Germany: Campus.

*Scherwitz, L. W., Brusis, O. A., Kesten, D., Safian, P. A., Hasper, E., Berg, A., & Siegrist, J. (1995). Lebenstiländerungen bei Herzinfarktpatienten im Rahmen der stationären und ambulanten Rehabilitation—Ergebnisse einer deutschen Pilotstudie [Lifestyle changes in heart attack patients involved in inpatient and outpatient rehabilitation—Results of a German pilot study]. *Zeitschrift für Kardiologie, 84,* 216–221.

*Scherwitz, L. W., Perkins, L. L., Chesney, M. A., & Hughes, G. H. (1991). Cook–Medley Hostility scale and subsets: Relationship to demographic and psychosocial characteristics in young adults in the CARDIA study. *Psychosomatic Medicine, 53,* 36–49.

Scherwitz, L. W., Perkins, L. L., Chesney, M. A., Hughes, G. H., Sidney, S., & Manolio, T. A. (1992). Hostility and health behaviors in young adults: The CARDIA Study. *American Journal of Epidemiology, 136,* 136–145.

Schilling, H. (1980). Projektive Verfahren zur psychologischen Anamnese [Projective techniques for psychological anamnesis]. In C. F. Fassbender & E. Mahler (Eds.), *Der Herzinfarkt als psychosomatische Erkrankung in der Rehabilitation* [Heart attack as a psychosomatic illness and rehabilitation] (pp. 125–135). Mannheim, Germany: Mannheimer Morgen.

Schleifer, S. J., Macari-Hinson, M. M., Coyle, D. A., Slater, W. R., Kahn, M., Gorlin, R., & Zucker, H. D. (1989). The nature and course of depression following myocardial infarction. *Archives of Internal Medicine, 149,* 1785–1789.

Schleifer, S. J., Slater, W. R., Macari-Hinson, M. M., Coyle, D. A., Kahn, M., Zucker, H. D., & Gorlin, R. (1991). Digitalis and β-blocking agents: Effects on depression following myocardial infarction. *American Heart Journal, 121,* 1397–1402.

Schlicht, W. (1994). *Sport und Primärprävention* [Sport and primary prevention]. Göttingen, Germany: Hogrefe.

Schlicht, W. (1996). *Wohlbefinden und Gesundheit durch Sport* [Well-being and health through sport]. Schorndorf, Germany: Hofmann.

Schlicht, W. (2000). Gesundheitsverhalten im Alltag: Auf der Suche nach einem Paradigma [Everyday behavioral health: In search of a new paradigm]. *Zeitschrift für Gesundheitspsychologie, 8,* 49–60.

Schliehe, F., & Haaf, H. -G. (1996). Zur Effektivität und Effizienz der medizinischen Rehabilitation [On the effectiveness and efficiency of medical rehabilitation]. *Deutsche Rentenversicherung, 10–11,* 666–689.

Schmid, S., Keller, S., Jäkel, C., Baum, E., & Basler, H.-D. (1999). Kognition und Motivation zu sportlicher Aktivität—eine Längsschnittstudie zum Transtheoretischen Modell [Cognition and the motivation to get involved in sports activities—A longitudinal study using a transtheoretical model]. *Zeitschrift für Gesundheitspsychologie, 7,* 21–26.

Schmidt, T. H., Dembroski, T. M., & Blümchen, G. (Eds.). (1986). *Biological and psychological factors in cardiovascular disease.* New York: Springer-Verlag.

Schnall, P. L., Belkić, K., Landsbergis, P., & Baker, D. (Eds.). (2000). The workplace and cardiovascular disease [Special issue]. *Occupational Medicine, 15*(1).

Schnall, P. L., Landsbergis, P., & Baker, D. (1994). Job strain and cardiovascular disease. *Annual Review of Public Health, 15,* 381–411.

Schnall, P. L., Schwartz, J. E., Landsbergis, P. A., Warren, K., & Pickering, T. G. (1998). A longitudinal study of job strain and ambulatory blood pressure: Results from a three-year follow-up. *Psychosomatic Medicine, 60,* 697–706.

Schocken, D. D., Greene, A. F., Worden, T. J., & Harrison, E. E. (1987). Effects of age and gender on the relationship between anxiety and coronary artery disease. *Psychosomatic Medicine, 49,* 118–126.

Schocken, D. D., Worden, T. J., Harrison, E. E., & Spielberger, C. D. (1984). Anxiety differences in patients with angina pectoris, non-anginal chest pain, and coronary heart disease. *Circulation, 70*(Suppl. 2), II-387.

Schott, T. (1987a). Frühberentung nach Herzinfarkt— Folgen und Auswirkungen auf Krankheitsbewältigung und Lebensqualität [Early retirement after a heart attack: The consequences and its effects on quality of life and the ability to overcome the illness]. In B. Badura, G. Kaufhold, H. Lehmann, H. Pfaff, T. Schott, & M. Waltz (Eds.), *Leben mit dem Herzinfarkt: Eine sozialepidemiologische Studie* [Living with a heart attack: A socioepidemiological study] (pp. 257–285). Berlin, Germany: Springer-Verlag.

Schott, T. (1987b). Die Rückkehr zur Arbeit [Return to work]. In B. Badura, G. Kaufhold, H. Lehmann, H. Pfaff, T. Schott, & M. Waltz (Eds.), *Leben mit dem Herzinfarkt: Eine sozialepidemiologische Studie* [Living with a heart attack: A socioepidemiological study] (pp. 179–203). Berlin, Germany: Springer-Verlag.

Schott, T., Iseringhausen, O., & vom Orde, A. (2002). Continuity and the quality of medical care for the cardiac patient: Cardiac rehabilitation and its interfaces to acute care (Phase I) and the process of coming back (Phase III). *Rehabilitation, 41,* 140–147.

Schröder, S., Baumbach, A., Herdeg, C., Oberhoff, M., Buchholz, O., & Karsch, K. R. (2000). Ergebnisse einer Befragung von 549 Patienten zum klinischen Langzeitverlauf und zur Lebensqualitätvier Jahre nach PTCA [Results of a survey of clinical outcomes and quality of life in 549 patients four years after PTCA]. *Medizinische Klinik, 95,* 130–135.

Schuler, G., Epstein, F. H., & Stransky, M. (1978). Brustschmerzen und kardiale Morbidität in zwei Zürcher Landgemeinden: Befragungsergebnisse 1974/75 [Chest pain and cardiac morbidity in two rural communities near Zurich: Survey results 1974/75]. *Sozial- und Praventivmedizin, 23,* 279.

Schuler, G., Hambrecht, R., & Schlierf, K. (1991). Progression der koronaeren Herzerkrankung unter koerperlichem Training und fettarmer Ernaehrung [The progression of coronary heart disease during physical training and adherence to a low-fat diet]. In U. Gleichmann, K. Mannebach, S. Gleichmann, & K. Held (Eds.), *Herausforderung Atherosklerose in den 90ern* [The challenge of atherosclerosis in the 90s] (pp. 29–34). Darmstadt, Germany: Steinkopff.

Schultheis, K. (1987). Psychological preparation for cardiac catheterization: An investigation of treatment and person variables. *Dissertation Abstracts International, 44*(10B), 3207.

Schulze, G. (2000). *Erlebnis-Gesellschaft* [The experiential society]. Frankfurt, Germany: Suhrkamp.

Schwarzer, R. (1987). Meta-Analysen: Methodik, Anwendungsbeispiel und Computerprogramm [Meta-analyses: Method, example, and computer program]. In D. Liepmann, G. Mohr, & R. Schwarzer (Eds.), *Arbeitsberichte des Instituts für Psychologie* (No. 7) [Working reports of the Institute for Psychology (No. 7)]. Berlin, Germany: Institut für Psychologie.

Schwarzer, R. (1996). *Psychologie des Gesundheitsverhaltens.* [The psychology of health behaviors]. Göttingen, Germany: Hogrefe.

Schwarzer, R., & Renner, B. (2000). Social cognitive predictors of health behavior: Action self efficacy and coping self efficacy. *Health Psychology, 19,* 487–495.

Schweizerische Arbeitsgruppe für kardiale Rehabilitation. (1998). *Kardiale Rehabilitation* [Cardiac rehabilitation]. Zurich, Switzerland: Höchst Marion Roussel AG.

Scott, I. A., Eyeson-Annan, M. L., Huxley, S. L., & West, M. J. (2000). Optimising care of acute myocardial infarction: Results of a regional quality improvement project. *Journal of Quality in Clinical Practice, 20,* 12–19.

Scott, R. R., Mayer, J. A., Denier, C. A., Dawson, B. L., & Lamparski, D. (1990). Long-term smoking status of cardiac patients following symptom-specific cessation advice. *Addictive Behaviors, 15,* 549–552.

Scottish Intercollegiate Guidelines Network. (2002). *Cardiac rehabilitation: A national clinical guideline.* Retrieved October 2002, from http://www.sign.ac.uk./pdf/sign57.pdf

Seemann, W. F. (1964). Verhaltensmerkmale von Kranken vor und nach einem Herzinfarkt [Behavioral characteristics of patients before and after a heart attack]. *Westfälisches Ärzteblatt, 5,* 320–326.

Selye, H. (1956). *The stress of life.* New York: McGraw-Hill.

Serebruany, V. L., O'Connor, C. M., & Gurbel, P. A. (2001). Effect of selective serotonin reuptake inhibitors on platelets in patients with coronary artery disease. *American Journal of Cardiology, 87,* 1398–1400.

Serlie, A. W., Duivenvoorden, H. J., Passchier, J., ten Cate, F. J., Deckers, J. W., & Erdman, R. A. (1996). Empirical psychological modeling of chest pain: A comparative study. *Journal of Psychosomatic Research, 40,* 625–635.

Serlie, A. W., Erdman, R. A., Passchier, J., Trijsburg, R. W., & ten Cate, F. J. (1995). Psychological aspects of non-cardiac chest pain. *Psychotherapy and Psychosomatics, 64,* 62–73.

Shalev, A. Y., Schreiber, S., Galai, T., & Melmed, R. (1993). Post traumatic stress disorder following medical events. *British Journal of Clinical Psychology, 32,* 352–357.

Shaper, A. G., Pocock, S. J., Walker, M., Phillips, A. N., Whitehead, T. P., & MacFarlane, P. W. (1985). Risk factors for ischaemic heart disease: The prospective phase of the British Regional Heart Study. *Journal of Epidemiology and Community Health, 39,* 197–209.

Shapiro, P. A., Lespérance, F., Frasure-Smith, N., O'Connor, C. M., Baker, B., Jiang, J. W., et al. (1999). An open-label preliminary trial of sertraline for treatment of major depression after acute myocardial infarction (the SADHART Trial). *American Heart Journal, 137,* 1100–1106.

Shaw, R. E., Cohen, F., Fishman Rosen, J., Murphy, M. C., Stertzer, S. H., Clark, D. A., & Myler, R. K. (1986). Psychologic predictors of psychosocial and medical outcomes in patients undergoing coronary angioplasty. *Psychosomatic Medicine, 48,* 582–597.

Sheehan, D. V., Ballenger, J., & Jacobsen, G. (1980). Treatment of endogenous anxiety with phobic, hysterical, and hypochondriacal symptoms. *Archives of General Psychiatry, 37,* 51–59.

*Sheffield, D., Krittayaphong, R., Cascio, W. E., Light, K. C., Golden, R. N., Finkel, J. B., et al. (1998). Heart rate variability at rest and during mental stress in patients with coronary artery disease: Differences in patients with high and low depression scores. *International Journal of Behavioral Medicine, 5,* 31–47.

Shekelle, R. B., Gale, M., & Norusis, M. (1985). Type A score (Jenkins Activity Survey) and risk of recurrent coronary heart disease in the aspirin myocardial infarction study. *American Journal of Cardiology, 56,* 221–225.

Shekelle, R. B., Gale, M., Ostfeld, A. M., & Paul, O. (1983). Hostility, risk of coronary heart disease, and mortality. *Psychosomatic Medicine, 45,* 109–115.

Shekelle, R. B., Hulley, S. B., Neaton, J. D., Billings, J. H., Borhani, N. O., Gerace, T. A., et al. (1986). Type A behavior and risk of coronary heart disease in the Multiple Risk Factor Intervention Trial. In T. H. Schmidt, T. M. Dembroski, and G. Blümchen (Eds.), *Biological and psychological factors in cardiovascular disease* (pp. 41–55). New York: Springer Verlag.

Shekelle, R. B., Vernon, S. W., & Ostfeld, A. M. (1991). Personality and coronary artery disease. *Psychosomatic Medicine, 53,* 176–184.

Shemesh, E., Rudnick, A., Kaluski, E., Milovanov, O., Salah, A., Alon, D., et al. (2002). A prospective study of posttraumatic stress symptoms and nonadherence in survivors of a myocardial infarction (MI). *General Hospital Psychiatry, 23,* 215–222.

*Sheps, D. S., Kaufmann, P. G., Sheffield, D., Light, K. C., McMahon, R. P., Bonsall, R., et al. (2001). Sex differences in chest pain in patients with documented coronary artery disease and exercise-induced ischemia: Results from the PIMI study. *American Heart Journal, 142,* 864–871.

*Sheps, D. S., Light, K. C., Bragdon, E. E., Herbst, M. C., & Hinderliter, A. L. (1989). Relationship between chest pain, exercise endorphin response and depression. *Circulation, 80,* II-591.

*Sheps, D. S., & Sheffield, D. (1997). Depressed mood is related to heart rate variability and ischemia during daily life. *Psychophysiology, 34*(Suppl. 1), S7.

*Siegman, A. W., Townsend, S. T., Blumenthal, R. S., Sorkin, J. D., & Civelek, A. C. (1998). Dimensions of anger and CHD in men and women: Self-ratings versus spouse ratings. *Journal of Behavioral Medicine, 21,* 315–336.

Siegrist, J. (1995). *Medizinische Soziologie* [Medical sociology]. Munich, Germany: Urban & Schwarzenberg.

Siegrist, J. (1996a). Adverse health effects of high-effort/low-reward conditions. *Journal of Occupational Health Psychology, 1,* 27–41.

Siegrist, J. (1996b). *Soziale Krisen und Gesundheit* [Social crisis and health]. Göttingen, Germany: Hogrefe.

Siegrist, J., & Matschinger, H. (1989). Restricted status control and cardiovascular risk. In A. Steptoe & A. Appels (Eds.), *Stress, personal control and health* (pp. 65–82). Chichester, England: Wiley.

Siegrist, J., Peter, R., Junge, A., & Cremer, P. (1990). Low status control, high effort at work and ischemic heart disease: Prospective evidence from blue-collar men. *Social Science & Medicine, 31,* 1127–1134.

Siegrist, J., Starke, D., Chandola, T., Godin, I., Marmot, M., Niedhammer, I., et al. (2004). The measurement of effort-reward imbalance at work: European comparisons. *Social Science & Medicine, 58,* 1483–1499.

*Siegrist, K., & Broer, M. (1997). Erwerbstätigkeit nach erstem Herzinfarkt und Rehabilitation [Employment status after a first heart attack and rehabilitation]. *Sozial- und Präventivmedizin, 42,* 358–366.

*Siegrist, K., Jürgensen, R., Bieber, G., & Halhuber, C. (1988). Zur Bedeutung der Sozialanamnese bei der Rehabilitation von Koronarkranken [On the significance of social anamnesis in the rehabilitation of coronary patients]. *Sozial- und Präventivmedizin 33,* 41–45.

Siepmann, F. (1980). Gesprächspsychotherapie mit Herzinfarkt-Patienten [Talk therapy with heart attack patients]. In C. F. Fassbender & E. Mahler (Eds.), *Der Herzinfarkt als psychosomatische Erkrankung in der Rehabilitation* [The heart attack as a psychosomatic illness in rehabilitation] (pp. 145–155). Mannheim, Germany: Mannheimer Morgen.

Sifneos, P. E. (1973). The prevalence of "alexithymic" characteristics in psychosomatic patients. *Psychotherapy and Psychosomatics, 22,* 255–262.

Sikes, W. W., & Rodenhauser, P. (1987). Rehabilitation programs for myocardial infarction patients: A national survey. *General Hospital Psychiatry, 9,* 182–187.

Silagy, C. (1998). Physician advice for smoking cessation. *The Cochrane Library.* Available at http://www.cochrane.org/reviews/clibintro.htm

Silagy, C., Mant, D., Fowler, G., & Lancaster, T. (1999). Nicotine replacement therapy for smoking cessation. *The Cochrane Library.* Available at http://www.cochrane.org/reviews/clibintro.htm

Silagy, C., Mant, D., Fowler, G., & Lodge, M. (1994). Meta-analysis on efficacy of nicotine replacement therapies in smoking cessation. *Lancet, 343,* 139–142.

Silbert, B. S., Santamaria, J. D., Kelly, W. J., O'Brien, J. L., Blyth, C. M., Wong, M. Y., & Allen, N. B. (2001). Early extubation after cardiac surgery: Emotional status in the early postoperative period.

Journal of Cardiothoracic and Vascular Anesthesia, 15, 439–444.

Siltanen, P., Lauroma, M., Nirkko, O., Punsar, S., Pyorala, K., Tuominen, H., et al. (1975). Psychological characteristics related to coronary heart disease. *Journal of Psychosomatic Research, 19,* 183–195.

Silverstone, P. H. (1987). Depression and outcome in acute myocardial infarction. *British Medical Journal (Clinical Research ed.), 294,* 219–220.

*Simson-Morton, D. G., Calfas, K. J., Oldenburg, B., & Burton, N. W. (1998). Effects of interventions in health care settings on physical activity or cardiorespiratory fitness. *American Journal of Preventive Medicine, 15,* 413–430.

Singer, B. A. (1987). The psychological impact of a myocardial infarction on the patient and family. *Psychotherapy in Private Practice, 5,* 53–63.

Singh-Manoux, A. (2003). Psychosocial factors and public health. *Journal of Epidemiology and Community Health, 57,* 553–556; discussion 554–555.

Sivarajan, E. S., Newton, K. M., Almes, M. J., Kempf, T. M., Mansfield, L. W., & Bruce, R. A. (1983). Limited effect of outpatient teaching and counseling after myocardial infarction: A controlled study. *Heart & Lung, 12,* 65–73.

Sivarajan Froehlicher, E. (1999). Multifactorial cardiac rehabilitation: Education, counseling, and behavioral interventions. In N. K. Wenger, L. K. Smith, E. S. Froelicher, & P. McCall Comoss (Eds.), *Cardiac rehabilitation: A guide to practice in the 21st century* (pp. 187–192). New York: Marcel Dekker.

Sjöland, H., Caidahl, K., Wiklund, I., Haglid, M., Hartford, M., Karlson, B. W., et al. (1997). Impact of coronary artery bypass grafting on various aspects of quality of life. *European Journal of Cardio-Thoracic Surgery, 12,* 612–619.

Skaggs, B. G., & Yates, B. C. (1999). Quality of life comparisons after coronary angioplasty and coronary artery bypass graft surgery. *Heart & Lung, 28,* 409–417.

Skevington, S. M. (1983). Chronic pain and depression: Universal or personal helplessness? *Pain, 15,* 309–317.

*Sloan, R. P., & Bigger, J. T., Jr. (1991). Biobehavioral factors in Cardiac Arrhythmia Pilot Study (CAPS): Review and examination. *Circulation, 83,* II-52–57.

*Smith, D. F., Sterndorff, B., Røpcke, G., Gustavsen, E. M., & Hansen, J. K. (1996). Prevalence and severity of anxiety, depression and Type A behaviors in angina pectoris. *Scandinavian Journal of Psychology, 37,* 249–258.

Smith, T. W., Follick, M. J., & Korr, K. S. (1984). Anger, neuroticism, Type A behaviour and the experience of angina. *British Journal of Medical Psychology, 57*(Part 3), 249–252.

*Söderman, E., & Lisspers, J. (1997). Diagnosing depression in patients with physical diseases using the Beck Depression Inventory (BDI). *Scandinavian Journal of Behavioral Therapy, 26,* 102–112.

Soejima, Y., Steptoe, A., Nozoe, S. I., & Tei, C. (1999). Psychosocial and clinical factors predicting resumption of work following acute myocardial infarction in Japanese men. *International Journal of Cardiology, 72,* 39–47.

Sokol, R. S., Folks, D. G., Herrick, R. W., & Freeman, A. M., III. (1987). Psychiatric outcome in men and women after coronary bypass surgery. *Psychosomatics, 28,* 11–16.

Soloff, P. H. (1978). Denial and rehabilitation of the post-infarction patient. *International Journal of Psychiatry in Medicine, 8,* 125–132.

Solomon, S. D., & Davidson, J. R. T. (1997). Trauma: Prevalence, impairment, service use, and cost. *Journal of Clinical Psychiatry, 58,* 5–11.

Song, J. K., Lee, S. J., Kang, D. H., Cheong, S. S., Hong, M. K., & Kim, J. J. (1996). Ergonovine echocardiography as a screening test for diagnosis of vasospastic angina before coronary angiography. *Journal of the American College of Cardiology, 27,* 1156–1161.

Southard, F. R., Certo, C., Comoss, P., Gordon, N. F., Herbert, W. G., Protas, E. J., et al. (1994). Core competencies for cardiac rehabilitation professionals: Position statement of the American Association of Cardiovascular and Pulmonary Rehabilitation. *Journal of Cardiopulmonary Rehabilitation, 14,* 87–92.

*Sparks, K. E., Shaw, D. K., Eddy, D., Hanigosky, P., & Vantrese, J. (1993). Alternatives for cardiac rehabilitation patients unable to return to a hospital-based program. *Heart & Lung, 22,* 298–303.

Sparrow, D., Dawber, T. R., & Colton, T. (1978). The influence of cigarette smoking on prognosis after first myocardial infarction: A report from the Framingham Study. *Journal of Chronic Disorders, 31,* 425–432.

Spencer, F. A., Salami, B., Yarzebski, J., Lessard, D., Gore, J. M., & Goldberg, R. J. (2001). Temporal trends and asssociated factors of inpatient cardiac rehabilitation in patients with acute myocardial infarction: A community-wide perspective. *Journal of Cardiopulmonary Rehabilitation, 21,* 377–384.

Spertus, J. A., McDonell, M., Woodman, C. L., & Fihn, S. D. (2000). Association between depression and worse disease-specific functional status in outpatients with coronary artery disease. *American Heart Journal, 140,* 105–110.

Spielberger, C. D., Gorsuch, R. L., & Lushene, R. H. (1970). *State–Trait Anxiety Inventory.* Palo Alto, CA: Consulting Psychologists Press.

Spinler, S. A., Hilleman, D. E., Cheng, J. W. M., Howard, P. A., Mauro, V. F., Lopez, L. M., et al. (2001). New recommendations from the 1999 American College of Cardiology/American Heart Association acute myocardial infarction guidelines. *Annals of Pharmacotherapy, 35,* 589–617.

Sprafka, J. M., Folsom, A. R., Burke, G. L., Hahn, L. P., & Pirie, P. (1990). Type A behavior and its association with cardiovascular disease prevalence in Blacks and Whites: The Minnesota Heart Survey. *Journal of Behavioral Medicine, 13,* 1–13.

Stansfeld, S. A., Bosma, H., Hemingway, H., & Marmot, M. G. (1998). Psychosocial work characteristics and social support as predictors of SF–36 health functioning: The Whitehall II study. *Psychosomatic Medicine, 60,* 247–255.

Stansfeld, S. A., Fuhrer, R., Shipley, M. J., & Marmot, M. G. (1999). Work characteristics predict psychiatric disorder: Prospective results from the Whitehall II Study. *Occupational and Environmental Medicine, 56,* 302–307.

Stansfeld, S. A., Head, J., & Marmot, M. G. (1998). Explaining social class differences in depression and well-being. *Social Psychiatry and Psychiatric Epidemiology, 33,* 1–9.

Statistisches Bundesamt. (1976). *Rehabilitationsmaßnahmen 1975* (Fachserie 13, Reihe 5.2) [Rehabilitation practice, 1975 (Special series 13, Vol. 5.2)]. Wiesbaden, Germany: Kohlhammer.

Statistisches Bundesamt. (1998). *Rehabilitationsmaßnahmen 1995* (Fachserie 13, Reihe 5.2). [Rehabilitation practice, 1995 (Special series 13, Vol. 5.2)]. Wiesbaden, Germany: Kohlhammer.

*Statistisches Bundesamt. (2000). *Herz-Kreislauferkrankungen* [Cardiovascular diseases]. Retrieved September 5, 2002, from http://www.gbe-bund.de:80/gbe/owa/

Statistisches Bundesamt. (2005). *Herz-Kreislauferkrankungen*[Cardiovascular diseases]. Retrieved September 10, 2005, from http://www.gbe-bund.de/cgi-express/oowaro/expsrv634/dbxwdevkit/xwd_init?isgbetolxs_start/393468854/96303444

Stead, L. F., & Lancaster, T. (1998). Group behavior therapy programs for smoking cessation. *The Cochrane Library.* Available at http://www.cochrane.org/reviews/clibintro.htm

Steenland, K., Fine, L., Belkić, K., Landsbergis, P., Schnall, P., Baker, D., et al. (2000). Research findings linking workplace factors to CVD outcomes. *Occupational Medicine, 15,* 7–68.

Steenland, K., Johnson, J., & Nowlin, S. (1997). A follow-up study of job strain and heart disease among males in the NHANES1 population. *American Journal of Industrial Medicine, 31,* 256–260.

*Steffens, D. C., O'Connor, C. M., Jiang, W. J., Pieper, C. F., Kuchibhatla, M. N., Arias, R. M., et al. (1999). The effect of major depression on functional status in patients with coronary artery disease. *Journal of the American Geriatric Society, 47,* 319–322.

*Stein, D., Troudart, T., Hymowitz, Z., Gotsman, M., & Kaplan de-Nour, A. (1990). Psychosocial adjustment before and after coronary artery bypass surgery. *International Journal of Psychiatric Medicine, 20,* 181–192.

*Stein, P. K., Carney, R. M., Freedland, K. E., Skala, J. A., Jaffe, A. S., Kleiger, R. E., & Rottman, J. N. (2000). Severe depression is associated with markedly reduced heart rate variability in patients with stable coronary heart disease. *Journal of Psychosomatic Research, 48,* 493–500.

Stephanos, S. (1973). *Analytisch-psychosomatische Therapie* [Analytic-psychosomatic therapy]. Bern, Switzerland: Huber.

Stephanos, S. (1979). Libidinal cathexis and emotional growth in the analytical treatment of psychosomatic patients. *Psychotherapy and Psychosomatics, 32,* 101–111.

Stephanos, S. (1982a). The contribution of psychoanalytic object theory to psychosomatic medicine. *Annals of Psychoanalysis, 10,* 187–204.

Stephanos, S. (1982b). Der Einfluss sozialer Sicherungssysteme auf die psychosomatischen Störungen am Beispiel des Krankheitsbildes "Herzinfarkt" [The influence of social security systems on psychosomatic problems in cases of "heart attack"]. *Praxis der Psychotherapie und Psychosomatik, 27,* 99–104.

Stephanos, S. (1982c). Der Herzinfarkt und seine Behandlung als analytisch-psychosomatische Aufgabe [Heart attack and its treatment as an analytic-psychosomatic problem]. *Jahrbuch der Psychoanalyse, 14,* 210–235.

Stern, T. A., Caplan, R. A., & Cassem, N. H. (1987). Use of benzodiazepines in a coronary care unit. *Psychosomatics, 28,* 19–23.

*Stern, M. J., & Cleary, P. (1982). The National Exercise and Heart Disease Project: Long-term psychosocial outcome. *Archives of Internal Medicine, 142,* 1093–1097.

Stern, M. J., Gorman, P. A., & Kaslow, L. (1983). The group counseling v. exercise therapy study: A controlled intervention with subjects following myocardial infarction. *Archives of Internal Medicine, 143,* 1719–1725.

Stern, M. J., Plionis, E., & Kaslow, L. (1984). Group process expectations and outcome with post-myocardial infarction patients. *General Hospital Psychiatry, 6,* 101–108.

Stewart, R. A., Sharples, K. J., North, F. M., Menkes, D. B., Baker, J., & Simes, J. (2000). Long-term assessment of psychological well-being in a randomized placebo-controlled trial of cholesterol reduction with pravastatin: The LIPID Study Investigators. *Archives of Internal Medicine, 160,* 3144–3152.

Stoiberer, I. A. M. (1984). *Stenocardien, Angina pectoris und Herzinfarkt Fallstudien im Spiegel des Thematischen Apperzeptionstestes mit biographischer Rueckblende* [Studies of stenocardia, angina pectoris, and heart attack as reflected in the Thematic Apperception Test by biographical view]. Unpublished doctoral dissertation, University of Salzburg, Salzburg, Austria.

Stone, J. A., Cyr, C., Friesen, M., Kennedy-Symonds, H., Stene, R., & Smilovitch, M. (2001). Canadian guidelines for cardiac rehabilitation and atherosclerotic heart disease prevention: A summary. *Canadian Journal of Cardiology, 17*(Suppl. B), 3–30.

Stone, S. V., & Costa, P. T. (1990). Disease-prone personality or distress-prone personality? The role of neuroticism in coronary heart disease. In H. S. Friedman (Ed.), *Personality and disease* (pp. 178–200). New York: Wiley.

Storment, C. T. (1951). Personality and heart disease. *Psychosomatic Medicine, 13,* 305–313.

Strasser, H. (1982). Psychosomatik und Rehabilitation [Psychosomaticism and rehabilitation]. *Rehabilitation, 21,* 21–28.

*Strauss, B., Paulsen, G., Strenge, H., Graetz, S., Regensburger, D., & Speidel, H. (1992). Preoperative and late postoperative psychosocial state following coronary artery bypass surgery. *Thoracic and Cardiovascular Surgery, 40,* 59–64.

Strauss, W., Fortin, T., Hartigan, P., Folland, E., & Parisi, A. (1995). Comparison of quality of life scores in patients with angina pectoris after angioplasty therapy compared with after medical therapy. *Circulation, 92,* 1710–1719.

Strik, J. J. M. H., Honig, A., Lousberg, R., Lousberg, A. H. P., Cheriex, E. C., Tuynman-Qua, H. G., et al. (2000). Efficacy and safety of fluoxetine in the treatment of patients with major depression after first myocardial infarction: Findings from a double-blind, placebo-controlled trial. *Psychosomatic Medicine, 62,* 783–789.

Suadicani, P., Hein, H. O., & Gyntelberg, F. (1993). Are social inequalities associated with the risk of ischaemic heart disease as a result of psychosocial working conditions? *Atherosclerosis, 101,* 165–175.

Sullivan, A. K., Holdright, D. R., Wright, C. A., Sparrow, J. L., Cunningham, D., & Fox, K. M. (1994). Chest pain in women: Clinical, investigative, and prognostic features. *British Medical Journal, 308,* 883–886.

Sullivan, M. D., LaCroix, A. Z., Russo, J., & Katon, W. J. (1998). Self-efficacy and self-reported functional status in coronary heart disease: A six-month prospective study. *Psychosomatic Medicine, 60,* 473–478.

Sullivan, M. D., LaCroix, A., Russo, J., Swords, E., Sornson, M., & Katon, W. (1999). Depression in coronary heart disease—What is the appropriate diagnostic threshold? *Psychosomatics, 40,* 286–292.

Sullivan, M. D., LaCroix, A. Z., Russo, J. E., & Walker, E. A. (2001). Depression and self-reported physical health in patients with coronary disease: Mediating and moderating factors. *Psychosomatic Medicine, 63,* 248–256.

Sunil Dath, N. N., Mishra, H., Kumaraiah, V., & Yavagal, S. T. (1997). Behavioural approach to coronary heart disease. *Journal of Personality and Clinical Studies, 13,* 29–33.

Susser, M., & Adelstein, A. (1975). An introduction to the work of William Farr. *American Journal of Epidemiology, 101,* 469–476.

Sutton, S. (1994). The past predicts the future: Interpreting behaviour-relationships in social-psychological models of health behaviours. In D. R. Rutter & L. Quine (Eds.), *Social psychology and health: European perspectives* (pp. 71–88). Aldershot, England: Avebury.

Suzuki, H., Takeyama, Y., Koba, S., Suwa, Y., & Katagiri, T. (1994). Small vessel pathology and coronary hemodynamics in patients with microvascular angina. *International Journal of Cardiology, 43,* 139–150.

*Swan, G. E., Carmelli, D., & Rosenman, R. H. (1986). Spouse-pair similarity on the California Psychological Inventory with reference to husband's coronary heart disease. *Psychosomatic Medicine, 48,* 172–186.

Sykes, D. H., Evans, A. E., Boyle, D. M., McIlmoyle, E. L., & Salathia, K. S. (1989). Discharge from a coronary care unit: Psychological factors. *Journal of Psychosomatic Research, 33,* 477–488.

Sylvén, C. (1986). Angina pectoris-like pain provoked by intravenous infusion of adenosine. *British Medical Journal (Clinical Research ed.), 293,* 1240.

Sylvén, C., Eriksson, B., Jensen, J., Geigant, E., & Hallin, R. G. (1996). Analgesic effects of adenosine during exercise-provoked myocardial ischaemia. *Neuroreport, 7,* 1521–1525.

Syme, S. L. (1996). Rethinking disease: Where do we go from here? *Annals of Epidemiology, 6,* 463–468.

Syme, S. L., & Balfour, J. L. (1997). Explaining inequalities in coronary heart disease [Comment]. *Lancet, 350,* 231–232.

Syme, S. L., & Balfour, J. L. (1998). Social determinants of disease. In R. B. Wallace (Ed.), *Maxcy-Rosenau-Last public health and preventive medicine* (14th ed., pp. 795–810). Stamford, CT: Appelton & Lange.

Tang, J. L., Law, M., & Wald, N. (1994). How effective is nicotine replacement therapy in helping people to stop smoking? *British Medical Journal, 308,* 21–26.

Tanus-Santos, J. E., Toledo, J. C. Y., Cittadino, M., Sabha, M., Rocha, J. C., & Moreno, H. (2001). Cardiovascular effects of transdermal nicotine in mildly hypertensive smokers. *American Journal of Hypertension, 14,* 610–614.

Task Force of the European Society of Cardiology and the North American Society of Pacing and Electrophysiology. (1996). Heart rate variability: Standards of measurement, physiological interpretation, and clinical use. *European Heart Journal, 17,* 354–381.

Tate Unger, B., & Warren, D. A. (1999). Case management in cardiac rehabilitation. In N. K. Wenger, L. K. Smith, E. S. Froelicher, & P. McCall Comoss (Eds.), *Cardiac rehabilitation: A guide to practice in the 21st century* (pp. 327–341). New York: Marcel Dekker.

Tavazzi, L., Boszormeny, E., & Broustet, J. P. (for the Task Force of the Working Group on Cardiac Rehabilitation of the European Society of Cardiology). (1992). Definition of cardiac rehabilitation. *European Heart Journal, 13*(Suppl. C), 1–45.

*Taylor, C. B., DeBusk, R. F., Davidson, D. M., Houston, N., & Burnett, K. (1981). Optimal methods for identifying depression following hospitalization for myocardial infarction. *Journal of Chronic Disease, 34,* 127–133.

Taylor, C. B., Houston-Miller, N., Haskell, W. L., & DeBusk, R. (1988). Smoking cessation after acute myocardial infarction: The effects of exercise training. *Addictive Behaviors, 13,* 331–335.

Taylor, C. B., Houston-Miller, N., Killen, J. D., & DeBusk, R. F. (1990). Smoking cessation after acute myocardial infarction: Effects of a nurse-managed intervention. *Annals of Internal Medicine, 113,* 118–123.

Taylor, R., & Rieger, A. (1985). Medicine as social science: Rudolf Virchow on the typhus epidemic in Upper Silesia. *International Journal of Health Services, 15,* 547–559.

Taylor, S. E. (1990). Health psychology: The science and the field. *American Psychologist, 45,* 40–50.

Teasley, D. (1982). Don't let cardiac catheterization strike fear in your patient's heart. *Nursing, 12,* 52–55.

*Tennant, C. C., & Langeluddecke, P. M. (1985). Psychological correlates of coronary heart disease. *Psychological Medicine, 15,* 581–588.

Tennant, C. C., Langeluddecke, P. M., Fulcher, G., & Wilby, J. (1987). Anger and other psychological factors in coronary atherosclerosis. *Psychological Medicine, 17,* 425–431.

Tennant, C., Mihailidou, A., Scott, A., Smith, R., Kellow, J., Jones, M., et al. (1994). Psychological symptom profiles in patients with chest pain. *Journal of Psychosomatic Research, 38,* 365–371.

*Tew, R., Guthrie, E. A., Creed, F. H., Cotter, L., Kisely, S., & Tomenson, B. (1995). A long-term follow-up study of patients with ischaemic heart disease versus patients with nonspecific chest pain. *Journal of Psychosomatic Research, 39,* 977–985.

*Theisen, M. E., MacNeill, S. E., Lumley, M. A., Ketterer, M. W., Goldberg, A. D., & Borzak, S. (1995). Psychosocial factors related to unrecognized acute myocardial infarction. *American Journal of Cardiology, 75,* 1211–1213.

Theorell, T., & Karasek, R. (1996). Current issues relating to psychological job strain and cardiovascular disease research. *Journal of Occupational Health Psychology, 1,* 9–26.

Theorell, T., Lind, E., & Floderus, B. (1975). The relationship of disturbing life-changes and emotions to the early development of myocardial infarction and other serious illnesses. *International Journal of Epidemiology, 4,* 281–293.

Theorell, T., Perski, A., Orth-Gomér, K., Hamsten, A., & de Faire, U. (1991). The effects of the strain of returning to work on the risk of cardiac death after a first myocardial infarction before the age of 45. *International Journal of Cardiology, 30,* 61–67.

Thiery, L. (1988). Physiopathology of leg pain. *Phlebologie, 41,* 624–634.

Thomas, R. J., Houston Miller, N., Lamendola, C., Berra, K., Hedbaeck, B., Durstine, J. L., & Haskell, W. (1996). National survey on gender differences in cardiac rehabilitation programs. *Journal of Cardiopulmonary Rehabilitation, 16,* 402–412.

Thomas, S. A., Friedmann, E., Wimbush, F., & Schron, E. (1997). Psychological factors and survival in the Cardiac Arrhythmia Suppression Trial (CAST): A reexamination. *American Journal of Critical Care, 6,* 116–126.

Thomassen, A., Nielsen, T. T., Bagger, J. P., Pedersen, A. K., & Henningsen, P. (1991). Antiischemic and metabolic effects of glutamate during pacing in patients with stable angina pectoris secondary to either coronary artery disease or Syndrome X. *American Journal of Cardiology, 68,* 291–295.

*Thompson, D. R. (1989). A randomized controlled trial of in-hospital nursing support for first time myocardial infarction patients and their partners: Effects on anxiety and depression. *Journal of Advanced Nursing, 14,* 291–297.

Thompson, D. R., & Bowman, G. S. (1998). Evidence for the effectiveness of cardiac rehabilitation. *Intensive and Critical Care Nursing, 14,* 36–48.

Thompson, D. R., Bowman, G. S., Kitson, A. L., de Bono, D. P., & Hopkins, A. (1996). Cardiac rehabilitation in the United Kingdom: Guidelines and audit standards. *Heart, 75,* 89–93.

Thompson, D. R., Bowman, G. S., Kitson, A. L., de Bono, D. P., & Hopkins, A. (1997). Cardiac rehabilitation services in England and Wales: A national survey. *International Journal of Cardiology, 59,* 299–304.

*Thompson, D. R., & Meddis, R. (1990). A prospective evaluation of in-hospital counselling for first time myocardial infarction men. *Journal of Psychosomatic Research, 34,* 237–248.

Thompson, D. R., & Webster, R. A. (1989). Effect of counselling on anxiety and depression in coronary patients. *Intensive Care Nursing, 5,* 52–54.

Thompson, D. R., & Webster, R. A. (1992). *Caring for the coronary patient.* Oxford, England: Butterworth-Heinemann.

*Thompson, D. R., Webster, R. A., Cordle, C. J., & Sutton, T. W. (1987). Specific sources and patterns of anxiety in male patients with first myocardial infarction. *British Journal of Medicine and Psychology, 60,* 343–348.

Thompson, R. N. (1999). Prediction of trauma responses following myocardial infarction. *Dissertation Abstracts International, 60,* 2965B.

Thoresen, C. E., Friedman, M., Gill, J. K., & Ulmer, D. K. (1982). The recurrent coronary prevention project: Some preliminary findings. *Acta Medica Scandinavica, 660*(Suppl.), 172–192.

Tjemsland, L., Soreide, J. A., & Malt, U. F. (1996). Traumatic distress symptoms in early breast cancer: I. Acute response to diagnosis. *Psychooncology, 5,* 1–8.

Timberlake, N., Klinger, L., Smith, P., Venn, G., Treasure, T., Harrison, M., & Newman, S. P. (1997). Incidence and patterns of depression following coronary artery bypass graft surgery. *Journal of Psychosomatic Research, 43,* 197–207.

Titscher, G., & Göbel-Bohrn, U. (1988). Themenzentrierte Gruppenarbeit bei Patienten mit aortokoronarem Bypass—Ein Erfahrungsbericht [Theme-oriented group therapy with patients who have undergone coronary artery bypass surgery—A report of experiences]. In H. C. Deter & W. Schüffel (Eds.), *Gruppen mit körperlich Kranken* [Support groups with the physically ill] (pp. 120–129). Berlin and Heidelberg, Germany: Springer.

Titscher, G., Huber, C., Ambros, O., Gruska, M., & Gaul, G. (1996). Psychosomatische Einflussgroessen auf die Restenosierung nach Percutaner Transluminaler Koronarangioplastie (PTCA) [The extent of psychosomatic influences on re-stenozation after percutaneous transluminal coronary angioplasty (PTCA)]. *Zeitschrift für Psychosomatische Medizin und Psychoanalyse, 42,* 154–168.

Titscher, G., & Schöppl, C. (2000). *Die Bedeutung der Paarbeziehung für Genese und Verlauf der koronaren Herzkrankheit* [The significance of one's relationship with one's partner for recovery and the trajectory of coronary heart disease]. Frankfurt, Germany: VAS.

Toivonen, L., Helenius, K., & Viitasalo, M. (1997). Electrocardiographic repolarization during stress from awakening on alarm call. *Journal of the American College of Cardiology, 30,* 774–779.

Tooth, L., & McKenna, K. (1995). Cardiac patient teaching: Application to patients undergoing coronary angioplasty and their partners. *Patient Education and Counseling, 25,* 1–8.

Tooth, L., McKenna, K., & Colquhoun, D. (1993). Prediction of compliance with a post-myocardial infarction home-based walking programme. *Australian Occupational Therapy Journal, 40,* 17–22.

Tooth, L. R., McKenna, K. T., & Maas, F. (1998). Preadmission education/counselling for patients undergoing coronary angioplasty: Impact on knowledge and risk factors. *Australian and New Zealand Journal of Public Health, 22,* 583–588.

Tooth, L. R., McKenna, K. T., & Maas, F. (1999). Prediction of functional and psychological status after percutaneous transluminal coronary angioplasty. *Heart & Lung, 28,* 276–283.

Tooth, L. R., McKenna, K., Maas, F., & McEniery, P. (1997). The effects of pre-coronary angioplasty education and counselling on patients and their spouses: A preliminary report. *Patient Education and Counselling, 32,* 185–196.

Torosian, T., Lumley, M. A., Pickard, S. D., & Ketterer, M. W. (1997). Silent versus symptomatic myocardial ischemia: The role of psychological and medical factors. *Health Psychology, 16,* 123–130.

*Travella, J. I., Forrester, A. W., Schultz, S. K., & Robinson, R. G. (1994). Depression following myocardial infarction: A nine year longitudinal study. *International Journal of Psychiatry in Medicine, 24,* 357–369.

*Trelawny-Ross, C., & Russell, O. (1987). Social and psychological responses to myocardial infarction: Multiple determinants of outcome at six months. *Journal of Psychosomatic Research, 31,* 125–130.

Trijsburg, R.W., Bal, J. A., Parsowa, W. P., Erdman, R. A., & Duivenvoorden, H. J. (1989). Prediction of physical indisposition with the help of a questionnaire for measuring denial and overcompensation. *Psychotherapy and Psychosomatics, 51,* 193–202.

Trijsburg, R. W., Erdman, R. A. M., Duivenvoorden, H. J., Thiel, J. H., & Verhage, F. (1987). Denial and overcompensation in male patients with myocardial infarction: An explorative study of the measurement of defense mechanisms by interpersonal comparison. *Psychotherapy and Psychosomatics, 47,* 22–28.

Trost, M. (1995). Nichtrauchertraining in Reha-Kliniken: Entwicklung eines Konzepts aufgrund einer Befragung von ehemaligen Rauchern [Nonsmoker training in rehabilitation hospitals: The development of a model based on a survey conducted with former smokers]. *Sucht, 1,* 43–52.

*Trzcieniecka Green, A., & Steptoe, A. (1996). The effects of stress management on the quality of life of patients following acute myocardial infarction or coronary bypass surgery. *European Heart Journal, 17,* 1663–1670.

*Tsouna-Hadjis, E., Kallergis, G., Agrios, N., Zakopoulos, N., Lyropoulos, S., Liakos, A., et al. (1998). Pain intensity in nondiabetic patients with myocardial infarction or unstable angina: Its association with clinical and psychological features. *International Journal of Cardiology, 67,* 165–169.

Tsutsumi, A., Kayaba, K., Theorell, T., & Siegrist, J. (2001). Association between job stress and depression among Japanese employees threatened by job loss in a comparison between two complementary job-stress models. *Scandinavian Journal of Work, Environment and Health, 27,* 146–153.

Tunstall-Pedoe, H., Woodward, M., Tavendale, R., A'Brook, R., & McCluskey, M. K. (1997). Comparison of the prediction by 27 different factors of coronary heart disease and death in men and women of the Scottish Heart Health Study: Cohort study. *British Medical Journal, 315,* 722–729.

Tverdal, A., Thelle, D., Stensvold, I., Leren, P. L., & Bjartveit, K. (1993). Mortality in relation to smoking history: 13 years' follow-up of 68,000 Norwegian men and women 35–49 years. *Journal of Clinical Epidemiology, 46,* 475–487.

Tzivoni, D., Keren, A., Meyler, S., Khoury, Z., Lerer, T., & Brunel, P. (1998). Cardiovascular safety of transdermal nicotine patches in patients with coronary artery disease who try to quit smoking. *Cardiovascular Drugs & Therapy, 12,* 239–244.

Uexküll, T. V. (Ed.). (2002). *Psychosomatische Medizin* (Psychosomatic medicine). Munich, Germany: Urban & Fisher.

Uhde, T. W., Boulenger, J. P., Roy-Byrne, P. P., Geraci, M. F., Vittone, B. J., & Post, R. M. (1985). Longitudinal course of panic disorder: Clinical and biological considerations. *Progress in Neuropsychopharmacology and Biological Psychiatry, 9,* 39–51.

Ullman, J. B. (1996). Structural equation modeling. In B. G. Tabachnik & L. S. Fidell (Eds.), *Using multivariate statistics* (pp. 709–811). New York: Harper-Collins College Publishers.

Ulvenstam, G., Aberg, A., Pennert, K., Vedin, A., & Wedel, H. (1985). Recurrent myocardial infarction: Two possibilities of prediction. *European Heart Journal, 6,* 303–311.

*Underwood, M. J., Firmin, R. K., & Jehu, D. (1993). Aspects of psychological and social morbidity in patients awaiting coronary bypass grafting. *British Heart Journal, 69,* 382–384.

Unverdorben, M., Brusis, O. A., & Rost, R. (1995). *Kardiologische Prävention und Rehabilitation* [Cardiac prevention and rehabilitation]. Cologne, Germany: Deutscher Ärzteverlag.

Unverdorben, M., Vallbracht, C., Gansser, R., Oster, H., Neuner, P., & Kunkel, B. (1996). Kardiovaskuläre Risiken der ambulanten kardiologischen Rehabilitation [Cardiovascular risks of outpatient cardiological rehabilitation]. *Herz-Kreislauf, 28,* 59–62.

U.S. Department of Health and Human Services. (1998). *Behavioral research in cardiovascular, lung, and blood health and disease.* Washington, DC: Public Health Service.

U.S. Department of Health and Human Services. (1999). *Promoting physical activity: A guide for community action.* Champaign, IL: Human Kinetics.

U.S. Department of Health and Human Services. (2000). *Clinical practice guideline: Treating tobacco use and dependence.* Washington, DC: Public Health Service.

*Uusküla, M. (1996). Psychological differences between young male and female survivors of myocardial infarction. *Psychotherapy and Psychosomatics, 65,* 327–330.

Vaglio, J., Jr., Conard, M., Poston, W. S., O'Keefe, J., Haddock, K., House, J., & Spertus, J. A. (2004). Testing the performance of the ENRCHD Social Support Instrument in cardiac patients. *Health and Quality of Life Outcomes, 2,* 24.

Valk, J. M., & Groen, J. J. (1967). Personality structure and conflict situation in patients with myocardial infarction. *Journal of Psychosomatic Research, 11,* 41–46.

*Valkamo, M., Hintikka, J., Honkalampi, K., Niskanen, L., Koivumaa-Honkanen, H., & Viinamaki, H. (2001). Alexithymia in patients with coronary heart disease. *Journal of Psychosomatic Research, 50,* 125–130.

van Dijl, H. (1982). Myocardial infarction patients and heightened aggressiveness/hostility. *Journal of Psychosomatic Research, 26,* 203–208.

*van Dijl, H., & Nagelkerke, N. (1980). Statistical discrimination of male myocardial infarction patients and healthy males by means of a psychological test and a tracing of basic dimensions of the infarction personality. *Psychotherapy and Psychosomatics, 34,* 196–203.

*van Dixhoorn, J., de Loos, J., & Duivenvoorden, H. J. (1983). Contribution of relaxation technique training to the rehabilitation of myocardial infarction patients. *Psychotherapy and Psychosomatics, 40,* 137–147.

van Domburg, R., Schmidt-Pedersen, S., & van den Brand, M. E. R. (2001). Feelings of being disabled as a predictor of mortality in men 10 years after percutaneous coronary transluminal angioplasty. *Journal of Psychosomatic Research, 51,* 469–477.

van Driel, R. C., & Op den Velde, W. (1995). Myocardial infarction and post-traumatic stress disorder. *Journal of Trauma and Stress, 8,* 151–159.

van Elderen, T., Maes, S., & Dusseldorp, E. (1999). Coping with coronary heart disease: A longitudinal study. *Journal of Psychosomatic Research, 47,* 175–183.

van Elderen, T., Maes, S., Seegers, G., Kragten, H., & Relik-van Wely, L. (1994). Effects of a post-hospitalization group health education programme for patients with coronary heart disease. *Psychology and Health, 9,* 317–330.

van Elderen-van Kemenade, T., Maes, S., & van den Broek, Y. (1994). Effects of a health education programme with telephone follow-up during cardiac rehabilitation. *British Journal of Clinical Psychology, 33,* 367–378.

Vanhees, L., McGee, H. M., Dugmore, L. D., Schepers, D., & van Daele, P. (2002). A representative study of cardiac rehabilitation activities in European Union member states. *Journal of Cardiopulmonary Rehabilitation, 22,* 264–272.

van Heijningen, K. (1960). Some notes on the psychiatric aspects of patients with coronary occlusion. *Advances in Psychosomatic Medicine, 1,* 294–298.

van Jaarsveld, C. H., Sanderman, R., Miedema, I., Ranchor, A. V., & Kempen, G. I. (2001). Changes in health-related quality of life in older patients with acute myocardial infarction or congestive heart failure: A prospective study. *Journal of the American Geriatric Society, 49,* 1052–1058.

van Melle, J. P., Winter, J. B., van den Brink, R. H. S., Spijkerman, T. S., Honig, A., Schene, A. H., et al. (2000). Study design of the Netherlands Heart Foundation Myocardial Infarction and Depression—Intervention Trial (MIND–IT). *European Heart Journal, 21*(Suppl. S), P1200.

Vantrappen, G. (1992). Critique of the session on diagnostic testing. *American Journal of Medicine, 92*(5A), 81S–83S.

*Vásquez-Barquero, J. L., Padierna Acero, J. A., Ochoteco, A., & Díez Manrique, J. F. (1985). Mental illness and ischemic heart disease: Analysis of psychiatric morbidity. *General Hospital Psychiatry, 7,* 15–20.

Vauthier, C. (1966). Réflexions sur la psychologie et la personnalité des grands coronariens [Reflections on the psychology and personality of large coronary]. *Médecine et Hygiene, 24,* 437–438.

Veith, R. C., Raskind, M. A., Caldwell, J. H., Barnes, R. F., Gumbrecht, G., & Ritchie, J. L. (1982). Cardiovascular effects of tricyclic antidepressants in depressed patients with chronic heart disease. *New England Journal of Medicine, 306,* 954–959.

*Verband Deutscher Rentenversicherungsträger. (1994). *VDR Statistik Rehabilitation des Jahres 1992* [VDR rehabilitation statistics for the year 1992] (Vol. 107). Frankfurt, Germany: Author.

*Verband Deutscher Rentenversicherungsträger. (1995). *VDR Statistik Rehabilitation des Jahres 1993* [VDR rehabilitation statistics for the year 1993] (Vol. 112). Frankfurt, Germany: Author.

*Verband Deutscher Rentenversicherungsträger. (1996). *VDR Statistik Rehabilitation des Jahres 1994* [VDR rehabilitation statistics for the year 1994] (Vol. 114). Frankfurt, Germany: Author.

*Verband Deutscher Rentenversicherungsträger. (2000). *VDR Statistik Rehabilitation (1995–1999).* [VDR rehabilitation statistics (1995–1999)]. Retrieved March 2002, from http://www.vdr.de/statistik

Verband Deutscher Rentenversicherungsträger, Reha-Kommission. (1992). *Empfehlungen zur Weiterentwicklung der medizinischen Rehabilitation in der gesetzlichen Rentenversicherung* [Recommendations for the further development of medical rehabilitation in statutory social security]. Frankfurt, Germany: Author.

Vidmar, P. M., & Rubinson, L. (1994). The relationship between self-efficacy and exercise compliance in a cardiac population. *Journal of Cardiopulmonary Rehabilitation, 14,* 246–254.

Vingerhoets, G. (1998). Perioperative anxiety and depression in open-heart surgery. *Psychosomatics, 39,* 30–37.

Virchow, R. (1968). *Mitteilungen über die in Oberschlesien herrschende Typhusepidemie* [Report on the typhus epidemic prevailing in Upper Silesia]. Darmstadt, Germany: Wissenschaftliche Buchgesellschaft. (Original work published 1849)

Virtanen, K. S. (1985). Evidence of myocardial ischaemia in patients with chest pain syndromes and normal coronary angiograms. *Acta Medica Scandinavica Supplements, 694,* 58–68.

*Visser, M. C., Koudstaal, P. J., Erdman, R.A., Deckers, J. W., Passchier, J., van Gijn, J., & Grobbee, D. E. (1995). Measuring quality of life in patients with myocardial infarction or stroke: A feasibility study of four questionnaires in the Netherlands. *Journal of Epidemiology and Community Health, 49,* 513–517.

Vlietstra, R. E., Kronmal, R. A., Oberman, A., Frye, R. L., & Killip, T. (1986). Effect of cigarette smoking on survival of patients with angiographically documented coronary artery disease. *JAMA, 255,* 1023–1027.

Vögele, C., & Steptoe, A. (1993). Ärger, Feindseligkeit und kardiovaskuläre Reaktivität: Implikationen für essentielle Hypertonie und koronare Herzkrankheit [Anger, hostility, and cardiovascular reactivity: Implications for high blood pressure and coronary disease]. In V. Hodapp & P. Schwenkmezger (Eds.), *Ärger und Ärgerausdruck* [Anger and the expression of anger] (pp. 169–191). Bern, Switzerland: Huber.

Völler, H. (1999). Auswirkung stationärer Rehabilitation auf kardiovaskuläre Risikofaktoren bei Patienten mit koronarer Herzerkrankung [The effects of inpatient rehabilitation on cardiovascular risk factors in patients with coronary heart disease]. *Deutsche Medizinische Wochenschrift, 124,* 817–823.

Völler, H., Dovifat, C., Rombeck, B., Binting, S., Hahmann, H., Klein, G., et al. (for the PIN-Studiengruppe). (1999). Ist eine dauerhafte Reduktion kardiovaskulärer Risikofaktoren nach stationärer Rehabilitation bei Koronarkranken möglich? [Is it possible to obtain a lasting reduction in cardiovascular risk factors for cardiac patients after inpatient rehabilitation?]. In Verband Deutscher Rentenversicherungsträger (Ed.), *8. Rehabilitationswissenschaftliches Kolloquium vom 8. Bis 10. März 1999 auf Norderney. Reha-Bedarf—Effektivität—Ökonomie. Tagungsband* [8th Rehabilitation Science Colloquium, 8th–10th March 1999, in Norderney. Rehabilitation needs—effectiveness—economy. Conference proceedings] (pp. 208–209). Frankfurt, Germany: Verband Deutscher Rentenversicherungsträger.

vom Orde, A., Schott, T., & Iseringhausen, O. (2002). Outcomes of cardiac rehabilitation treatment and cost-effectiveness relations—A comparison between inpatient and outpatient rehabilitation programmes. *Rehabilitation, 41,* 119–129.

*von Troschke, J., Klaes, L., & Maschewsky-Schneider, U. (Eds.). (1991). *Erfolge gemeindebezogener Prävention: Ergebnisse aus der Deutschen Herz-Kreislauf-Präventionsstudie (DHP)* [Successes in community-based prevention: Results from the German Cardiovascular Prevention Study]. St. Augustin, Germany: Asgard.

Voors, A. A., van Brussel, B. L., Plokker, H. W., Ernst, S. M., Ernst, N. M., Koomen, E. M., et al. (1996). Smoking and cardiac events after venous coronary bypass surgery. A 15-year follow-up study. *Circulation, 93,* 42–47.

Wachter, V. M., Jünger, S., Renz, D., Wollthan, S., Sim, H., Hendrischke, A., et al. (2000). Psychosoziale Belastung und Inanspruchnahme medizinischer Leistungen nach koronarer Bypassoperation [Psychosocial stress and utilization of medical services after coronary bypass operation]. *Gesundheitswesen, 62,* 451–456.

Wade, J., Dougherty, L., Hart, R., Rafii, A., & Price, D. (1992). A canonical correlation analysis of the influence of neuroticism and extraversion on chronic pain, suffering, and pain behavior. *Pain, 51,* 67–73.

Währborg, P. (1990). Coronary Angioplasty Versus Bypass Revascularization Investigation. *European Heart Journal, 20,* 653–658.

Währborg, P. (1999). Quality of life after coronary angioplasty or bypass surgery: 1-year follow-up in the Coronary Angioplasty Versus Bypass Revascularization Investigation (CABRI) trial. *European Heart Journal, 20,* 653–658.

Walling, A. D., & Crawford, M. H. (1993). Exercise testing in women with chest pain: Applications and limitations of computer analysis. *Coronary Artery Disease, 4,* 783–789.

Wamala, S. P., Mittleman, M. A., Horsten, M., Schenck-Gustafsson, K., & Orth-Gomér, K. (2000). Job stress and the occupational gradient in coronary heart disease risk in women: The Stockholm Female Coronary Risk Study. *Social Science & Medicine, 51,* 481–489.

Wardwell, W. I., Bahnson, C. B., & Caron, H. S. (1963). Social and psychological factors in coronary heart disease. *Journal of Human Behavior, 4,* 154–165.

Ware, J. E., Jr., & Sherbourne, D. C. (1992). The MOS 36-item Short-Form Health Survey (SF-36): I. Conceptual framework and item selection. *Medical Care, 30,* 473–483.

*Watkins, L. L., & Grossman, P. (1999). Association of depressive symptoms with reduced baroreflex cardiac control in coronary artery disease. *American Heart Journal, 137,* 453–457.

Weaver, C. A., Ko, Y. H., Alexander, E. R., Pao, Y. L., & Ting, N. (1980). The Cornell Medical Index as a predictor of health in a prospective cardiovascular study in Taiwan. *American Journal of Epidemiology, 111,* 113–124.

Weber, M. (1968). *Economy and society.* New York: Bedminster Press. (Original work published 1922)

Weed, D. L. (1986). On the logic of causal inference. *American Journal of Epidemiology, 123,* 965–979.

Weidemann, H. (1996). Kardiologische Rehabilitation: Eine orientierende Übersicht [Cardiac rehabilitation: An overview]. *Zeitschrift für Ärztliche Fortbildung, 90,* 479–486.

Weidemann, H., Gerdes, N., Halhuber, C., Undeutsch, K., Schering, C., & Zwingmann, E. (1999). Ergebnisse der stationären Rehabilitation von Herzkranken im Rahmen einer prospektiven, therapiezielorientierten Studie (PROTOS-Studie) zur Messung von kurz-, mittel- und längerfristigen

Reha-Effekten mit validierten Untersuchungsinstrumenten [Results of the inpatient rehabilitation of heart patients in the context of a prospective, therapy-goal-oriented study (PROTOS study) to measure short-, medium- and long-term rehabilitation effects with validated research instruments]. *Perfusion, 12,* 162–168.

Weidemann, H., Halhuber, M. J., Gehring, J., Keck, M., Matthes, P., Hofmann, H., et al. (1991). Die Komponenten einer umfassenden kardiologischen Rehabilitation in der Phase II nach WHO [Components of a comprehensive cardiac rehabilitation program, Phase II, following WHO guidelines]. *Herz-Kreislauf, 23,* 337–341.

Weidemann, H., & Meyer, K. (1991). *Lehrbuch der Bewegungstherapie mit Herzkranken—Pathophysiologie Trainingslehre Praxis* [Textbook of movement therapy with cardiac patients—Pathophysiology, training, and practice]. Darmstadt, Germany: Steinkopff.

Weinblatt, E., Ruberman, W., Goldberg, J. D., Frank, C. W., Shapiro, S., & Chaudhary, B. S. (1978). Relation of education to sudden death after myocardial infarction. *New England Journal of Medicine, 299,* 60–65.

Weinstein, E. J., & Au, P. K. (1991). Use of hypnosis before and during angioplasty. *American Journal of Clinical Hypnosis, 34,* 29–37.

Weinstein, N. D. (1988). The precaution adoption process. *Health Psychology, 17,* 445–453.

Weinstein, N. D. (1998). Stage theories of health behavior: Conceptual and methodological issues. *Health Psychology, 17,* 290–299.

Weiss, E., Dlin, B. M., Rollin, H. R., Fischer, H. K., & Bepler, C. R. (1957). Emotional factors in coronary occlusion. *Archives of Internal Medicine, 99,* 628–641.

Weiss, E., & English, O. S. (1957). *Psychosomatic medicine: A clinical study of psychophysiologic reactions* (3rd ed.). Philadelphia: W. B. Saunders.

Weissman, M. M. (1990). The hidden patient: Unrecognized panic disorder. *Journal of Clinical Psychiatry, 51*(Suppl.), 5–8.

Weizsäcker, V. (1950). *Der Gestaltkreis. Theorie der Einheit von Wahrnehmen und Bewegen* [The Gestaltkreis. Theory of the unit of perception and motion]. Leipzig, Germany: Thieme.

Welin, C., Lappas, G., & Wilhelmsen, L. (2000). Independent importance of psychosocial factors for prognosis after myocardial infarction. *Journal of Internal Medicine, 247,* 629–639.

*Wells, K. B., Rogers, W., Burnam, M. A., & Camp, P. (1993). Course of depression in patients with hypertension, myocardial infarction, or insulin-dependent diabetes. *American Journal of Psychiatry, 150,* 632–638.

Wenger, N. K. (1976). Cardiac rehabilitation: The United Kingdom and the United States. *Annals of Internal Medicine, 84,* 214–216.

Wenger, N. K. (1989). Cardiac rehabilitation services in the U.S. *Giornale Italiano di Cardiologia, 19,* 173–174.

Wenger, N. K. (1992). Rehabilitation of the coronary patient in the 21st century: Challenges and opportunities. In N. K. Wenger & H. K. Hellerstein (Eds.), *Rehabilitation of the coronary patient* (pp. 581–592). New York: Churchill Livingstone.

Wenger, N. K. (1993). Modern coronary rehabilitation. *Coronary Rehabilitation, 94,* 131–141.

Wenger, N. K. (1999). Overview: Charting the course for cardiac rehabilitation into the 21st century. In N. K. Wenger, L. K. Smith, E. S. Froelicher, & P. McCall Comoss (Eds.), *Cardiac rehabilitation: A guide to practice in the 21st century* (pp. 1–7). New York: Marcel Dekker.

Wenger, N. K., Froelicher, E. S., Smith, L. K., Ades, P. A., Berra, K., Blumenthal, J., et al. (1995). *Cardiac rehabilitation* (Clinical Practice Guidelines No. 17; AHCPR Publication No. 96-0672). Rockville, MD: U.S. Department of Health and Human Services, Public Health Service, Agency for Health Care Policy and Research and National Heart, Lung, and Blood Institute.

Wenger, T. L., Cohn, J. B., & Bustrack, J. (1983). Comparison of the effects of bupropion and amitriptyline on cardiac conduction in depressed patients. *Journal of Clinical Psychiatry, 44,* 174–175.

Wenger, T. L., & Stern, W. C. (1983). The cardiovascular profile of bupropion. *Journal of Clinical Psychiatry, 44,* 176–182.

Westin, L., Carlsson, R., Erhardt, L., Cantor, G. E., & McNeil, T. (1999). Differences in quality of life in men and women with ischemic heart disease: A prospective controlled study. *Scandinavian Cardiovascular Journal, 33,* 160–165.

Westin, L., Carlsson, R., Israelsson, B., Willenheimer, R., Cline, C., & McNeil, T. F. (1997). Quality of life in patients with ischaemic heart disease: A prospective controlled study. *Journal of Internal Medicine, 242,* 239–247.

White, A. R., Rampes, H., & Ernst, E. (1999). Acupuncture for smoking cessation. *The Cochrane Library.* Available at http://www.cochrane.org/reviews/clibintro.htm

White, P. D. (1951). The psyche and the soma; the spiritual and physical atributes of the heart. *Annals of Internal Medicine, 35,* 129.

White, R. E., & Frasure-Smith, N. (1995). Uncertainty and psychologic stress after coronary angioplasty and coronary bypass surgery. *Heart & Lung, 24,* 19–27.

Whitehead, A., & Whitehead, J. (1991). A general parametric approach to the meta-analysis of randomized clinical trials. *Statistics and Medicine, 10,* 1665–1677.

*Wiklund, I., & Welin, C. (1992). A comparison of different psychosocial questionnaires in patients with myocardial infarction. *Scandinavian Journal of Rehabilitation Medicine, 24,* 195–202.

Wilhelmsson, C., Vedin, J. A., Elmfeldt, D., Tibblin, G., & Wilhelmsen, L. (1975). Smoking and myocardial infarction. *Lancet, 1,* 415–419.

Wilkinson, R. G. (1996). *Unhealthy societies: The afflictions of inequality.* London: Routledge.

Wilkinson, R. G. (1999). Income inequality, social cohesion, and health: Clarifying the theory—A reply to Muntaner and Lynch. *International Journal of Health Services, 29,* 525–543.

Wilkinson, R. G. (2000). Inequality and the social environment: A reply to Lynch et al. *Journal of Epidemiology and Community Health, 54,* 411–413.

Willett, W. C., Green, A., Stampfer, M. J., Speizer, F. E., Colditz, G. A., Rosner, B., et al. (1987). Relative and absolute excess risks of coronary heart disease among women who smoke cigarettes. *New England Journal of Medicine, 317,* 1303–1309.

Williams, H. (1950). Coronary occlusions in relation to ambitious strivings. *Bulletin of the Menninger Clinic, 14,* 108–110.

Williams, R. B. (1987). Refining the Type A hypothesis: Emergence of the hostility complex. *American Journal of Cardiology, 60,* 27J–32J.

Williams, R. B., Barefoot, J., Califf, R., Haney, T., Saunders, W., Pryor, D., et al. (1992). Prognostic importance of social and economic resources among medically treated patients with angiographically documented coronary heart disease. *JAMA, 267,* 520–524.

Williams, R. B., Barefoot, J. C., Haney, T. L., & Harrell, F. E. (1988). Type A behavior and angiographically documented coronary atherosclerosis in a sample of 2,289 patients. *Psychosomatic Medicine, 50,* 139–152.

Williams, R. B., Haney, T. L., Lee, K. L., Kong, Y., Blumenthal, J. A., & Whalen, R. E. (1980). Type A behavior, hostility, and coronary atherosclerosis. *Psychosomatic Medicine, 42,* 539–549.

Wilson, D. K., Wallston, K. A., & King, J. E. (1990). Effects of contract framing, motivation to quit, and self-efficacy on smoking reduction. *Journal of Applied Social Psychology, 20,* 531–547.

Wilson, D. K., Wallston, K. A., King, J. E., Smith, M. S., & Heim, C. (1993). Validation of smoking abstinence in newly diagnosed cardiovascular patients. *Addictive Behaviors, 18,* 421–429.

Wilson, J. P., & Lindy, J. D. (1994). *Countertransference in the treatment of PTSD.* New York: Guilford Press.

Wilson, K., Gibson, N., Willan, A., & Cook, D. (2000). Effect of smoking cessation on mortality after myocardial infarction: Meta-analysis of cohort studies. *Archives of Internal Medicine, 160,* 939–944.

*Winefield, H. R., & Martin, C. J. (1981–82). Measurement and prediction of recovery after myocardial infarction. *International Journal of Psychiatry and Medicine, 11,* 145–154.

Winkleby, M. A., Ragland, D. R., Fisher, J. M., & Syme, S. L. (1988). Excess risk of sickness and disease in bus drivers: A review and synthesis of epidemiological studies. *International Journal of Epidemiology, 17,* 255–262.

Wise, T. N. (2001). George L. Engel: A tribute and farewell. *Psychosomatics, 42,* 93.

Wishnie, H. A., Hackett, T. P., & Cassem, N. H. (1971). Psychological hazards of convalescence following myocardial infarction. *Journal of the American Medical Association, 215,* 1292–1296.

Wolf, S. (1967). Short communication: The end of the rope: The role of the brain in cardiac death. *Canadian Medical Association Journal, 97,* 1022–1025.

Wolfe, L. A., Dafoe, W. A., Hendren-Roberge, E. A., & Goodman, L. S. (1990). Cardiovascular rehabilitation in Ontario (Canada). *Journal of Cardiopulmonary Rehabilitation, 10,* 130–140.

Wolfe, L. A., Herbert, W. G., Miller, J., & Miller, D. S. (1987). Status of cardiovascular rehabilitation in Virginia. *Journal of Cardiopulmonary Rehabilitation, 7,* 42–50.

Woll, A., & Bös, K. (1994). *Gesundheit zum Mitmachen—Projektbericht Gesundheitsförderung in der Gemeinde Bad Schönborn.* [Do It for Health—A project report on health promotion in the Bad Schönborn community]. Hofmann, Germany: Schorndorf.

Woodward, M., Moohan, M., & Tunstall-Pedoe, H. (1999). Self-reported smoking, cigarette yields and inhalation biochemistry related to the incidence of coronary heart disease: Results from the Scottish Heart Health Study. *Journal of Epidemiology and Biostatistics, 4,* 285–295.

Working Group for the Study of Transdermal Nicotine in Patients With Coronary Artery Disease. (1994). Nicotine replacement therapy for patients with coronary artery disease. *Archives of Internal Medicine, 154,* 989–995.

World Health Organization. (1969). *Rehabilitation of patients with cardiovascular disease* (Report on a seminar). Copenhagen, Denmark: WHO Regional Office for Europe.

World Health Organization. (1991). *International classification of diseases* (10th revision). Geneva, Switzerland: Author.

World Health Organization. (1993). *Needs and action priorities in cardiac rehabilitation and secondary prevention in patients with CHD.* Copenhagen, Denmark: WHO Regional Office for Europe.

World Health Organization. (2003). *WHO statistical information system.* Retrieved March 2003 from http://www.who.int/whosis

Wray, L., Herzog, A. R., Willis, R., & Wallace, R. B. (1998). The impact of education and heart attack on smoking cessation among middle-aged adults. *Journal of Health and Social Behavior, 39,* 271–294.

Writing Committee for the ENRICHD Investigators. (2003). Effects of treating depression and low perceived social support on clinical events after myocardial infarction: The Enhancing Recovery in Coronary Heart Disease patients (ENRICHD) randomized trial. *JAMA, 289,* 3106–3116.

Wulsin, L. R., & Singal, B. M. (2003). Do depressive symptoms increase the risk for the onset of coronary disease? A systematic quantitative review. *Psychosomatic Medicine, 65,* 201–210.

Wulsin, L. R., Vaillant, G. E., & Wells, V. E. (1999). A systematic review of the mortality of depression. *Psychosomatic Medicine, 61,* 6–17.

Wurtele, S. K., & Maddux, J. E. (1987). Relative contributions of protection motivation theory components in predicting exercise intentions and behavior. *Health Psychology, 6,* 453–466.

Wyss, W. H. V. (1924). Über den Einfluß psychischer Vorgänge auf die Innervation von Herz und Gefäßen [The influence of psychological process on the innervation of the heart and vascular system]. *Schweizer Archiv für Neurologie und Psychiatrie, 14,* 30–33.

Wyss, W. H. V. (1927). Herz und Psyche in ihren Wechselwirkungen [The interplay of heart and mind]. *Schweizerische Medizinische Wochenschrift, 57,* 433–436.

Wyss, W. H. V. (1931). *Körperlich–seelische Zusammenhänge in Gesundheit und Krankheit* [Physical–mental connections in health and illness]. Leipzig, Germany: Thieme.

Yalom, I. D. (1975). *Theory and practice of group therapy.* New York: Basic Books.

Yingling, K. W., Wulsin, L. R., Arnold, L. M., & Rouan, G. W. (1993). Estimated prevalences of panic disorder and depression among consecutive patients seen in an emergency department with acute chest pain. *Journal of General Internal Medicine, 8,* 231–235.

Yoshida, T., Yoshida, K., Yamamoto, C., Nagasaka, M., Tadaura, H., Meguro, T., et al. (2001). Effects of a two-week, hospitalized phase II cardiac rehabilitation program on physical capacity, lipid profiles and psychological variables in patients with acute myocardial infarction. *Japanese Circulation Journal, 65,* 87–93.

Young, D. R., Haskell, W. L., Taylor, C. B., & Fortmann, S. P. (1996). Effects of community health education on physical activity knowledge, attitudes, and behavior—The Stanford Five-City Project. *American Journal of Epidemiology, 144,* 264–274.

Young, L. D., Barboriak, J. J., Hoffman, R. G., & Anderson, A. J. (1984). Coronary-prone behavior attitudes in moderate to severe coronary artery occlusion. *Journal of Behavioral Medicine, 7,* 205–215.

Yusuf, S., Cairns, J. A., Camm, A. J., Fallen, E. L., & Gersh, B. J. (1998). *Evidence-based cardiology.* London: BMJ Publishing Group.

Zachariae, R., Melchiorsen, H., Frøbert, O., Bjerring, P., & Bagger, J. P. (2001). Experimental pain and psychologic status of patients with chest pain with normal coronary arteries or ischemic heart disease. *American Heart Journal, 142,* 63–71.

Zeiher, A. M., Krause, T., Schachinger, V., Minners, J., & Moser, E. (1995). Impaired endothelium-dependent vasodilation of coronary resistance vessels is associated with exercise-induced myocardial ischemia. *Circulation, 91,* 2345–2352.

Ziegelstein, R. C., Fauerbach, J. A., Stevens, S. S., Romanelli, J., Richter, D. P., & Bush, D. E. (2000). Patients with depression are less likely to follow recommendations to reduce cardiac risk during recovery from a myocardial infarction. *Archives of Internal Medicine, 160,* 1818–1823.

*Ziemann, K. M., & Dracup, K. (1990). Patient–nurse contracts in critical care: A controlled trial. *Progress in Cardiovascular Nursing, 5,* 98–103.

Zigmond, A. S., & Snaith, R. P. (1983). The Hospital Anxiety and Depression Scale. *Acta Psychiatrica Scandinavica, 67,* 361–370.

*Zotti, A. M., Bettinardi, O., Soffiantino, F., Gavazzi, L., & Steptoe, A. (1991). Psychophysiological stress testing in postinfarction patients: Psychological correlates of cardiovascular arousal and abnormal cardiac responses. *Circulation, 83,* 1125–1135.

Zung, W. K. (1965). A self-rating depression scale. *Archives of General Psychiatry, 12,* 63–70.

Zyzanski, S. J., & Jenkins, C. D. (1970). Basic dimensions within the coronary-prone behavior pattern. *Journal of Chronic Diseases, 22,* 781–795.

Author Index

Aaronson, N. K., 213
Abbot, E. C., 192
Abbot, N. C., 102
Abbott, R. D., 164, 166
Abel, T., 17
Aberg, A., 91, 92
Abrahamsen, A. M., 91
A'Brook, R., 88
Adam, M., 211
Adelstein, A., 14
Ades, P. A., 114, 231, 259, 268, 276, 277
Adsett, C. A., 71
Agarwal, A., 193
Agmon, Y., 192
Ahern, D. K., 145–147, 174
Ahlbom, A., 24, 25
Ahn, D. K., 136
Ahto, M., 130
Ainsworth, B. E., 109
Ajzen, I., 115, 116
Albrecht, D., 215, 220
Alderman, M. H., 155
Alexander, E. R., 189
Alexander, F., 48
Alfredsson, L., 24, 25
Allan, R., 33, 60, 62, 63, 74, 75
Allen, J. K., 87, 93, 95–97, 105, 216
Allert, T., 75
Allison, T. G., 221
Alonzo, A. A., 60, 62
Alpert, A., 204
Alpert, J. S., 201
Altenhöner, T., 264
Alter, C. L., 63
Alterman, T., 24, 25
Althaus, U., 76
Altman, I., 186

Altmann-Herz, U., 66
Alvarez, W., 62
Ambros, O., 218
American Association of Cardiovascular and Pulmonary Rehabilitation, 258–262
American College of Cardiology, 101
American College of Sports Medicine, 107
American Heart Association, 101, 107, 110, 255, 256
American Psychiatric Association, 60, 128, 154, 155, 246
Amey, M. C., 270, 271
Amick, B. C., 3rd, 27
Amoroso, P. J., 104
Amos, C. I., 25, 166
Amsterdam, E., 204
Anderson, A. J., 164, 215
Anderson, J. E., 100
Anderson, K. O., 222, 223, 226
Andreasen, F., 192
Andreotti, F., 179
Andrew, G. M., 114
Andrew, M. J., 134, 140
Andrykowski, M. A., 63
Angelico, F., 167
Angelino, P. F., 87, 92
Antonovsky, A., 17
Appels, A. P. W. M., 46, 80, 148, 164, 172, 173, 216, 218, 221, 223
Applebaum, I. L., 53
Arendt-Nielsen, L., 193
Aresin, L., 80
Arlow, J. A., 42, 44, 47, 51, 78, 80
Armstrong, K. L., 270, 271
Arnaot, M. R., 100
Arnesen, E., 88

Arnold, L. M., 196
Arntz, A., 189
Aronow, E., 51
Arsenault, A., 128, 129
Artalejo, F., 18
Arthur, R. J., 52
Assael, M., 54, 79
Assmann, G., 89
Au, P. K., 221, 224
Aust, B., 17, 22, 28, 31
Avierinos, C., 46

Baboriak, J. J., 215
Babyak, M. A., 132, 243–245
Badura, B., 108, 110, 111, 118, 251, 260, 263, 264, 274
Baer, F. W., 46, 216
Bagger, J. P., 128, 192, 193
Bahnson, C. B., 43, 44
Baillie, A. J., 103
Bak, P., 193
Baker, D., 17, 22, 24, 25, 126
Baker, M., 221
Baker, R. A., 134
Baker, T. B., 97, 98, 100
Bal, J. A., 45
Balady, G. J., 259–261
Balfour, J. L., 18, 32
Balint, M., 57
Ballenger, J., 201
Bandura, A., 113, 116
Banwart, L., 227
Bär, F. W., 46, 218, 216, 218, 221
Bär, J., 46
Barboriak, J. J., 164
Bardé, B., 13, 53, 60, 62, 68, 70, 118
Barefoot, J. C., 18, 32, 131, 132, 148, 151, 162, 166, 167, 172, 175, 177, 180, 181

347

Subject Index

About the Editors

Jochen Jordan, PhD, Dipl.-Psychologist, worked from 1975 through 2006 at the Clinic for Psychosomatic Medicine and Psychotherapy in the hospital of the University of Frankfurt, Frankfurt, Germany. He is now director of Germany's first clinic devoted to psychocardiology, the Kerckhoff Clinic, Bad Nauheim, Germany. He has studied education science and psychology at the University of Gießen, Gießen, Germany, and the University of Heidelberg, Heidelberg, Germany. He has won awards for the promotion of scientific work from the Deutsche Herzstiftung and for the promotion of scientific cardiac work from the Deutsche Gesellschaft für Prävention und Rehabilitation von Herz-Kreislauferkrankungen (German Society for Prevention and Rehabilitation of Heart and Circulatory Diseases). Other areas of specialization include psychodynamic individual and group therapy, therapy of couples with sexual functional disorders, and body therapy. His primary working areas are in psychocardiology, coping, and the process of psychotherapy.

Benjamin Bardé, PhD, Dipl.-Psychologist, Dipl.-Sociologist, practices psychoanalysis in Frankfurt, Germany. He has studied philosophy, sociology, and psychology and has received postgraduate training in behavior therapy, psychoanalysis, and group therapy. His areas of research interest have included psychocardiology, psychotherapy, trauma (posttraumatic stress disorder), analysis, and development of social organizations.

Andreas Michael Zeiher, PhD, MD, obtained his medical degree in 1981 after studying at the Medical School at Albert-Ludwigs University, Freiburg, Germany. His medical training continued in the Division of Cardiology at the University of Freiburg, Freiburg, Germany, where he became associate professor of medicine in 1990 and was the director of interventional cardiology from 1990 to 1995. Since 1995, Dr. Zeiher has held the position of Chairman of the Department of Internal Medicine in the Division of Cardiology/Nephrology/Angiology at the J. W. Goethe University, Frankfurt, Germany. He is also currently the vice chairman of the board of directors at J. W. Goethe University and is the past chairman of the Working Group on Interventional Cardiology of the European Society of Cardiology. His research is focused on novel diagnostic and therapeutic strategies for coronary artery disease, including identification of innovative biomarkers for disease activity and clinical application of regenerative cardiovascular therapies using stem cells. He has published more than 200 original papers.